HIV: Challenges and Concerns

HIV: Challenges and Concerns

Edited by Chris Stinson

hayle
medical
New York

Hayle Medical,
750 Third Avenue, 9th Floor,
New York, NY 10017, USA

Visit us on the World Wide Web at:
www.haylemedical.com

ISBN: 978-1-63241-501-1

The publisher's policy is to use permanent paper from mills that operate a sustainable forestry policy. Furthermore, the publisher ensures that the text paper and cover boards used have met acceptable environmental accreditation standards.

Printed in China.

Cataloging-in-Publication Data

HIV : challenges and concerns / edited by Chris Stinson.
p. cm.
Includes bibliographical references and index.
ISBN 978-1-63241-501-1
1. HIV (Viruses). 2. HIV infections. I. Stinson, Chris.
RC606.6 .H58 2018
616.979 2--dc23

Table of Contents

Preface

HIV and AIDS are diseases that currently have no cure. Therapies that slow down the effects of the disease as well as its progression into AIDS are proving to be very successful. Drugs that can combat HIV viruses are collectively called antiretroviral therapies. These can reduce the multiplication of the virus by blocking its mutation. The concept of "treatment as prevention" has also become a recommended practice to reduce cross-infection. The topics covered in this book offer the readers new insights in this field. It is a vital tool for all researching or studying HIV treatment and therapies as it gives incredible insights into emerging trends and concepts.

This book unites the global concepts and researches in an organized manner for a comprehensive understanding of the subject. It is a ripe text for all researchers, students, scientists or anyone else who is interested in acquiring a better knowledge of this dynamic field.

I extend my sincere thanks to the contributors for such eloquent research chapters. Finally, I thank my family for being a source of support and help.

Editor

1

Baseline CD4 Cell Counts of Newly Diagnosed HIV Cases in China

Houlin Tang[1], Yurong Mao[1], Cynthia X. Shi[1,2], Jing Han[1], Liyan Wang[3], Juan Xu[1], Qianqian Qin[3], Roger Detels[4], Zunyou Wu[1]*

1 Division of Integration and Evaluation, National Center for AIDS/STD Control and Prevention, Chinese Center for Disease Control and Prevention, Beijing, China, **2** Department of Epidemiology, School of Public Health, Harvard University, Boston, Massachusetts, United States of America, **3** Division of Epidemiology, National Center for AIDS/STD Control and Prevention, Chinese Center for Disease Control and Prevention, Beijing, China, **4** Department of Epidemiology, School of Public Health, University of California at Los Angeles, California, United States of America

Abstract

Background: Late diagnosis of HIV infection is common. We aim to assess the proportion of newly diagnosed HIV cases receiving timely baseline CD4 count testing and the associated factors in China.

Methods: Data were extracted from the Chinese HIV/AIDS Comprehensive Response Information Management System. Adult patients over 15 years old who had been newly diagnosed with HIV infection in China between 2006 and 2012 were identified. The study cohort comprised individuals who had a measured baseline CD4 count.

Results: Among 388,496 newly identified HIV cases, the median baseline CD4 count was 294 cells/μl (IQR: 130–454), and over half (N = 130,442, 58.8%) were less than 350 cells/μl. The median baseline CD4 count increased from 221 (IQR: 63–410) in 2006 to 314 (IQR: 159–460) in 2012. A slight majority of patients (N = 221,980, 57.1%) received baseline CD4 count testing within 6 months of diagnosis. The proportion of individuals who received timely baseline CD4 count testing increased significantly from 20.0% in 2006 to 76.9% in 2012. Factors associated with failing to receiving timely CD4 count testing were: being male (OR: 1.17, 95% CI: 1.15–1.19), age 55 years or older (OR:1.03, 95% CI: 1.00–1.06), educational attainment of primary school education or below (OR: 1.30, 95% CI: 1.28–1.32), infection with HIV through injection drug use (OR: 2.07, 95% CI: 2.02–2.12) or sexual contact and injection drug use (OR: 1.87, 95% CI: 1.76–1.99), diagnosis in a hospital (OR: 1.91, 95% CI: 1.88–1.95) or in a detention center (OR: 1.75, 95% CI: 1.70–1.80), and employment as a migrant worker (OR:1.55, 95% CI:1.53–1.58).

Conclusion: The proportion of newly identified HIV patients receiving timely baseline CD4 testing has increased significantly in China from 2006–2012. Continued effort is needed for further promotion of early HIV diagnosis and timely baseline CD4 cell count testing.

Editor: Barbara Ensoli, Istituto Superiore di Sanità, Italy

Funding: The authors report funding from the National Health and Family Planning Commission of the People's Republic of China (grant#131-11-0001-0501), and the US National Institutes of Health (grant# U2RTW06918). The funders had no role in study design, data collection and analysis, decision to publish, or preparation of the manuscript.

Competing Interests: The authors have declared that no competing interests exist.

* E-mail: wuzy@263.net

Introduction

CD4 cell count is a major indicator of human immunodeficiency virus (HIV) infection disease progression [1,2]. Patients who receive a late diagnosis, defined as a baseline CD4 cell count<200 cells/μl, have significantly poorer responses to antiretroviral therapy (ART) and worse prognoses [3,4,5,6]. The proportion of patients who present late to diagnosis and treatment remains unacceptably high [7,8,9,10]. Internationally, the observed proportion of patients with late diagnoses is stable or worsening [7]. Although it is recommended that CD4 cell count testing should be carried out promptly after diagnosis, many patients fail to receive on-time testing [11,12]. In the United States, an ongoing outpatient study in eight cities found that 78% of patients had a measured CD4 count within 3 months of HIV diagnosis [7]. This proportion was significantly lower in developing countries. Studies in Thailand, Vietnam, and South Africa reported that only 34%, 49%, and 62.6% of patients, respectively, received CD4 count assessment with 6 months of HIV diagnosis [13,14,15].

In 2002, China implemented the National Free Antiretroviral Therapy Program (NFATP) to address the issue of poor access to HIV/AIDS treatment. Patients who meet the national treatment criteria of a CD4 count ≤200 cells/μl (revised to ≤350cells/μl in 2008) are eligible for ART at no cost to the patient [16]. The program has contributed to a dramatic reduction in mortality among patients receiving HIV treatment [17]. In order to expand NFATP coverage, the government has increased HIV screening access, leading to a rise in the number of people diagnosed with HIV [18]. After the diagnosis of HIV infection, timely CD4 cell count testing is a crucial step in determining whether the patient meets criteria for ART initiation and engaging the patient in appropriate care and treatment [19,20]. From 2007, the national HIV/AIDS program set quantitative targets of core indicators to monitor progress in key areas of HIV work. From 2007 to 2009, the proportion of CD4 cell count monitoring for people diagnosed with HIV and AIDS increased from 45.3% and 10.1% in 2007 to 54.2% and 62.5% in 2009, respectively [21].

However, past studies have indicated that many patients are lost or delayed along the continuum of care. A study in Guangxi and Yunnan found that only 37% of patients who were diagnosed with HIV from 2005 to 2009 received baseline CD4 testing within 6 months [20]. The proportion increased dramatically from 7% in 2005 to 62% in 2009. A separate study noted that in 2009, approximately 30% of the ART-initiated patients who received baseline CD4 testing had CD4 <50 cells/µl, indicating that many patients were being diagnosed and treated late [22,23]. Prompt baseline CD4 testing is a critical step in successful linkage to HIV treatment.

By using data extracted from the Chinese HIV/AIDS Comprehensive Response Information Management System (CRIMS) [24], we aimed to identify trends in the proportion of individuals who received timely baseline CD4 cell count testing within 6 months of HIV diagnosis in China from 2006 to 2012. We also sought to determine changes in median baseline CD4 cell counts over time and factors associated with failing to receive CD4 cell count testing.

Methods

Data source

Data were collected from CRIMS, a web-based real-time database system managed by the National Centre for AIDS/STD Control and Prevention (NCAIDS), Chinese Center for Disease Control and Prevention (CDC). CRIMS was developed in 2005 and has previously been described elsewhere [24]. Local CDC staffs, who are trained on data upload and management, create electronic records in CRIMS for each patient who tests positive for HIV. Staffs receive annual refresher training. Patient records contain information on demographic characteristics, contact information (including both permanent and temporary residential addresses), sexual and drug use risk behaviors, likely transmission routes, medical histories, and laboratory test results [24]. For this study, we included all adult individuals (over 15 years old) who received a confirmed HIV diagnosis between January 1, 2006 and December 31, 2012. All HIV screening is done in accordance with national HIV policy. Provider-initiated testing and counseling (PITC) has been in place in hospitals since 2007.

Data analysis

The primary outcome of interest was the proportion of newly diagnosed HIV/AIDS individuals who received baseline CD4 cell count testing within 6 months of diagnosis. Data were described by the median (interquartile range, IQR) and the distribution across four CD4 cell count categories (<200, 200–349, 350–500, and ≥ 500). Demographic characteristics were analyzed using chi-squared statistics for dichotomous and categorical variables. Univariate and multivariate logistic regression models were used to assess the factors associated with not receiving a timely CD4 cell count. Variables with $p<0.10$ under univariate analysis were retained for multivariate modeling using stepwise selection, and 95% confidences intervals were estimated using these models. Results with a two-sided $p<0.01$ were considered statistically significant. All data analyses were performed using SAS Version 9.3 (SAS Institute, Cary, NC, USA).

Ethics statement

This study was a secondary data analysis using existing Chinese government HIV/AIDS CRIMS data. All subjects signed a general informed consent upon enrollment to CRIMS indicating that their data, after removing personal identifiers, could be used in statistical analyses and/or epidemiological research studies. Therefore, no additional study specific informed consent was necessary for this current study. Patient records and information were de-identified prior to analysis. This study protocol was reviewed and approved by the Institutional Review Board of the National Center for AIDS/STD Control and Prevention, Chinese Center for Disease Control and Prevention (approval #X130205248).

Results

Between January 1, 2006 and December 31, 2012, there were 394,294 individuals newly diagnosed with HIV infection in China. Patients under 15 years of age (N = 5,798) were excluded from the study cohort. Of the remaining 388,496 newly diagnosed individuals, 221,980 (57.1%) patients received a baseline CD4 cell count within 6 months of HIV diagnosis over the six-year study period (Table 1).

The number of newly identified HIV cases with measured baseline CD4 counts more than doubled between 2006 and 2012, increasing from 35,087 to 81,416. The proportion of newly diagnosed individuals who received a baseline CD4 cell count test within 6 months increased from 20.0% in 2006 to 76.9% in 2012. National policies recommend CD4 cell count testing within 14 days after diagnosis of HIV infection. Our study found that the proportion of newly diagnosed individuals who received baseline CD4 cell count testing within 14 days increased from 10.9% in 2006 to 46.1% in 2012 (Table 1).

The median baseline CD4 cell count of individuals who received timely testing over the study period was 294 cells/µl (IQR: 130–454). Over half of the patients (N = 130,442, 58.8%) had baseline CD4 cell counts <350 cells/µl, and 76,582 patients (34.5%) had baseline CD4 cell counts <200 cells/µl. Less than a quarter of patients (N = 43,547, 19.6%) had baseline CD4 cell counts ≥500 cells/µl (Table 1).

The median baseline CD4 cell count increased slightly by each calendar year over the study period from 221 cells/µl (IQR: 63–410) in 2006 to 314 cells/µl (IQR: 159–460) in 2012. The percentage of individuals with baseline CD4 cell counts <200 cells/µl, indicating advanced disease, decreased from 46.9% in 2006 to 30.7% in 2012. The percentage of individuals diagnosed with baseline CD4 cell counts ≥500 cells/µl, indicating a recent acquisition of HIV infection, has remained relatively stable (Table 1).

Characteristics associated with receiving baseline CD4 cell count testing within 6 months were being female, being married, having attained middle school education or higher, having acquired HIV through male-to-male sexual contact or commercial blood plasma donation, and being diagnosed with HIV infection at a voluntary counseling and testing (VCT) clinic (Table 2). A total of 34,248 newly diagnosed individuals (8.8%) died within 6 months after HIV diagnosis. Of these individuals, 23,661 (69.1%) had not received CD4 cell count testing.

In the univariate logistic regression model, factors associated with baseline CD4 cell count testing within 6 months of HIV diagnosis were age group, gender, marital status, education level, ethnicity, employment as a migrant worker, route of HIV transmission, site of HIV diagnosis, and year of HIV diagnosis (Table 2).

Table 1. Baseline CD4 cell counts (within 6 months of diagnosis) of HIV individuals in China: 2006–2012.

	2006	2007	2008	2009	2010	2011	2012	Total
Total No.	**35087**	**40491**	**47675**	**54552**	**58109**	**71166**	**81416**	**388496**
No. (%) of subjects with baseline CD4 cells counts within one year								
<15 days	3812 (10.9)	7021 (17.3)	12038 (25.3)	16332 (29.9)	20544 (35.4)	29437 (41.1)	37561 (46.1)	126745 (32.6)
<30 days	4608 (13.1)	8472 (20.9)	14538 (30.5)	20172 (37.0)	25372 (43.7)	36712 (51.6)	46753 (57.4)	156627 (40.3)
<90 days	5893 (16.8)	10949 (27.0)	18340 (38.5)	25434 (46.6)	32467 (55.9)	46623 (65.5)	57773 (71.0)	197479 (50.8)
<180 days	7030 (20.0)	13125 (32.4)	21122 (44.3)	29078 (53.3)	37081 (63.8)	51957 (73.0)	62587 (76.9)	221980 (57.1)
Median (IQR) baseline CD4 cell count	221(63–410)	252(80–429)	280(106–448)	287(116–454)	295(130–459)	299(140–454)	314(159–460)	294(130–454)
No. (%) of subjects with CD4 cell counts (cells/μl)								
<200	3298 (46.9)	5552 (42.3)	7851 (37.2)	10620 (36.5)	12751 (34.4)	17266 (33.2)	19244 (30.7)	76582 (34.5)
200–349	1476 (21.0)	2941 (22.4)	5062 (24.0)	6858 (23.6)	9062 (24.4)	12877 (24.8)	15584 (24.9)	53860 (24.3)
350–499	1066 (15.2)	2299 (17.5)	4092 (19.4)	5802 (20.0)	7800 (21.0)	11691 (22.5)	15241 (24.4)	47991 (21.6)
≥500	1190 (16.9)	2333 (17.8)	4117 (19.5)	5798 (19.9)	7468 (20.1)	10123 (19.5)	12518 (20.0)	43547 (19.6)

Table 2. Factors associated with baseline CD4 cell counts (within 6 months of diagnosis) of HIV individuals in China: 2006–2012, based on multivariate logistic regression analysis.

	No. of new cases	No. (%) of subjects with baseline CD4 cell count	Unadjusted OR (95% CI)	P-value	Adjusted OR (95% CI)	P-value
Year of HIV diagnosis						
2006	35087	7030 (20.0)	1.00		1.00	
2007	40491	13125 (32.4)	0.52 (0.51–0.54)	<0.01	0.57 (0.55–0.59)	<0.01
2008	47675	21122 (44.3)	0.32 (0.31–0.33)	<0.01	0.39 (0.38–0.40)	<0.01
2009	54552	29078 (53.3)	0.22 (0.21–0.23)	<0.01	0.28 (0.27–0.29)	<0.01
2010	58109	37081 (63.8)	0.14 (0.14–0.15)	<0.01	0.19 (0.18–0.20)	<0.01
2011	71166	51957 (73.0)	0.09 (0.09–0.10)	<0.01	0.13 (0.12–0.13)	<0.01
2012	81416	62587 (76.9)	0.08 (0.07–0.08)	<0.01	0.11 (0.10–0.11)	<0.01
Gender						
Female	113340	67460 (59.5)	1.00		1.00	
Male	275156	154520 (56.2)	1.15 (1.13–1.16)	<0.01	1.17 (1.15–1.19)	<0.01
Age (years)						
15–24	58323	31195 (53.5)	1.00		1.00	
25–34	132737	70982 (53.5)	1.00 (0.98–1.02)	0.96	0.82 (0.80–0.84)	<0.01
35–44	101295	58885 (58.1)	0.83 (0.81–0.85)	<0.01	0.80 (0.78–0.82)	<0.01
45–54	43726	28773 (65.8)	0.60 (0.58–0.61)	<0.01	0.80 (0.78–0.83)	<0.01
55+	52415	32145 (61.3)	0.73 (0.71–0.74)	<0.01	1.03 (1.00–1.06)	0.03
Marital status						
Single, divorced, or widowed	175776	101301 (57.6)	1.00		1.00	
Married or lives with partner	201596	119162 (59.1)	0.94 (0.93–0.95)	<0.01	0.87 (0.86–0.89)	<0.01
Education						
Middle school or above	231092	145738 (63.1)	1.00		1.00	
Primary school or below	145077	75502 (52.0)	1.57 (1.55–1.60)	<0.01	1.30 (1.28–1.32)	<0.01
Occupation						
Other*	210105	119033 (56.7)	1.00	<0.01	1.00	
Farmer or rural laborer	178391	102947 (57.7)	0.96 (0.95–0.97)		0.99 (0.97–1.00)	0.15
Ethnicity						
Minority group	117896	53500 (45.4)	1.00		1.00	
Han	270600	168480 (62.3)	0.50 (0.50–0.51)	<0.01	0.76 (0.74–0.77)	<0.01
Route of HIV infection						
Heterosexual contact	222148	143431 (64.6)	1.00		1.00	
Male-to-male sexual contact	44840	35277 (78.7)	0.49 (0.48–0.51)	<0.01	0.62 (0.60–0.64)	<0.01
Injection drug use	76815	26791 (34.9)	3.40 (3.34–3.46)	<0.01	2.07 (2.02–2.12)	<0.01
Sexual contact and injection drug use	5030	2111 (42.0)	2.52 (2.38–2.67)	<0.01	1.87 (1.76–1.99)	<0.01
Blood (plasma) donation	17204	10429 (60.6)	1.18 (1.15–1.22)	<0.01	0.83 (0.81–0.87)	<0.01
Site of HIV diagnosis						
VCT centers	110360	73316 (66.4)	1.00		1.00	
Hospitals	153367	87886 (57.3)	1.48 (1.45–1.50)	<0.01	1.91 (1.88–1.95)	<0.01
Detention centers	47218	14846 (31.4)	4.32 (4.22–4.42)	<0.01	1.75 (1.70–1.80)	<0.01
Others**	77551	45932 (59.2)	1.36 (1.34–1.39)	<0.01	1.42 (1.39–1.46)	<0.01
Migrant worker***						
No	294016	177081 (60.2)	1.00		1.00	
Yes	94480	44899 (47.5)	1.67 (1.65–1.70)	<0.01	1.55 (1.53–1.58)	<0.01
Total	388496	221980 (57.1)	-	-	-	-

*Includes laborer, unemployed, businessman, student, public servant, and unclear.
**Includes targeted intervention project, physical examination for sex workers, and unclear.
***Defined as having migrated from the registered region of residence to another region for at least six months.

In the multivariate logistic regression model (Table 2), predictors for not receiving CD4 cell count testing with 6 months included being male (OR: 1.17, 95% CI: 1.15–1.19), age 55 years or older (OR: 1.03, 95% CI: 1.00–1.06), educational attainment of primary school or below (OR: 1.30, 95% CI: 1.28–1.32), occupation as a farmer or rural laborer (OR: 1.16, 95% CI: 1.15–1.18), route of HIV transmission classified as injecting drug use (OR: 2.07, 95% CI: 2.02–2.12) or sexual contact and injecting drug use (OR: 1.87, 95% CI: 1.76–1.99), HIV diagnosis in a hospital (OR: 1.91, 95% CI: 1.88–1.95) or a detention center (OR: 1.75, 95% CI: 1.70–1.80), and being a migrant worker (OR: 1.55, 95% CI: 1.53–1.58). Factors associated with timely CD4 testing included being married or cohabiting with a partner (OR: 0.87, 95% CI: 0.86–0.89), being of Han ethnicity (OR: 0.76, 95% CI: 0.74–0.77), and route of HIV transmission classified as male-to-male sexual contact (OR: 0.62, 95% CI: 0.60–0.64) or commercial blood plasma donation (OR: 0.83, 95% CI: 0.81–0.87).

Baseline CD4 cell counts were also analyzed by the route of HIV infection and the year of reporting (Table 3). There were significant differences in the distributions of CD4 cell counts by the routes of HIV infection and by the year of HIV diagnosis (heterosexual contact: $\chi^2 = 119.63$, $p<0.01$; male-to-male sexual contact: $\chi^2 = 21.07$, $p<0.01$; IDUs: $\chi^2 = 191.85$, $p<0.01$; and commercial blood plasma donation: $\chi^2 = 66.95$, $p<0.01$). Individuals infected through heterosexual contact and commercial blood plasma donation were more likely to have baseline CD4 cell counts <200 cells/µl than individuals infected by male-to-male sexual contact, injection drug use, or sexual contact and injection drug use.

The median baseline CD4 cell counts for all age groups increased slightly from 2006 to 2012 (Figure 1). However, the median baseline CD4 cell count for patients 45 years and older remained below 250 cells/µl over the study period. The median baseline CD4 cell counts of patients by route of transmission show none-to-little increase over the study period (Figure 2). Individuals infected through heterosexual contact and through commercial blood plasma donation had considerably lower median baseline CD4 cell counts than other subgroups.

Discussion

The aim of our study was to identify the proportion of HIV-positive individuals in China who received baseline CD4 testing within 6 months and characteristics associated with failing to receive testing within 6 months. CD4 cell count measurements are a standard component of HIV testing algorithms to monitor disease progression. Few past studies in China [20] have evaluated access to baseline CD4 cell count testing, and this is the first study to present results on a national scale.

In the era of "Treatment as Prevention," early HIV detection, timely monitoring of disease progression, and early linkage to ART are critical steps to curbing the spread of HIV [25,26,27,28]. In the United States, about 77% of HIV-diagnosed individuals are linked to care within 3–4 months, and 51% were retained in ongoing care [29]. With effective interventions such as the addition of case management, the proportion of HIV-positive patients linked to ongoing care can be significantly increased compared to those who receive the standard of care [30]. As China continues to develop and expand its national AIDS programs, including the NFATP, it will be critical to have regular assessment and monitoring of the programs' ability to link newly identified HIV-positive individuals to timely CD4 testing and treatment initiation.

To monitor the implementation of the national AIDS programs, NCAIDS developed annual quantitative targets of core program elements, including the "proportion of people known to be living with HIV whose CD4 cell counts were monitored at least once a year, to determine anti-retroviral therapy eligibility" [21]. For individuals nationwide diagnosed with HIV and AIDS, this proportion rose from 45.3 and 10.1% in 2007 to 54.2 and 62.5% in 2009, respectively [21]. Expanding on this previous finding, this current study shows that significant progress has also been made in increasing baseline CD4 cell count testing among HIV newly diagnosed individuals, as evidenced by the increase in CD4 cell count testing within 6 months from 20.0% in 2006 to 76.9% in 2012. The increases in CD4 monitoring of both new HIV cases and previously diagnosed cases were facilitated by structural expansions of the national AIDS programs and increases in the availability of testing materials/equipment [20,31].

National policies recommend that the blood draw for the baseline CD4 cell count test should be completed at the first follow-up visit, which is scheduled at 14 days following the diagnosis. In our study, about 53.7% of individuals diagnosed in 2012 did not receive baseline CD4 cell count testing by the 14-day benchmark, and 23.1% did not receive CD4 cell count testing within 6 months. We identified several individual-level risk factors for failing to receive CD4 cell count testing within 6 months: age 55 years or older, male, primary school education or below, route of HIV transmission categorized as injection drug use or combined sexual contact and injection drug use, being diagnosed at a hospital or a detention center, and being a migrant worker. Some population-level factors are also likely to influence the obtainment and timing of CD4 testing. Until recent years, many county hospitals did not have the CD4 cell count testing equipment. In several regions with very low HIV prevalence, some counties and municipalities only had one CD4 detection machine for the entire area. This was likely to have delayed CD4 cell count testing for a small propotion of newly diagnosed HIV-positive individuals. Other population-level factors may include stigma and long distances between residences and clinics [32].

In our study, the majority of newly HIV diagnosed individuals were infected through heterosexual contact (Table 2). This is in accordance with recent literature indicating that sexual transmission has become the dominant mode of HIV transmission in China [23,33,34]. Over 60% of these individuals had baseline CD4 cell counts <350 cells/µl over the study period (Table 3), which is a higher proportion than those infected by male-to-male sexual contact or injection drug use. While HIV in China was historically driven by epidemics among injection drug users (IDUs), China will need to adjust to the challenges of facing an HIV epidemic that is predominantly spread by sexual contact. The group with the highest proportion (over 75%) of CD4 cell counts <350 cells/µl were individuals infected through commercial blood plasma donation. In the mid-1990s, there were major outbreaks of HIV through unsafe commercial blood and plasma donations [35,36]. The extent of the epidemic was identified through large-scale targeted screening interventions among former paid plasma donors [37].

The two populations who had the highest median baseline CD4 counts were IDUs and men who have sex with men (MSM). This suggests that outreach efforts to reach these high-risk populations have produced some success in promoting early and regular HIV screening. However, MSM had the highest percentage of timely CD4 testing (78.7%) while IDUs had the lowest percentage (34.9%) when comparing subpopulations by route of transmission. Past research studies have similarly noted that MSM present with higher median CD4 levels compared to other risk groups [7]. In

Table 3. Number and percentage of newly HIV-diagnosed adults receiving baseline CD4 cell count testing within 6 months of diagnosis in China: 2006–2012, by routes of HIV transmission.

		2006		2007		2008		2009		2010		2011		2012		χ^2
	Total	No.	%	No.	%	No.	%	No.	%	No.	%	No.	%	No.	%	P-value
Heterosexual contact																
<200	54579	1519	46.0	3043	42.0	4863	39.3	7229	39.7	9459	38.7	13277	37.7	15189	35.6	
200–349	35232	712	21.5	1686	23.2	3015	24.4	4279	23.5	6031	24.7	8870	24.7	10639	24.9	$\chi^2 = 119.63$
350–500	28918	522	15.8	1282	17.7	2298	18.6	3426	18.8	4674	19.1	7225	19.1	9491	22.3	$p<0.01$
≥500	24702	552	16.7	1240	17.1	2202	17.8	3274	18.0	4261	17.4	5839	17.4	7334	17.2	
Male-to-male sexual contact																
<200	6622	70	28.7	165	24.6	371	18.3	662	18.3	1059	18.8	1822	19.6	2473	18.0	
200–349	9274	65	26.6	182	27.1	575	28.4	1019	28.1	1525	27.0	2348	25.2	3560	25.9	$\chi^2 = 21.07$
350–500	10438	54	22.1	183	27.2	568	28.1	1033	28.5	1651	29.2	2763	29.7	4186	30.4	$p<0.01$
≥500	8943	55	22.5	142	21.1	511	25.2	910	25.1	1413	25.0	2383	25.6	3529	25.7	
Injection drug use																
<200	6635	549	33.1	867	30.5	1006	27.5	1115	26.4	1051	23.3	1100	21.4	947	19.9	
200–349	6158	375	22.6	660	23.2	840	23.0	991	23.5	1015	22.5	1209	23.5	1068	22.5	$\chi^2 = 191.81$
350–500	6277	305	18.3	601	21.1	802	22.0	901	21.3	1072	23.8	1312	25.5	1284	27.0	$p<0.01$
≥500	7721	431	26.0	715	25.2	1003	27.5	1213	28.8	1373	30.4	1530	29.7	1456	30.6	
Sexual contact and injection drug use																
<200	566	8	40.0	19	35.8	90	24.9	140	32.9	94	20.8	126	29.2	89	24.3	
200–349	482	5	25.0	10	18.9	95	26.2	86	20.2	98	21.7	92	21.3	96	26.2	$\chi^2 = 0.85$
350–500	461	3	15.0	7	13.2	78	21.5	86	20.2	106	23.5	89	20.6	92	25.1	$p = 0.36$
≥500	602	4	20.0	17	32.1	99	27.3	113	26.6	154	34.1	125	28.9	90	24.5	
Blood (plasma) donation																
<200	6502	1030	66.3	1215	68.3	1129	60.6	1046	63.2	824	61.4	773	56.5	485	55.8	
200–349	1867	274	17.6	290	16.3	364	19.5	281	17.0	241	17.9	247	18.1	170	19.6	$\chi^2 = 66.95$
350–500	1152	149	9.6	143	8.0	192	10.3	178	10.8	153	11.4	198	14.5	139	16.0	$p<0.01$
≥500	908	100	6.4	131	7.4	177	9.5	150	9.0	125	9.3	150	11.0	75	8.6	

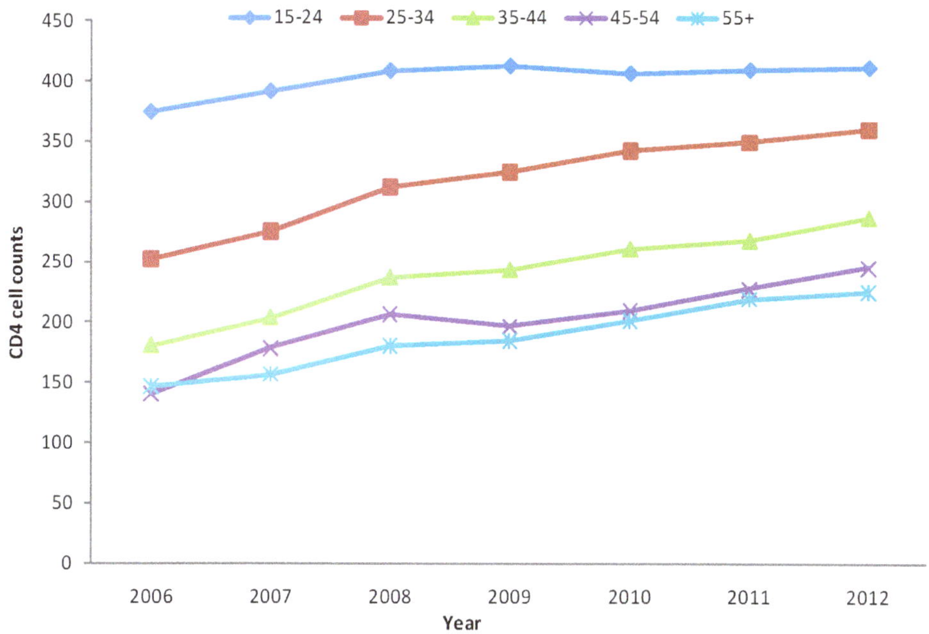

Figure 1. Median baseline CD4 cell counts (within 6 months of diagnosis) of newly diagnosed HIV individuals in China from 2006 to 2012, stratified by age group. The median baseline CD4 cell counts, stratified by age group, increased each year from 2006 to 2012. Older age groups were associated with lower median baseline CD4 cell counts.

our study cohort, the relative success in linking HIV-positive MSM to timely CD4 testing may also be due to a comprehensive prevention and control program in sixty-one cities from 2008 to 2009 targeted towards MSM. This program was carried out with the support of MSM community groups. This program led to policies and additional ongoing intervention programs that address

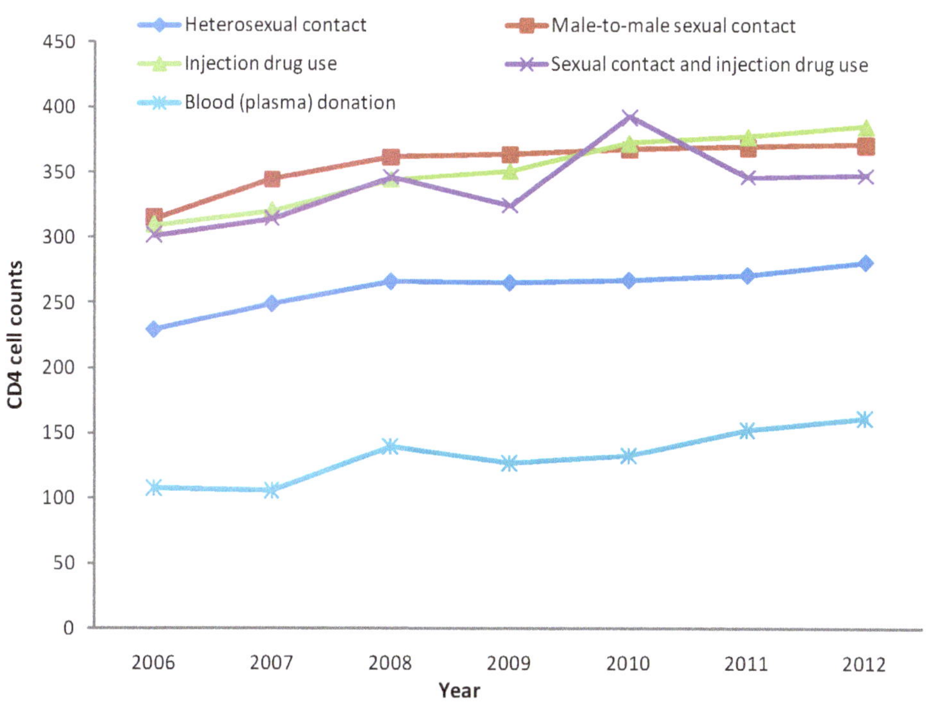

Figure 2. Median baseline CD4 cell counts (within 6 months of diagnosis) of newly diagnosed HIV individuals in China from 2006 to 2012, stratified by routes of infection. The median baseline CD4 cell counts, stratified by route of transmission, increased each year from 2006 to 2012. Subjects infected through injection drug use, male-to-male sexual contact, or sexual contact and injection drug use were consistently associated with higher median baseline CD4 cell counts compared to those infected through heterosexual contact or infected through blood (plasma) donation.

HIV prevention, HIV diagnosis and CD4 cell count testing among MSM.

The barriers for IDUs to access medical care are well-documented [38]. In China, many IDUs are engaged in migrant work, have unstable lifestyles, experience stigma and discrimination from health providers, and face the fear of arrest due to the illegality of drug use in China [19]. Our study noted a slight increase of CD4 cell count levels in IDUs over the study period. In recent years, several intervention measures been taken to decrease illicit drug use and to strengthen prevention and control of HIV transmission among IDUs [39,40]. Another significant strategy for engaging the HIV-positive IDU population in regular care is to expand access to methadone maintenance treatment, which has been shown to independently promote linkage to HIV care and treatment [41].

Our study found that older patients were more likely to present at late disease stages, which has been noted previously in the literature [42]. There is currently very limited research [43,44] on elderly HIV patients in China, who are not typically considered a vulnerable population for contracting HIV. According to data in CRIMS, the number of newly diagnosed individuals who were 55 years old or older has significantly increased in recent years [unpublished data, NCAIDS, 2013], as it has in the United States. Further studies are needed to explore issues related to the diagnosis and treatment of elderly HIV-positive patients in China.

Perhaps due to the implementation of the national AIDS programs [21] the proportion of patients with advanced HIV disease (CD4 count <200 cells/μl) has declined slightly since 2007. Of the 221,963 individuals who received timely baseline CD4 testing, the proportion of patients diagnosed late with HIV has declined slightly over the study period from 2006 to 2012. In our study cohort, 34.5% of individuals (N = 76580) had baseline CD4 counts of <200 cells/μl and 58.8% (N = 130434) had baseline CD4 counts of <350 cells/μl (Table 1). Late diagnosis and late ART initiation are strongly associated with negative health outcomes, including suboptimal CD4 increases with treatment, a high rate of opportunistic infections, and increased risk of mortality [45]. Early identification of HIV and prompt monitoring are critical to improving patient outcomes and reducing disease transmission.

Our study has several limitations. First, all data is reported by local providers and may have not been uploaded to the national databases in a timely manner. While providers and CDC staff review the data for completeness and accuracy, there may be some errors in the database. Second, in most cases, the route of infection was self-reported by the individual, and some misreporting may have occurred due to stigma, particularly for the categories of male-to-male sexual contact and injection drug use. Third, while we attempted to reduce the influence of confounding variables by using multivariate analysis, it remains possible that there was confounding by unmeasured variables. Fourth, our study analysis did not assess disease progression of the newly diagnosed HIV/AIDS patients by clinical staging or viral load testing. This information is available elsewhere in CRIMS; however, a full discussion of monitoring strategies over the study period is beyond the scope of this paper. Finally, our study did not exclude individuals who died between their diagnosis and the 6-month benchmark for timely CD4 testing. These patients were included in the 8% of the study cohort who were indicated as lost to follow-up and subsequently categorized as not having received timely CD4 testing. A study that only assesses individuals who were still living 6 months after HIV diagnosis may produce higher rates of timely CD4 testing.

The risk factors identified in this study should guide future intervention strategies to increase early HIV diagnosis and CD4 cell count testing among key populations. In recent years, an increasing number of HIV cases have been identified at VCT clinics at local CDC sites, which have higher rates of linkage to baseline CD4 testing. Regional strategies that have achieved success in reducing loss to follow up and increasing linkage to care have included in-parallel Western blot confirmation testing and baseline CD4 testing (Yunnan) and compressing the timeframe from screening, confirmation, and CD4 testing (Guangxi).

This study's evaluation of baseline CD4 cell count testing after HIV diagnosis provides a valuable reference for further increasing testing coverage and linkage to care. Despite significant improvement, a high proportion (23.1%) of HIV-positive patients still failed to receive timely CD4 count testing in 2012, the last year of the study. To shorten the time to CD4 cell count testing and to improve access to regular testing and treatment, there should be efforts to dramatically improve referrals and integration of patient tracking between the health facilities responsible for patient follow-up, CD4 cell count testing, and ART delivery.

Acknowledgments

The authors thank all of the health care and laboratory staff who participated in data collection for this study and conducted CD4 baseline testing.

Disclaimer: The opinions expressed herein reflect the collective views of the co-authors and do not necessarily represent the official position of the National Center for AIDS/STD Control and Prevention, Chinese Center for Diseases Control and Prevention. Funding organizations had no role in the design and conduct of the study; collection, management, analysis, and interpretation of the data; and preparation, review, or approval of the manuscript.

Author Contributions

Conceived and designed the experiments: HT YM ZW. Performed the experiments: HT JH JX LW QQ. Analyzed the data: HT. Contributed reagents/materials/analysis tools: HT JH JX LW QQ. Wrote the paper: HT CS ZW. Intepreted results: RD. Edited and revised manuscript: RD.

References

1. Mellors JW, Muñoz A, Giorgi JV, Margolick JB, Tassoni CJ, et al. (1997) Plasma viral load and CD4+ lymphocytes as prognostic markers of HIV-1 infection. Annals of Internal Medicine 126: 946–954.
2. Hogg RS, Yip B, Chan KJ, Wood E, Craib KJ, et al. (2001) Rates of disease progression by baseline CD4 cell count and viral load after initiating triple-drug therapy. JAMA 286: 2568–2567.
3. Dybul M, Bolan R, Condoluci D, Cox-Iyamu R, Redfield R, et al. (2002) Evaluation of initial CD4+ T cell counts in individuals with newly diagnosed human immunodeficiency virus infection, by sex and race, in urban settings. Journal of Infectious Diseases 185: 1818–1821.
4. Hammer SM, Squires KE, Hughes MD, Grimes JM, Demeter LM, et al. (1997) A controlled trial of two nucleoside analogues plus indinavir in persons with human immunodeficiency virus infection and CD4 cell counts of 200 per cubic millimeter or less. AIDS Clinical Trials Group 320 Study Team. N Engl J Med 337: 725–733.
5. Chaisson RE, Keruly JC, Moore RD (2000) Association of initial CD4 cell count and viral load with response to highly active antiretroviral therapy. JAMA 284: 3128–3129.
6. Chadborn TR, Delpech VC, Sabin CA, Sinka K, Evans BG (2006) The late diagnosis and consequent short-term mortality of HIV-infected heterosexuals (England and Wales, 2000–2004). AIDS 20: 2371–2379.
7. Buchacz K, Armon C, Palella FJ, Baker RK, Tedaldi E, et al. (2012) CD4 Cell Counts at HIV Diagnosis among HIV Outpatient Study Participants, 2000–2009. AIDS Res Treat 2012: 869841.
8. Ogbuanu IU, Torres ME, Kettinger L, Albrecht H, Duffus WA (2009) Epidemiological characterization of individuals with newly reported HIV

infection: South Carolina, 2004–2005. American Journal of Public Health 99 Suppl 1: S111–117.
9. Gardner EM, McLees MP, Steiner JF, Del Rio C, Burman WJ (2011) The spectrum of engagement in HIV care and its relevance to test-and-treat strategies for prevention of HIV infection. Clinical Infectious Diseases 52: 793–800.
10. Althoff KN, Gange SJ, Klein MB, Brooks JT, Hogg RS, et al. (2010) Late presentation for human immunodeficiency virus care in the United States and Canada. Clinical Infectious Diseases 50: 1512–1520.
11. Easterbrook PJ, Yu LM, Goetghebeur E, Boag F, McLean K, et al. (2000) Ten-year trends in CD4 cell counts at HIV and AIDS diagnosis in a London HIV clinic. AIDS 14: 561–571.
12. CD4 Collaborative Group (1992) Use of monitored CD4 cell counts: predictions of the AIDS epidemic in Scotland. AIDS 6: 213–222.
13. Thanawuth N, Chongsuvivatwong V (2008) Late HIV diagnosis and delay in CD4 count measurement among HIV-infected patients in Southern Thailand. AIDS Care 20: 43–50.
14. Tran DA, Shakeshaft A, Ngo AD, Rule J, Wilson DP, et al. (2012) Structural Barriers to Timely Initiation of Antiretroviral Treatment in Vietnam: Findings from Six Outpatient Clinics. PloS one 7: e51289.
15. Kranzer K, Zeinecker J, Ginsberg P, Orrell C, Kalawe NN, et al. (2010) Linkage to HIV Care and Antiretroviral Therapy in Cape Town, South Africa. PloS one 5: e13801.
16. Zhang F, Dou Z, Ma Y, Zhang Y, Zhao Y, et al. (2011) Effect of earlier initiation of antiretroviral treatment and increased treatment coverage on HIV-related mortality in China: a national observational cohort study. Lancet Infect Dis 11: 516–524.
17. Zhang F, Dou Z, Ma Y, Zhao Y, Liu Z, et al. (2009) Five-year outcomes of the China National Free Antiretroviral Treatment Program. Annals of Internal Medicine 151: 241–251, W-252.
18. Wu Z, Wang Y, Detels R, Rotheram-Borus MJ (2010) China AIDS policy implementation: reversing the HIV/AIDS epidemic by 2015. International Journal of Epidemiology 39 Suppl 2: ii1–3.
19. Zhang F, Haberer JE, Wang Y, Zhao Y, Ma Y, et al. (2007) The Chinese free antiretroviral treatment program: challenges and responses. AIDS 21: S143–148.
20. Zhang Y, Lu L, Li HQ, Liu W, Tang ZR, et al. (2011) Engaging HIV-infected patients in antiretroviral therapy services: CD4 cell count testing after HIV diagnosis from 2005 to 2009 in Yunnan and Guangxi, China. Chinese Medical Journal 124: 1488–1492.
21. Liu Y, Wu Z, Mao Y, Rou K, Wang L, et al. (2010) Quantitatively monitoring AIDS policy implementation in China. International Journal of Epidemiology 39 Suppl 2: ii90–96.
22. Wen Y, Zhao D, Ma Y, Zhao Y, Lu L, et al. (2011) Some patient-related factors associated with late access to ART in China' s free ART program. AIDS Care 23: 1226–1235.
23. Dou Z, Chen RY, Xu J, Ma Y, Jiao JH, et al. (2010) Changing baseline characteristics among patients in the China National Free Antiretroviral Treatment Program, 2002–09. International Journal of Epidemiology 39 Suppl 2: ii56–64.
24. Mao Y, Wu Z, Poundstone K, Wang C, Qin Q, et al. (2010) Development of a unified web-based national HIV/AIDS information system in China. International Journal of Epidemiology 39 Suppl 2: 79–89.
25. Galvan FH, Bing EG, Bluthenthal RN (2000) Accessing HIV testing and care. Journal of Acquired Immune Deficiency Syndromes 25 Suppl 2: S151–156.
26. García F, de Lazzari E, Plana M, Castro P, Mestre G, et al. (2004) Long-term CD4+ T-cell response to highly active antiretroviral therapy according to baseline CD4+ T-cell count. Journal of Acquired Immune Deficiency Syndromes 36: 702–713.
27. UNAIDS (2012) Global report 2012: UNAIDS report on the global AIDS epidemic. Geneva: UNAIDS.
28. Hull MW, Wu Z, Montaner JS (2012) Optimizing the engagement of care cascade: a critical step to maximize the impact of HIV treatment as prevention. Curr Opin HIV AIDS 7: 579–586.
29. Centers for Disease Control and Prevention (CDC) (2011) Vital signs: HIV prevention through care and treatment—United States. MMWR Morbidity and Mortality Weekly Report 60: 1618–1623.
30. Gardner LI, Metsch LR, Anderson-Mahoney P, Loughlin AM, del Rio C, et al. (2005) Efficacy of a brief case management intervention to link recently diagnosed HIV-infected persons to care. AIDS 19: 423–431.
31. Jiang Y, Qiu M, Zhang G, Xing W, Xiao Y, et al. (2010) Quality assurance in the HIV/AIDS laboratory network of China. International Journal of Epidemiology 39 Suppl 2: ii72–78.
32. Govindasamy D, Ford N, Kranzer K (2012) Risk factors, barriers and facilitators for linkage to antiretroviral therapy care: a systematic review. AIDS 26: 2059–2067.
33. Wu Z (2011) New challenge and complex situation on HIV/AIDS control and prevention in China (in Chinese). Chin J Public Health 27: 1505–1507.
34. Wang N, Wang L, Wu Z, Guo W, Sun X, et al. (2010) Estimating the number of people living with HIV/AIDS in China: 2003–2009. International Journal of Epidemiology 39 Suppl 2: ii21–ii28.
35. Wu Z, Liu Z, Detels R (1995) HIV-1 infection in commercial plasma donors in China. Lancet 346: 61–62.
36. Wu Z, Sullivan SG, Wang Y, Rotheram-Borus MJ, Detels R (2007) Evolution of China's response to HIV/AIDS. Lancet 369: 679–690.
37. Wu Z, Rou K, Detels R (2001) Prevalence of HIV infection among former commercial plasma donors in rural eastern China. Health Policy and Planning 16: 41–46.
38. Celentano DD, Galai N, Sethi AK, Shah NG, Strathdee SA, et al. (2001) Time to initiating highly active antiretroviral therapy among HIV-infected injection drug users. AIDS 15: 1707–1715.
39. Yin W, Hao Y, Sun X, Gong X, Li F, et al. (2010) Scaling up the national methadone maintenance treatment program in China: achievements and challenges. International Journal of Epidemiology 39 Suppl 2: ii29–37.
40. Smith K, Bartlett N, Wang N (2012) A harm reduction paradox: comparing China's policies on needle and syringe exchange and methadone maintenance. Int J Drug Policy 23: 327–332.
41. Zhao Y, Shi CX, McGoogan JM, Rou K, Zhang F, et al. (2013) Predictors of accessing antiretroviral therapy among HIV-infected drug users in China's National Methadone Maintenance Treatment Program. Addiction Forthcoming.
42. Mugavero MJ, Castellano C, Edelman D, Hicks C (2007) Late diagnosis of HIV infection: the role of age and sex. American Journal of Medicine 120: 370–373.
43. Liu H, Lin X, Xu Y, Chen S, Shi J, et al. (2012) Emerging HIV epidemic among older adults in Nanning, China. Aids Patient Care and STDS 26: 565–567.
44. Chen X, Zheng J, He JM, Qin B, Hu Y, et al. (2011) Unusual increase in reported HIV/AIDS cases among older persons in western Hunan province, China. Sexually Transmitted Infections 87: 538.
45. Lawn SD, Little F, Bekker LG, Kaplan R, Campbel E, et al. (2009) Changing mortality risk associated with CD4 cell response to antiretroviral therapy in South Africa. AIDS 23: 335–342.

2

Scale-Up, Retention and HIV/STI Prevalence Trends among Female Sex Workers Attending VICITS Clinics in Guatemala

Sonia Morales-Miranda[1]*, Jerry O. Jacobson[1], Itzel Loya-Montiel[1], Ricardo Mendizabal-Burastero[1], César Galindo-Arandi[1], Carlos Flores[2], Sanny Y. Chen[3]

1 Center for Health Studies, Universidad del Valle de Guatemala, Guatemala City, Guatemala, **2** National STI/HIV/AIDS Program, Ministry of Public Health, Guatemala City, Guatemala, **3** Division of Global HIV/AIDS, Centers for Disease Control and Prevention – Central America Regional Office, Guatemala City, Guatemala

Abstract

Background: Since 2007, Guatemala integrated STI clinical service with an HIV prevention model into four existing public health clinics to prevent HIV infection, known as the VICITS strategy. We present the first assessment of VICITS scale-up, retention, HIV and STI prevalence trends, and risk factors associated with HIV infection among Female Sex Workers (FSW) attending VICITS clinics in Guatemala.

Methods: Demographic, behavioral and clinical data were collected using a standardized form. Data was analyzed by year and health center. HIV and STI prevalence were estimated from routine visits. Retention was estimated as the percent of new users attending VICITS clinics who returned for at least one follow-up visit to any VICITS clinic within 12 months. Separate multivariate logistic regression models were conducted to investigate factors associated with HIV infection and program retention.

Results: During 2007–2011 5,682 FSW visited a VICITS clinic for the first-time. HIV prevalence varied from 0.4% to 5.8%, and chlamydia prevalence from 0% to 14.3%, across sites. Attending the Puerto Barrios clinic, having a current syphilis infection, working primarily on the street, and using the telephone or internet to contact clients were associated with HIV infection. The number of FSW accessing VICITS annually increased from 556 to 2,557 (361%) during the period. In 2011 retention varied across locations from 7.7% to 42.7%. Factors negatively impacting retention included current HIV diagnosis, having practiced sex work in another country, being born in Honduras, and attending Marco Antonio Foundation or Quetzaltenango clinic sites. Systematic time trends did not emerge, however 2008 and 2010 were characterized by reduced retention.

Conclusions: Our data show local differences in HIV prevalence and clinic attendance that can be used to prioritize prevention activities targeting FSW in Guatemala. VICITS achieved rapid scale-up; however, a better understanding of the causes of low return rates is urgently needed.

Editor: Julian W. Tang, Alberta Provincial Laboratory for Public Health/University of Alberta, Canada

Funding: This project was supported by the President's Emergency Plan for AIDS Relief (PEPFAR) through the Centers for Disease Control and Prevention under the terms of the Cooperative Agreement #GH000011 with Del Valle University of Guatemala. DISCLAIMER: The findings and conclusions in this paper are those of the authors and do not necessarily represent the official position of the Centers for Disease Control and Prevention. Use of trade names and commercial sources are for identification purposes only and does not imply endorsement by the Public Health Service or the U.S. Department of Health and Human Services. The funders had no role in study design, data collection and analysis, decision to publish, or preparation of the manuscript.

Competing Interests: SC is an employee of CDC, part of US Government. JJ is an independent consultant. There are no patents, products in development or marketed products to declare.

* Email: smorales@ces.uvg.edu.gt

Introduction

Guatemala has a concentrated epidemic of human immunodeficiency virus (HIV) with prevalence greater than 5% in at-risk groups, such as men who have sex with men (MSM) and male and female sex workers (MSW, FSW) [1]. Sexual transmission accounts for 93% of the HIV transmission in Guatemala [2]. In 1998, the first study of FSW reported an HIV prevalence of 4.7% (n = 470) in Guatemala City, 11.1% (n = 117) in Puerto Barrios, Izabal (Honduras border), and 2.4% (n = 210) in Escuintla and Puerto San José [3]. In 2003, HIV prevalence was reported at 4.3% in Guatemala City (n = 309) and Puerto Barrios (n = 98) and 2.4% in Escuintla and Puerto San José [4]. In 2006, a study of 300 FSW in Puerto Barrios, Quetzaltenango, Coatepeque, Zacapa, and Guatemala City found an HIV prevalence of 1.1% [5], and in 2010, another study of FSW from 17 departmental areas in the country reported an HIV prevalence of 3.8% [6]. The behavioral surveillance survey from 2012 reported an HIV prevalence of 1.1% (95% CI 0.5–2.4; n = 607) in Guatemala City, 3.7% (95% CI 1.8–6.5; n = 299) in Escuintla/Puerto San José, and 2.0% (CI

95% 0.7–4.3; n = 296) in Malacatán and Tecún Umán (Mexico border) [7].

The potential for sexually transmitted infections (STIs) to facilitate HIV transmission has been widely documented [8]. Data have shown that the control of STI can prevent the acquisition of HIV infection. In 2007, the Guatemala Ministry of Public Health (MSPAS) implemented the Sentinel Surveillance of HIV/STI (VICITS) strategy in existing public health clinics–a strategy that lies within the framework of second-generation HIV surveillance that utilizes STI and behavioral data to inform, prevent, and control the HIV epidemic in key populations in Guatemala. The VICITS clinics serve the general population and key populations such as MSM, FSW, and transgender individuals. They provide more extensive services for the prevention, diagnosis, care, and treatment of STIs to FSW than the general population. These specific services include a comprehensive physical examination with gynecological and anal examinations, laboratory diagnosis of STIs, STI counseling, and access to STI medications and condoms. Currently, there are four VICITS clinics that serve FSW: STI health center in Zone 3 in Guatemala City (since 2007), health center in the city of Puerto Barrios in Izabal bordering Honduras (since 2008), health clinic at Marco Antonio Foundation (FMA), non-governmental organization (NGO) in Guatemala City (since 2010), and a health center in Quetzaltenango, the second largest city in Guatemala (since 2010).

By law, FSW working in Guatemala must register routine visits to health centers in an official booklet to certify that they do not have an STI infection [9]. Since 2007, MSPAS has obtained sentinel surveillance data for HIV, syphilis, chlamydia, and gonorrhea among FSW through the VICITS strategy. In addition to providing sentinel surveillance data for MSPAS program use and action, the VICITS strategy also provides behavioral interventions for the prevention and control of STIs among FSW, such as increasing the knowledge of HIV and STI transmission, encouraging consistent condom use, and distributing condoms at each visit. Specialized counseling for FSW is also provided by health personnel who receive periodic trainings in stigma and discrimination and who have an awareness and understanding of the implication of stigma in creating obstacles to effective HIV prevention.

In the absence of reliable data sources to characterize the HIV and STI epidemic among FSW, the VICITS strategy presents a promising option for lower-middle income countries with limited resources. The VICITS model, which integrates provision of STI diagnostic and treatment services, HIV prevention including condom promotion and behavioral interventions, and routine monitoring of clinical, behavioral, and laboratory data for surveillance purposes, was first implemented in Bolivia [10]. Although on-going collection of HIV and STI sentinel surveillance data among FSW has been conducted in Guatemala since 2007, no analyses have been conducted to explore HIV and STI trends over time or to describe performance in terms of scale-up and retention outcomes.

We analyzed risk behaviors and the prevalence of HIV and STI infection over a 5-year period (2007–2011), and investigated risk factors for HIV infection among FSW attending four VICITS clinics in Guatemala. Additionally, as measures of success of the VICITS strategy, we investigated scale-up, retention, and factors associated with retention at four clinics.

Methods

VICITS clinics

We included the four existing VICITS clinics in our analyses: STI health center No. 2 located in zone 3 in Guatemala City (Zone 3); a health center in Puerto Barrios, Izabal (PB); FMA located in zone 4 in Guatemala City; and a health center in Quetzaltenango city.

FSW VICITS attendees

Women 18 years of age or older who presented for a routine medical visit at one of the four VICITS clinics, who reported exchanging sex for money in the last 12 months, and who agreed to provide consent were recruited into the VICITS program.

Comprehensive HIV/STI prevention strategy (or VICITS services)

Clinic attendees who met the inclusion criteria received the following services at the first visit: pre-test counseling for HIV/STI including promotion of condom use, physical evaluation (including vaginal and anal exams), HIV testing and etiologic diagnosis of syphilis, genital infection with *Neisseria gonorrhoeae* or *Chlamydia trachomatis*, and syndromic management of STIs, treatment of STIs, as indicated, post-test counseling for HIV, and free condoms. The attending physician or nurse collected data using a standard medical record form from a face-to-face interview on patient demographics, sexual relationships, medical history, and findings from the physical evaluation and laboratory test results at each visit. Demographic information, and alcohol and illicit drug use were assessed during the first visit only. Laboratory test results were assessed every three and six months. After the initial visit, FSW with symptoms or signs of an STI were evaluated at least every 15 days and received presumptive treatment and a reference card for free treatment of their partners at VICITS clinics. FSW who tested positive for HIV were referred to the MSPAS Comprehensive Care Unit for follow up and treatment if indicated.

Laboratory tests

HIV was diagnosed using rapid tests (Determine) on-site in accordance with the national algorithm for HIV screening and confirmed with Enzyme-Linked Immuno Sorbent Assay (ELISA) at the National Reference Laboratory [11]. Syphilis was diagnosed with reactive Venereal Disease Research Laboratory (VDRL) with *hiso end-point dilution* titer ≥1:8 and confirmed with treponema rapid test or *Treponema pallidum* particle agglutination (TPPA) at the local laboratory and with ELISA at the National Health Laboratory. Genital infection with *Neisseria gonorrhoeae* or *Chlamydia trachomatis* was diagnosed with PACE2 test (Gen-Probe) at VICITS clinic Zone 3. All STI testing procedures followed the national algorithm [11]. Syphilis and HIV results were delivered 45 minutes after samples were collected. Quality control procedures were performed every three months on 100% of the HIV-positive samples and 10% of the HIV-negative samples at the National Reference Laboratory.

Statistical analysis

Following each visit, data from the form were entered into an Epi-Info database. The unique patient identifier was an alphanumeric code comprising initials of first and last names, sex, and birth date. In a given year, an active patient was defined as a FSW with at least one registered consultation to a VICITS clinic during the year. The number of FSW attending VICITS clinics each year

Table 1. Sociodemographic and behavioral characteristics of FSW attending VICITS clinics for the first time by clinic, Guatemala, 2007–2011 (N = 5,682).

Clinic	Zone 3	FMA	Puerto Barrios	Quetzaltenango	P value**	Total
	n (%)	n (%)	n (%)	n (%)		n (%)
	N = 3,928	N = 597	N = 575	N = 523		N = 5,623
Year of first visit						
2007	556(14.1)	0	0	0	<.001	556(9.9)
2008	952(24.2)	0	45(7.8	0		997(17.7)
2009	1,119(28.5)	0	186(32.3)	0		1,305(23.2)
2010	748(19.0)	206(34.5)	183(31.8)	10(1.9)		1,147(20.4)
2011	553(14.1)	391(65.5)	161(28.0)	513(98.1)		1,618(28.8)
Median age in years (IQR)	26(22–30)	27(23–34)	25(22–30)	25(22–30)	<.01	26(22–31)
Marital status*					<.001	
Single	2,905(78.6)	412(69.5)	494(85.9)	420(80.3)		4,231(78.6)
Married/cohabiting	500(13.5)	172(29.0)	40(7.0)	53(10.1)		765(14.2)
Separated/Widowed	289(7.8)	9(1.5)	41(7.1)	50(9.6)		389(7.2)
Highest level of education completed*					<.001	
<Primary	1,483(37.7)	311(52.1)	222(38.6)	113(21.6)		2,129(37.9)
Primary	814(20.7)	152(25.5)	165(28.7)	109(20.8)		1,240(22.0)
≥HS	1,631(41.5)	134(22.4)	188(32.7)	301(57.5)		2,254(40.1)
Nationality					<.001	
Guatemala	2,616(66.6)	467(78.2)	258(44.9)	364(69.6)		3,705(65.9)
El Salvador	481(12.2)	88(14.7)	31(5.4)	62(11.8)		662(11.8)
Nicaragua	527(13.4)	19(3.2)	37(6.4)	50(9.6)		633(11.3)
Honduras	289(7.4)	19(3.2)	247(43.0)	42(8.0)		597(10.6)
Other	15(0.4)	4(0.7)	2(0.3)	5(1.0)		26(0.5)
Pregnant					<.001	
Median age at first sexual intercourse (IQR)	16(15–17)	15(14–17)	15(14–17)	16(15–17)		16(14–17)
Age at first sexual intercourse					<.001	
<15	883(23.6)	197(33.0)	180(31.4)	110(21.0)		1,370(25.2)
15–17	2,076(55.5)	289(48.4)	303(52.8)	301(57.5)		2,969(54.6)
≥18	782(20.9)	111(18.6)	91(15.8)	112(21.4)		1,096(20.2)
Time in sex work*					<.001	
≤1 year	2,295(64.6)	128(33.2)	359(63.1)	212(40.6)		2,994(59.5)
>1 year	1,257(35.4)	257(66.7)	210(36.9)	310(59.4)		2,034(40.4)
Ever practiced sex work in another country	206(6.0)	17(4.3)	75(13.6)	41(7.8)	<.001	339(6.9)
Median number of clients in the past 7 days	10(5–24)	15(7–25)	4(2–7)	15(10–20)		10(5–20)
Consistent condom use with clients in the past 30 days*	3,650(97.0)	524(91.4)	533(95.5)	509(98.4)	<.001	5,216(96.4)
Sex work location*					<.001	
Strip club	1,693(43.1)	8(1.3)	59(10.3)	339(64.8)		2,099(37.3)
Bar	1,051(26.8)	83(13.9)	480(83.5)	124(23.7)		1,738(30.9)
Street	263(6.7)	338(56.7)	2(0.3)	6(1.1)		609(10.8)
Brothels based at residential homes	791(20.1)	14(2.3)	24(4.2)	39(7.5)		868(15.4)
Other	130(3.3)	153(25.7)	10(1.7)	15(2.9)		308(5.5)
Tested for HIV in the last 12 months	1,075(38.4)	458(77.0)	551(95.8)	474(90.6)	<.001	2,558(57.0)

Table 1. Cont.

Clinic	Zone 3	FMA	Puerto Barrios	Quetzaltenango	P value**	Total
	n (%)	n (%)	n (%)	n (%)		n (%)
	N = 3,928	N = 597	N = 575	N = 523		N = 5,623
Know HIV positive status in the first visit	4(0.4)	7(1.5)	14(2.0)	1(0.2)	<.001	26(1.0)
Ever used drugs	922(26.0)	68(11.5)	154(26.8)	17(3.2)	<.001	1,161(22.2)
STI diagnosis in the past 12 months	420(10.7)	55(9.2)	28(4.9)	87(6.6)	<.001	590(10.5)

*Totals do not add up due to missing observations.
**Chi-square test for categorical variables and Mann-Whitney-Wilcoxon test for continuous variables.

during 2007–2011 was calculated for each VICITS clinic. We analyzed socio-demographic characteristics (age, marital status, literacy, nationality) and behavioral variables (age at first sexual intercourse, number of years in sex work, number of clients within the past week, consistent condom use with clients in the past 30 days, sex work location (e.g. bar, strip club, brothel or street), tested for HIV in the past 12 months, lifetime drug use, and STI diagnosis in the past 12 months).

Prevalence of HIV and STIs among active FSW in VICITS during 2007–2011 was estimated annually. Prevalence of HIV infection included laboratory results up to and including the respective year. Time trends in STI prevalence were assessed using person-level logistic regression models estimated separately for each VICITS location. The models regressed laboratory-confirmed infection status on year of first visit to identify time trends in prevalence. Transforms of year (square, cubed, square root) were also examined. Time trends in demographic and behavioral characteristics of VICITS clients were assessed similarly. Discrete quantitative variables (e.g. number of partners) were assessed using normal instead of logistic regression models. Separately, person-level logistic regression models controlling for facility assessed factors associated with HIV infection and retention among first-time VICITS clinic attendees. Only known confounders and variables that were statistically significant ($p<.10$) in univariate analyses were included in the multivariate model. The final model includes adjusted odds ratio significant at the 10% level.

Scale-up of services and retention of clients over time were also assessed as indicators of program performance. Retention was defined as the percentage of patients who returned for one or more follow-up visits to the same or a different clinic within 12 months of the initial visit. Because systematic patterns in retention are relevant to interpreting trends in infection prevalence among active patients, a logistic regression predicting retention was fit to health center, socio demographic characteristics, and behavioral variables. Year of visit was also examined as a covariate in order to estimate trends in retention unexplained by changes in patient characteristics over time. Diagnosis of HIV prior to entering VICITS and during the first VICITS visit was also examined.

Ethical statements

This is a secondary data analysis, not associated with patient identification data. The protocol was approved by Del Valle University and Centers for Disease Control and Prevention (CDC) Atlanta Ethics Committee.

Results

Characteristics of FSW seeking health services at VICITS clinics for the first-time

A total of 5,682 FSW visited one of four VICITS clinics for the first-time from 2007 through 2011. The majority of the FSWs were seen at Zone 3 (Table 1). The median age at all four clinics was 26 years (IQR 22–31), 78.6% were single, 37.9% had less than primary education completed, and 65.9% reported being born in Guatemala. However, at the Puerto Barrios (PB) clinic, which borders Honduras, we observed a higher percentage of FSW of Honduran nationality compared to other clinics. The median number of clients in the past seven days at all clinics was 10 (IQR 5–20), 59.5% reported practicing sex work for less than a year, and 3.6% reported inconsistent condom use with clients in the past 30 days. Approximately 84% reported working primarily at venue-based locations (i.e. strip clubs, brothels based at residential homes or bars) and only 10.8% reported working at street locations. Of note, FSW attending the FMA clinic had different characteristics than other clinics with 29.0% reported being married or cohabitating with a partner, 52.1% having less than primary education completed, 56.7% working primarily on the streets, and 9.6% using condoms inconsistently with clients in the past 30 days (Table 1).

Prevalence of HIV and other STI

Annual HIV prevalence at each of the clinics is shown in Table 2. HIV prevalence was greatest among FSW seen at the PB site, with no statistical difference over the years. *Chlamydia* had the highest prevalence of all other STIs at all four clinics. The annual chlamydia and syphilis prevalence in Zone 3 and PB remained constant over time while the prevalence of gonorrhea increased in PB (0% in 2009, 0% in 2010, 4.4% in 2011; $p = .04$) and remained constant in Zone 3.

In multivariate analysis, risk factors for HIV infection during 2007–2011 included attending the PB clinic (adjusted odds ratio [AOR] 4.52, 95% CI 2.09–9.78), having less than primary education vs. primary education (AOR 1.96, 95% CI 1.08–3.57), current syphilis infection (AOR 4.32, 95% CI 1.46–12.81), working primarily on the street (AOR 4.14, 95% CI 1.60–10.69), and using the telephone or internet to contact clients (AOR 3.40, 95% CI 1.11–10.38) (Table 3).

Scale-up

The four project sites initially experienced significant growth in the number of active (first-time and returning) FSW clients

Table 2. Prevalence of HIV and other STI among FSW attending VICITS clinics for the first-time by clinic, Guatemala, 2007–2011.

Clinic	2007		2008		2009		2010		2011		
	n/N	%	n/N	%	n/N	%	n/N	%	n/N	%	P value
Zone 3											
Chlamydia	6/168	3.6	20/414	4.8	9/138	6.5	13/221	5.9	0/43	0.0	0.74
Gonorrhea	0/168	0.0	6/414	1.4	2/138	1.4	0/221	0.0	0/43	0.0	0.46
Syphilis	8/507	1.6	10/698	1.4	5/692	0.7	3/546	0.5	5/464	1.1	0.15
HIV	5/509	1.0	10/715	1.4	6/703	0.9	2/547	0.4	7/462	1.5	0.85
FMA											
Syphilis	-	-	-	-	-	-	8/185	4.3	6/287	2.1	0.19
HIV	-	-	-	-	-	-	3/187	1.6	9/382	2.4	0.56
Puerto Barrios											
Chlamydia	-	-	-	-	4/28	14.3	8/98	8.2	3/45	6.7	0.27
Gonorrhea	-	-	-	-	0/28	0.0	0/98	0.0	2/45	4.4	0.04
Syphilis	-	-	0/5	-	2/70	2.9	5/118	4.2	1/104	1.0	0.46
HIV	-	-	0/5	-	4/86	4.7	4/117	3.4	6/102	5.8	0.56
Quetzaltenango											
HIV	-	-	-	-	-	-	0/2	-	2/259	0.8	-

Notes: HIV measure takes into account tests prior to and including the respective year; other STI measures include results during the year. Results not shown for n<25. Chlamydia and gonorrhea results not available at Quetzaltenango and FMA clinics. Syphilis results not available at the Quetzaltenango clinic.

Table 3. Risk factors associated with HIV infection among FSW attending VICITS clinics for the first time, Guatemala, 2007–2011 (N = 4,021).

Variable	OR (95% CI)	AOR (95% CI)
Age		
18–24	1.00	
25–34	1.09 (0.61–1.95)	
≥35	2.10 (1.04–4.24)	
Clinic		
Zone 3	1.00	1.00
FMA	2.09 (1.06–4.10)	0.73 (0.31–1.71)
Puerto Barrios	4.58 (2.40–8.74)	4.52 (2.09–9.78)
Quetzaltenango	0.75 (0.18–3.15)	1.11 (0.26–1.71)
Highest level of education completed		
<Primary	1.00	1.00
Primary	0.44 (0.24–0.81)	0.51 (0.28–0.93)
≥HS	0.54 (0.26–1.11)	0.73 (0.35–1.54)
Current syphilis infection	6.13 (2.13–17.59)	4.32 (1.46–12.81)
Sex work location		
Strip club	1.00	1.00
Bar	2.42 (1.17–5.02)	1.37 (0.61–3.11)
Street	3.69 (1.67–8.18)	4.14 (1.60–10.69)
Brothels based at residential homes	0.94 (0.33–2.72)	1.01 (0.35–2.94)
Other (telephone or internet)	3.13 (1.15–8.54)	3.40 (1.11–10.38)

(Figure 1). At the Zone 3 site, the number of FSW increased at an annual average of 85% from 2007 to 2009 and subsequently decreased at 8% annually during 2010 and 2011. At the PB site (on the Caribbean coast bordering Honduras), VICITS scaled up from 356% since the first year and by 19% annually thereafter.

Retention

Overall, retention (FSW returning to the same or different clinic within 12 months) was low across all four sites during 2007 through 2011. Quetzaltenango had the lowest retention rate in 2011, followed by FMA and PB. Our data show an increase in retention from 39.4% in 2007 to 42.7% in 2011 at the Zone 3 site and a decrease from 48.9% in 2008 to 37.3% in 2011 at PB (Table 4). In a multivariate logistic regression model controlling for age and education, factors associated with negatively impacting retention included having a current HIV diagnosis, ever practicing sex work in another country, being born in Honduras, presenting for the first consultation to VICITS at the FMA or Quetzaltenango clinic sites, and visiting a VICITS clinic for the first-time in 2008 or 2010 (Table 5). Systematic time trends with respect to retention were not detected (Table 5).

Discussion

Our data show local differences in HIV prevalence, patients characteristics, and clinic attendance that can be used to prioritize prevention activities targeting FSW in Guatemala. We found a low prevalence of HIV and other STIs among FSW attending VICITS clinics during 2007–2011. This trend was consistent with the findings from the behavioral surveillance survey implemented in 2012, which reported an HIV prevalence of 1.1% (95% CI. 5%–2.4%) in Guatemala City [7].

Also, we found no statistically significant differences in the prevalence of chlamydia, gonorrhea, syphilis, and HIV over time at the longest running VICITS clinic (Zone 3). These findings contrast with the report from the UALE project, another sentinel surveillance project implemented in Guatemala. They found a significant decline in gonorrhea, chlamydia, trichomoniasis, and candidiasis in follow-up visit during a 3.5 year period in Escuintla Guatemala. However, this finding could be attributed to the differences in demographic characteristics of FSW enrolled in the UALE project (e.g., higher illiterate rate among FSW in UALE compared to FSW in Zone 3) [12]. The PB site, which borders Honduras, reported the highest proportion of immigrant FSW. This group of FSW showed the highest HIV and chlamydia prevalence across VICITS clinics, but lower than the data reported by a similar sentinel strategy in Honduras [13]. The correlation of border and high STI prevalence was also described in another study conducted near the border of Guatemala and Mexico [14].

We also found that the VICITS surveillance and prevention strategy achieved rapid scale-up during 2007–2011. Although all four sites experienced a substantial increase in the number of FSW attending VICITS clinics for the first-time after the first year of implementation, we have observed a gradual decrease in the number of new VICITS clinic attendees at the longest running clinic in Guatemala City (Zone 3) since 2010. The opening of a second VICITS clinic in Guatemala City in 2010 can partially explain for this decrease at Zone 3, as both clinics serve FSW in Guatemala City. These findings suggest that the VICITS strategy is feasible and well accepted, at least initially, by FSW.

Low retention figures were found is all sites, but Quetzaltenango showed lowest retention rate across the four clinics. These results might be influenced by the mobility of the population and the lack

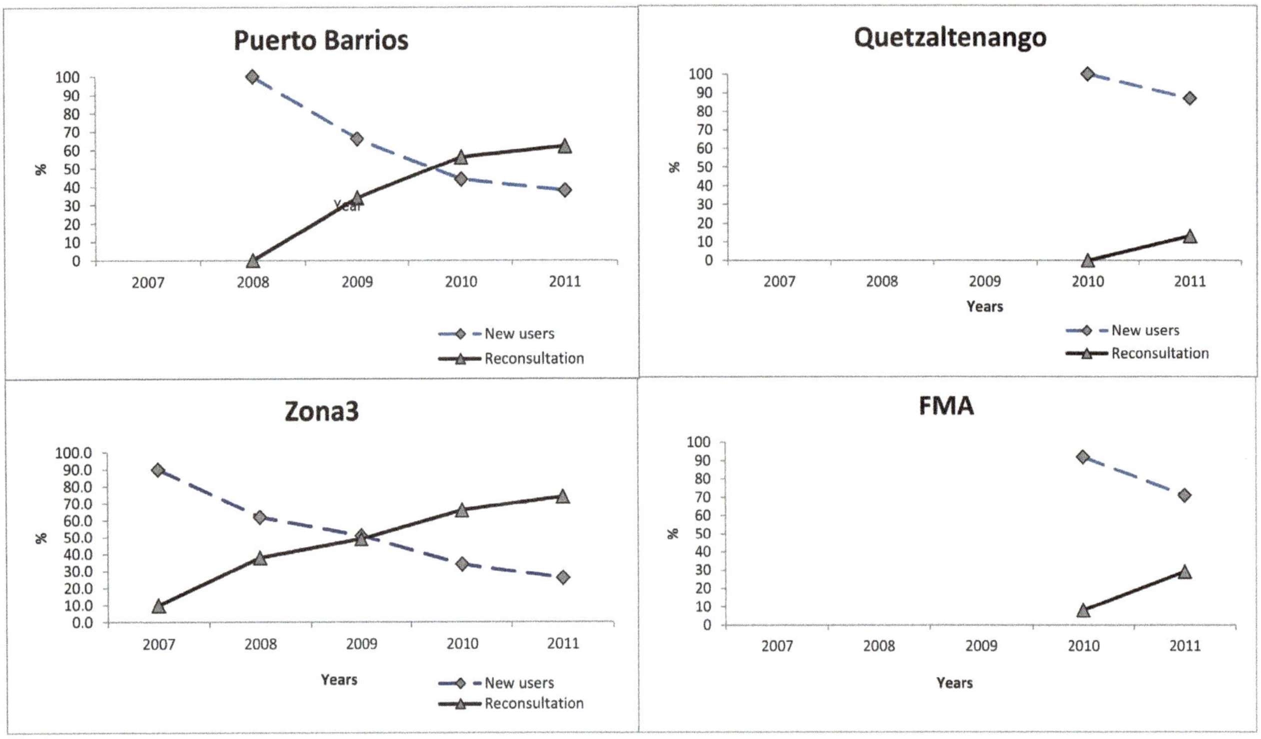

Figure 1. Number of active FSW attending VICITS clinics over time by clinic, Guatemala, 2007–2011.

of data from regular STI services in the country. However, these finding were similar to the data from Honduras that showed nearly half of FSW returning to follow up visits [13]. As we explore other methods to increase retention at VICITS sites, the experience and data from Peru suggests that the use of mobile clinics might increase the reach and retention of FSW at VICITS clinics [15].

Results from multivariate logistic regression showed that FSW who were diagnosed with an HIV infection at first-visit were less likely to return to the same or different VICITS clinic (retention) for re-testing and follow up. In Guatemala, national guidelines for HIV diagnosis makes obligatory reference to clinical care units for HIV follow up, but common illness, such as STIs, should continue to be treated at secondary care level (where VICITS clinics are). The loss of follow up of these patients might be due to this duality, but it might be also explained by dissatisfaction of public health services, as reported by other studies in Guatemala [16]. The VICITS strategy needs to focus in strengthening close follow up in order to improve retention, or in improving newer methodologies to reach and retain FSW. A better understanding of the causes of low return rates by first-time users at all clinics are urgently needed to enhance accuracy of sentinel surveillance data collected and to improve VICITS program retention.

Our findings are subject to several limitations. First, FSW attending VICITS clinics may not be representative of the FSW population in Guatemala. However, these estimates only reflect FSW attending VICITS clinics located in Guatemala's largest cities. Second, only FSW seeking health services at VICITS clinics are included in the analysis. Although all FSW must register routine visits in an official booklet, they can be seen at any health center of the MSPAS. Individuals who promote the VICITS strategy coordinate outreach activities with local NGOs, conduct weekly visits to places where FSW solicit business, and monitor social networking sites that promote the VICITS strategy on a weekly basis. They contact FSW and encourage them to seek health services at VICITS sites to increase testing coverage of the FSW population. Third, data are self-reported and social desirability may underestimate the reporting of stigmatized behaviors [11]. Counselors and clinical staff at VICITS clinics

Table 4. Distribution of FSW who returned for a follow-up visit within 1 year of initial visit by clinic, Guatemala, 2007–2011.

Clinic	2007	2008	2009	2010	2011
	% (n)	**% (n)**	**% (n)**	**% (n)**	**% (n)**
Zone 3	39.4 (554)	33.1 (949)	40.5 (1136)	34.5 (751)	42.7 (368)
Puerto Barrios	-	48.9 (45)	40.9 (186)	32.8 (183)	37.3 (110)
FMA	-	-	-	11.7 (206)	33.5 (275)
Quetzaltenango	-	-	-	0.0 (10)	7.7 (377)

Note: Data include patients with initial visits up to August 20, 2011.

Table 5. Factors associated with retention among FSW attending VICITS clinics for the first-time, Guatemala, 2007–2011 (N = 4,449).

Variable	OR (95% CI)	AOR (95% CI)
Facility		
Zone 3	1.00	1.00
FMA	0.53 (0.43–0.66)	0.38 (0.27–0.52)
Quetzaltenango	0.14 (0.09–0.20)	0.11 (0.07–0.17)
Puerto Barrios	1.02 (0.85–1.23)	1.06 (0.85–1.32)
Year of first visit		
2007	1.00	1.00
2008	0.79 (0.63–0.98)	0.77 (0.62–0.97)
2009	1.05 (0.86–1.29)	1.01 (0.82–1.25)
2010	0.66 (0.53–0.81)	0.76 (0.60–0.95)
2011	0.61 (0.49–0.75)	1.12 (0.87–1.45)
Age	1.09 (0.96–1.23)	1.01 (1.00–1.02)
Highest level of education completed		
<Primary	1.00	1.00
Primary	1.03 (0.91–1.17)	1.02 (0.88–1.18)
≥HS	0.79 (0.67–0.93)	0.85 (0.71–1.02)
Nationality		
Guatemala	1.00	1.00
El Salvador	1.02 (0.85–1.23)	1.00 (0.82–1.24)
Nicaragua	1.08 (0.90–1.29)	1.05 (0.86–1.28)
Honduras	0.84 (0.69–1.02)	0.77 (0.61–0.97)
Other	0.48 (0.18–1.28)	0.50 (0.17–1.53)
Ever practiced sex work in another country	0.77 (0.60–0.99)	0.75 (0.57–0.98)
Current HIV diagnosis	0.43 (0.21–0.90)	0.39 (0.18–0.85)
Ever used drugs	1.14 (0.99–1.31)	
Sex work location		
Strip club	1.00	
Bar	1.09 (0.95–1.26)	
Street	1.06 (0.86–1.31)	
Brothels based at residential homes	1.13 (0.95–1.34)	
Other*	0.68 (0.52–0.90)	

*Telephone or internet contacts.

are trained to reduce stigma and discrimination towards key populations. Fourth, we did not collect information on sex behavior with type of partner, which might explain the dynamics of HIV and STI transmission in Guatemala.

Despite these limitations, we contend that our VICITS strategy increases access to HIV and STI testing, thus increasing the possibility of early diagnosis of HIV-positive FSW and linking them successfully to care and treatment. In the current context of HIV surveillance and prevention in Guatemala, the VICITS strategy provides critical preventive and care services to key populations, while simultaneously monitoring the epidemic through the systematic collection of routine and programmatic data at existing public health clinics, without the need to conduct separate surveillance activities over time. This strategy provides timely surveillance data and important behavioral information for the design of new prevention activities that can strengthen existing prevention strategies to reduce HIV transmission in Guatemala.

Acknowledgments

The authors would like to thank the National HIV/AIDS Program, VICITS clinical and administrative staff from Zone 3, Puerto Barrios, Marco Antonio Foundation, and Quetzaltenango for their contribution to this work.

Author Contributions

Conceived and designed the experiments: SMM. Performed the experiments: SMM CGA. Analyzed the data: SMM JJ SC RMB. Contributed reagents/materials/analysis tools: CF SC. Wrote the paper: SMM JJ ILM RMB CGA CF SC.

References

1. ONUSIDA/OPS/UNICEF (2009) Retos planteados por la epidemia de VIH en América Latina y el Caribe. Peru.
2. MSPAS/CNE (2012) Estimaciones y proyecciones del VIH y VIH avanzado Guatemala. Guatemala.
3. Hernandez B, Arana B (2000) Prevalencia de VIH en poblaciones de alto y bajo riesgo. Guatemala.
4. Pinzon Z, Soto RJ, Aguilar S (2003) Estudio Multicéntrico Centroamericano de Prevalencia de VIH/ITS y Comportamientos en Trabajadoras Comerciales del Sexo en Guatemala. Guatemala.
5. VM (2006) Estudio de Línea de Base Proyecto Intensificación de las acciones de prevención y atención integral del VIH/SIDA en poblaciones y áreas prioritarias de Guatemala. Guatemala.
6. VM (2010) Informe de Linea Final de Evalaución: Proyecto "Intensificación de las acciones de prevención y atención integral de VIH/Sida grupos vulnerables y áreas prioritarias de Guatemala. Guatemala.
7. Morales-Miranda S, Alvarez-Rodriguez B, Arambu N, Aguilar J, Huamán B, et al. (2013) Encuesta de Vigilancia de Comportamiento Sexual y Prevalencia del VIH e ITS, en poblaciones vulnerables y poblaciones clave. Ciudad de Guatemala.
8. WHO (2012) Prevention and treatment of HIV and other sexually transmitted infections for sex workers in low- and middle-income countries: recommendations for a public health approach. Geneva.
9. MSPAS (1986) Acuerdo Gubernativo 342–86: Reglamento para el control de las enfermedades de transmisión sexual. Guatemala.
10. Levine WC, Revollo R, Kaune V, Vega J, Tinajeros F, et al. (1998) Decline in sexually transmitted disease prevalence in female Bolivian sex workers: impact of an HIV prevention project. AIDS 12. Available: http://journals.lww.com/aidsonline/Fulltext/1998/14000/Decline_in_sexually_transmitted_disease_prevalence.22.aspx.
11. PNS (2008) Lineamientos para la orientación en ITS, VIH y SIDA. Guatemala.
12. Sabidó M, Giardina F, Hernández G, Fernández VH, Monzón JE, et al. (2009) The UALE Project: decline in the incidence of HIV and sexually transmitted infections and increase in the use of condoms among sex workers in Guatemala. J Acquir Immune Defic Syndr 51 Suppl 1: S35–41. Available: http://www.ncbi.nlm.nih.gov/pubmed/19384099.
13. Tinajeros F, Miller WM, Castro L, Artiles N, Flores F, et al. (2012) Declining sexually transmitted infections among female sex workers: the results of an HIV and sexually transmitted infection prevention strategy in Honduras, 2006–08. Int J STD AIDS 23: 88–93. Available: http://www.ncbi.nlm.nih.gov/pubmed/22422681.
14. Uribe-Salas F, Conde-Glez CJ, Juárez-Figueroa L, Hernández-Castellanos A (2003) Sociodemographic Dynamics and Sexually Transmitted Infections in Female Sex Workers at the Mexican–Guatemalan Border. Sex Transm Dis 30(3): 266–71. Available: http://journals.lww.com/stdjournal/Fulltext/2003/03000/Sociodemographic_Dynamics_and_Sexually_Transmitted.18.aspx.
15. Campos PE, Buffardi AL, Cárcamo CP, García PJ, Buendia C, et al. (2013) Reaching the unreachable: providing STI control services to female sex workers via mobile team outreach. PLoS One 8: e81041. Available: http://www.pubmedcentral.nih.gov/articlerender.fcgi?artid=3839873&tool=pmcentrez&rendertype=abstract. Accessed 5 February 2014.
16. Porras C, Sabidó M, Fernández-Dávila P, Fernández VH, Batres A, et al. (2008) Reproductive health and healthcare among sex workers in Escuintla, Guatemala. Cult Health Sex 10: 529–538. Available: http://www.ncbi.nlm.nih.gov/pubmed/18568874. Accessed 13 February 2014.

3

Temporal Trends in the Swedish HIV-1 Epidemic: Increase in Non-B Subtypes and Recombinant Forms over Three Decades

Ujjwal Neogi[1]*, Amanda Häggblom[2,3], Michele Santacatterina[4], Göran Bratt[5], Magnus Gisslén[6], Jan Albert[7], Anders Sonnerborg[1,2]

1 Division of Clinical Microbiology, Department of Laboratory Medicine, Karolinska Institutet, Stockholm, Sweden, 2 Unit of Infectious Diseases, Department of Medicine Huddinge, Karolinska Institutet, Stockholm, Sweden, 3 Department of Infectious Diseases, County Council of Gävleborg, Gävle, Sweden, 4 Unit of Biostatistics, Institute of Environmental Medicine, Karolinska Institutet, Stockholm, Sweden, 5 Department of Clinical Science and Education, Venhälsan, Stockholm South General Hospital, Stockholm, Sweden, 6 Department of Infectious Diseases, University of Gothenburg, Gothenburg, Sweden, 7 Department of Microbiology, Tumor and Cell Biology, Karolinska Institutet, Stockholm, Sweden

Abstract

Background: HIV-1 subtype B (HIV-1B) still dominates in resource-rich countries but increased migration contributes to changes in the global subtype distribution. Also, spread of non-B subtypes within such countries occurs. The trend of the subtype distribution from the beginning of the epidemic in the country has earlier not been reported in detail. Thus the primary objective of this study is to describe the temporal trend of the subtype distribution from the beginning of the HIV-1 epidemic in Sweden over three decades.

Methods: HIV-1 *pol* sequences from patients (n = 3967) diagnosed in Sweden 1983– 2012, corresponding to >40% of patients ever diagnosed, were re-subtyped using several automated bioinformatics tools. The temporal trends of subtypes and recombinants during three decades were described by a multinomial logistic regression model.

Results: All eleven group M HIV-1 subtypes and sub-subtypes (78%), 17 circulating recombinant forms (CRFs) (19%) and 32 unique recombinants forms (URF) (3%) were identified. When all patients were analysed, there was an increase of newly diagnosed HIV-1C (RR, 95%CI: 1.10, 1.06–1.14), recombinants (1.20, 1.17–1.24) and other pure subtypes (1.11, 1.07–1.16) over time compared to HIV-1B. The same pattern was found when all patients infected in Sweden (n = 1165) were analysed. Also, for MSM patients infected in Sweden (n = 921), recombinant forms and other pure subtypes increased.

Significance: Sweden exhibits one of the most diverse subtype epidemics outside Africa. The increase of non-B subtypes is due to migration and to a spread among heterosexually infected patients and MSM within the country. This viral heterogeneity may become a hotspot for development of more diverse and complex recombinant forms if the epidemics converge.

Editor: Dimitrios Paraskevis, University of Athens, Medical School, Greece

Funding: Funding provided by Swedish International Developing Agency, CHAIN FP7 EU, the Swedish Civil Contingencies Agency [SWE-2009-151], and the Swedish Research Council [521-2012-3476 and 2007-7092]. The funders had no role in study design, data collection and analysis, decision to publish, or preparation of the manuscript.

Competing Interests: The authors have declared that no competing interests exist.

* E-mail: ujjwal.neogi@ki.se

These authors contributed equally to this work.

Introduction

Significant disparity is observed in the global distribution of human immunodeficiency virus type 1 (HIV-1) subtypes [1]. The greatest viral diversity is found in west and central Africa, while the epidemic is largely mono-phylogenetic in other regions, e.g. South Africa, Ethiopia, and India where HIV-1 subtype C (HIV-1C) dominates [2–5]. In resource rich areas, the epidemic was driven during the first decades by HIV-1 subtype B (HIV-1B) [6–8], but an increase of non-B subtypes in Western Europe has been reported [9,10]. However, cross-sectional data across 20 European countries show that HIV-1B is still predominant in all of the countries, ranging from 45% to 90% [7].

Representative information on the HIV-1 subtype distribution is valuable for tracking the epidemiology and understanding the evolutionary trajectory of the virus. With the advance of automated subtyping tools, the accuracy of subtype prediction and the feasibility to analyse large datasets have increased.

However, subtyping of viral recombinant forms needs more stringent analysis and the use of atleast two of the bioinformatics tools available is recommended [11].

Sweden has a low prevalence (0.06%) and incidence of HIV-1 infection and the migration from high prevalence countries has therefore played an important role in the increased diversity of the subtypes since the 1990s [12]. Our previous study of patients diagnosed 1980–1993, showed that almost exclusively HIV-1B was circulating up to the end of the 1980s [12]. An increasing trend with non-B subtypes was thereafter observed with 30% of newly diagnosed cases in 1993 and we predicted that the HIV-1 subtype distribution would become even more diverse [12]. A more recent study confirmed that HIV-1B has decreased over time in patients who were diagnosed between 2003 and 2010 in Sweden [13].

Although the HIV-1 epidemic in Sweden thus shifted from a mono-phylogenetic HIV-1B epidemic to a more diverse pattern over time [12,13], the detailed changes since the start of the epidemic up to now have not yet been described. We therefore re-subtyped all available sequences from HIV-1 infected individuals diagnosed in Sweden between 1983 and 2012, and described the temporal trends the HIV-1 subtypes and recombinants over three decades.

Material and Methods

Patients and dataset

The data were derived from the Swedish InfCare HIV database, which at the 31st December 2012 included >99% of living adult Swedish residents with confirmed HIV infection (n = 6374), and the majority of all patients diagnosed 1983–2012 (n = 9146), at 30 clinics from all regions of the country. The Public Health Agency of Sweden report 10332 individuals with HIV diagnosis during this time period (http://folkhalsomyndigheten.se/about-folkhalso myndigheten-the-public-health-agency-of-sweden/) but in the official statistics the numbers are over reported due to duplicates. Of the 9146 individuals, 7068 (77%) subjects have been exposed to combined antiretroviral therapy (ART) with three drugs or more from 1996, and at 31st of December 2012, 5872 (92.1%) were active on ART. Since 1983, 747 patients have left the country, 61 have been reported missing and 1813 patients have died, as reported in the database.

The database contains demographic data, clinical data, treatment history and the results of almost all routine genotypic resistance testing (GRT) ever performed, including the viral sequences, starting in 1992 [14]. In the national guidelines, routine GRT has been recommended for patients who fail ART and for newly diagnosed patients since 2001 [15]. In 587 out of the 2501 (23%) patients who were diagnosed between 1981 and 1991, the viruses have been sequenced retrospectively. Of the remaining patients from the 1980s, >700 subjects have earlier been serotyped and/or genotyped as belonging to mainly HIV-1B [12]. After excluding 33 HIV-2 patients, 253 patients with no registered date of HIV-1 diagnosis and 4925 patients with no sequence available in the database for re-subtyping, the present dataset included sequences from 3967 HIV-1 infected individuals (Table 1). The year wise HIV-1 diagnosis among the different transmission risk group is presented in table S1. Among the patients without sequences diagnosed before 1992, 49.7% were men who have sex with men (MSM), 21.8% were intra-venous drug users (IVDU), 18.5% were heterosexually infected and 10% were others/unknown. From 1992 up to 2012, the corresponding proportions were MSM: 20%; IVDU: 6.9%; heterosexually infected: 58.2% and others/unknown: 14.9%.

Sequences and subtyping

For accurate identification of recombinant forms only partial *pol* sequences that had a minimum length of 500 nucleotides (nt) were used. For patients with multiple sequences (1253/3967; 32%), the oldest sequence was used for subtyping and the most recent sequence was used to verify the subtype.

HIV-1 subtyping was inferred initially by two methods: i) REGA subtyping tool version 3 (REGA v3), which uses an improved decision-tree algorithm and has greater sensitivity for identification of pure subtypes and recombinants [11]; and ii) COMET (http://comet.retrovirology.lu/), which uses context-based modelling for expeditious typing of HIV-1 viruses. Both the tools showed best performances for pure subtypes and CRFs [11]. Additionally we used Recombinant identification program version 3 (RIP 3.0) with 200 nt window size, which determines recombination in shorter sequences (<700 nt) [http://www.hiv.lanl.gov/content/sequence/RIP/RIPexplain.html]; and HIV-1 BLAST, available in the HIV Los Alamos Database [http://www.hiv.lanl.gov/content/sequence/BASIC_BLAST/basic_blast.html], to identify the nearest HIV-1 sequences from different geographical proximity. Due to limitations such as differences in the length of the sequences, the presence of degenerate bases "N" inside the sequences (especially older sequences), thus detailed phylogenetic analysis was not done. Further, the presence of drug resistance mutations can affect the phylogenetic inference but not affect subtyping and the length of the sequences could be adjusted in the alignment in the automated tools. However, the REGA v3 uses phylogenetic methods to identify the subtype of a specific sequence.

A sequence was designated as a particular subtype if two of the three tools (REGA, COMET or RIP) determined it. The sequences were designated as pure subtype [A (A1 and A2), B, C, D, F (F1 and F2), G, H, J, and K], circulating recombinant forms (CRFs) [CRF01 to CRF49 as of May 2013], and unique recombinant forms (URFs). The URFs were further characterised using bootscan analysis incorporated in the Rega v3 tool and validated in the SimPlot v3 software [16].

Statistical analysis

Demography and clinical parameters were assessed by Kruskal-Wallis equality-of-populations rank test for continuous variables and χ^2 test for categorical variables. To assess trends of the HIV-1 subtypes, a multinomial logistic regression model [17] was used for the 3967 patients with HIV diagnosis between 1983 and 2012. The outcome (the HIV-1 subtypes) was grouped into HIV-1B (reference group), HIV-1C, recombinants, and other pure subtypes. The year of HIV-1 diagnosis was the only covariate considered within the model. Square root of year of diagnosis was also added in the model to test for non-linearity, but was not significant. As sensitivity analysis and to get a more detailed description of which strains were primarily imported to Sweden and which strains actually have spread in Sweden, we performed analyses restricted to: 1) All patients infected in Sweden (n = 1551); 2) Patients heterosexually infected in Sweden (n = 307); 3) MSM infected in Sweden (n = 921); 4) All patients born and infected in Sweden (n = 1165); 5) All patients infected outside of Sweden (n = 2161); 6) All patients born in Sweden and infected outside of Sweden (n = 455); 7) Patients born and infected outside of Sweden (n = 1699). Statistical analyses were performed using Stata version 12.1 SE (StataCorp LP, USA)

Ethical considerations

The study was approved by Regional Ethics Committée Stockholm (2005/1167–31/3). The patient information was anonymised and de-identified prior to analysis. The authors

Table 1. Demographics of individuals diagnosed with HIV-1 during 1983–2012 in Sweden, included in the study (n = 3967).

		B	C	Subtype Recombinant	Other Pure	All	P-value
Female	N (%)	206(11.0)	414(57.0)	380(44.2)	277(54.0)	1277(32.2)	<0.001**
CD4/μl at diagnosis	Median (IQR)	410 (243–593)	289 (161–440)	310 (140–510)	330 (180–500)	352 (189–534)	<0.001*
Year of diagnosis	Median (IQR)	2000 (1991–2007)	2005 (2000–2009)	2007 (2004–2010)	2005 (1998–2009)	2004 (1996–2008)	<0.001*
Year of sequence	Median (IQR)	2003 (1998–2008)	2007 (2003–2010)	2008 (2005–2010)	2007 (2003–2010)	2006 (2001–2009)	<0.001*
Route of transmission* **							
IVDU	N (%)	218(11.7)	2(0.3)	96(11.2)	11(2.1)	327(8.2)	
Hetero Male	N (%)	130(7.0)	227(31.3)	262(30.5)	160(31.2)	779(19.6)	
Hetero Female	N (%)	127(6.8)	341(47.0)	314(36.5)	228(44.4)	1010(25.5)	
MSM	N (%)	1334(71.4)	21(2.9)	98(11.4)	38(7.4)	1491(37.6)	
Other	N (%)	59(3.2)	135(18.6)	90(10.5)	76(14.8)	360(9.1)	
Total	N (%)	1868(100)	726(100)	860(100)	513(100)	3967(100)	<0.001**
Country of birth******							
Sweden	N (%)	1239(68.2)	82(11.4)	307(36.1)	97(19.1)	1725(44.3)	
Africa - East and Southern	N (%)	20(1.1)	459(64.0)	42(4.9)	197(38.8)	718(18.4)	
Africa - West and Central	N (%)	9(0.5)	74(10.3)	164(19.3)	65(12.9)	312(8.0)	
Asia and Pacific	N (%)	75(4.1)	11(1.5)	218(25.6)	19(3.7)	323(8.3)	
Caribbean	N (%)	25(1.4)	0(0)	3(0.4)	1(0.2)	29(0.8)	
Eastern Europe and Central Asia	N (%)	69(3.8)	2(0.3)	35(4.1)	51(10.0)	157(4.0)	
Latin America	N (%)	119(6.6)	2(0.3)	16(1.9)	11(2.2)	148(3.8)	
North Africa and Middle East	N (%)	57(3.1)	75(10.5)	29(3.4)	47(9.2)	208(5.3)	
Other	N (%)	204(11.2)	12(1.8)	36(4.2)	20(3.9)	272(7.0)	
Total	N (%)	1817(100)	717(100)	850(100)	508(100)	3892(100)	<0.001**
Country of transmission******							
Sweden	N (%)	1160(70.4)	73(11.0)	236(29.2)	82(17.6)	1551(43.3)	
Africa - East and Southern	N (%)	21(1.3)	408(61.6)	38(4.7)	181(38.8)	648(18.1)	
Africa - West and Central	N (%)	1(0.06)	67(10.1)	156(19.3)	62(13.3)	286(8.0)	
Asia and Pacific	N (%)	80(4.9)	13(2.0)	308(38.2)	22(4.7)	423(11.8)	
Caribbean	N (%)	6(0.4)	0(0)	2(0.2)	0(0)	8(0.2)	
Eastern Europe and Central Asia	N (%)	21(1.3)	1(0.2)	18(2.2)	46(9.9)	86(2.4)	
Latin America	N (%)	62(3.8)	1(0.2)	8(1.0)	4(0.9)	75(2.1)	
North Africa and Middle East	N (%)	24(1.5)	75(11.3)	16(2.0)	34(7.3)	149(4.2)	
Other	N (%)	272(16.5)	24(3.6)	25(3.1)	35(7.5)	356(9.9)	
Total	N (%)	1647(100)	662(100)	807(100)	466(100)	3582(100)	<0.001**

*Kruskal-Wallis equality-of-populations rank test; **Chi2 test: ***Intravenous drug users: IVDU; Hetero: heterosexually infected; MSM: men who have sex with men; Others: blood products or unknown; ****The countries were divided into categories based on the UNAIDS definition (http://www.unaids.org/en/regionscountries/countries/).

confirm that there are some restrictions on the data underlying the conclusions in the manuscript. Anonymized sequences may be accessed via Genbank (accession numbers, JQ698667–JQ698874) [13]. The sequences that were analysed are representative of the entire country thereby, in principle, allow for the reconstruction of the transmission network. The entire dataset is available upon request from the steering committee of InfCare HIV.

Results

Patient dataset

Patient's demographics are presented in Table 1. Self-reported country of infection was available for 91% (3600/3967) of the patients. Among them, 43% (1551/3600) of the transmission events had occurred in Sweden. The median year of diagnosis differed between the subtypes (HIV-1B: 2000; HIV-1C: 2005; other pure subtypes: 2005; recombinants: 2007) ($p<0.001$). Compared to HIV-1B, non-B subtypes had a lower median CD4+ T-cell count at diagnosis (B: 410/µl; C: 289/µl; other pure: 310/µl; recombinants: 330/µl) ($p<0.001$). Also, patients with non-B subtypes were more frequently late presenters than patients with HIV-1B (<200 cells/mm^3: 27–34% versus 20%; <350 cells/mm^3: 53–62% versus 40%).

Diversified presence of HIV-1 subtypes

All eleven pure subtypes and sub-subtypes within HIV-1 group M (3107/3967; 78%), 17 CRFs (757/3967; 19%), and 32 URFs (103/3967; 3%) were identified (Figure 1). HIV-1B dominated (47%) followed by HIV-1C (18%) and CRF01_AE (12%). HIV-1B dominated in MSM (91%) and IVDU (66%). Among IVDU, 27% were infected with CRF01_AE. A diverse pattern was seen in heterosexually infected patients among whom HIV-1C dominated (31%). The city wise major pure subtypes HIV-1B and HIV-1C along with major CRFs 01_AE and 02_AG was presented in table S2.

Subtype predictions using different tools

The REGA v3 and COMET showed 96% concordance to determine the subtypes and recombinants forms. The majority of the discordance was observed between RIP 3.0 versus REGA v3 and BLAST on subtyping of CRFs (mainly 01_AE and 02_AG). REGA v3 improved thus the identification of 02_AG compared to the RIP 3.0 tool, as reported earlier [11]. The highest concordance was observed between REGA v3 and BLAST (97%). For the patients for whom there was more than one sequence, a 98% (1207/1230) concordance was observed. The 2% discordance was due to read-length variations, mainly in the terminal region, which limited the possibility to identify recombinants. The median length of the sequences were 1058 nt (range: 551–1758 nt).

Temporal trends of HIV-1 subtypes and recombinants

There was a significant increase of newly diagnosed HIV-1C, recombinants, and other pure subtypes over time compared to HIV-1B (set as reference) ($p<0.01$) (Figure 2). The multinomial regression model was adjusted for year of diagnosis tested for non-linearity however it was not significant. By extending the graph, the model predicts the exceed of recombinant forms by 2015. In the sensitivity analysis of year of HIV-1 diagnosis, an increase of HIV-1C, recombinant forms and other pure subtypes, using HIV-1B as a reference, was seen for all patients (n = 1551) who were reported to be infected in Sweden. The relative risk ratio (RRR) for HIV-1C was 1.10 (95%CI: 1.06–1.14), for recombinants 1.20 (95%CI: 1.17–1.24) and for other pure subtypes 1.11 (95%CI: 1.07–1.16) (Table 2). The same pattern was seen for patients born and infected in Sweden (n = 1165) (HIV-1C: 1.06, 1.02–1.11; recombinants: 1.22, 1.17–1.27; other pure subtypes: 1.10, 1.05–1.17) and for patients heterosexually infected in Sweden (n = 307) (HIV-1C: 1.12, 1.06–1.18; recombinants: 1.19, 1.13–1.27; other pure subtypes: 1.14, 1.08–1.20). For MSM patients infected in Sweden (n = 921), recombinant forms (1.27, 0.99–1.19) and other pure subtypes (1.1, 1.05–1.17) increased significantly compared to HIV-1B, but not HIV-1C (1.08, 0.99–1.19).

In the second sensitivity analysis of the year of diagnosis restricted to the patients infected outside Sweden (Table 3), a significant increase of HIV-1C (1.07, 1.06–1.09), recombinant forms (1.15, 1.12–1.17) and other pure subtypes was seen (1.05; 1.04–1.07) when all patients (n = 2161) were analysed as well as for patients (n = 1699) who were born and infected outside Sweden (HIV-1C: 1.08, 1.05–1.11; recombinant forms: 1.14, 1.11–1.17; other pure subtypes: 1.05, 1.03–1.07). For patients (n = 455) born in Sweden but infected outside, recombinants (1.16, 1.11–1.20) and other pure subtypes (1.08, 1.03–1.13) were significantly increased, but not HIV-1C (1.03, 0.02–1.07).

Mosaic pattern of URFs

A total of 103 patients (3%) were infected by URFs. Recombinants between HIV-1A1 and D (A1D) were the most common (n = 21), followed by A1C (n = 12), A1G (n = 11), BC (n = 10), BF1, BD, CD, and complex triple recombinants (n = 7, each) (Figure 3A). Further major URFs (A1C, A1D, BC, A1G) which have HXB2 positions 2253 to 3260 and had minimum degenerate bases (≤5) were used for bootscan analysis (n = 43) implemented in Rega v3 with 400 bp window size and 20 bp step size and SimPlot analysis with 300 bp window size and 20 bp step size. The breakpoint analysis showed 33 different mosaic patterns of recombinants (Figure 3B), indicating a presence of diverse recombinants in the country.

Movement of major HIV-1 subtypes and recombinant forms

Based on the self-reported country of transmission along with the migration history in the country and probable geographic linkages of the sequences using BLAST analysis, the predicted movements of the HIV-1 strains were described. HIV-1C entered from three different regions: East Africa, Southern Africa and West-Central Africa (Burundi and Congo). CRF01_AE migrated from mainly Thailand and CRF02_AG from West-Central Africa. A fraction of 06_cpx migrated from Eastern Europe - Central Asia. HIV-1B was mainly introduced from Latin America, United States and Western Europe, although a small fraction was introduced from Thailand.

Discussion

The Swedish HIV-1 epidemic started in December 1979 in Stockholm with an outbreak of HIV-1B infection among MSM [18]. We describe now the changes of the diversity of the HIV-1 subtypes during three decades, using viral sequences from nearly 4000 patients, representing almost half of all diagnosed patients in Sweden ever. Our analysis shows that all eleven group M pure subtypes and sub-subtypes, 17 CRFs and several URFs have been introduced into the country and that there is a trend of increasing new diagnosis of HIV-1C and CRFs, as compared to HIV-1B.

The initial spread of HIV-1 in Western Europe was driven by HIV-1B [19]. Although, HIV-1B was still predominant among the MSM and the IVDUs in the present study, as also observed in a cross-sectional multinational European study [20], the prediction of a further diversification of HIV-1 subtypes in Sweden due

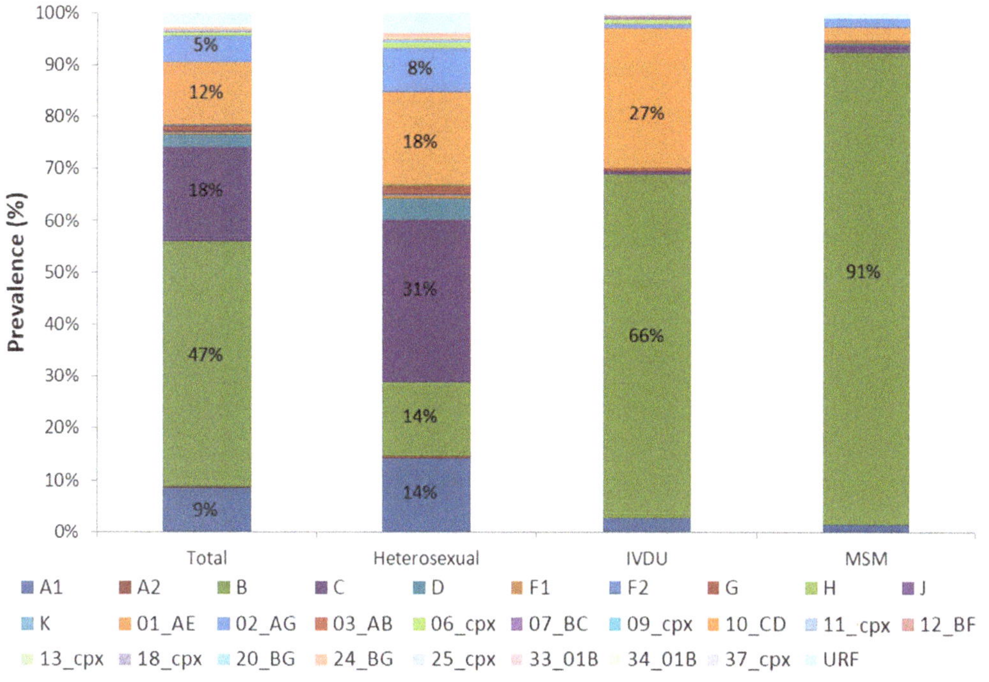

Figure 1. Distribution of HIV-1 subtypes in Sweden between 1983 and 2012. Final dataset included *pol* sequences (length >500 nt) from 3967 HIV-1 infected patients. HIV-1 subtyping was determined by three methods (see method section). The sequences were designated as pure subtypes [A (A1 and A2), B, C, D, F (F1 and F2), G, H, J, and K], circulating recombinant forms (01_AE, 02_AG, 03_AB, 06_cpx, 10_CD, 11_cpx, 12_BF, 13_cpx, 18_cpx, 20_BG, 24_BG, 25_cpx, 33_01B, 34_01B, 37_cpx) and unique recombinant forms (URFs).

migration was confirmed [12]. When virus sequences from all patients were analysed, increasing trends of HIV-1C, recombinants (CRFs and URFs) and other pure subtypes were thus observed. This strong increase of viral diversity at the national level was to a large extent due to human mobility from high prevalence countries, both from those where such a viral heterogeneity pattern prevails and from countries where the epidemics are largely mono-phylogenetic, such as Ethiopia and Thailand.

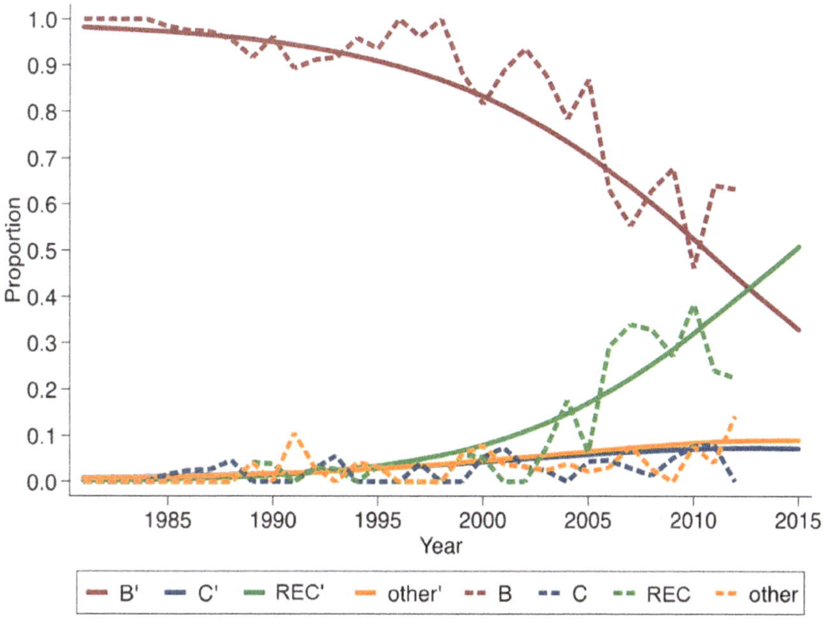

Figure 2. Proportions and predicted proportions of newly diagnosed HIV-1 subtype B (B), subtype C (C), recombinant forms (REC) and other subtypes (other) by year of diagnosis. Dotted lines represent actual prevalence in each year, while the smooth lines represent the predicted prevalence. Multinomial logistic regression model adjusted for year of diagnosis was used.

Table 2. Patients infected in Sweden - sensitivity analysis of year of HIV-1 diagnosis and the trends in subtype pattern during 1983–2012, using subtype B (HIV-1B) as reference.

	All patients infected in Sweden		Patients born and infected in Sweden		MSM infected in Sweden		Heterosexually infected in Sweden	
	(n = 1551)		(n = 1165)		(n = 921)		(n = 307)	
	RRR (95% CI)	p-value	RRR (95% CI)	p-value	RRR (95% CI)	p-value	RRR (95% CI)	p-value
HIV-1B	Ref.		Ref.		Ref.		Ref.	
HIV-1C								
Year of diagnosis	1.10 (1.06–1.14)	<0.001	1.06 (1.02–1.11)	0.007	1.08 (0.99–1.19)	0.096	1.12 (1.06–1.18)	<0.001
Recombinants								
Year of diagnosis	1.20 (1.17–1.24)	<0.001	1.22 (1.17–1.27)	<0.001	1.27 (1.17–1.37)	<0.001	1.19 (1.13–1.27)	<0.001
Other								
Year of diagnosis	1.11 (1.07–1.16)	<0.001	1.10 (1.05–1.17)	<0.001	1.22 (1.07–1.38)	0.003	1.14 (1.08–1.20)	<0.001

An multinomial logistic regression model [17] was used. The outcome (the HIV-1 subtypes) was grouped into HIV-1B (reference group), HIV-1C, recombinants and other pure subtypes. Relative risk ratio and 95% confidence intervals were determined. RRR represents relative risk ratio.

In addition to the migration of already HIV-1 infected individuals, we found that patients who were born and infected in Sweden contributed to the changing HIV-1 subtypes as well as those born abroad but reported to be infected in Sweden, as suggested by our sensitivity analysis. This was true also for MSM infected in Sweden where an increase of CRFs and other pure subtypes was described. Thus, the changing Swedish HIV-1 subtype pattern is not only due to migration of persons who were infected at arrival, but also to a spread of non-subtype B strains among migrants after arrival to the country and MSM. It shall be noted that the country of infection was self-reported and data collected this way are likely to underestimate the proportion of migrants infected after arrival to a country [21]. It is therefore not unlikely that the infection with non-B subtypes among persons living in Sweden is even higher than reported in the present study. Our finding of an increase of HIV-1C infections among those reported to have become infected in Sweden is line with the reports that in other regions where HIV-1C has been introduced, its prevalence has increased gradually. E.g. in Brazil, a temporal increase in the prevalence of HIV-1C and related recombinants has been observed over time [22,23].

A contribution to the relative increase in non-HIV-1B infections among newly diagnosed patients in Sweden could be that undiagnosed HIV-1 infection is more common among migrants, as compared to MSM [24]. The time of diagnosis is shifted away from time of infection towards more recent years. Thus, the T-cell counts at diagnosis were lower among non-B infected patients and late presentation was more common compared to HIV-1B infected subjects. Also, differences in the coverage rate and efficacy of ART may lead to a relative decrease in the number of persons infected by HIV-1B strains within the country since undetectable viremia due to ART is associated with minimal contagiousness [25]. Thus, although the general coverage rate in Sweden is presently high, >90%, the proportion of successfully treated MSM is even higher than among heterosexually infected individuals [24]. Considering the actual change in proportions over calendar years and the analysis predictions, the recombinant forms will probably dominate by the year 2015 among newly diagnosed patients in Sweden. But it is obvious that the development will still be highly dependent on the migration patterns for the coming years.

There are some caveats that need to be mentioned. Half of the patients had not sequences available for subtyping, among whom MSM dominated among those diagnosed before 1992 and migrants among those diagnosed later. However, there was no difference in gender and mode of transmission between those having sequences and those who did not have sequences. Also, most of these patients were diagnosed during the 1980s and we have earlier shown that the vast majority of patients during this time period were infected by HIV-1B [12]. At least 491 patients entered into the cohort when they were on therapy and due to non-detectable viral load, genotyping was not performed. However, the majority of these patients were migrants from Africa. Altogether, the trend in increase of non-HIV-1B is unlikely to be over-estimated, rather the opposite. Another caveat is that the country of infection was assessed through self-reports, but this bias would also rather result in an underestimation of non-HIV-1B [21]. It shall however be noted that it is not uncommon the migrants visit their home country and that they might become infected there [21]. Thus, our study cannot precisely define the actual spread of non-B strains within Sweden. It is also likely that the prevalence of recombinant forms was underestimated since only the *pol* region was sequenced, as earlier described for the Indian HIV-1 epidemic when only one gene was analysed [3].

Table 3. Patients infected outside of Sweden - sensitivity analysis of year of HIV-1 diagnosis and the trends in subtype pattern during 1983–2012, using subtype B (HIV-1B) as reference.

	All patients infected outside Sweden		**Patients born in Sweden and infected outside Sweden**		**Patients born and infected outside Sweden**	
	(n = 2161)		**(n = 455)**		**(n = 1699)**	
	RRR (95% CI)	p-value	RRR (95% CI)	p-value	RRR (95% CI)	p-value
HIV-1B	Ref.		Ref.		Ref.	
HIV-1C						
Year of diagnosis	1.07 (1.06–1.09)	<0.001	1.03 (0.02–1.07)	0.216	1.08 (1.05–1.1)	<0.001
Recombinants						
Year of diagnosis	1.15 (1.12–1.17)	<0.001	1.16 (1.11–1.20)	<0.001	1.14 (1.11–1.17)	<0.001
Other						
Year of diagnosis	1.05 (1.04–1.07)	<0.001	1.08 (1.03–1.13)	<0.001	1.05 (1.03–1.07)	<0.001

An univariate multinomial logistic regression model [17] was used. The outcome (the HIV-1 subtypes) was grouped into HIV-1B (reference group), HIV-1C, recombinants, and other pure subtypes. Relative risk ratio and 95% confidence intervals were determined. RRR represents relative risk ratio.

Despite these caveats, we believe that the strength of the study is that it covers data from the beginning of HIV epidemic till date and includes almost all sequences performed in routine diagnostics in Sweden, corresponding to almost 4000 individuals.

In conclusion, this is the first comprehensive study to describe the trends of the HIV-1 subtype distribution in Sweden since the beginning of the pandemic. To best of our knowledge, the epidemic is one of the most diverse epidemics outside west-central

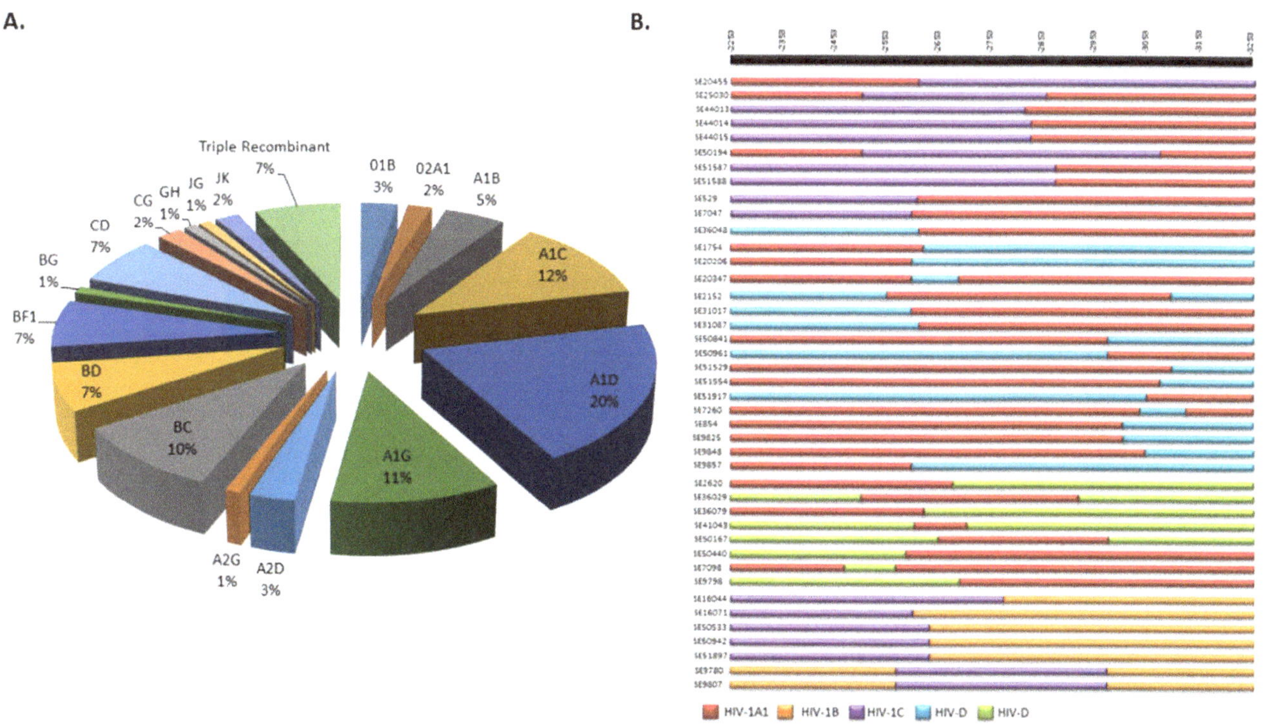

Figure 3. Types and mosaic pattern of HIV-1 unique recombinant forms identified in Sweden. A. Proportion of recombinant forms was identified based on REGAv3, COMET and RIP 3.0 followed by bootscan analysis incorporated in REGAv3 and SimPlot analysis. **B. Mosaic pattern of URFs identified by REGAv3 and SimPlot.** Major URFs (A1C, A1D, BC, A1G) which have HXB2 positions 2253 to 3260 and had minimum degenerate bases (≤5) were used for bootscan analysis (n = 43) implemented in Rega v3 with 400 bp window size and 20 bp step size and SimPlot analysis with 300 bp window size and 20 bp step size. The reference sequences were selected for SimPlot analysis is based on the recombinant pattern. Upper bar presents HXB2 co-ordinate.

Africa with presence of all pure HIV-1 M group subtype, 17 CRFs and 32 URFs. Countries such as Portugal, Belgium, Switzerland and more recently, UK and Germany are having similar trends with an increasing of non-B subtypes [20,26,27]. Presently, there seems to be no or limited transmission of HIV-1 between the major populations at risk but if sexual intermingling increases in the future, the viral heterogeneity may become a hotspot for diverse and complex URFs. Such a scenario is supported by the spreading of novel recombinants across multiple risk groups in the United Kingdom [28] and that several triple URFs already are circulating in Sweden. Apart from that HIV-1B was also found to be Continual molecular surveillance is recommended to understand the changing nature of the epidemic and the mobility of the HIV-1 strains.

Supporting Information

Table S1 The Table describes the number of newly diagnosed patients whose virus was sequenced each year from 1983 to 2012, both in total and for the different categories of patients. IVDU: intravenous drug users; MSM: men who have sex with men; Others: infected through blood products and unknown.

Table S2 The table describes the city wise distribution of HIV-1 major subtypes and recombinants (HIV-1B, HIV-1C, 01_AE and 02_AG) analysed in this study.

Author Contributions

Conceived and designed the experiments: UN AH AS. Performed the experiments: UN AH MS. Analyzed the data: UN AH. Contributed reagents/materials/analysis tools: MS GB MG JA AS. Contributed to the writing of the manuscript: UN AH AS MS GB MG JA.

References

1. Hemelaar J, Gouws E, Ghys PD, Osmanov S,C W-UNHI (2011) Global trends in molecular epidemiology of HIV-1 during 2000–2007. AIDS 25: 679–689.
2. Delatorre EO, Bello G (2012) Phylodynamics of HIV-1 subtype C epidemic in east Africa. PLoS One 7: e41904.
3. Neogi U, Bontell I, Shet A, De Costa A, Gupta S, et al. (2012) Molecular epidemiology of HIV-1 subtypes in India: origin and evolutionary history of the predominant subtype C. PLoS One 7: e39819.
4. Lihana RW, Ssemwanga D, Abimiku A, Ndembi N (2012) Update on HIV-1 diversity in Africa: a decade in review. AIDS Rev 14: 83–100.
5. Kassu A, Fujino M, Matsuda M, Nishizawa M, Ota F, et al. (2007) Molecular epidemiology of HIV type 1 in treatment-naive patients in north Ethiopia. AIDS Res Hum Retroviruses 23: 564–568.
6. Pyne MT, Hackett J Jr, Holzmayer V, Hillyard DR (2013) Large-scale analysis of the prevalence and geographic distribution of HIV-1 non-B variants in the United States. J Clin Microbiol.
7. Frentz D, Wensing AM, Albert J, Paraskevis D, Abecasis AB, et al. (2013) Limited cross-border infections in patients newly diagnosed with HIV in Europe. Retrovirology 10: 36.
8. Paraskevis D, Pybus O, Magiorkinis G, Hatzakis A, Wensing AM, et al. (2009) Tracing the HIV-1 subtype B mobility in Europe: a phylogeographic approach. Retrovirology 6: 49.
9. Frange P, Galimand J, Vidal N, Goujard C, Deveau C, et al. (2008) New and old complex recombinant HIV-1 strains among patients with primary infection in 1996–2006 in France: the French ANRS CO06 primo cohort study. Retrovirology 5: 69.
10. Fox J, Castro H, Kaye S, McClure M, Weber JN, et al. (2010) Epidemiology of non-B clade forms of HIV-1 in men who have sex with men in the UK. AIDS 24: 2397–2401.
11. Pineda-Pena AC, Faria NR, Imbrechts S, Libin P, Abecasis AB, et al. (2013) Automated subtyping of HIV-1 genetic sequences for clinical and surveillance purposes: Performance evaluation of the new REGA version 3 and seven other tools. Infect Genet Evol.
12. Sonnerborg A, Durdevic S, Giesecke J, Sallberg M (1997) Dynamics of the HIV-1 subtype distribution in the Swedish HIV-1 epidemic during the period 1980 to 1993. AIDS Res Hum Retroviruses 13: 343–345.
13. Karlsson A, Bjorkman P, Bratt G, Ekvall H, Gisslen M, et al. (2012) Low prevalence of transmitted drug resistance in patients newly diagnosed with HIV-1 infection in Sweden 2003–2010. PLoS One 7: e33484.
14. Bontell I, Haggblom A, Bratt G, Albert J, Sonnerborg A (2013) Trends in antiretroviral therapy and prevalence of HIV drug resistance mutations in Sweden 1997–2011. PLoS One 8: e59337.
15. Sandstrom E, Uhnoo I, Ahlqvist-Rastad J, Bratt G, Berglund T, et al. (2003) Antiretroviral treatment of human immunodeficiency virus infection: Swedish recommendations. Scand J Infect Dis 35: 155–167.
16. Lole KS, Bollinger RC, Paranjape RS, Gadkari D, Kulkarni SS, et al. (1999) Full-length human immunodeficiency virus type 1 genomes from subtype C-infected seroconverters in India, with evidence of intersubtype recombination. J Virol 73: 152–160.
17. Lee K, Ahn H, Moon H, Kodell RL, Chen JJ (2013) Multinomial logistic regression ensembles. J Biopharm Stat 23: 681–694.
18. Von Krogh G, Brostrom C, Hermanson J, Von Sydow M, Biberfeld G, et al. (1987) The introduction of HIV during 1979–80 in a sexually active homosexual population of Stockholm. Scand J Infect Dis 19: 285–288.
19. Vangroenweghe D (2001) The earliest cases of human immunodeficiency virus type 1 group M in Congo-Kinshasa, Rwanda and Burundi and the origin of acquired immune deficiency syndrome. Philos Trans R Soc Lond B Biol Sci 356: 923–925.
20. Abecasis AB, Wensing AM, Paraskevis D, Vercauteren J, Theys K, et al. (2013) HIV-1 subtype distribution and its demographic determinants in newly diagnosed patients in Europe suggest highly compartmentalized epidemics. Retrovirology 10: 7.
21. Rice BD, Elford J, Yin Z, Delpech VC (2012) A new method to assign country of HIV infection among heterosexuals born abroad and diagnosed with HIV. AIDS 26: 1961–1966.
22. Alcantara KC, Reis MN, Cardoso LP, Bello G, Stefani MM (2013) Increasing heterosexual transmission of HIV-1 subtype C in Inland Central Western Brazil. J Med Virol 85: 396–404.
23. Almeida SE, de Medeiros RM, Junqueira DM, Graf T, Passaes CP, et al. (2012) Temporal dynamics of HIV-1 circulating subtypes in distinct exposure categories in southern Brazil. Virol J 9: 306.
24. Helleberg M, Haggblom A, Sonnerborg A, Obel N (2013) HIV care in the Swedish-Danish HIV cohort 1995–2010, closing the gaps. PLoS One 8: e72257.
25. Cohen MS, Chen YQ, McCauley M, Gamble T, Hosseinipour MC, et al. (2011) Prevention of HIV-1 infection with early antiretroviral therapy. N Engl J Med 365: 493–505.
26. Palma AC, Araujo F, Duque V, Borges F, Paixao MT, et al. (2007) Molecular epidemiology and prevalence of drug resistance-associated mutations in newly diagnosed HIV-1 patients in Portugal. Infect Genet Evol 7: 391–398.
27. von Wyl V, Kouyos RD, Yerly S, Boni J, Shah C, et al. (2011) The role of migration and domestic transmission in the spread of HIV-1 non-B subtypes in Switzerland. J Infect Dis 204: 1095–1103.
28. Foster GM, Ambrose JC, Hue S, Delpech VC, Fearnhill E, et al. (2014) Novel HIV-1 Recombinants Spreading across Multiple Risk Groups in the United Kingdom: The Identification and Phylogeography of Circulating Recombinant Form (CRF) 50_A1D. PLoS One 9: e83337.

4

A Toolbox for Tuberculosis (TB) Diagnosis: An Indian Multi-Centric Study (2006-2008); Evaluation of Serological Assays Based on PGL-Tb1 and ESAT-6/CFP10 Antigens for TB Diagnosis

Philippe H. Lagrange[1]*, Satheesh K. Thangaraj[2], Rajeshwar Dayal[3], Alaka Deshpande[4], Nirmal K. Ganguly[5], Enrico Girardi[6], Beenu Joshi[7], Kiran Katoch[7], Vishwa M. Katoch[7], Manoj Kumar[8], Vemu Lakshmi[9], Marc Leportier[2], Christophe Longuet[10], Subbalaxmi V. S. Malladi[9], Deepali Mukerjee[5], Deepthi Nair[11], Alamelu Raja[12], Balambal Raman[12], Camilla Rodrigues[13], Pratibha Sharma[11], Amit Singh[3], Sarman Singh[8], Archana Sodha[13], Basirudeen Syed Ahamed Kabeer[12], Guy Vernet[10], Delia Goletti[6]

1 Service de Microbiologie, Hôpital Saint Louis, Paris, France, **2** BioMérieux, Marcy-l'Etoile, France and New Delhi, India, **3** SN Medical College, Agra, India, **4** Sir J.J. Group of Govt Hosp. & Grant Medical College, Mumbai, India, **5** Indian Council of Medical Research, New Delhi, India, **6** Department of Epidemiology and Preclinical Research, L. Spallanzani National Institute for Infectious Diseases, Rome, Italy, **7** National JALMA Institute of Leprosy & Other Mycrobacterial Diseases, Agra, India, **8** All India Institute of Medical Sciences, New Delhi, India, **9** Nizam's Institute of Medical Sciences, Hyderabad, India, **10** Fondation Mérieux, Lyon, France, **11** Safdarjung Hospital, New Delhi, India, **12** National Institute for Research in Tuberculosis (formerly Tuberculosis Research Center), Chetput, Chennai, India, **13** Microbiology Section, P D Hinduja Hospital & Medical Research Centre, Veer Savarkar Marg Mahim, Mumbai, India

Abstract

Background: The aim of this multi-centric prospective study in India was to assess the accuracy of a serological test as an additional tool for diagnosing active tuberculosis (ATB). In particular, an assay based on ELISA using a phenolic glycolipid (PGL-Tb1) or a fusion protein (ESAT-6/CFP10) was compared to the tuberculin skin test (TST) and the microbiological results according to HIV status.

Methods: Individuals with and without ATB and HIV infection were enrolled. Serology and TST results were analyzed *per se* and in combination with the microbiological data.

Results: Among the 778 ATB patients, 102 were HIV-infected, 316 HIV-uninfected and 360 had an HIV-unknown status. Of the 945 non-ATB subjects, 559 were at low risk (community adults) and 386 at high risk of *M. tuberculosis* exposure. Among those with ATB, the sensitivity of ELISA-PGL-Tb1 for ATB was higher than that of ELISA-ESAT-6/CFP10, both in HIV-infected (72.3% versus 63.7%, $p = 0.29$) and HIV-uninfected/HIV-unknown groups (40.5% versus 28.6%; $p < 0.0001$), whereas the specificity was around 91% for both tests. Sensitivity for ATB increased when the results of the two ELISA were combined, reaching 75.5% in the HIV-infected and 50.9% in the group of HIV-uninfected/HIV-unknown ATB, with a significant decrease of the global specificity (83.9%). Analyzing the ELISA results with the microbiological results, we observed that the sensitivity of both serology tests was independent of the ATB patients' smear microscopy (SM) status and grade. Combining the results of SM with both ELISA, the detection of ATB patients significantly increased ($p < 0.0001$), particularly in those with extrapulmonary TB (up to 45.1%) or HIV infection (up to 83.3%). No significant association was observed between TST and serology results.

Conclusions: In this prospective multi-centric study, the combination of two rapid tests, such as SM and serology, might be useful in detecting ATB, especially in HIV-infected patients.

Editor: Jean Louis Herrmann, Hopital Raymond Poincare - Universite Versailles St. Quentin, France

Funding: Fondation Merieux funded the study. In addition "Ricerca Corrente" from the Italian Ministry of Health partially funded the study. The funders had no role in study design, data collection and analysis, decision to publish, or preparation of the manuscript.

Competing Interests: The authors have read the journal's policy and have the following conflicts: One co-author (ST) is an employee of BioMérieux and another co-author (ML) was an employee of BioMérieux when the study was designed and developed. One co-author (CL) is an employee of Fondation Mérieux which is the foundation of BioMérieux that supported the study. Another coauthor (GV) has since March 2012 been an employee of the Fondation Mérieux.

guide for authors.

* E-mail: plagrange@sfr.fr

Introduction

Diagnosing active tuberculosis (ATB) accurately and rapidly is a key challenge for eradicating the TB epidemic [1,2]. Sputum smear microscopy (SM), currently the only diagnostic test in most TB-endemic areas, has several limitations; in particular, the sensitivity compared with culture is variable [2–4], multiple patient visits are required [5–7], considerable technical training is necessary and the procedure is labor-intensive [1,8].

Antibody detection tests (serological tests), used for the diagnosis of several infectious diseases, may potentially improve TB diagnosis. These tests measure the presence of specific antibodies (mostly IgG) directed against immunodominant antigens of the investigated pathogen. Compared to SM, antibody detection methods may enable rapid TB diagnosis, as these tests have the advantages of being quick (results can be available within hours) and technologically easy, requiring minimal training. In addition, these tests could be adapted to point-of-care formats that can be implemented at lower levels of health services in low- and middle-income countries [8–11].

The serology tests used for diagnosing TB have a long record in the TB literature, but have never been well-developed, due to their low diagnostic values with poor specificity and sensitivity [12]. Since the 1990s, newer approaches have been chosen using enzyme-linked immunosorbent assays (ELISA) and highly purified antigens or recombinant proteins [9,13]. Improvement of their performances has been obtained by using several different antigens simultaneously [14,15]. However, several assessments of these serological tests in Human Immunodeficiency Virus-infected (HIV) patients have been at best inconclusive [16,17] mainly because HIV-TB co-infected patients have been shown to be poor serological responders to protein antigens [18–22].

Serological tests based on ELISA using a panel of non-protein antigens such as glycolipids specific for *M. tuberculosis* have been developed [23,24] and evaluated [13,25–31]. About 65–70% of HIV-TB co-infected patients had serum reactivity to at least one glycolipid antigen and maintained the diverse antibody repertoire previously observed in HIV-uninfected TB patients [32]. The reason why such antibody response is preserved, despite the decline of CD4 T-lymphocyte counts in HIV-TB patients, has been related to the novel CD1-restricted lipid antigen presentation pathway [33,34]. This is in sharp contrast to the classical response to T-cell-dependent peptide antigens which are MHC restricted [35,36].

A remaining key question is, to what extent can the disappointing performance of current serological tests be associated with a high background prevalence of latent TB infection (LTBI) in the evaluated settings? A partial answer has been reported showing that the fusion protein of ESAT-6/CFP10 has variable diagnostic values among subjects from low (Denmark), moderate (Brazil) and high TB incidence countries (Tanzania and Ethiopia) [37]. Furthermore, it has been reported that the levels of antibodies against several protein antigens, including the ESAT-6/CFP10, might increase before the occurrence of clinical symptoms and microbiological confirmation of ATB in HIV-TB co-infected patients [38]; similar results have also been observed using glycolipid antigens such as PGL-Tb1 [39]. A specific remark also concerns the recent findings that an additional cell-surface glycolipid, the lipoarabinomannan (LAM), can be detected in the concentrated urines of ATB patients with advanced HIV disease [40]. In these patients with low CD4 cell counts, the sensitivity of this LAM-based assay was significantly higher than the SM (around 25%).

Although *in vitro* amplification of mycobacterial target DNA by PCR-based methods can provide rapid results, until recently the technology was not fully standardized. It is now suitable for routine clinical practice for diagnosing PTB [41]. However, a high proportion of negative results to the GeneXpert Technology were observed in SM/culture-negative extrapulmonary TB [42]. SM-negative PTB are frequently found in HIV-infected patients who require invasive procedures to confirm a diagnosis [1].

In a recent meta-analysis, inconsistent estimates of sensitivity and specificity of serology tests for ATB diagnosis have been described [43–45]. It was reported that none of the serology tests achieved sufficient sensitivity to replace SM, but the combination of serology tests based on selected antigens was shown to provide higher sensitivities than single antigens. The authors also recommended that further research be done to determine whether combinations of SM and antibody detection with multiple antigens could improve case findings in high prevalence countries.

A single rapid assay for TB diagnosis, such as the SM, PCR or serology, will not detect all ATB cases, thus we studied new algorithms in an attempt to increase the ATB cases detection rate. In an effort to find the best approach for TB diagnosis in a TB-endemic country, as India, we enrolled subjects with or without active TB and tried to identify the right combination of diagnostic tools for the toolbox. The first part of our multi-centric prospective study was to assess the diagnostic value of several microbiological tools [46], whereas the aim of the second part was to assess the performance of the QFT-GIT and TST, in addition to microbiological results, as contributors for diagnosing ATB according to HIV status [47]. The aim of this third part was to assess the performance of a serological test based on ELISA using a phenolic glycolipid or recombinant fusion protein, in addition to microbiological and TST results, as contributors for detecting ATB, stratifying by HIV status.

Materials and Methods

Study populations

Patients with ATB and individuals without ATB were prospectively enrolled from January 2006 to July 2008 at different medical centers as described [46]. Written informed consent was obtained from all subjects before enrollment. The study was approved by the local ethical committees: the Institutional Ethical Committee of the Tuberculosis Research Centre in Chennai (TRC-IEC No: 2006005), the Institutional Review Board at Hinduja Hospital, Mumbai (No: 316-05-CR), the Institutional Ethical Committee of AIIMS, New Delhi (AIIMS-IEC No: A-35:05/10/2005), the Institutional Ethical Committee of the Safdarjung Hospital, New Delhi (No Sur./1/2007), the NIMS Institutional Ethics Committee (No. EC/264 (A)/2005) and the Ethical Committee of National JALMA Institute for Leprosy and other Mycobacterial Diseases, Agra (minutes: 27/04/2006).

In brief, clinical symptoms and radiological findings of the patients were first assessed independently by each clinician taking part in the enrollment. Three sputum samples were collected and processed. The SM was stained using the hot Ziehl-Neelsen method and the semi-quantitative yield of acid-fast-bacilli (AFB) was recorded according to WHO recommendations [48]. The 3 sputum samples were cultured in solid and liquid medium and the presence of *M.tuberculosis* in the positive culture samples was further confirmed by molecular Gen-probe based PCR. The number of days to obtain a positive culture was also recorded [46].

Non-ATB individuals were also enrolled as controls: blood donors, healthy community adults (HCA), healthy family contacts

(HFC), health care workers (HCW-laboratory staff and nurses), hospitalized non-ATB patients and cured TB patients. Because the different areas of recruitment are highly endemic for TB, all subjects (except the blood donors) were asked to give one to three sputum samples and were subjected to radiological examinations to rule out the suspicion of ATB. All enrolled healthy individuals were stratified by risk for TB exposure. Subjects at high TB risk were included only if they agreed to participate in a six month follow-up to exclude ATB occurrence.

Each individual's data were then recorded at each site using a standardized questionnaire involving 3 files (clinical/radiological evaluation, clinical/radiological follow-up and laboratory analysis) for both ATB patients and non-ATB individuals. An individual clinical suspicion of TB score (CSTB) was given for each patient; this was made by the clinician in charge of the patient at the time of inclusion in the study and before knowing any microbiological and immunological results. Included individuals were classified into 3 categories: very high, high, and low, as previously reported [46]. CSTB was used as a pre-test evaluation before enrollment. However, the study and the data analysis were performed using samples with a definite diagnosis of "ATB" or "non-ATB".

Serological assays for HIV diagnosis

The presence of HIV infection was diagnosed or ruled out by two commercial ELISA in serum (Retroquic Comb Aids-RS, Span Diagnostics India; HIV TRI-DOT, J. Mitra & Co, India). The results were scored as positive when the serum was positive by both tests. If a serum was reactive in only one ELISA, HIV-Western Blot was performed as a confirmatory test to rule out a false ELISA result.

Serology tests for TB diagnosis

The complete ELISA protocol standardization and buffer formulations were made by one of us (TS) in the R&D Immunoassay Laboratory (R&D lab), bioMérieux SA, France [49]. In brief, assay standardization was made using a unique specific wash buffer formulated for the PGL-Tb1 glycolipid and the ESAT-6/CFP10 fusion protein. All the ELISA plate coating and reagent preparations were made centrally in the R&D lab and then distributed to each microbiology laboratory associated with the enrollment sites. The tests were performed after specific training conducted by one of us (TS). Testing for each serum sample was performed in duplicate wells: ELISA for the separate detection of anti-PGL-Tb1 and anti-ESAT6-CFP10 IgG antibody (with a common newly formulated protocol). A positive control, negative control and calibrator were included for each ELISA plate to avoid inter plate variation. Any serum with discordant results higher than 10% between the 2 results from the duplicate was re-tested. The mean optical density (OD) from the 2 wells was recorded for each serum. We then calculated the median OD plus inter-quartile range (IQR) for each group of ATB patients and non-ATB individuals. No ELISA results were communicated to the physician in charge of the patients before the end of the study, and the laboratory technicians performing the serum ELISA were not informed of the medical status of the patient whose sample was tested.

Antigens

PGLTb1: purification of PGLTb1 was performed using column chromatography as described earlier [50]. A new method of purification was designed to improve the purity of PGL-Tb1. This part of the work was done by one of us (TS) in the R&D Lab, and is described in his PhD thesis [49]. ESAT-6/CFP10: this antigen is a recombinant fusion protein and was provided by P. Andersen (Staten Serum Institute, Copenhagen. Denmark).

Data collection

After collection, the data were subsequently transferred to EPIINFO files by one of the authors (TS). Each file included the patient's characteristics, risk of TB, clinical symptoms, whether TST was performed or not, chest X-ray findings, the effect of a 10 day antibiotic trial, the final clinical diagnosis, CSTB, the final therapeutic intervention with the therapy initiation date and the anti-TB drugs prescribed. The last part of the file consisted of the treatment outcome obtained during the 6 to 9 month follow-up of each individual with ATB and the absence of clinical symptoms in the non-ATB control groups. Patients with both pulmonary and extrapulmonary localizations (infiltrate and pleural effusion, for instance) were classified as pulmonary TB. The specific biological file consisted of the microbiological and the immunological results: HIV status (HIV-infected, HIV-uninfected or HIV-unknown), and in a subgroup of HIV-infected patients, the number of CD4 and CD8 cell counts/µL; OD values obtained by the ELISA using the PGL-Tb1 antigen and fusion protein ESAT-6/CFP10.

ATB was defined as "confirmed" either microbiologically (after identification of *M.tuberculosis* in LJ and/or in BacT/ALERT MP culture and molecular tests) or by histology. Conversely, patients were classified as having "clinical" ATB if the diagnosis was only based on clinical and radiological criteria (after excluding other diseases), including appropriate responses to anti-tuberculous therapy.

Statistical data analysis

The Mann-Whitney test was used to compare the OD values to understand the significance of difference, while the Fisher exact test and Chi-Square test were used to evaluate the significance of difference between the numbers of positives of different serology tests [51,52].The Pearson correlation was used to evaluate the correlation between the OD values of different ELISA and also to understand the impact of parameters like age, sex, SM grade and time to positivity (TTP) of the liquid culture upon the individual OD values. A Receiver Operative Characteristic (ROC) analysis was performed to measure the diagnostic efficiency of the ELISA to each antigen and also to find the best OD cut-off value [53–55]. Sensitivity, specificity, positive predictive value (PPV), negative predictive value (NPV) and the likelihood ratio (LR) were calculated as recommended [56]. The analysis was carried out with SPSS v 20 for Windows (SPSS Italia SRL, Bologna, Italy), GraphPad Prism 6.0 software and EPIINFO 3.2.2 (CDC, Atlanta, USA).

Results

Populations enrolled and characteristics

We enrolled 2,213 individuals in the 2-year period. We deleted 75 patient files because they were incomplete. Additionally, 272 children were evaluated separately [57], and 143 subjects belonging to a satellite study without any serology test were excluded (partial results already reported) [58–60].

As shown in **Figure 1**, the remaining files correspond to 778 adult patients with ATB: 102 HIV-infected, 316 HIV-uninfected and 360 with an unknown HIV status. Based on the HIV status subgroup, the ATB patients were further stratified by TB localization (pulmonary and disease). The 945 individuals without ATB were further stratified by their relative risk of TB exposure: those at low risk of LTBI [459 healthy blood donors and 100 healthy community adults(HCA)] and those at high risk of LTBI

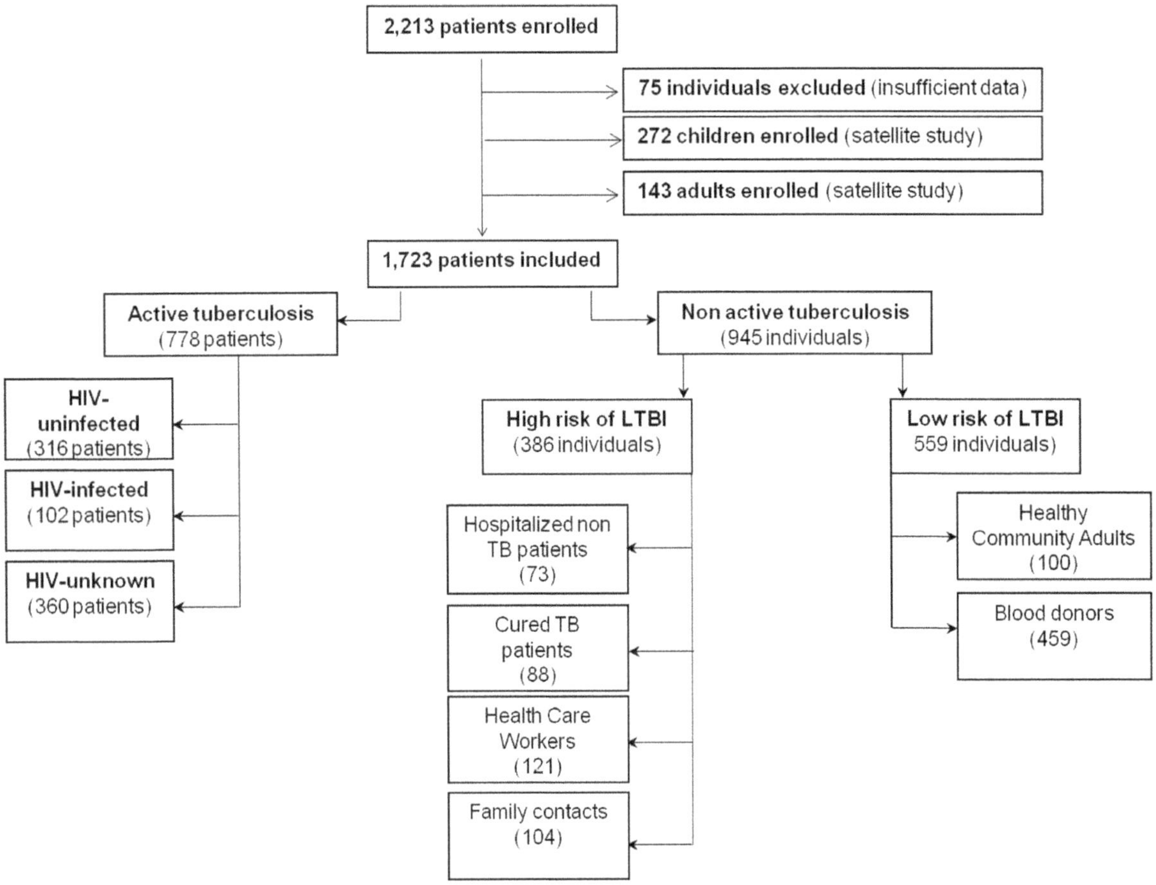

Figure 1. Flow chart of patients recruited to the multi-centric study stratified by active tuberculosis and non-active tuberculosis patient subgroups. Footnotes: HIV: Human Immunodeficiency Virus; LTBI: latent tuberculosis infection.

[73 hospitalized non-active TB patients, 88 cured TB patients, 121 Health Care Workers (HCW), 104 Healthy Family contacts (HFC)].

Serology results: quantitative ELISA results

The median anti-PGL-Tb1 and anti-ESAT6/CFP10 antibody levels were significantly higher in the different groups of ATB than in the low risk of LTBI group ($p<0.0001$) and the high risk LTBI group ($p<0.0001$) (**Table 1, Figure 2**), independent of the HIV status. The median anti-PGL-Tb1 and anti-ESAT6/CFP10 antibody levels were not significantly different between pulmonary and extrapulmonary ATB, independent of the HIV status, as shown in **Table 1, Figure 3**. When stratified by HIV status, the median anti-PGL-Tb1 and anti-ESAT6/CFP10 antibody levels were significantly higher among the 102 HIV-infected ATB patients than among the 316 HIV-uninfected ($p<0.0001$) or 360 HIV-unknown ($p<0.0001$) ATB patients. It is worthy to note that the median anti-PGL-Tb1 and anti-ESAT-6/CFP10 antibody levels between the HIV-unknown and the HIV-uninfected ATB patients were not statistically different ($p=0.0501$ and $p=0.3173$, respectively).

Among the individuals at high risk of LTBI, the cured-TB patients had significantly higher anti-PGL-Tb1 and anti-ESAT-6/CFP10 antibody levels than the hospitalized non-TB patients ($p=0.0004$ and $p=0.0088$), HCW ($p<0.0001$ and $p<0.0001$) and HFC ($p=0.0059$ and $p<0.0001$) (**Table 1, Figure 4**). Considering the groups at high or low risk as a whole, the median anti-PGL-Tb1 and anti-ESAT-6/CFP10 antibody levels were significantly higher in the 386 individuals at high risk of LTBI (**Table 1, Figure 2**) than among the 559 individuals at low risk of LTBI ($p<0.0001$). It is important to note that the anti-PGL-Tb1 and anti-ESAT-6/CFP10 antibody levels were significantly lower for all the subgroups at high risk of LTBI compared to the ATB patients with unknown HIV status ($p<0.0001$), except for the group of cured-TB patients and HIV-unknown ATB patients, where no significant difference was observed ($p=0.99$ and 0.19, respectively).

According to the relative clinical, radiological and microbiological variability observed in populations recruited at the different sites [46], the antibody responses were further evaluated in ATB patients and non-ATB individuals stratified by the enrolment center. Given that TB localization, as shown above (**Table 1, Figure 3**), was not influencing the anti-PGL-Tb1 and anti-ESAT-6/CFP10 antibody levels, we then investigated the effect of the site of recruitment upon the antibody levels of the whole group of ATB patients stratified by HIV status: the HIV-infected group versus the group of subjects defined as HIV-uninfected and the HIV-unknown (grouped together), since these two groups had serology results with comparable antibody levels.

The results are shown in **Table 2**. Among the HIV-infected patients, the anti-PGL-Tb1 and anti-ESAT-6/CFP10 antibody levels were not influenced by the site of recruitment and no significant difference was observed among each considered group (**Table 3**), except for the patients recruited at AIIMS who showed

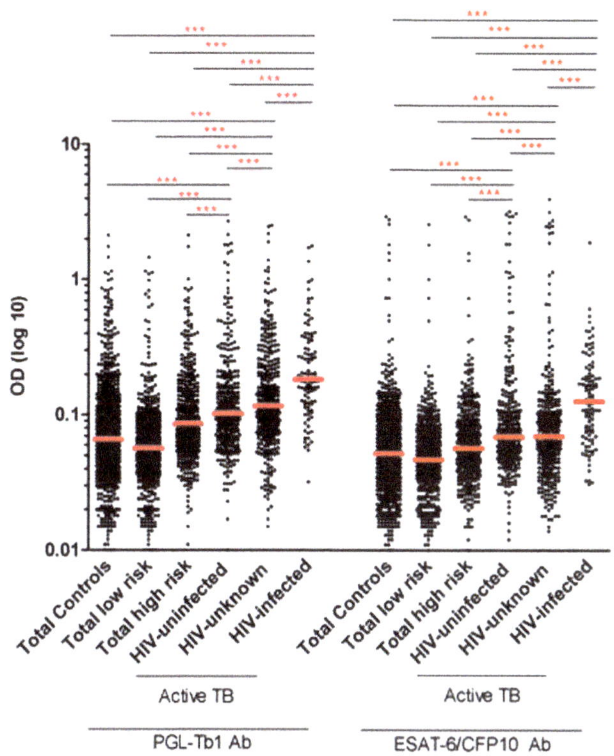

Figure 2. Individual IgG antibody levels against PGL-Tb1 and ESAT-6/CFP10 in subjects with or without active tuberculosis disease stratified by HIV status. Dot plot indicates the single antibody level per subject analyzed; median is indicated by the red line. ***: p<0.0001. **Footnotes**: HIV: Human Immunodeficiency Virus; LTBI: latent tuberculosis infection; OD: optical density.

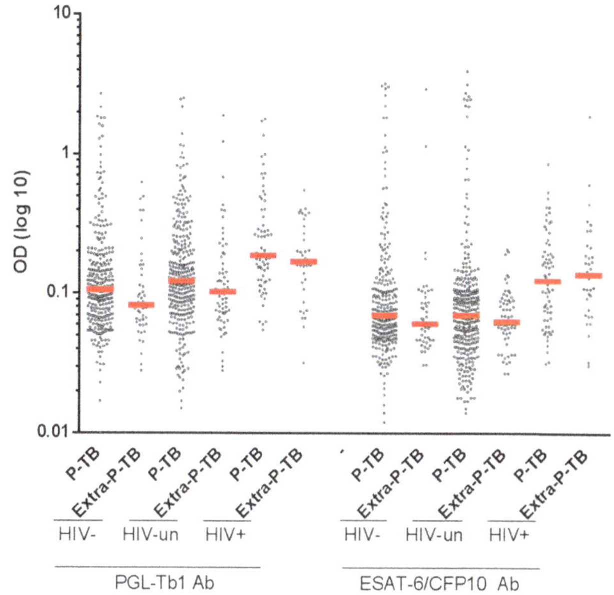

Figure 3. Individual IgG antibody levels against PGL-Tb1 and ESAT-6/CFP10 in subjects with active tuberculosis disease stratified by HIV status and disease localization (pulmonary and extrapulmonary). Dot plot indicates the single antibody level per subject analyzed; median is indicated by the red line. ***: p<0.0001. **Footnotes**: HIV: Human Immunodeficiency Virus; P-TB: pulmonary tuberculosis; Extra P-TB: extrapulmonary tuberculosis; OD: optical density.

significantly higher anti-PGL-Tb1 levels (p = 0.0073). Differently, among the HIV-uninfected/HIV-unknown subgroup, significantly higher anti-PGL-Tb1 antibody levels were observed among the ATB patients recruited at AIIMS and JALMA compared to the other groups (**Table 4**). Similarly, significantly higher anti-ESAT-6/CFP10 antibody levels were observed among the ATB patients recruited at Hinduja and AIIMS compared to the other groups (**Table 4**).

The antibody level variability among the different groups of non-ATB individuals recruited at the different sites and stratified by LTBI risk is shown in **Table 5**.

Among the low risk of LTBI group, the blood donors and the HCA enrolled at Hinduja showed similar anti-PGL-Tb1 and anti-ESAT-6/CFP10 antibody levels (p = 0.90 and p = 0.07, respectively), however these levels were significantly higher than those observed among the blood donors recruited at AIIMS (<0.0001) or at NIMS ($p<0.0001$).

Among the different subgroups of individuals at high risk for LTBI, there was an important variability associated with the antibody levels considered and the site of recruitment. For instance, the 30 hospitalized patients with lepromatous leprosy enrolled at JALMA showed significantly lower anti-ESAT-6/CFP10 antibody levels than the 47 hospitalized non-ATB patients enrolled at Hinduja ($p<0.0001$), but no significant difference was observed for the anti-PGL-Tb1 antibody levels (p = 0.25). Among the HCW group, the antibody levels against both antigens in those enrolled at Hinduja and at AIIMS were not statistically different ($p = 0.92$). In contrast, those enrolled at TRC presented higher anti-PGL-Tb1 and anti-ESAT-6/CFP10 antibody levels compared to the HCW enrolled at the 2 other centers, but the difference was significant only for the anti-PGL-Tb1 when compared with those enrolled at AIIMS ($p = 0.0187$). Among the HFC group, significantly higher anti-PGL-Tb1 and anti-ESAT-6/CFP10 antibody levels were found in those enrolled at TRC, compared to those enrolled at JALMA ($p = 0.0199$, $p<0.0001$, respectively).

Qualitative ELISA results and diagnostic values for ATB. ROC curve analysis

Based on the significant difference found in the quantitative analysis of serological tests, we performed an ROC analysis to evaluate its potentials for TB diagnostics, stratifying by HIV status.

For this purpose, at the beginning we used ATB HIV-infected, HIV-uninfected or HIV-unknown individuals as the "diseased group" and the blood donors as the "control group". In a further analysis of those with ATB, we combined the serological data from patients without HIV infection with those with an unknown HIV status.

Significant area under the curve (AUC) analysis results were obtained, independent of the antigen used and HIV status. It is important to note that the results obtained with anti-PGL-Tb1 antigen demonstrated a significantly higher discriminative ability in the group of HIV-infected ATB patients compared to the results obtained in the combined group (HIV-uninfected and HIV-unknown ATB patients), with higher AUC values (0.901 and 0.780). Similarly, for the results obtained with the ESAT-6/CFP10 antigen, a significantly higher discriminative ability was found in the HIV-infected ATB patients than in the combined group (HIV-uninfected and HIV-unknown ATB patients), with higher AUC values (0.869 and 0.713). Similar results were observed when HIV-

Table 1. Quantitative levels of anti-PGL-Tb1 and anti-ESAT-6/CFP10 antibodies (median) as measured by optical density in different groups of active TB patients according to their HIV status, disease localization and in individuals without active TB according to their risk of TB infection.

Active TB	**HIV-infected**			**HIV-uninfected**			**HIV-unknown**		
	N	**Median OD (IQR)**		**N**	**Median OD (IQR)**		**N**	**Median OD (IQR)**	
		PGL-Tb1	**ESAT-6/CFP10**		**PGL-Tb1**	**ESAT-6/CFP10**		**PGL-Tb1**	**ESAT-6/CFP10**
Pulmonary (P)	68	0.189	0.126	270	0.107	0.071	293	0.123	0.071
		(0.126–0.388)	(0.070–0.202)		(0.069–0.188)	(0.051–0.116)		(0.078–0.226)	(0.045–0.108)
Extrapulmonary (EP)	34	0.170	0.140	46	0.083	0.062	67	0.103	0.064
		(0.102–0.315)	0.077–0.221)		(0.062–0.152)	(0.047–0.097)		(0.073–0.163)	(0.053–0.090)
p P versus EP		*0.1895*	*0.6367*		*0.0549*	*0.1804*		*0.0886*	*0.4387*
All patients	102	0.185*	0.130*	316	0.103*	0.069*	360	0.117**	0.070**
		(0.124–0.347)	(0.074–0.208)		(0.067–0.172)	(0.049–0.108)		(0.076–0.214)	(0.046–0.105)
No active TB									
	N	Median OD (IQR)				**N**	Median OD (IQR)		
Low risk of LTBI		**PGL-Tb1**		**ESAT-6/CFP10**	***High risk of LTBI***		**PGL-Tb1**	**ESAT-6/CFP10**	
Blood donors	459	0.056		0.045	Hospitalized patients	73	0.077	0.060	
		(0.039–0.082)		(0.034–0.063)			(0.055–0.146)	(0.034–0.103)	
Healthy Community Adults	100	0.067		0.059	Health Care Workers	121	0.072	0.052	
		(0.046–0.100)		(0.043–0.080)			(0.052–0.106)	(0.039–0.081)	
					Healthy Family Contacts	104	0.089	0.053	
	-			-			(0.059–0.160)	(0.042–0.076)	
	-			-	Cured TB patients	88	0.112****	0.076****	
							(0.080–0.203)	(0.052–0.120)	
Total	559	0.057		0.047	Total	386	0.086***	0.057***	
		(0.040–0.085)		(0.035–0.067)			(0.057–0.149)	(0.041–0.087)	

Footnotes: TB: tuberculosis; HIV: human immunodeficiency virus; LTBI: latent tuberculosis infection; N; number of serum tested; OD: optical density; * HIV-infected versus HIV-uninfected, versus HIV-unknown: $p<0.0001$; ** HIV-uninfected versus HIV-unknown: $p>0.05$; *** Low risk versus high risk individuals: $p < 0.0001$;****Cured TB patients versus other HR of LTBI: $p<0.01$; IQR (interquartile range).

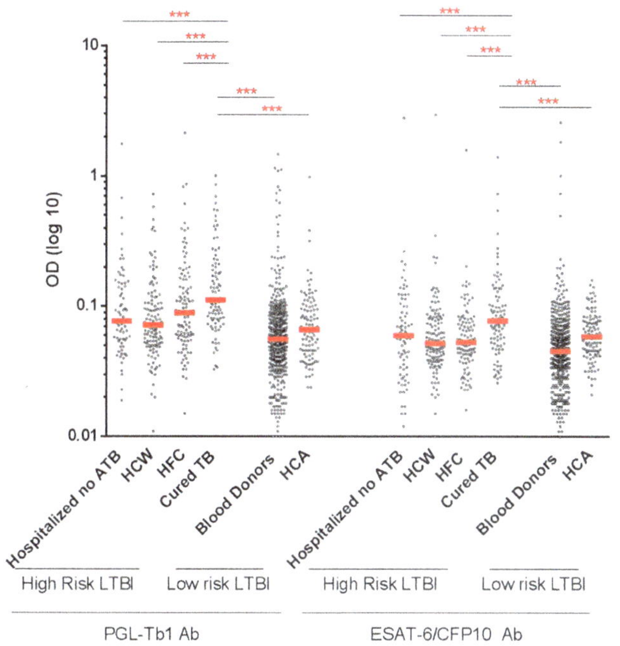

Figure 4. Individual IgG antibody levels against PGL-Tb1 and ESAT-6/CFP10 in subjects without active tuberculosis disease stratified by the risk of tuberculosis infection. Dot plot indicates the single antibody level per subject analyzed; median is indicated by the red line. ***: p<0.0001. **Footnotes**: LTBI: latent tuberculosis infection; Ab: antibody; ATB: active tuberculosis; HCW: health care workers; HFC: healthy family contacts; HCA: healthy community adults; OD: optical density.

uninfected and HIV-unknown groups were considered separately, **Table 6, Figure 5**).

Diagnostic values: overall sensitivity for ATB diagnosis

By ROC analysis we found that the OD cut-off point of 0.130 for the PGL-Tb1 antigen (with an LR of 8.05 and 4.55 for the HIV-infected and HIV-non infected ATB patients, respectively) and an OD of 0.100 for the ESAT-6/CFP10 antigen (with an LR of 7.70 and 3.45 for the HIV-infected and HIV-non infected ATB patients, respectively) predicted ATB with the sensitivity and specificity indicated in **Table 7**.

The sensitivity of the ELISA varied according to the tested populations and the antigen used. Such variability indicates the heterogeneity of the serological response, as already described [17,61].

Independent of HIV status, the sensitivity of the ELISA using the PGL-Tb1 was significantly higher than that obtained with the ESAT6/CFP10 antigen for the entire group of ATB individuals (p<0.0001) and for the pulmonary ATB individuals (p<0.0001), but the difference was not significant for the extrapulmonary ATB Individuals (p = 0.1422). Similarly, the sensitivity of the ELISA using the PGL-Tb1 was significantly higher than that obtained with the ESAT6/CFP10 antigen for the entire group of HIV-uninfected (p<0.0001) or HIV-unknown (p<0.0001), but was not significantly higher when compared with the entire group of HIV-infected ATB patients (p = 0.2948).

The cumulative sensitivity obtained with the combination of the positive scores obtained by the two serology tests was significantly higher than the sensitivity obtained with each single test for all the ATB patients (p = 0.0003 and p<0.0001), and pulmonary ATB patients (p = 0.0007 and p = <0.0001). The difference varied more for the extrapulmonary ATB patients (PGL-Tb1: p = 0.1956 and ESAT6/CFP10: p = 0.0040).

Using the combined ELISA positive results from each antigen, the cumulative results showed that as a group, the overall sensitivity was significantly higher in the HIV-infected (75.5%) than in the HIV-uninfected (48.4%) (p<0.0001) or HIV-unknown (53.1%) ATB patients (p<0.0001), and there was no significant difference between the HIV-uninfected and HIV-unknown ATB patients (p = 0.2477). Regarding TB localization, the sensitivity was not statistically different in pulmonary (76.5%) or extrapulmonary (73.5%) HIV-infected ATB patients (p = 0.8088). The sensitivity was lower in the HIV-uninfected patients with extrapulmonary TB compared to those with pulmonary TB (43.5% and 49.3%, respectively) or in HIV-unknown patients (37.3% and 56.7%, respectively). The difference was not significant for the former (p = 0.5248), but statistically significant for the latter (p = 0.0045). When the whole group of HIV-uninfected and HIV-unknown patients was considered, the sensitivity was significantly higher in those with pulmonary ATB than extrapulmonary ATB (53.1% and 39.8%, respectively; p = 0.0131).

Table 2. Evaluation of the quantitative level of anti-PGL-Tb1 and anti-ESAT-6/CFP10 antibodies in patients with active TB stratified by HIV status and center of enrolment.

	HIV-infected			HIV-non-infected*		
		Median OD (IQR)			Median OD (IQR)	
Center	**N**	**PGL-Tb1**	**ESAT-6/CFP10**	**N**	**PGL-Tb1**	**ESAT-6/CFP10**
Hinduja	50	0.161 (0.119–0.260)	0.140 (0.084–0.203)	190	0.107 (0.075–0.160)	**0.085** (0.060–0.109)
AIIMS	29	**0.280** (0.169–0.458)	0.127 (0.066–0.247)	94	**0.124** (0.071–0.441)	**0.079** (0.049–0.146)
Safdarjung	1	0.845 (0.845–0.845)	0.310 (0.310–0.310)	119	**0.096** (0.055–0.182)	0.062 (0.035–0.091)
JALMA	0	NA	NA	99	**0.144** (0.091–0.255)	0.063 (0.038–0.101)
NIMS	4	0.301 (0.107–0.664)	0.133 (0.068–0.250)	49	0.118 (0.060–0.210)	0.054 (0.032–0.107)
TRC	18	0.173 (0.088–0.417)	0.094 (0.058–0.192)	125	0.103 (0.069–0.172)	0.067 (0.52–0.090)

Footnotes: TB: tuberculosis; HIV: human immunodeficiency virus; LTBI: latent tuberculosis infection; N; number of serum tested; OD: optical density; IQR (interquartile range).
*HIV non-infected corresponds to the true HIV-uninfected and HIV-unknown patients with active TB.

Table 3. Evaluation of the statistical difference of PGL-Tb1 and anti-ESAT-6/CFP10 antibodies in HIV-infected active TB patients stratified by the center of enrolment (as reported in Table 2).

Centers	Centers: Hinduja	AIIMS	Safdarjung	JALMA	NIMS	TRC	Centers	Centers: Hinduja	AIIMS	Safdarjung	JALMA	NIMS	TRC
	p value for PGL-Tb1 antibodies							*p value for ESAT6/CFP10 antibodies*					
Hinduja	NA	*0.0073*	NA	NA	*0.5385*	*0.9314*	Hinduja	NA	*0.5223*	NA	NA	*0.7351*	*0.1085*
AIIMS	-	NA	NA	NA	*0.8155*	*0.0810*	AIIMS	-	NA	NA	NA	*0.9316*	*0.3418*
Safdarjung	-	-	NA	NA	NA	NA	Safdarjung	-	-	NA	NA	NA	NA
JALMA	-	-	-	NA	NA	NA	JALMA	-	-	-	NA	NA	NA
NIMS	-	-	-	-	NA	*0.4971*	NIMS	-	-	-	-	NA	*0.5843*
TRC	-	-	-	-	-	NA	TRC	-	-	-	-	-	NA

Footnotes: p value was evaluated by comparing the quantitative levels of antibodies obtained in the different tests by the Mann-Whitney test.

Table 4. Evaluation of the statistical difference of PGL-Tb1 and anti-ESAT-6/CFP10 antibodies in HIV-uninfected and unknown active TB patients stratified by the center of enrolment (as reported in Table 2).

Antigen	Centers	Centers: Hinduja	AIIMS	Safdarjung	JALMA	NIMS	TRC	Antigen	Centers	Centers: Hinduja	AIIMS	Safdarjung	JALMA	NIMS	TRC
		p value for PGL-Tb1 antibodies								*p value for ESAT6/CFP10 antibodies*					
PGL-Tb1		**Hinduja**	**AIIMS**	**Safdarjung**	**JALMA**	**NIMS**	**TRC**	**ESAT6/CFP10**		**Hinduja**	**AIIMS**	**Safdarjung**	**JALMA**	**NIMS**	**TRC**
	Hinduja	NA	*0.0461*	*0.1282*	*0.0005*	*0.8466*	*0.7251*		**Hinduja**	NA	*0.8400*	*<0.0001*	*0.0002*	*0.0005*	*0.0006*
	AIIMS	-	NA	*0.0027*	*0.6982*	*0.1778*	*0.0639*		**AIIMS**	-	NA	*0.0003*	*0.0039*	*0.0061*	*0.0532*
	Safdarjung	-	-	NA	*0.0002*	*0.3139*	*0.2016*		**Safdarjung**	-	-	NA	*0.3706*	*0.7169*	*0.0752*
	JALMA	-	-	-	NA	*0.0699*	*0.0018*		**JALMA**	-	-	-	NA	*0.3546*	*0.1968*
	NIMS	-	-	-	-	NA	*0.8253*		**NIMS**	-	-	-	-	NA	*0.0604*
	TRC	-	-	-	-	-	NA		**TRC**	-	-	-	-	-	NA

Footnotes: p value was evaluated by comparing the quantitative levels of antibodies obtained in the different tests by the Mann-Whitney test.

Table 5. Evaluation of quantitative levels of anti-PGL-Tb1 and anti-ESAT-6/CFP10 antibodies (medians) in individuals with varying risk of latent tuberculosis infection stratified by the center of enrolment.

Antigen	Center	High risk controls							
		Hospitalized non-ATB Patients		Heath Care Workers		Healthy Family Contacts		Cured TB Patients	
		N	OD median (IQR)	N	OD median (IQR)	N	OD median (IQR)	N	OD median (IQR)
PGL-Tb1	**Hinduja**	40	0.078 (0.057–0.157)	38	0.064 (0.052–0.093)	0	NA	0	NA
	AIIMS	2	0.104 (0.067–0.140)	34	0.064 (0.051–0.088)	0	NA	0	NA
	Safdarjung	1	0.171	0	NA	0	NA	0	NA
	JALMA	30	0.076 (0.049–0.106)	0	NA	48	0.083 (0.045–0.118)	0	NA
	TRC	0	NA	49	**0.095*** (0.053–0.173)	56	**0.098*** (0.063–0.187)	90	0.112 (0.080–0.203)
ESAT-6/CFP10	**Hinduja**	42	0.074 (0.055–0.124)	38	0.046 (0.038–0.070)	0	NA	29	NA
	AIIMS	2	1.419 (0.056–2.781)	34	0.054 (0.042–0.078)	0	NA	5	NA
	Safdarjung	1	0.070	0	NA	0	NA	0	NA
	JALMA	30	**0.030*** (0.025–0.061)	0	NA	48	0.044 (0.028–0.060)	0	NA
	TRC	0	NA	49	**0.055** (0.040–0.109)	56	**0.064*** (0.048–0.084)	90	0.076 (0.052–0.120)
Low risk controls									
		Blood donors (BD)		Healthy Community Adults (HCA)					
		N	OD median (IQR)	N	OD median (IQR)		*p* value BD versus HCA		*p value BD from Hinduja vs BD from other sites*
PGL-Tb1	**Hinduja**	199	0.065 (0.049–0.090)	100	0.067 (0.046–0.100)		*0.9000*		*NA*
	AIIMS	200	**0.051** (0.035–0.076)	0	NA		*NA*		*0.0003*
	NIMS	60	**0.039** (0.020–0.056)	0	NA		*NA*		*<0.0001*
ESAT-6/CFP10	**Hinduja**	199	0.057 (0.042–0.081)	100	0.059 (0.043–0.080)		*0.0737*		*NA*
	AIIMS	200	**0.042** (0.029–0.053)	0	NA		*NA*		*<0.0001*
	NIMS	69	**0.027** (0.018–0.041)	0	NA		*NA*		*<0.0001*

Footnotes: N= number of serum tested; NA: not applicable because no individual has been recruited at that center;* p<0.01.

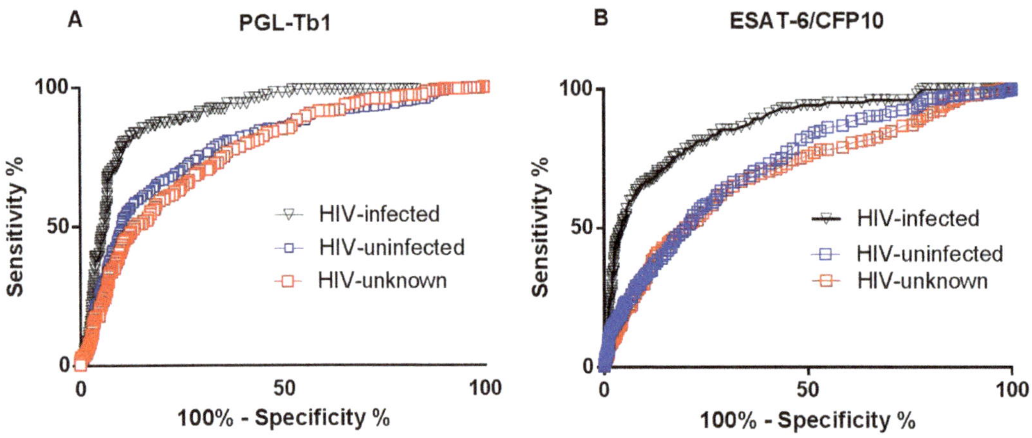

Figure 5. Receiving operative curves of a serology test for active tuberculosis in patients stratified by HIV status. Receiving operative curves calculated in HIV-uninfected (blue spot), HIV-unknown (red spot) or HIV-infected (black spot) patients with active TB and in healthy individuals with low risk of latent TB infection for antibodies: A. against PGL-Tb1 (left graph); B. ESAT-6/CFP10 (right graph) antigens. **Footnotes**: HIV: Human Immunodeficiency Virus.

Overall specificity for ATB diagnosis

The specificity for ATB diagnosis of the ELISA was almost 90.0% and quite similar for the 2 antigens considered when evaluated either in the blood donors or in the HCA group, with no significant difference observed between the two ELISA and the population tested (**Table 8**). To note: when the serology results from the two low risk populations were combined, the overall specificity for the PGL-Tb1 antigen (90.9%) was not significantly different than that obtained with the ESAT-/CFP10 antigen (91.4%) ($p = 0.8334$).

When the cumulative serology-positive results were used, the respective specificity declined significantly from 91.1% and 91.7% to 84.8% among the blood donors ($p = 0.0044$ and $p = 0.0014$), and from 90.0% to 80.0% among the HCA group, but the difference was not statistically significant ($p = 0.0734$). The overall specificity using the cumulative positive ELISA results of both groups and both antigens declined significantly from 90.9% and 91.4% to 83.9% ($p = 0.0006$ and $p = 0.0002$, respectively); these 3 values were used to determine the respective diagnostic values of each ELISA and their cumulative results.

Performances of the two ELISA for the diagnosis of ATB

The diagnostic values (PPV and NPV and LR) of each serological test and their cumulative results have been calculated and the results are shown in **Table 9**. The NPV and the positive LR were significantly higher among the HIV-infected compared to the HIV-non-infected ATB patients using the PGL-Tb1, ESAT-/CFP10, or using the cumulative results. By contrast, the PPV and the negative LR were significantly lower among the HIV-infected than the HIV-non-infected ATB patients using the PGL-Tb1, ESAT-/CFP10, or using the 2 antigens.

ELISA diagnostic values compared to Smear Microscopy (SM) results

In general, the serological tests have been described as having a very low diagnostic value for detecting SM-negative pulmonary TB patients [43,62], therefore the sensitivity of the serology using ELISA based on two single antigens and their cumulative results was further evaluated in the ATB patients stratified by the SM results, HIV status and TB localization (**Table 10**).

It is clearly shown that the serology using each antigen performed equally well in SM-negative compared to SM-positive

Table 6. Evaluation of areas under the curve of the Receiver Operating Characteristic (ROC) of anti-PGL-Tb1 and anti-ESAT6/CFP10 antibodies of 102 HIV-infected, 316 HIV-uninfected, 360 HIV-unknown active TB patients and additional subjects without active TB (459 healthy subjects as in the blood donors).

Antigen	HIV-infected	HIV-uninfected	HIV-unknown	HIV-non-infected*	HIV-uninfected versus HIV-unknown	HIV-infected versus HIV-non-infected
	areas under the curve of the Receiver Operating Characteristic (95%CI)					
PGL-Tb1	0.901±0.015	0.770±0.017	0.790±0.016	0.780±0.014	*p = 0.40*	*p<0.0001*
	(0.870–0.931)	(0.736–0.803)	(0.758–0.822)	(0.753–0.808)	*p = 0.40*	*p<0.0001*
	p<0.0001	*p*<0.0001	*p*<0.0001	*p*<0.0001		
ESAT-6/CFP10	0.869±0.019	0.730±0.018	0.699±0.019	0.713±0.015	*p = 0.23*	*p<0.0001*
	(0.830–0.907)	(0.694–0.766)	(0.662–0.735)	(0.683–0.743)	*p = 0.23*	*p<0.0001*
	p<0.0001	*p*<0.0001	*p*<0.0001	*p*<0.0001		

Footnotes: TB: tuberculosis; HIV: human immunodeficiency virus; * HIV-non-infected corresponds to the true HIV-uninfected and HIV-unknown patients with active Tuberculosis.

Table 7. Sensitivity of the serology test using ELISA based on the PGL-Tb1 or the ESAT-6/CFP10 antigen and their cumulative results in the different groups of active TB enrolled patients stratified by HIV status and TB localization.

Antigen	HIV status	n/N	Pulmonary ATB	n/N	Extrapulmonary ATB%	Pulmonary versus extrapulmonary	n/N	All ATB%
			% (95% CI)		% (95% CI)			% (95% CI)
PGL-Tb1 *	Infected	50/68	**73.5** (61.4–83.5)***	23/34	**67.7** (49.5–82.6)***	*P* = 0.6423	73/102	**72.3** (62.4–80.7)***
	Uninfected	104/270	38.5 (32.7–44.6)	13/46	28.3 (16.0–43.5)	*P* = 0.2472	117/316	37.0 (31.7–42.6)
	Unknown	136/293	46.4 (40.6–52.3)	22/67	32.8 (21.9–45.4)	*P* = 0.0556	158/360	43.6 (38.4–48.9)
	Uninfected +unknown	240/563	42.6 (38.5–46.8)	35/113	31.0 (22.6–40.4)	*P* = 0.0213	275/676	40.5 (36.8–44.3)
	Total	290/631	**46.0** (42.0–49.9)	58/147	**39.5** (31.5–47.8)	*P* = 0.1675	348/778	**44.7** (41.2–48.3)
ESAT-6/CFP10**	Infected	42/68	**61.8** (49.2–73.3)***	23/34	**67.7** (49.5–82.6)***	*P* = 0.6639	65/102	**63.7** (53.6–78.0)***
	Uninfected	82/270	30.4 (24.9–36.2)	11/46	23.9 (12.6–38.8)	*P* = 0.4841	93/316	29.4 (24.5–34.8)
	Unknown	89/293	31.0 (25.8–36.7)	11/67	16.4 (8.5–27.5)	*P* = 0.0162	100/360	27.8 (23.2–32.7)
	Uninfected +unknown	171/563	30.6 (26.8–34.5)	22/113	19.5 (12.6–28.0)	*P* = 0.0169	193/676	28.6 (25.2–32.1)
	Total	213/631	**33.9** (30.2–37.8)	45/147	**30.6** (23.3–38.7)	*P* = 0.4966	258/778	**33.2** (29.9–36.6)
Both antigens	Infected	52/68	**76.5** (64.6985.9)***	25/34	**73.5** (55.6–87.1)***	*P* = 0.8088	77/102	**75.5** (66.0–83.5)***
	Uninfected	133/270	49.3 (43.2–55.4)	20/46	43.5 (28.9–58.9)	*P* = 0.5248	153/316	48.4 (42.8–54.1)
	Unknown	166/293	56.7 (50.8–62.4)	25/67	37.3 (25.8–50.0)	*P* = 0.0045	191/360	53.1 (47.8–58.3)
	Uninfected +unknown	299/563	53.1 (48.9–57.3)	45/113	39.8 (30.7–49.5)	*P* = 0.0131	344/676	50.9 (47.1–54.7)
	Total	351/631	**55.6** (51.7–59.6)	70/147	**47.6** (39.3–56.0)	*P* = 0.0816	421/778	**54.1** (50.5–57.7)

Footnotes: TB: tuberculosis; HIV: human immunodeficiency virus; n/N = number of positive tests/number of tested sera in each group; * Cut-off value for PGL-Tb1: OD = 0.130; ** Cut-off value for ESAT-6/CFP10: OD = 0.100; *** HIV-infected versus HIV-uninfected or HIV-unknown: $p<0.0001$;

Table 8. Specificity of the serology test based on the ELISA using the PGL-Tb1 or the ESAT-6/CFP10 antigens and their cumulative results in the different groups of individuals classified as low risk of TB infection.

Antigen	n/N	Blood donors	n/N	Healthy subjects	*p* value of blood donors versus Healthy subjects	n/N	Total
	Percentage (95% CI)						
PGL-Tb1*	418/459	**91.1** (88.0–93.4)	90/100	**90.0** (82.4–94.5)	*p* = 0.7038	508/559	**90.9** (88.2–93.1)
ESAT-6/CFP10**	421/459	**91.7** (88.8–94.0)	90/100	**90.0** (82.4–94.5)	*p* = 0.5573	511/559	**91.4** (88.7–93.5)
PGL-Tb1 versus ESAT-/CFP10 (*p* value)		*p* = 0.8141		*p* = 1.000			*p* = 0.8334
Both antigens	389/459	**84.8** (81.1–87.9)	80/100	**80.0** (70.9–86.8)	*p* = 0.2336	469/559	**83.9** (80.6–86.9)

Footnotes: n/N = number of negative tests/number of tested sera in each group; * Cut-off value for PGL-Tb1: OD = 0.130; ** Cut-off value for ESAT-6/CFP10: OD = 0.100.

ATB patients, independent of their HIV status and TB localization (**Table 10**). To note: among the HIV-infected in whom the proportion of SM-positive results was very low (pulmonary TB: 41.2% and extrapulmonary TB: 11.8%), the cumulative ELISA results were able to detect 82.5% of the pulmonary cases and 73.3% of the extrapulmonary TB cases.

The combinations of results from SM status and combined serology tests were shown to improve the ATB case findings significantly, but varied according to the HIV status and TB disease localization (**Table 11**). The overall TB detection rate reached nearly 80% among the total ATB population, and the increased capacity to detect ATB was higher in extrapulmonary (+ 41.1%) compared to pulmonary TB patients (+14.9%). The increasing capacity to detect ATB patients was even higher among the HIV-infected than among the HIV-uninfected or HIV-unknown ATB patients. The highest case finding was obtained among both the pulmonary (89.7%) and extrapulmonary HIV-infected ATB patients (79.4%). Similar results were also observed using the results obtained with single antigens (data not shown).

The increasing capacity to detect ATB patients using the combination of the results from SM and serology in ATB patients appeared to be related to the independence of the antibody production relative to the TB localization as shown in **Table 1 and Table 10**.

This increased capacity to detect ATB patients might be also coupled with the absence of relationship between the antibody production and yield of mycobacteria in the patients' specimens. The yield of mycobacteria in the patients' specimens was measured as SM grade and the Time to Positivity (TTP) of the liquid culture [46]. As shown in **Figure 6A**, there was no correlation between the TTP (the number of days has been shown to be inversely related to the mycobacterial yield in the specimens) and the individual serum anti-PGL-Tb1 antibody level ($R^2 = 0.0007$, $p = 0.5449$), or the anti-ESAT-6/CFP10 antibody level ($R2 = 0.0005$, $p = 0.6013$) among the groups of HIV-uninfected and HIV-unknown pulmonary TB patients. This absence of correlation was further demonstrated at each center and was independent of TB localization (data not shown). Similarly, the same absence of relationship (**Figure 6B**) was observed among the HIV-infected ATB patients: PGL-Tb1 ($R^2 = 0.0002$, $p = 0.9018$), ESAT-6/CFP10 ($R^2 = 0.0189$, $p = 0.2786$). Accordingly, we observed an absence of impact of the SM grade on the sensitivity of the serology tests in pulmonary TB patients, independent of the HIV status, as shown in **Table 12**.

Among the 56 HIV-infected ATB patients with reported concomitant CD4 cell counts [median (IQR): 179.0 cells/µl (93.75-211.8)], it was shown that the individual antibody level against both the anti-PGL-Tb1 and anti-EST-6/CFP10 antigen was not influenced by the degree of immunosuppression (**Figure 7A**). There was no correlation between the individual CD4 cell counts with the anti-PGL-Tb1 ($R^2 = 0.00103$; $p = 0.8141$), or anti-ESAT-6/CFP10 ($R^2 = 0.01574$; $p = 0.3569$) antibody levels. As shown in **Figure 7B**, similar anti-PGL-Tb1 antibody levels were found in HIV-infected ATB patients with CD4 cell counts higher or lower than 200/µl (OD = 0.171; 0.115-0.263 versus 0.190; 0.117-379, respectively; p = 0.6529). However, a lower anti-ESAT-6/CFP10 antibody level was found in HIV-infected ATB patients with CD4 cell counts less than 200/µl (OD = 0.110; 0.073-0.183) compared to those with CD4 cell counts higher than 200/µl (OD = 0.189; 0.080–0.312), but the difference was not statistically significant (p = 0.1824). Accordingly, the serology sensitivity among the HIV-infected ATB was not significantly different when patients were stratified by their CD4 cell counts using a threshold at 200/µl (**Table 13**).

Table 9. Accuracy of active tuberculosis diagnosis by the serology test based on the ELISA using the PGL-Tb1, ESAT-6/CFP10 or both antigens in ATB patients (pulmonary and extrapulmonary TB) stratified by HIV status.

PGL-Tb1*	HIV-infected	HIV-infected + HIV-unknown	Total
Sensitivity (95% CI)	72.3 (62.4–80.7)	40.5 (36.8–44.3)	44.7 (41.2–48.3)
Specificity (95% CI)	90.9 (88.2–93.1)	90.9 (88.2–93.1)	90.9 (88.2–93.1)
PPV (95% CI)	58.9 (49.7-67.6)	84.3 (79.9–88.1)	87.2 (83.5–90.3)
NPV (95% CI)	94.8 (92.5–96.5)	55.8 (52.5–59.1)	54.2 (50.9–57.4)
LR+	7.93	4.44	4.90
LR-	3.31	1.53	1.65
ESAT-6/CFP10**	**HIV-infected**	**HIV-infected + HIV-unknown**	**Total**
Sensitivity (95% CI)	63.7 (53.6–78.0)	28.6 (25.2–32.1)	33.2 (29.9–36.6)
Specificity (95% CI)	91.4(88.8–93.6)	91.4(88.8–93.6)	91.4(88.8–93.6)
PPV (95% CI)	57.5 (47.9–66.8)	80.1 (74.5–84.9)	84.3 (79.9–88.2)
NPV (95% CI)	93.3 (90.8–95.2)	51.4 (48.3–54.6)	49.6 (46.5–52.7)
LR+	7.42	3.33	3.86
LR-	2.52	1.07	1.37
Both antigens	**HIV-infected**	**HIV-infected + HIV-unknown**	**Total**
Sensitivity (95% CI)	75.5 (66.0–83.5)	50.9 (47.14–54.7)	54.1 (50.5–57.7)
Specificity (95% CI)	83.9 (80.6–86.9)	83.9 (80.6–86.9)	83.9 (80.6–86.9)
PPV (95% CI)	46.1 (38.4–54.0)	79.3 (75.1–83.0)	82.4 (78.8-85.6)
NPV (95% CI)	94.9 (92.6–96.7)	58.6 (55.1–62.0)	56.8 (53.3–60.2)
LR+	4.69	3.16	3.36
LR-	3.43	1.71	1.83

Footnotes: TB: tuberculosis; HIV: human immunodeficiency virus; n/N = number of positive tests/number of tested sera in each group; * Cut-off value for PGL-Tb1: OD = 0.130; ** Cut-off value for ESAT-6/CFP10: OD = 0.100; CI: confidence interval; PPV: positive predictive value; NPV: negative predictive value; LR+: positive likelihood ratio; LR-: negative likelihood ratio.

Comparison of the sensitivity of TST and ELISA for diagnosis of active TB

TST is the single diagnostic reference test for LTBI and cannot be used as a diagnostic test for ATB although it usually performed as a diagnostic adjunct tool for SM-negative patients with a high suspicion of ATB. We have compared the quantitative results of the two tests among the 277 ATB patients with concomitant TST and serology results.

As shown in **Figure 8A**, there was no significant correlation between the individual TST diameter and anti-PGL-Tb1 ($R^2 = 0.003504$, $p = 0.3800$), or anti-ESAT-/CFP10 antibody levels ($R^2 = 0.002088$, $p = 0.4972$) among the HIV-uninfected and HIV-unknown ATB patients. Similarly, there was also no significant correlation between the individual TST and PGL-Tb1 ($R^2 = 0.002048$, $p = 0.8123$), or anti-ESAT-/CFP10 antibody levels ($R^2 = 0.005193$, $p = 0.7051$) among the HIV-infected ATB patients (**Figure 8B**).

Diagnostic values according to the clinical suspicion of TB (CSTB)

It was also interesting to evaluate the association between the two serological tests based on ELISA results and the CSTB described in ATB patients stratified by HIV status and TB localization; however, no impact of the CSTB on the serology results was observed in pulmonary or extrapulmonary ATB, independent of their HIV status (data not shown).

Discussion

We are presenting the results of the serology study using an ELISA format based on a phenolic glycolipid (PGL-Tb1) or fusion protein (ESAT6/CFP10). This study was the third part of a prospective multi-centric trial designed to investigate the performance of a diagnostic toolbox for ATB in India, a highly TB-endemic country. The two previous reports involved different diagnostic tools such as the clinical and radiological findings, microbiological results [46], and *in vitro* cell-mediated immune responses as measured by the QuantiFERON-TB Gold in Tube and TST [47]. Using the same populations of ATB patients and non-ATB individuals, our aim was to assess the accuracy of two serological tests *per se* and as additional tools to support ATB diagnosis.

Although no current guideline recommends the use of serological assays for detecting ATB, dozens of commercial kits are sold, mostly in developing countries [63]. Scientific evidence of published data on commercial serological tests for both pulmonary and extrapulmonary TB diagnosis reported inconsistent estimates of sensitivity and specificity [43,44]. Moreover, poor overall quality of these tests has been attributed to an unsatisfactory patient selection methodology [64]. Based on these findings, cost-effective data and expert opinion, the World Health Organization (WHO) has issued a recommendation against the use of currently available serological tests for TB diagnosis, but has stressed the importance of continued research on these and other tests that could provide quick and accurate TB diagnosis [65].

Table 10. Sensitivity of the serology test based on the ELISA using the PGL-Tb1 and ESAT-6/CFP10 antigens and their cumulative results in active TB patients stratified by Smear Microscopy (SM), TB localization and HIV status.

Antigen	HIV status	Pulmonary				p value SM(−) versus SM(+)	Extrapulmonary				p valueSM(−) versus SM(+)
		n/N	SM-negative	n/N	SM-positive		n/N	SM-negative	n/N	SM-positive	
			% (95% CI)		% (95% CI)			% (95% CI)		% (95% CI)	
PGLTb1*	Infected	31/40	77.5 (61.6–89.2)	19/28	67.9 (47.7–84.1)	*0.4130*	22/30	73.3 (54.1–87.7)	2/4	50.0 (9.6–93.2)	*0.5636*
	Uninfected	19/64	29.7 (18.9–42.4)	85/206	41.3 (34.5–48.3)	*0.1072*	11/37	29.0 (15.4–45.9)	2/9	22.2 (2.8–60.0)	*1.0000*
	Unknown	49/113	43.4 (34.1–53.0)	87/180	48.3 (40.855.9)	*0.4704*	19/55	34.6 (22.2–48.6)	3/12	25.0 (5.5–57.2)	*0.7371*
	Uninfected +unknown	68/177	38.4 (31.2–46.0)	172/386	44.6 (39.5–49.7)	*0.1989*	30/92	32.3 (22.9–42.8)	5/21	23.8 (8.2–47.2)	*0.6022*
	Total	**99/217**	**45.6 (38.9–52.5)**	**191/414**	**46.1 (41.3–51.1)**	***0.9331***	**52/122**	**42.3 (33.4–51.5)**	**7/25**	**28.0 (12.1–49.4)**	***0.2626***
ESAT6/CFP10**	Infected	28/40	70.0 (53.5–83.4)	14/28	50.9 (30.7–69.4)	*0.1294*	20/30	66.7 (47.2–82.7)	3/4	75.0 (19.4–99.4)	*1.0000*
	Uninfected	21/64	32.8 (21.6–45.7)	62/206	30.1 (23.9–36.9)	*0.7567*	9/37	24.3 (11.8–41.2)	2/9	22.2 (2.8–60.0)	*1.0000*
	Unknown	30/113	26.6 (18.7–35.7)	59/180	32.8 (26.0–40.2)	*0.2972*	9/55	16.4 (7.7–28.8)	2/12	16.7 (2.1–48.4)	*1.0000*
	Uninfected +unknown	51/177	28.8 (22.3–36.1)	121/386	31.4 (26.8–36.2)	*0.5563*	18/92	19.6 (12.0–29.2)	4/21	19.1 (5.5–41.9)	*1.0000*
	Total	**79/217**	**36.4 (30.0–43.2)**	**135/414**	**32.6 (28.1–37.4)**	***0.3761***	**38/122**	**31.2 (23.1–40.2)**	**7/25**	**28.0 (12.1–49.4)**	***0.8166***
Both antigens	Infected	33/40	82.5 (67.2–92.7)	19/28	67.9 (47.7–84.4)	*0.2451*	23/30	73.3 (54.1–87.7)	3/4	75.0 (19.4–99.4)	*1.0000*
	Uninfected	28/64	43.8 (31.4–56.7)	104/102	50.5 (43.5–57.5)	*0.3914*	16/37	43.2 (27.1–60.5)	4/9	44.4 (13.7–78.8)	*1.0000*
	Unknown	56/113	49.6 (40.0–59.1)	111/180	61.7 (54.1–68.8)	*0.0523*	22/55	40.0 (27.0–54.1)	3/12	25.0 (5.5–57.2)	*0.5120*
	Uninfected +unknown	84/177	47.5 (39.9–55.1)	215/386	55.7 (50.6–61.7)	*0.0699*	38/92	46.3 (35.3–57.7)	7/21	33.3 (14.6–57.0)	*0.3313*
	Total	**117/217**	**53.9 (47.0–60.7)**	**234/414**	**56.6 (51.6–61.4)**	***0.5554***	**61/122**	**50.0 (40.8–59.2)**	**10/25**	**40.0 (23.1–61.3**	***0.3884***

Footnotes: TB: tuberculosis; HIV: human immunodeficiency virus; n/N = number of positive tests/number of tested sera in each group; SM: smear microscopy; * Cut-off value for PGL-Tb1: OD = 0.130; ** Cut-off value for ESAT-6/CFP10: OD = 0.100; CI: confidence interval.

Table 11. Sensitivity of the SM test and combined sensitivity of the SM with the serology results based on the cumulative anti-PGL-Tb1 and anti-ESAT-6/CFP10 ELISA positive data among the SM-negative (serology positive) active TB patients stratified by disease localization and HIV status.

HIV status	test	n/N	Pulmonary TB	n/N	Extrapulmonary TB	n/N	All forms of TB
			% (95% CI)		% (95% CI)		% (95% CI)
Infected	SM (+)	28/68	41.2 (29.4–53.8)	4/34	11.8 (3.3–27.5)	32/102	31.4 (22.6–41.3)
	SM(+) + ELISA (+)	61/68	**89.7** (79.9–95.8)	27/34	**79.4** (62.1–91.3)	88/102	**86.3** (78.0–92.3)
	SM+ versus SM+ELISA+		*p <0.0001*		*p <0.0001*		*p <0.0001*
Uninfected	SM (+)	206/270	76.3 (70.6–81.2)	9/46	19.6 (9.4–33.9)	215/316	68.0 (62.6–73.2)
	SM(+) + ELISA (+)	234/270	**86.7** (82.2–90.5)	25/46	**54.4** (39.0–69.1)	259/316	**82.0** (77.3–86.0)
	SM+ versus SM+ELISA+		*p =0.0027*		*p =0.0010*		*p <0.0001*
Unknown	SM (+)	180/293	61.4 (55.6–67.0)	12/67	17.9 (9.6–29.2)	192/360	53.3 (48.0–58.6)
	SM(+) + ELISA (+)	236/293	**80.5** (75.5–84.9)	34/67	**50.8** (38.2–63.2)	270/360	**75.0** (70.2–79.4)
	SM+ versus SM+ELISA+		*p <0.0001*		*p =0.0001*		*p <0.0001*
Uninfected +Unknown	SM (+)	386/563	68.6 (64.6–72.4)	21/113	18.6 (11.9–27.0)	407/676	60.2 (56.4–63.9)
	SM(+) + ELISA (+)	470/563	**83.5** (80.2–86.5)	59/113	**52.2** (42.6–61.7)	529/676	**78.3** (80.0–81.3)
	SM+ versus SM+ELISA+		*p <0.0001*		*p <0.0001*		*p <0.0001*
Total	SM (+)	414/631	65.6 (61.8–69.3)	25/147	17.0 (11.3–24.1)	439/778	56.4 (52.9–60.0)
	SM(+) + ELISA (+)	531/631	**84.2** (81.1–86.9)	86/147	**58.1** (49.7–66.2)	617/778	**79.3** (76.3–82.1)
	SM+ versus SM+ELISA+		*p <0.0001*		*p <0.0001*		*p <0.0001*

Footnotes: TB: tuberculosis; HIV: human immunodeficiency virus; n/N = number of positive tests/number of tested sera in each group; SM: smear microscopy; Cut-off value for PGL-Tb1: OD = 0.130; ESAT-6/CFP10: OD = 0.100.

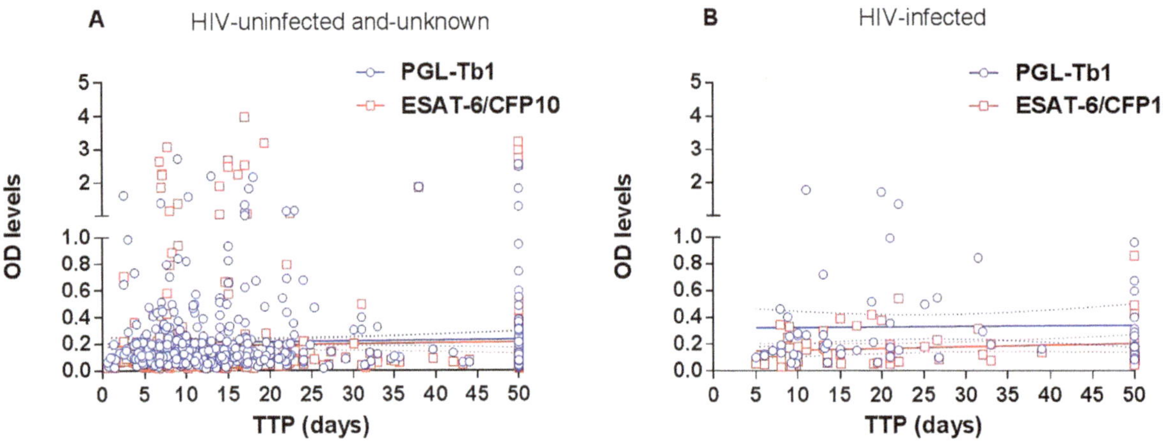

Figure 6. Impact of mycobacterial load and antibody responses stratified by HIV status. Relationship between individual time to positivity (TTP in days) of a liquid culture and individual serological tests based on optical density values against PGL-Tb1 antigen (blue spot) or ESAT-6/CFP10 (red spot) antigen in (A) the whole group of 270 HIV-uninfected and 293 HIV-unknown patients and in (B) the group of 68 HIV-infected patients with active pulmonary TB. The continuous lines represent the linear regression curve for anti-PGL-Tb1 antibody or for anti-ESAT-6/CFP10 antibody tested individuals; the hatched lines represent the 95% confidence intervals. **Footnotes**: HIV: Human Immunodeficiency Virus; OD: optical density; TTP: time to positivity.

Insufficient serological results are available for ATB sputum smear-negative patients with HIV co-infection [45,66–73]. Moreover, these results are based on the use of protein antigens that may affect the accuracy of the assays. The approach of using non-protein antigens (phosphoglycolipid, lipo-oligosaccharide, diacyl-trehalose or phenolic glycolipid) may overcome this drawback [32]. In fact, in HIV–TB co-infected patients from low TB endemic countries, the sensitivity of a serological test based on an ELISA using a glycolipid was similar [14] or even higher compared to an assay based on protein antigens [39,74]. Moreover, these mycobacterial-derived products seem to be species specific, without any influence from previous BCG vaccination [75] or co-existing mycobacteriosis due to non-tuberculosis mycobacteria infection [13].

In our current multi-centric study performed in India, we confirmed the data generated in non-endemic TB countries showing a high potential of serological tests with one glycolipid antigen (PGL-Tb1) in HIV-TB co-infected patients [39]. In addition, our present data showed that in ATB patients, the IgG antibody levels to one single antigen (PGL-Tb1 or ESAT-6/CFP10) were independent of the SM status and grade and were significantly higher than the levels observed in all healthy controls at relatively low and high risk of LTBI, except the cured TB patients. Nonetheless, the IgG antibody levels against both the PGL-Tb1 and ESAT-6/CFP10 antigen in the healthy controls varied according to the site of recruitment and the extent of *M. tuberculosis* exposure. As reported previously, the varying degree of TB infectiousness was demonstrated among the ATB patients enrolled at the different sites of recruitment [46], and consequently, a higher prevalence of LTBI, as measured with the TST and QFT-GIT responses, was observed in the close contacts recruited at the sites where the ATB patients were more infectious [47]. This indicates that the ATB incidence in a given country and region has a marked influence on the cell-mediated responses and antibody responses to *M.tuberculosis* specific antigens reflecting repeated exposure to the pathogen [37].

Among the groups of ATB patients, there was no significant difference of antibody levels or test sensitivity between the HIV-uninfected and HIV-unknown ATB patients. This is most likely due to the fact that these two populations of ATB patients were similar regarding their HIV status, as previously reported [46,47].

In contrast, the anti-PGL-Tb1 and anti-ESAT6/CFP10 antibody levels were significantly higher in HIV-infected sera than in HIV-uninfected ($p<0.0001$), or in HIV-unknown ($p<0.0001$) sera from ATB patients. Thus, although the majority of HIV-infected ATB patients in our study had advanced immunosuppression, it was shown that the anti-PGL-Tb1 antibody production was not dependent on the degree of immunosuppression. On the other hand, there was a trend for the anti-ESAT-6/CFP10 fusion protein antibody response to be more dependent on the degree of immunosuppression (higher antibody levels were found in HIV-TB co-infected patients with more than 200/µl CD4 cell counts compared to those with lower counts). However, the difference was not significant, probably due to the low number of patients with available CD4 counts.

As recently demonstrated, the absence of effect upon the anti-PGL-Tb1 response could be linked to the glycolipid structure of the PGL-Tb1 antigen and its presentation via the CD1 pathway for lymphocyte activation [33,34]. Indirect evidence that the canonical presentation pathway involving CD4T-lymphocytes is not involved in the anti-glycolipid antibody response is illustrated by the absence of a direct correlation between the CD4 T-lymphocyte counts and the individual IgG antibody production, as shown in our study. Likewise, evidence has been published demonstrating that a subpopulation of CD4 T-lymphocytes involved in the CD1-restricted glycolipid antigen presentation pathway in leprosy [76] and TB patients [77,78] persists in patients with AIDS [79]. T-lymphocyte independence of the antibody response to another specific mycobacterial phenolic glycolipid antigen (the PGL-1 antigen being specific for *M.leprae*) has been shown in lepromatous leprosy patients, also when very high anti-PGL-1 antibody levels (both IgM and IgG) were found in the absence of a specific T-cell mediated immune response [80]. It was also shown there was no relationship between TST results and anti-PGL-Tb1 antibody levels in ATB patients, similar to the results shown in the present study (**Fig.8**). In the lepromatous leprosy patients, a good correlation between IgM and IgG anti-PGL-1 antibody levels and bacteriological yield (as expressed by the bacteriological index performed in skin biopsies) has been also

Table 12. Sensitivity of the serology test based on the ELISA using the PGL-Tb1 and ESAT-6/CFP10 antigens and their cumulative results in active pulmonary TB patients stratified by SM grade and HIV status.

HIV status	n/N	SM (-)	n/N	SM scanty	n/N	SM (+)	n/N	SM (++)	n/N	SM (+++)
		% (95% CI)		% (95% CI)		% (95% CI)		% (95% CI)		% (95% CI)
HIV-infected										
PGL-Tb1	31/40	**77.5** (61.6–89.2)	4/4	**100** (39.8–100)	5/7	**71.4** (29.0–96.3)	6/10	**60.0** (26.2–87.8)	4/7	**57.1** (18.4–90.1)
p SM (-) versus others				*0.56*		*0.66*		*0.42*		*0.35*
ESAT6/CFP10	28/40	**70.0** (53.5–83.4)	2/4	**50.0** (68.0–93.2)	3/7	**42.9** (10.0–81.6)	6/10	**60.0** (26.2–87.8)	3/7	**42.9** (10. –81.6)
p SM (-) versus others				*0.58*		*0.21*		*0.71*		*0.21*
Both antigens	33/40	**82.5** (67.2–92.7)	4/4	**100** (39.8–100)	5/7	**71.4** (29.0–96.3)	6/10	**60.0** (26.2–87.8)	4/7	**57.1** (18.4–90.1)
p SM (-) versus others				*1.00*		*0.61*		*0.20*		*0.16*
HIV-uninfected										
PGL-Tb1	19/64	**29.7** (18.9–42.4)	9/24	**37.5** (18.8–59.4)	20/53	**37.7** (24.8–52.1)	20/50	**40.0** (26.4–54.8)	36/79	**45.6** (34.3–57.2)
p SM (-) versus others				*0.60*		*0.43*		*0.32*		*0.06*
ESAT6/CFP10	21/64	**32.8** (21.6–45.7)	6/24	**25.0** (9.8–46.7)	18/53	**34.0** (21.5–48.3)	13/50	**26.0** (14.6–40.3)	25/79	**31.7** (21.6–43.1)
p SM (-) versus others				*0.61*		*1.00*		*0.54*		*1.00*
Both antigens	28/64	**43.8** (31.4–56.7)	12/24	**50.0** (29.1–70.9)	26/53	**49.1** (35.1–63.2)	23/50	**46.0** (31.8–60.7)	43/79	**54.4** (42.8–65.7)
p SM (-) versus others				*0.64*		*0.58*		*0.85*		*0.24*
HIV-unknown										
PGL-Tb1	49/113	**43.4** (34.1–53.0)	9/14	**64.3** (35.1–87.2)	30/52	**57.7** (43.2–71.3)	11/39	**28.2** (15.0–44.9)	37/75	**49.3** (37.6–61.1)
p SM (-) versus others				*0.16*		*0.10*		*0.13*		*0.46*
ESAT6/CFP10	30/113	**26.6** (18.7–35.7)	6/14	**42.9** (17.7–71.1)	18/52	**34.6** (22.0–49.1)	12/39	**30.8** (17.0–47.6)	23/75	**30.7** (20.5–42.4)
p SM (-) versus others				*0.22*		*0.36*		*0.68*		*0.62*
Both antigens	56/113	**49.6** (40.0–59.1)	10/14	**71.4** (41.9–91.6)	36/52	**69.2** (54.9–81.3)	20/39	**51.3** (34.8–67.8)	45/75	**60.0** (48.4–71.2)
p SM (-) versus others				*0.16*		*0.0196*		*1.00*		*0.18*

Footnotes: TB: tuberculosis; HIV: human immunodeficiency virus; n/N = number of positive tests/number of tested sera in each group; SM: smear microscopy; Cut-off value for PGL-Tb1: OD = 0.130; Cut-off value for ESAT-6/CFP10: OD = 0.100; CI: confidence interval.

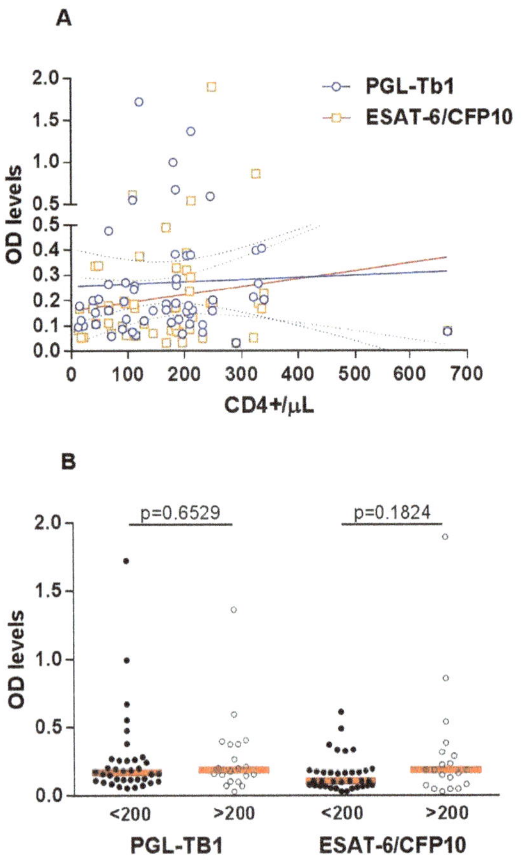

Figure 7. Impact of CD4 counts on antibody responses in HIV-infected active tuberculosis patients A. Correlation between individual CD4 cell counts and individual serological tests based on optical density values of ELISA against PGL-Tb1 antigen (blue spot) ($R^2 = 0.00103$; $p = 0.8141$) or ESAT-6/CFP10 antigen (red spot) ($R^2 = 0.01574$; $p = 0.3569$) in 53 HIV-infected ATB patients. The continuous lines represent the linear regression curve for anti-PGL-Tb1 antibody or for anti-ESAT-6/CFP10 antibody tested individuals; the hatched lines represent the 95% confidence intervals. B. Anti-PGL-Tb1 and anti-ESAT-6/CFP10 antibody levels stratified by CD4 cell counts among the 56 HIV-infected ATB patients. Horizontal red lines indicate the median value. **Footnotes**: OD: optical density.

described [81]. However in the context of pulmonary TB, no significant association between the proportion of anti-PGL-Tb1 positive results and bacillary load was found. Our results confirmed the absence of a relationship between the bacillary load and antibody levels: no significant correlation was observed between the Time to Positivity (in days) of a liquid culture and the anti-PGL-Tb1 or anti-ESAT-6/CFP10 antibody levels in the same ATB patients, independent of the HIV status. Similarly, the sensitivity of the serological test based on an ELISA using each antigen was not influenced by the SM status or grade evaluated among the specimen samples of the pulmonary ATB patients.

With an overall specificity of around 90%, the sensitivity of the two serological tests, using either the PGL-Tb1 or the ESAT-6/CFP10 antigen, was statistically higher in the HIV-TB co-infected patients compared to the HIV-uninfected or HIV-unknown TB patients, independent of the disease localization [39]. The overall sensitivity for ATB using the cumulative results obtained with the two antigens was always higher than using one single antigen, but with a statistical significant reduction of specificity, confirming previous studies [14,45,61]. Nevertheless, the sensitivity of the serological tests for ATB in HIV-infected subjects was 75.5% with a significant negative LR (94.9%). Lower sensitivity was shown among the HIV-uninfected (50.9%) and HIV-unknown ATB patients (54.1%).

The sensitivity of the SM for diagnosing ATB was variable and dependent on the HIV status and localization of the disease, being very low among the whole group of extrapulmonary ATB (17%) and among the whole group of HIV-infected ATB patients (31.4%). In the present study, the serology using either the glycolipid or the fusion protein antigen was able to detect an equal number of ATB patients, independent of SM score and HIV status. Thus, the combination of SM-positive results with the serological tests based on single or multiple antigens (cumulative results) improved the case findings in ATB patients. This higher sensitivity could be related to the independence of antibody production of disease localization, mycobacterial load of the ATB patient's specimens and the degree of immunosuppression.

The varying degree of the physicians' clinical suspicion of TB did not influence the accuracy of the two serological tests and other immunological tools [47], in contrast to the clinical symptoms, radiological findings and microbiological tools [46]. These results might be associated with the absence of impact of duration and severity of TB disease on the B-cell immune responses in ATB patients.

Table 13. Comparison of the sensitivity of the TST and the serology test based on ELISA using each antigen and their cumulative results in HIV-infected active TB patients stratified by CD4 cell counts/µL (lower or above 200/µL).

	Percentage (95% CI)				
	n/N	<200 CD4 cell counts/µL	n/N	>200 CD4 cell counts/µL	*P*
		% (95% CI)		% (95% CI)	
ELISA					
PGL-Tb1	22/36	61.1 (43.5–76.9)	15/20	75.0 (50.9–91.3)	*0.3824*
ESAT-6/CFP10	22/36	61.1 (43.5–76.9)	14/20	70.0 (45.7–88.1)	*0.5713*
Both antigens	24/36	66.7 (49.0–81.4)	15/20	75.0 (50.9–91.3)	*0.5613*
TST	9/11	81.8 (48.2–97.7)	3/4	75.0 (19.4–99.4)	*1.000*

Footnotes: TB: tuberculosis; HIV: human immunodeficiency virus; n/N = number of positive tests/number of tested sera in each group; TST: tuberculin skin test (cut-off 5 mm); Cut-off value for PGL-Tb1: OD = 0.130; Cut-off value for ESAT-6/CFP10: OD = 0.100; CI: confidence interval.

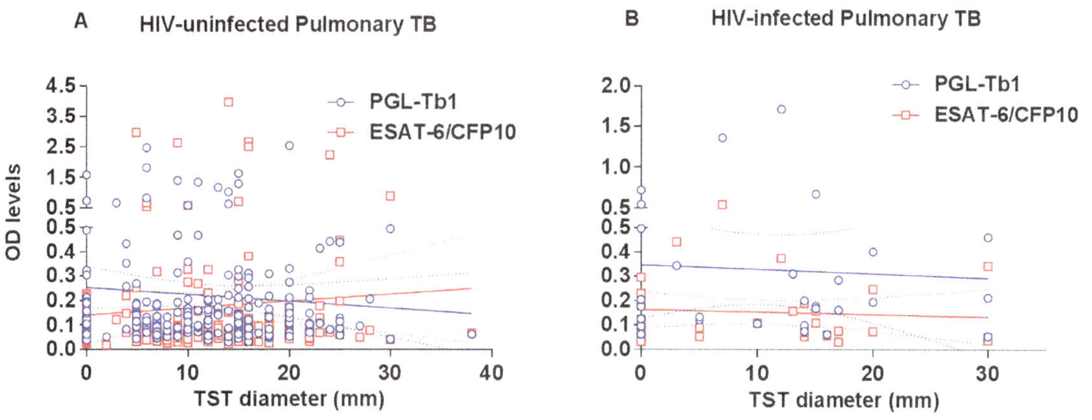

Figure 8. Correlation between the tuberculin skin test and antibody responses in active tuberculosis patients stratified by HIV status. Correlation between the individual tuberculin skin test diameter (in mm) and the individual serological tests based on optical density values of the ELISA against PGL-Tb1 antigen (blue spot) and ESAT-6/CFP10 (red spot) antigen in (A) the whole group of 127 HIV-uninfected and 119 HIV-unknown patients and in (B) the group of 30 HIV-infected patients with active pulmonary TB. The continuous lines represent the linear regression curve for anti-PGL-Tb1 antibody or for anti-ESAT-6/CFP10 antibody tested individuals; the hatched lines represent the 95% confidence intervals. **Footnotes**: HIV: Human Immunodeficiency Virus; TB: tuberculosis; TST: tuberculin skin test; OD: optical density.

In conclusion, from a clinical viewpoint, our study showed that the combined use of the SM test and the two serological tests led to an increase of sensitivity for ATB diagnosis in those with extrapulmonary localization and HIV co-infection. Therefore, serological assays using the cumulative results obtained with both a phenolic glycolipid antigen such as the PGL-Tb1 and a fusion protein such as the ESAT-6/CFP10 may be evaluated as a potentially interesting additional tool for diagnosing ATB in HIV-infected patients in high TB-endemic countries.

Author Contributions

Conceived and designed the experiments: PHL DM NKG. Performed the experiments: BSAK A. Sodha BJ VK MK VL DN PS A. Singh AD SVSM CR AR BR. Analyzed the data: DG EG PHL. Contributed reagents/materials/analysis tools: ML GV CL. Wrote the paper: PHL DG. Indian supervisor of the study: ST. Performed all the quality controls of the data: ST. Enrolled patients: AR CR A. Sodha RD BJ KK VK VL DN AD SMVS SS. Supervised the experiments: AR CR.

References

1. Keeler E, Perkins MD, Small P, Hanson C, Reed S, et al. (2006) Reducing the global burden of tuberculosis: The contribution of improved diagnostics. Nature 444 Suppl 1: 49–57.
2. Young DB, Perkins MD, Duncan K, Barry CE 3rd (2008) Confronting the scientific obstacles to global control of tuberculosis. J Clin Invest 118: 1255–1265.
3. Siddiqi K, Lambert ML, Walley J (2003) Clinical diagnosis of smear-negative pulmonary tuberculosis in low-income countries: The current evidence. Lancet Infect Dis 3: 288–296.
4. Steingart KR, Ng V, Henry M, Hopewell PC, Ramsay A, et al. (2006) Sputum processing methods to improve the sensitivity of smear microscopy for tuberculosis: A systematic review. Lancet Infect Dis 6: 664–674.
5. Mase SR, Ramsay A, Ng V, Henry M, Hopewell PC, et al. (2007) Yield of serial sputum specimen examinations in the diagnosis of pulmonary tuberculosis: A systematic review. Int J Tuberc Lung Dis 11: 485–495.
6. Squire SB, Belaye AK, Kashoti A, Salaniponi FM, Mundy CJ, et al. (2005) 'Lost' smear-positive pulmonary tuberculosis cases: Where are they and why did we lose them? Int J Tuberc Lung Dis 9: 25–31.
7. World Health Organization (2003) Treatment of tuberculosis: Guidelines for national programmes; WHO 3rd ed. WHO/CDS/TB: 313.
8. Perkins MD, Roscigno G, Zumla A (2006) Progress towards improved tuberculosis diagnostics for developing countries. Lancet 367: 942–943.
9. Daniel TM (1988) Antibody and antigen detection for the immunodiagnosis of tuberculosis: Why not? what more is needed? where do we stand today? J Infect Dis 158: 678–680.
10. Daniel TM, Debanne SM (1987) The serodiagnosis of tuberculosis and other mycobacterial diseases by enzyme-linked immunosorbent assay. Am Rev Respir Dis 135: 1137–1151.
11. Menzies D (2004) What is the current and potential role of diagnostic tests other than sputum microscopy and culture? in frieden T (ed.), Toman's tuberculosis: Case detection, treatment, and monitoring – questions and answers. WHO Geneva 2nd ed, vol. /2004.334: 87–91.
12. Gennaro ML (2000) Immunologic diagnosis of tuberculosis. Clin Infect Dis 30 Suppl 3: S243–6.
13. Bothamley GH (1995) Serological diagnosis of tuberculosis. Eur Respir J Suppl 20: 676s–688s.
14. Simonney N, Molina JM, Molimard M, Oksenhendler E, Perronne C, et al. (1995) Analysis of the immunological humoral response to mycobacterium tuberculosis glycolipid antigens (DAT, PGLTb1) for diagnosis of tuberculosis in HIV-seropositive and -seronegative patients. Eur J Clin Microbiol Infect Dis 14: 883–891.
15. Lyashchenko K, Colangeli R, Houde M, Al Jahdali H, Menzies D, et al. (1998) Heterogeneous antibody responses in tuberculosis. Infect Immun 66: 3936–3940.
16. Verbon A, Weverling GJ, Kuijper S, Speelman P, Jansen HM, et al. (1993) Evaluation of different tests for the serodiagnosis of tuberculosis and the use of likelihood ratios in serology. Am Rev Respir Dis 148: 378–384.
17. Wilkins E (1994) The serodiagnosis of tuberculosis. In: Davies PDO, editor Clinical tuberculosis London: Chapman & Hall Medical: 367–380.
18. Chan ED, Heifets L, Iseman MD (2000) Immunologic diagnosis of tuberculosis: A review. Tuber Lung Dis 80: 131–140.
19. Daniel TM, Sippola AA, Okwera A, Kabengera S, Hatanga E, et al. (1994) Reduced sensitivity of tuberculosis serodiagnosis in patients with AIDS in uganda. Tuber Lung Dis 75: 33–37.
20. McDonough JA, Sada DE, Sippola AA, Ferguson LE, Daniel TM (1992) Microplate and dot immunoassays for the serodiagnosis of tuberculosis. J Lab Clin Med 120: 318–322.
21. Talbot EA, Hay Burgess DC, Hone NM, Iademarco MF, Mwasekaga MJ, et al. (2004) Tuberculosis serodiagnosis in a predominantly HIV-infected population of hospitalized patients with cough, botswana, 2002. Clin Infect Dis 39: e1–7.
22. van der Werf TS, Das PK, van Soolingen D, Yong S, van der Mark TW, et al. (1992) Sero-diagnosis of tuberculosis with A60 antigen enzyme-linked immunosorbent assay: Failure in HIV-infected individuals in ghana. Med Microbiol Immunol 181: 71–76.
23. Papa F, Cruaud P, David HL (1989) Antigenicity and specificity of selected glycolipid fractions from mycobacterium tuberculosis. Res Microbiol 140: 569–578.
24. Cruaud P, Yamashita JT, Casabona NM, Papa F, David HL (1990) Evaluation of a novel 2,3-diacyl-trehalose-2'-sulphate (SL-IV) antigen for case finding and diagnosis of leprosy and tuberculosis. Res Microbiol 141: 679–694.
25. Torgal-Garcia J, David HL, Papa F (1988) Preliminary evaluation of a mycobacterium tuberculosis phenolglycolipid antigen in the serologic diagnosis of tuberculosis. Ann Inst Pasteur Microbiol 139: 289–294.
26. Saltini C, Amicosante M, Girardi E, Antonucci G, Ippolito G, et al. (1993) Early abnormalities of the antibody response against mycobacterium tuberculosis in human immunodeficiency virus infection. J Infect Dis 168: 1409–1414.

27. Savage C, Vincent P, Leclerc H (1993) Serodiagnosis of tuberculosis. evaluation of a sulpholipid antigen. Zentralbl Bakteriol 278: 49–57.
28. Daleine G, Lagrange PH (1995) Preliminary evaluation of a mycobacterium tuberculosis lipooligosaccharide (LOS) antigen in the serological diagnosis of tuberculosis in HIV seropositive and seronegative patients. Tuber Lung Dis 76: 234–239.
29. Boggian K, Fierz W, Vernazza PL (1996) Infrequent detection of lipoarabinomannan antibodies in human immunodeficiency virus-associated mycobacterial disease. swiss HIV cohort study. J Clin Microbiol 34: 1854–1855.
30. Simonney N, Molina JM, Molimard M, Oksenhendler E, Lagrange PH (1996) Comparison of A60 and three glycolipid antigens in an ELISA test for tuberculosis. Clin Microbiol Infect 2: 214–222.
31. Mathur ML, LoBue PA, Catanzaro A (1999) Evaluation of a serologic test for the diagnosis of tuberculosis. Int J Tuberc Lung Dis 3: 732–735.
32. Colangeli R, Antinori A, Cingolani A, Ortona L, Lyashchenko K, et al. (1999) Humoral immune responses to multiple antigens of mycobacterium tuberculosis in tuberculosis patients co-infected with the human immunodeficiency virus. Int J Tuberc Lung Dis 3: 1127–1131.
33. De Libero G, Mori L (2005) Recognition of lipid antigens by T cells. Nat Rev Immunol 5: 485–496.
34. Lang ML, Glatman-Freedman A (2006) Do CD1-restricted T cells contribute to antibody-mediated immunity against mycobacterium tuberculosis? Infect Immun 74: 803–809.
35. Kroon FP, van Dissel JT, Labadie J, van Loon AM, van Furth R (1995) Antibody response to diphtheria, tetanus, and poliomyelitis vaccines in relation to the number of CD4+ T lymphocytes in adults infected with human immunodeficiency virus. Clin Infect Dis 21: 1197–1203.
36. Laal S SY (2005) Immune-based methods. In Cole ST (ed), Tuberculosis and the tubercle bacillus, ASM Press, Washington, DC,: 71–83.
37. Hoff ST, Abebe M, Ravn P, Range N, Malenganisho W, et al. (2007) Evaluation of mycobacterium tuberculosis—specific antibody responses in populations with different levels of exposure from tanzania, ethiopia, brazil, and denmark. Clin Infect Dis 45: 575–582.
38. Gennaro ML, Affouf M, Kanaujia GV, Brusasca PN, Mangura B, et al. (2007) Antibody markers of incident tuberculosis among HIV-infected adults in the USA: A historical prospective study. Int J Tuberc Lung Dis 11: 624–631.
39. Simonney N, Chavanet P, Perronne C, Leportier M, Revol F, et al. (2007) B-cell immune responses in HIV positive and HIV negative patients with tuberculosis evaluated with an ELISA using a glycolipid antigen. Tuberculosis (Edinb) 87: 109–122.
40. Dheda K, Davids V, Lenders L, Roberts T, Meldau R, et al. (2010) Clinical utility of a commercial LAM-ELISA assay for TB diagnosis in HIV-infected patients using urine and sputum samples. PLoS One 5: e9848.
41. Steingart KR, Sohn H, Schiller I, Kloda LA, Boehme CC, et al. (2013) Xpert(R) MTB/RIF assay for pulmonary tuberculosis and rifampicin resistance in adults. Cochrane Database Syst Rev 1: CD009593.
42. Vadwai V, Boehme C, Nabeta P, Shetty A, Alland D, et al. (2011) Xpert MTB/RIF: A new pillar in diagnosis of extrapulmonary tuberculosis? J Clin Microbiol 49: 2540–2545.
43. Steingart KR, Henry M, Laal S, Hopewell PC, Ramsay A, et al. (2007) Commercial serological antibody detection tests for the diagnosis of pulmonary tuberculosis: A systematic review. PLoS Med 4: e202.
44. Steingart KR, Henry M, Laal S, Hopewell PC, Ramsay A, et al. (2007) A systematic review of commercial serological antibody detection tests for the diagnosis of extrapulmonary tuberculosis. Thorax 62: 911–918.
45. Steingart KR, Dendukuri N, Henry M, Schiller I, Nahid P, et al. (2009) Performance of purified antigens for serodiagnosis of pulmonary tuberculosis: A meta-analysis. Clin Vaccine Immunol 16: 260–276.
46. Lagrange PH, Thangaraj SK, Dayal R, Despande A, Ganguly NK, et al. (2012) A toolbox for tuberculosis diagnosis: An indian multicentric study (2006–2008): Microbiological results. PLoS One 7: e43739.
47. Lagrange PH, Thangaraj SK, Dayal R, Deshpande A, Ganguly NK, et al. (2013) A toolbox for tuberculosis (TB) diagnosis: An indian multicentric study (2006–2008). evaluation of QuantiFERON-TB gold in tube for TB diagnosis. PLoS One 8: e73579.
48. Enarson D, Rieder H, Arnadottir T, Trébucq A (2000) Management of tuberculosis: A guide for low-income countries. 5th ed Int Union against Tuberculosis and Lung Disease, Paris.
49. Thangaraj Satheesh K (2008.) Study on selected *M.tuberculosis* specific antigens for IgG antibody response for the development of ELISA based diagnostic test for tuberculosis. Nizam's Institute of Medical Sciences, University Hyderabad, A P, India April.
50. Daffe M, Lacave C, Laneelle MA, Laneelle G (1987) Structure of the major triglycosyl phenol-phthiocerol of mycobacterium tuberculosis (strain canetti). Eur J Biochem 167: 155–160.
51. Pal N, Sarkar S (2005) Statistics: Concepts and applications. Prentice-Hall of India Private Limited, New Delhi.
52. [Anonymous] (2003) Basic statistics-electronic stat book. stat soft inc. www.statsoft.com/textbook/.
53. Zweig MH, Campbell G (1993) Receiver-operating characteristic (ROC) plots: A fundamental evaluation tool in clinical medicine. Clin Chem 39: 561–577.
54. Altman DG, Bland JM (1994) Diagnostic tests 3: Receiver operating characteristic plots. BMJ 309: 188.
55. Thompson ML (2003) Assessing the diagnostic accuracy of a sequence of tests. Biostatistics 4: 341–351.
56. Banoo S, Bell D, Bossuyt P, Herring A, Mabey D, et al. (2006) Evaluation of diagnostic tests for infectious diseases: General principles. Nat Rev Microbiol 4: S20–32.
57. Dayal R, Verma V, Sharma B, Kumar G, Kumar N, et al. (2012) Diagnostic value of interferon- gamma release assays (QuantiFERON-TB gold(R) in tube) in childhood tuberculosis. Indian J Pediatr 79: 183–187.
58. Goletti D, Raja A, Ahamed Kabeer BS, Rodrigues C, Sodha A, et al. (2010) IFN-gamma, but not IP-10, MCP-2 or IL-2 response to RD1 selected peptides associates to active tuberculosis. J Infect 61: 133–143.
59. Goletti D, Raja A, Syed Ahamed Kabeer B, Rodrigues C, Sodha A, et al. (2010) Is IP-10 an accurate marker for detecting M. tuberculosis-specific response in HIV-infected persons? PLoS One 5: e12577.
60. Kabeer BS, Raja A, Raman B, Thangaraj S, Leportier M, et al. (2011) IP-10 response to RD1 antigens might be a useful biomarker for monitoring tuberculosis therapy. BMC Infect Dis 11: 135-2334-11-135.
61. Kunnath-Velayudhan S, Gennaro ML (2011) Immunodiagnosis of tuberculosis: A dynamic view of biomarker discovery. Clin Microbiol Rev 24: 792–805.
62. Pai M, Kalantri S, Dheda K (2006) New tools and emerging technologies for the diagnosis of tuberculosis: Part II. active tuberculosis and drug resistance. Expert Rev Mol Diagn 6: 423–432.
63. Steingart KR, Ramsay A, Pai M (2007) Commercial serological tests for the diagnosis of tuberculosis: Do they work? Future Microbiol 2: 355–359.
64. Steingart KR, Flores LL, Dendukuri N, Schiller I, Laal S, et al. (2011) Commercial serological tests for the diagnosis of active pulmonary and extrapulmonary tuberculosis: An updated systematic review and meta-analysis. PLoS Med 8: e1001062.
65. World Health Organization (2011) Commercial serodiagnostic tests for diagnosis of tuberculosis: Policy statement.geneva. WHO.
66. Ratanasuwan W, Kreiss JK, Nolan CM, Schaeffler BA, Suwanagool S, et al. (1997) Evaluation of the MycoDot test for the diagnosis of tuberculosis in HIV seropositive and seronegative patients. Int J Tuberc Lung Dis 1: 259–264.
67. Somi GR, O'Brien RJ, Mfinanga GS, Ipuge YA (1999) Evaluation of the MycoDot test in patients with suspected tuberculosis in a field setting in tanzania. Int J Tuberc Lung Dis 3: 231–238.
68. Theuer C, Chaisson R, Elias D, Schecter G, Glassroth J (1989) Detection of circulating antibodies to purified protein derivative in tuberculosis patients with or without human immunodeficiency virus infection. Am Rev Respir Dis 139 (suppl 4): ABSTRACT 395.
69. Antunes A, Nina J, David S (2002) Serological screening for tuberculosis in the community: An evaluation of the mycodot procedure in an african population with high HIV-2 prevalence (republic of guinea-bissau). Res Microbiol 153: 301–305.
70. Barrera L, de Kantor I, Ritacco V, Reniero A, Lopez B, et al. (1992) Humoral response to mycobacterium tuberculosis in patients with human immunodeficiency virus infection. Tuber Lung Dis 73: 187–191.
71. Pouthier F, Perriens JH, Mukadi Y, Kayembe T, St Louis ME, et al. (1994) Anti-A60 immunoglobulin G in the serodiagnosis of tuberculosis in HIV-seropositive and seronegative patients. AIDS 8: 1277–1280.
72. Thybo S, Richter C, Wachmann H, Maselle SY, Mwakyusa DH, et al. (1995) Humoral response to mycobacterium tuberculosis-specific antigens in african tuberculosis patients with high prevalence of human immunodeficiency virus infection. Tuber Lung Dis 76: 149–155.
73. Schleicher GK, Feldman C, Vermaak Y, Verschoor JA (2002) Prevalence of anti-mycolic acid antibodies in patients with pulmonary tuberculosis co-infected with HIV. Clin Chem Lab Med 40: 882–887.
74. Harrington JJ, 3rd, Ho JL, Lapa e Silva JR, Conde MB, Kritski AL, et al. (2000) Mycobacterium tuberculosis lipid antigens: Use of multi-antigen based enzyme immunoassay for free and complex dissociated antibodies. Int J Tuberc Lung Dis 4: 161–167.
75. Das S, Cheng SH, Lowrie DB, Walker KB, Mitchison DA, et al. (1992) The pattern of mycobacterial antigen recognition in sera from mantoux-negative individuals is essentially unaffected by bacille calmette-guerin (BCG) vaccination in either south india or london. Clin Exp Immunol 89: 402-406.
76. Sieling PA, Ochoa MT, Jullien D, Leslie DS, Sabet S, et al. (2000) Evidence for human CD4+ T cells in the CD1-restricted repertoire: Derivation of mycobacteria-reactive T cells from leprosy lesions. J Immunol 164: 4790–4796.
77. Stenger S, Modlin RL (1999) T cell mediated immunity to mycobacterium tuberculosis. Curr Opin Microbiol 2: 89–93.
78. Stenger S (2001) Cytolytic T cells in the immune response to mycobacterium tuberculosis. Scand J Infect Dis 33: 483–487.
79. Gong J, Stenger S, Zack JA, Jones BE, Bristol GC, et al. (1998) Isolation of mycobacterium-reactive CD1-restricted T cells from patients with human immunodeficiency virus infection. J Clin Invest 101: 383–389.
80. David HL, Papa F, Cruaud P, Berlie HC, Maroja MF, et al. (1992) Relationships between titers of antibodies immunoreacting against glycolipid antigens from mycobacterium leprae and M. tuberculosis, the mitsuda and mantoux reactions, and bacteriological loads: Implications in the pathogenesis, epidemiology and serodiagnosis of leprosy and tuberculosis. Int J Lepr Other Mycobact Dis 60: 208–224.
81. Lyons NF, Shannon EJ, Ellis BP, Naafs B (1988) Association of IgG and IgM antibodies to phenolic glycolipid-1 antigen of mycobacterium leprae with disease parameters in multibacillary leprosy patients. Lepr Rev 59: 45–52.

The Cost-Effectiveness of Different Feeding Patterns Combined with Prompt Treatments for Preventing Mother-to-Child HIV Transmission in South Africa: Estimates from Simulation Modeling

Wenhua Yu[¶], **Changping Li**[¶], **Xiaomeng Fu**[¶], **Zhuang Cui, Xiaoqian Liu, Linlin Fan, Guan Zhang, Jun Ma***

Department of Health Statistics, College of Public Health, Tianjin Medical University, Tianjin, China

Abstract

Objectives: Based on the important changes in South Africa since 2009 and the Antiretroviral Treatment Guideline 2013 recommendations, we explored the cost-effectiveness of different strategy combinations according to the South African HIV-infected mothers' prompt treatments and different feeding patterns.

Study Design: A decision analytic model was applied to simulate cohorts of 10,000 HIV-infected pregnant women to compare the cost-effectiveness of two different HIV strategy combinations: (1) Women were tested and treated promptly at any time during pregnancy (Promptly treated cohort). (2) Women did not get testing or treatment until after delivery and appropriate standard treatments were offered as a remedy (Remedy cohort). Replacement feeding or exclusive breastfeeding was assigned in both strategies. Outcome measures included the number of infant HIV cases averted, the cost per infant HIV case averted, and the cost per life year(LY) saved from the interventions. One-way and multivariate sensitivity analyses were performed to estimate the uncertainty ranges of all outcomes.

Results: The remedy strategy does not particularly cost-effective. Compared with the untreated baseline cohort which leads to 1127 infected infants, 698 (61.93%) and 110 (9.76%) of pediatric HIV cases are averted in the promptly treated cohort and remedy cohort respectively, with incremental cost-effectiveness of $68.51 and $118.33 per LY, respectively. With or without the antenatal testing and treatments, breastfeeding is less cost-effective ($193.26 per LY) than replacement feeding ($134.88 per LY), without considering the impact of willingness to pay.

Conclusion: Compared with the prompt treatments, remedy in labor or during the postnatal period is less cost-effective. Antenatal HIV testing and prompt treatments and avoiding breastfeeding are the best strategies. Although encouraging mothers to practice replacement feeding in South Africa is far from easy and the advantages of breastfeeding can not be ignored, we still suggest choosing replacement feeding as far as possible.

Editor: Julian W. Tang, Alberta Provincial Laboratory for Public Health/University of Alberta, Canada

Funding: This study was not only supported by the grants from China's ministry of health, bureau of education of science and technology (201202017), and China's Ministry of Education, Humanities and Social Sciences Project (11YJCZH022, 11YJCZH080), but also partially sponsored by National Natural Science Foundation of China (NSFC, 71373175). The funders had no role in study design, data collection and analysis, decision to publish, or preparation of the manuscript.

Competing Interests: The authors have declared that no competing interests exist.

* Email: junma@tijmu.edu.cn

¶ These authors contributed equally to this work.

Introduction

Identification of human immunodeficiency virus (HIV) infection is critical from both clinical and public health perspectives. Antenatal HIV testing is undertaken primarily to offer interventions to reduce the risk of HIV transmission from mother to child. Globally, about 40% of pregnant women in low- and middle-income countries received HIV testing and counseling in 2012, up from 26% in 2009 [1].These prevention of Mother-to-child transmission (PMTCT) services in low- and middle-income countries have prevented approximately 409,000 children from acquiring HIV [2]. Around 330,000 children were HIV-infected prenatally in 2011, which represented a decline of 24% since 2009 in sub-Saharan Africa [2]. Especially the implementation of South Africa's massive HIV testing and counseling campaign between April 2010 and June 2011,which urged everyone in 12–60 years old to be tested [3], caused the national testing coverage to exceed 95% in 2012 [2].

However, there are the persons who are tested late or are unaware of their infection until relatively late in their disease course, as a result, missing the opportunity of getting prompt intervention. A World Health Organization (WHO) study of HIV diagnoses in Georgia in 2009–2011 found that 64% of new HIV diagnoses could be considered 'late' and that the reasons for the high rates of late diagnosis included lack of access to acceptable HIV testing and counseling services [2]. An interview study of 760 HIV-infected persons in Los Angeles County suggested that many persons reported with Acquired Immune Deficiency Syndrome (AIDS) were unaware of their infection until relatively late in their disease course. Of particular concern is that almost half (46%) of the reported respondents did not seek testing until they were ill [4]. A study based in two Durban clinics found most patients were tested at a late stage of infection with over 60% of CD4 counts below 200 cells/mm^3.Of those who were eligible for treatment, more than a fifth died, mostly before any treatment [5]. A survey had suggested that late HIV diagnosis may lead to accelerted progression and that some of the patients in the survey developed AIDS within a year of HIV infection[6]. These findings are in excellent agreement with those reported by other researchers [7].

Since the first report of transmission of HIV through breastfeeding was published in 1985 [8], avoidance of breastfeeding has remained an important component of efforts to prevent mother-to-child transmission (MTCT) of HIV [9]. There is no doubt that breastfeeding is risky for MTCT [8,10] and approximately 5%–20% of babies infected through MTCT acquire HIV infection via breastfeeding [2], but breastfeeding may be associated with other factors. Breastfeeding is particularly important in resource-poor regions of the world, where limited access to clean water increases the risk of diarrhea if replacement feeding is used, and many mothers do not have the means to afford the cost of formula [11]. Infant morbidity and mortality rates are generally decreased by breastfeeding, which provides optimal nutrition and partially protects against common childhood infections [11–13,20].

On account of realistic public health considerations, in 2010, WHO issued its first guidelines [14] that allowed new recommendations on antiretroviral (ARV) prophylaxis to either the mother or infant during breastfeeding in areas where breastfeeding was judged to be the most appropriate choice of infant feeding for HIV-infected women. In addition, guidelines were developed to provide international standards to reduce the risk of MTCT from a background risk of 35% to less than 5% (or even lower) in breastfeeding populations [14]. Exclusive breastfeeding for the first few months of life can be successfully supported in HIV-infected women [2] and if replacement feeding is not available [15], one alternative is to provide antiretroviral prophylaxis (ART) to the mother or child during breastfeeding [16–19].

HIV/AIDS in South Africa is a prominent health concern [21]. The Joint United Nations Programme on HIV and AIDS (UNAIDS) report estimated that 5,700,000 South Africans had HIV/AIDS, with HIV prevalence in pregnant women at 28% [22], or just under 12% of South Africa's population of 48 million in 2007 [23]. However, important changes have occurred in the country since 2009 [24]. Government funding in South Africa increased for expansion of antiretroviral therapy, scaling up of PMTCT programmes, promotion of HIV and tuberculosis treatment integration, and increased investments in HIV prevention [25]. South Africa now has the world's largest programme of antiretroviral therapy, with about 1.8 million people estimated to be taking antiretroviral. HIV prevention has received increasing attention [24].

Breastfeeding is the norm in South Africa, but the percentage of exclusive breastfeeding for 6 months among South African HIV infected mothers is one of the lowest in the world, at 8% in 2003 [26,27]. However, the situations have been changed since 2010 when the infants feeding patterns shifted the emphasis to exclusive breastfeeding [24], and as a result, South Africa has had one of the sharpest declines in new infections among children [28]. Yearly infections in children have dropped from 56,500 in 2009 to 29,100 in 2011. [29] A cohort study of 1032 HIV-infected mothers showed that 40% of women reported to exclusive breastfeeding [30].There were approximately 45% of HIV mothers reported as exclusive breastfeeding in another Kesho Bora study [16].

It should be noted that the cost of drugs to HIV are usually borne by the government, whereas formula is usually paid for by the individual. Meanwhile, encouraging HIV mothers to practice exclusive breastfeeding is also far from easy. Breast milk provides all of the fluids and nutrients that a young baby requires, so it means that even water should be avoided [31,32]. However, in many societies, it is normal for a baby to be given water, tea, porridge or other foods as well as breast milk, even during the first few weeks of life [33,34]. The HIV-infected mothers assigned to the formula feeding often experience community, family, or spousal pressure to breastfeed and are sometimes concerned about maintaining the confidentiality of their HIV status; further, formula-feeding logistics are more difficult than those for breastfeeding, particularly in resource-poor areas [14].

Numerous simulations [35,36] have been conducted to prevent MTCT. However, most of them explored the effect of only a single intervention. For example, some studies evaluated the cost - effectiveness of antenatal HIV testing but the remedial measures for untested or testing late HIV-infected mothers were not included [37–40]. Neil Soderlund et al. simulated the cost-effectiveness of four feeding strategies and three antiretroviral interventions but the interventions were considered separately [40]. In practice, however, interventions should not be implemented individually and several interventions can be implemented simultaneously or consecutively. Based on the important changes in South Africa [24] and the South African Antiretroviral Treatment Guideline 2013 recommendations [26], we explored different strategy combinations rather than a single intervention according to the South African HIV-infected mothers' varying status and different designs of feeding patterns. We simulated the different status(prompt treatment, remedial treatments or neither) of HIV infected mothers based on the characters of South African pregnant women in Kesho Bora study and others[16,30,41,42], and we aimed to assess the cost-effectiveness of the feeding patterns of HIV-exposed infants (exclusive breastfeeding or replacement feeding) in light of the mothers' status.

Materials and Methods

Model framework

We developed a decision analytic model using the TreeAge Pro 2011 software package (TreeAge Software, Inc, Williamstown, MA) [45] to compare the cost-effectiveness of two different HIV strategy combinations given only to HIV positive mothers: (1) HIV positive pregnant mothers were tested and treated promptly at any time during pregnancy. They knew their HIV status after antenatal HIV testing in time and received an ARV intervention or standard ART recommended by WHO on the basis of eligibility (Promptly treated cohort). (2) Pregnant mothers did not get tested or treated until after delivery. They presented late in labor without having a diagnosis of their HIV status and thus missed the window of opportunity for prompt interventions. A course of fixed dose combination (FDC) and other treatments were offered as a remedy (Remedy cohort). The first strategy was the gold standard, whereas the second one was remedial when the first wasn't available. The non-responders were assigned as untreated in the two cohorts, and replacement feeding or exclusive breastfeeding was assigned in the two strategies. We evaluated interventions against a 'no intervention' scenario (the mothers'

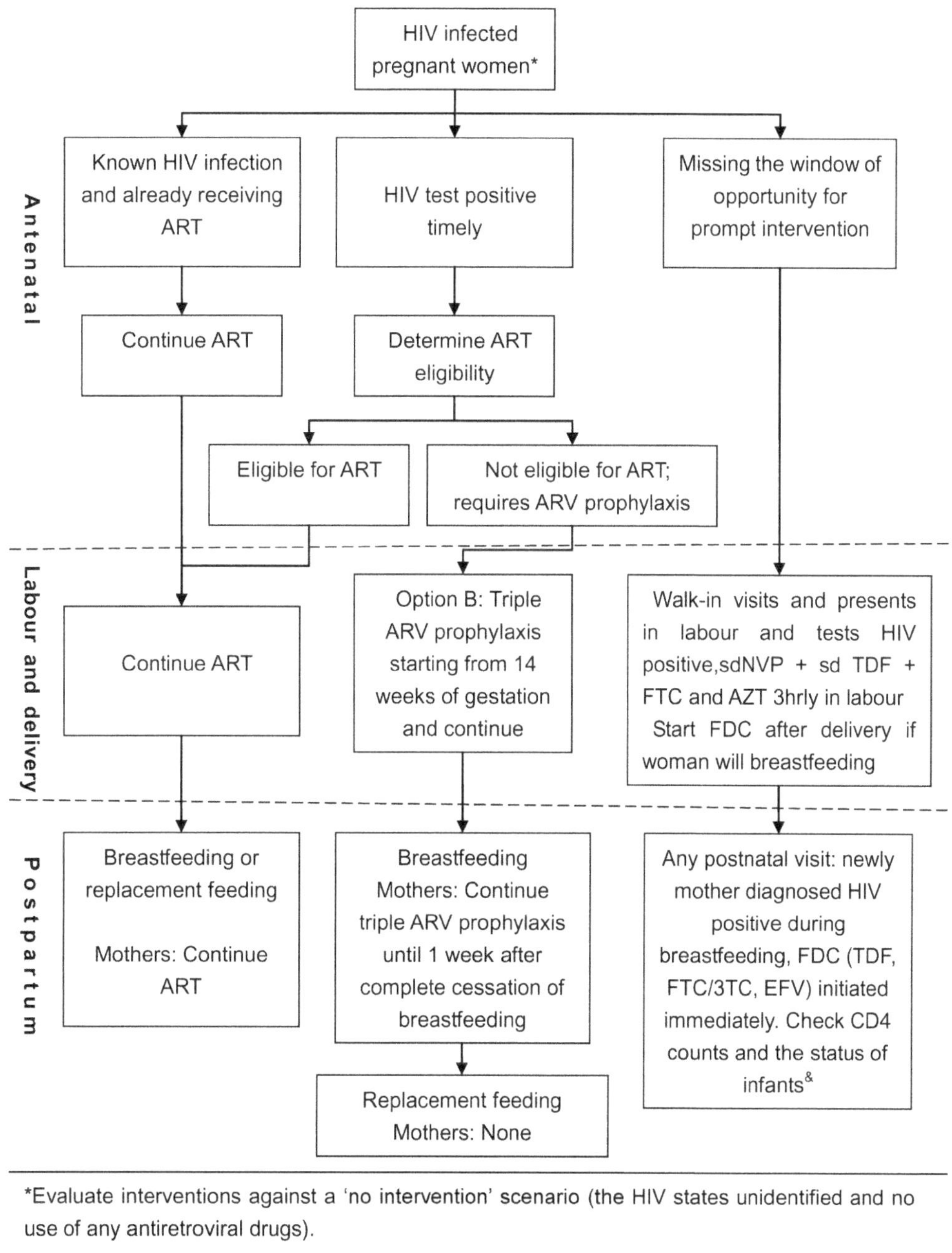

Figure 1. Decision analytic model schematic. & Irrespective of mode of feeding patterns, infants accepted NVP promptly and daily for 6 weeks. ART, antiretroviral therapy; ARV, antiretroviral prophylaxis; sdNVP, single dose nevirapine; sdTDF, single dose Tenofovir; FTC,emtricitabine; AZT, Zidovudine; FDC, fixed dose combination,(TDF, FTC/3TC, EFV); 3TC,Lamivudine; EFV, Efavirenz.

HIV status unidentified and no use of any antiretroviral drugs). The model structures are showed in Figure 1 and Figure 2.

We presented key model outcomes, including the number of infant HIV cases averted, the number of infant life years (LY) saved, the cost per infant HIV case averted, and the cost per LY [40,45] saved from the interventions.

Intervention and settings

The decision analytic model was created to simulate 3–6 cohorts. We used the Monte Carlo simulation method to simulate 10,000 HIV-infected pregnant women from South Africa (average age is 27 years old) in each cohort [16]. The distribution of the pregnant mothers' age, the CD4 counts and other parameters were all based on the characters of South African pregnant women in Kesho Bora study and others [16,30,41,42]. We simulated the severity and progression of the maternal HIV disease, infants' HIV infections and the time that mothers' highly active antiretroviral therapy (HAART) treatments started based on mothers' CD4 counts during pregnancy. The median CD4 cell count was assumed to be 360×10^6 cells/mm^3. The square root of CD4 count is assumed to be normally distributed within a 95th percentile range of 43 to 984 cells/mm^3 [37]. We assumed that HIV-infected, pregnant women who have CD4 cell counts less than 350 cells/mm^3 received HAART during pregnancy, as the WHO

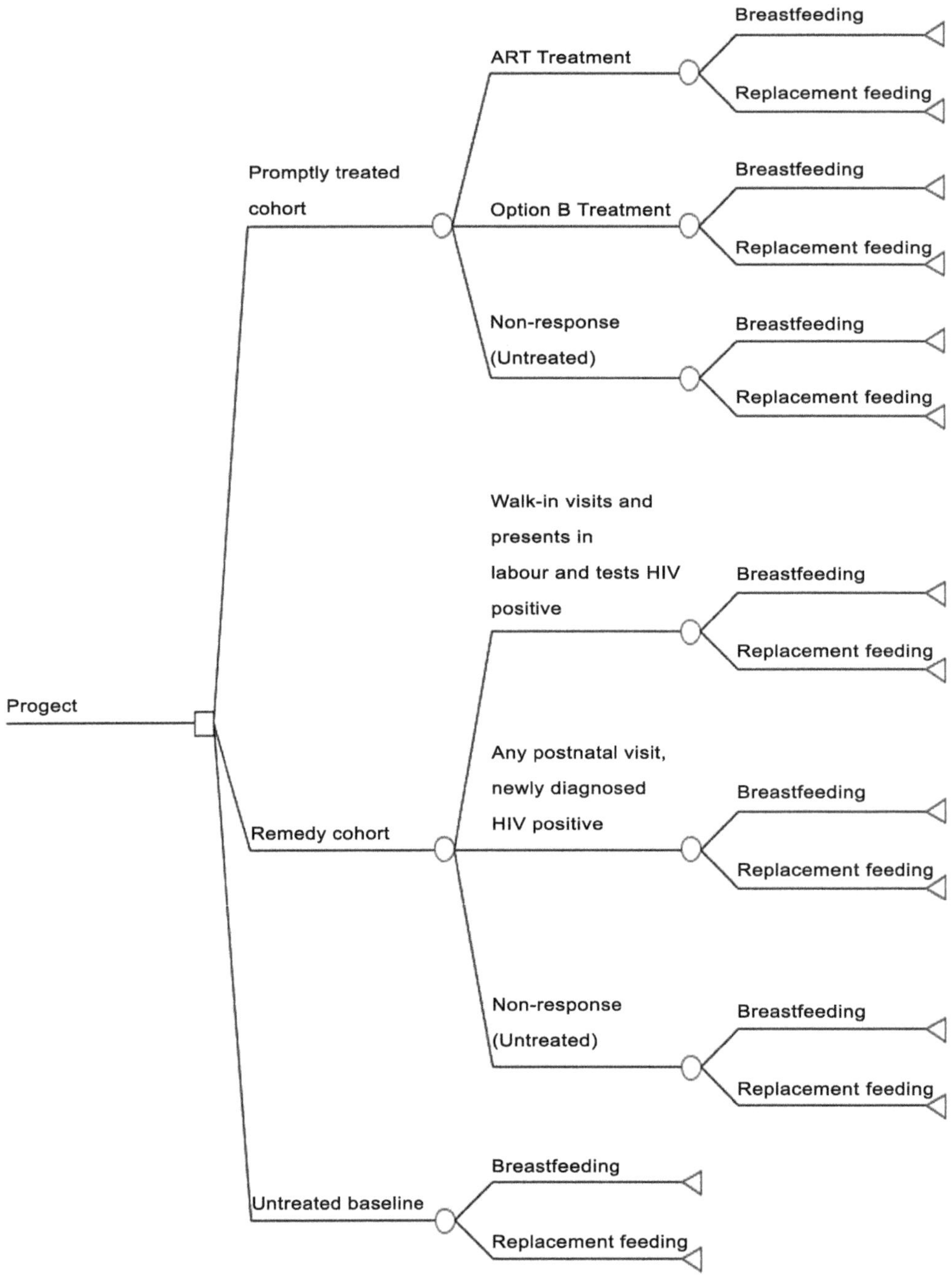

Figure 2. Structure of decision analytic model. ART, antiretroviral therapy.

recently recommended [14]. The intervention approaches assumed that maternal antepartum daily ART continued during pregnancy, delivery, and thereafter. For women who were not eligible for ART, the model used implementation of triple antiretroviral prophylaxis (Zidovudine (AZT) + Lamivudine (3TC) + lopinavir (LPV)) [14], as did the Kesho Bora study conducted in South Africa [16]. Triple ARV prophylaxis started as early as 14 weeks of gestation and continued until delivery; if breastfeeding was applied, it continued until cessation of breastfeeding at 6 months postpartum. All the infants received daily nevirapine (NVP) from birth until age 6 weeks, regardless of the mode of infant feeding.

For HIV-infected mothers who missed the window of opportunity for prompt intervention, some of them were unable to realize their HIV infectious status, which resulted in walk-in labour visits and delayed HIV testing; single-dose nevirapine (sdNVP) + single dose Tenofovir (sdTDF) + emtricitabine (FTC) + Zidovudine (AZT) were then offered at the onset of labor as a remedy, and NVP was also given to their newborn babies daily for 6 weeks [26]. A course of fixed dose combination (FDC) was started after delivery if the woman was assigned to breastfeeding. For others who were diagnosed HIV-positive during breastfeeding at any postnatal visit, FDC (TDF, FTC/3TC, Efavirenz (EFV)) was initiated immediately, and the mothers' CD4 counts and their infants' HIV status were checked. All the interventions mentioned above were in line with recommendations by the South African Antiretroviral Treatment Guideline 2013 [26]. We identified these detailed interventions to ensure the accuracy of the intervention cost and effect.

We also assumed a standard testing strategy consisting of a serum enzyme-linked immunosorbent assay followed by confirmatory Western blotting. We presumed infants complied with exclusive breastfeeding from ages of about 6 weeks to 6 months if their mothers intended to breastfeed, as the WHO recommended [44].

Probabilities

The probabilities and ranges used in the model were derived from published studies of large, population-randomized, controlled trials and published, updated meta-analyses [11,12,15,16,41,43]. We obtained estimates for the model's parameters from South African data when available. Otherwise, we used data from international literatures in an attempt to use estimates from other resource-limited countries. A function to convert annual probability into 18-month probability was used, as follows:

$$P_{18\text{months}} = 1\text{-}e^{\ln(1\text{-}P\text{year}) \times 1.5} [45]$$

The base rates of MTCT were estimated from a randomized controlled trial conducted in Kenya and South Africa by the Kesho Bora study group [16]. In a group of those eligible for ART, the average HIV-positive rate in infants who were breastfed for 18 months was 7.5% (compared with 0.75% in the replacement-feeding group). A range of 3.5%–14.76% was included in the sensitivity analyses, taking the impact of CD4 counts into account. In the group of mothers whose CD4 counts were ≥350 cells/mm^3 and who were assigned to breastfeeding, the converted 18-month infection rate was 6.97% (95% confidence interval (CI) 3.58%–13.62%). The sensitivity analysis includes a lower transmission rate of 1%, derived from an 18-month follow-up study of HIV–infected mothers whose CD4 counts were ≥500 cells/mm^3 in the Kesho Bora study [16,41]. The risk of MTCT was 2% with the use of antiretroviral medicines and avoidance of breastfeeding [43]. 19.5% of exclusively breastfed infants were infected with HIV by 6 months, a figure derived from a intervention cohort study of 1132 HIV positive pregnant women [30]. We used the vertical MTCT rate of HIV infection during postpartum of 15.81% (95% CI 10.7%–21.02%) and 29.03% (95% CI 22.98%–35.26%) without interventions to prevent transmission when the mother was assigned to breastfeeding or replacement feeding, respectively [13,78].

On average, 59% (95% CI 53%–64%) of pregnant women living with HIV were estimated to be eligible for ART on the basis of those with CD4 counts <350 cells/mm^3 receiving lifelong ART [1]. The 83% and 67% South African coverage rates of ART among adults and children (aged 0–14 years), respectively, were assumptions made on the basis of the WHO's Global Update on HIV Treatment 2013 Report [1]. The latest data from 23 countries indicated that the average retention rates for people on ART decrease over time (from about 86% at 12 months to 82% at 24 months) [1]. We assigned 40% and 15.4% as the percentage of women who were selected to exclusive breastfeeding and replacement feeding respectively [30]. Since data to measure precisely the efficacy of remedial intervention in labor and that of FDC during postpartum care are not available, we estimated the variable efficacy of the remedial intervention in labor as 62.75% (95% CI 40.76%–84.74%), derived from data of the Petra study [46,47]. We rounded the efficacy of FDC to 47.91% (95% CI 43.57%–51.92%), this figure came from a research of 2,127 electronic medical records between July 1999 to June 2006.The hazard ratio (HR) of FDC was 0.92 [48]. In addition, we assumed that the converted 18-month mortality in exclusive breastfeeding infants was 18.9% versus 15.4% in infants given replacement feeds [49], and calculated the adjusted mortality rate which represents the unrelated HIV infection mortality by deducting the under-five mortality rate (42.15/1000 in 2013) [50]. The input probabilities for our decision tree are displayed in Table 1.

Cost estimates

The input cost estimates for our decision tree are presented in Table 2. Cost and utility estimates were also derived from published literatures when necessary. All cost was expressed in 2012 US dollars and South African prices. The total cost included the cost of ART and ARV treatments, the cost of visiting, counseling and testing and the cost of breastfeeding and formula milk [58]. We calculated the cost of mothers from the moment when treatments begin until 1 week after cessation of breastfeeding and the cost during the first 18 months of life for the HIV-exposed infants. The cost-effectiveness was calculated relative to the control group as (IC+NC−HC)/(LS*LE−LL*LE) [40]; where IC = intervention costs, NC = health care costs because of additional morbidity in formula fed children not infected with HIV, HC = costs of HIV related care avoided by preventing infections, LS = lives saved by prevention of HIV infection, LL = lives lost because of formula feeding in children not infected with HIV, and LE = life expectancy. Cost estimates for antiretroviral drugs were based on the Clinton Health Access Initiative (CHAI)'s ceiling price list [51]. The average of the two most common first-line regimens (zidovudine/lamivudine/nevirapine or tenofovir/lamivudine/efavirenz, $146.50/year) were used as the cost of triple ARV during pregnancy [42]. The cost of HAART during pregnancy and lactation were estimated as $76.82 and $50.65, respectively [53,79]. We estimated the baseline cost of a single rapid HIV testing as $2.36 and $6.30, when the testing was negative or positive, respectively [53]. In case of a positive testing, additional confirmatory testing was needed. The cost of CD4 testing was estimated as $5.43 per unit [43,52]. Cost ware discounted by 3% per year [45].

Estimation of life years saved

We focused our analysis on the effectiveness for HIV-exposed infants and estimated the effect using the life years saved. To estimate the number of LY saved induced by the intervention, life expectancy in South Africa at birth was estimated from a review of available demographic data [24], and the base-case calculation used a life expectancy of 60 years. For a child with perinatal transmission of HIV who goes on HAART for life, we estimated a life expectancy approximately two-thirds that of a child without HIV [53,54]. The model used a disease progression scenario in which 25%, 80%, and 100% of children progress to AIDS at 12, 60, and 120 months, respectively. Children were assumed to live for an average of 12 months after progression to AIDS [55,56].

We used the same weights for all infants, irrespective of age. When children were aged less than 5 years, irrespective of their CD4 counts, we assumed they were eligible to start ART. Children aged greater than 5 years were monitored for ART by CD4 testing each year [26]. The parameters are presented in Table 1.

Table 1. References and input probabilities for the decision analytic model.

Reference	Probability Variable	Details	Circumstances	Value	Range
[16]	positive rate of HIV in 18 months	Breastfeeding	ART	7.50%	(3.50%–14.76%)
[16][32]			ARV	6.97%	(1.00%–13.62%)
[13][11]			None treatment	29.03%	(22.98%–35.26%)
[43]		Replacement feeding	ART	0.75%	(0.75%–1.50%)
[43]			ARV	2.00%	-
[13] [78]			None treatment	15.81%	(10.70%–21.02%)
[30]	Efficacy	Using sdNVP + sdTDF + FTC and AZT 3hrly	In labour as a remedy	62.75%	(40.76%–84.74%)
[48]		Initiating FDC immediately	Breastfeeding during postpartum care	47.91%	(43.57%–51.92%)
[2]	Rate of coverage	ART	Among pregnant women	83.00%	(79.00%–87.00%)
		ART	Among infected infants	67.00%	(60.00%–75.00%)
[2]		HIV testing and counseling	Among pregnant women	95.00%	(90.00%–98.00%)
Assumed, [16][27][30]		Exclusive breast feeding	In HIV infected women	40.00%	(8.00%–44.68%)
[30]		Replacement feeding	In HIV infected women	15.4%	-
[2]	Rates of average retention	ART	In 12 months	86.00%	-
			In 24 months	82.00%	-
[13]	Estimated rate of transmission	Breast milk		19.50%	(6.50%–24.90%)
[2]	Average rate of being eligible for ART	Based on CD4<350	Mothers living with HIV	59.00%	(53.00%–64.00%)
Assumed [60],	Proportion of HIV	Infected women among the unidentified	Presented in labor	18.52%	(5.00%–50.00%)
			Diagnosed at postnatal visit	22.22%	(5.00%–50.00%)
[24]	Life experience(year)	Child	Without HIV	60	-
[53] [54]			With prenatal HIV on HAART	40	-
[55]			With prenatal HIV if no no antiretroviral	10	-
[42] [43]			With AIDS	1	-
[50]		Under-five mortality rate		42.15‰	-
[49]	Motility rate of infants in 18 months	Breastfeed		18.9%	-
[49]		Replacement feeding		15.4%	-

ART, antiretroviral therapy; ARV, antiretroviral prophylaxis; sdNVP, single dose nevirapine; sdTDF, single dose Tenofovir; FTC, emtricitabine; AZT, Zidovudine; FDC, (TDF, FTC/3TC, EFV); 3TC,Lamivudine; EFV, Efavirenz; HAART, highly active antiretroviral therapy.

Sensitivity and uncertainty analyses

In the sensitivity analyses, the uncertain assumptions about the input cost and behavioral impacts of interventions were varied. An aggregate model was developed using the highest and lowest values and the best fitting parameter. The model's epidemiological values were point estimates and 95% CI for parameters based on published study results. We conducted additional univariate sensitivity analyses with values of cost estimate from one-third to 3 times of their baseline estimates. We also tested the sensitivity of the rankings to variation of the assumptions regarding key parameters.

Results

Three theoretical cohorts(the promptly treated cohort, the remedy cohort and the no intervention control cohort) were applied in our analytic model, all of which were based on estimates of 40% breast feeding coverage and 15.4% replacement feeding rate during postpartum. It is found that the incremental cost per infant HIV case averted were $2063.05 and $3579.66 for the promptly treated cohort and remedy cohort, respectively. Tables 3 reported on the incremental cost-effectiveness ratios (ICER) for interventions, which were listed in the descending order of the infant HIV cases averted. Figure 3 showed an expansion path graphically, with the slope of the line joining any two points indicating the ICER for the more costly option [57]. The remedy strategy did not particularly cost-effective. Compared with the 'no intervention' scenario which leaded to 1127 infected infants, 698 (61.93%) and 110 (9.76%) of pediatric HIV cases were averted in the promptly treated cohort and remedy cohort respectively, with incremental cost-effectiveness of $68.51 and $118.33 per LY, respectively (Figure 3.A).

Because all the HIV-exposed mothers among the two cohorts were designed to have different feeding patterns, we also

Table 2. References and input cost estimates for the decision analytic model.

Reference	Composition of cost	Items	Value($)(year = 2012)
[43][52]	Testing cost	CD4 testing	5.43
[53]		ELISA testing	2.10
[53]		Positive rapid HIV testing	2.36
[53]		ELISA testing and Weston blotting	6.30
[53][79]	HAART cost	HAART in pregnancy	76.82
[53][79]		HAART during lactation	50.65
[2]		ART (first-line regimens)	186.00
[43]	ARV cost	Triple ARV in pregnancy(first-line regimens)	146.50
[51]		sdNVP+sdTDF+FTC and AZT in labor per unit	0.44
[51][43]		FDC(TDF+FTC/3TC+EFV) per year	159.00
[58]	Counseling and Health care cost	Cost of behavior counseling	3.74
[58]	Feeding cost	Breastfeeding (6 month)	153.98
[58]		Formula feeding (6 month)	310.82

ELISA, enzyme-linked immunosorbent assay; HAART, highly active antiretroviral therapy; ART, antiretroviral prophylaxis; ARV, antiretroviral prophylaxis; sdNVP, single dose nevirapine; sdTDF, single dose Tenofovir; FTC, emtricitabine; AZT, Zidovudine; FDC, (TDF, FTC/3TC, EFV); 3TC,Lamivudine; EFV, Efavirenz.

conducted a subgroup analysis according to the feeding patterns, using the untreated cohort (Untreated mothers who were assigned to breastfeeding) for comparison. Compared with the untreated cohort, assigning promptly treated cohort to the replacement feeding strategy was the more cost-effective ($134.88 per infant LY saved), followed by the promptly treated cohort being assigned to breastfeeding ($193.26 infant LY saved), as showed in Figure 3.B. With or without the antenatal testing and treatments, breastfeeding was less cost-effective than replacement feeding strategies.

Sensitivity Analysis

Since the actual values can vary in different settings, both one-way and multivariate sensitivity analyses were conducted to examine the factors that account for the variation in the cost per LY saved. The promptly treated cohort retained a cost-effectiveness ratio lower than $120 per LY in all one-variable sensitivity analyses. When we varied our uncertain assumptions regarding the input parameters, the ranking of interventions remained stable.

If the treatment efficacy of FDC ranged from 25% to 75%, the cost per LY would range $76.5–$223.8 in the remedy cohort. Although the ranking of interventions remained stable under these assumptions, the treatment efficacy of FDC in postnatal intervention significantly influenced the results.

When we decreased the rate of breastfeeding coverage in HIV-infected women from 100% to 5%, the incremental cost-effective per LY increased from $39.02 to $52.95 and from $67.97 to $406.94 in the prompt treated cohort and remedy cohort, respectively. Breastfeeding had a stronger influence on the remedy cohort than the promptly treated cohort. When the rate of breastfeeding coverage in HIV-infected women was reduced by 5% each time, about 57 and 19 infants might be avoided in the promptly treated cohort and remedy cohort, respectively.

Variation in the proportion of newly HIV-infected women presenting in labor and at postnatal visits also substantially affected the result of the remedy cohort. The proportion of HIV-infected women presenting in labor was set to vary by up to 3 times of the point estimate which could entail a ratio as high as 32% of the point estimate ($157 per LY) in the remedy cohort. Similarly, when the proportion of HIV-infected women treated during the postnatal visits increased from the base-case value of 22% to 80%, the cost per LY increased from $59.20 to $95.15 per LY in the remedy cohort. In conclusion, without consideration of willingness to pay, remedial treatments both in labor and at postnatal visits were worthwhile.

Discussion

In this study, we developed a decision analytic model for prevention of mother-to-child HIV transmission and applied it to discuss the cost-effectiveness of antenatal HIV testing and treatments recommended by WHO versus the interventions used as a remedy in labor and the postpartum period after missing the window of opportunity for prompt intervention.

Early knowledge of HIV status may enable women to make more appropriate decisions with regard to their own health and that of their unborn children [59]. Our study reveals that antenatal testing and prompt treatment will prevent more than half of pediatric HIV cases. Knowledge of the mother's infection status can save an additional 5.9 pediatric LY [37]. There was a correlation coefficient of .66 between the period of confirmed HIV status and receipt of ARV, which illustrated that later confirmation of HIV-infected status led to less possibility of receiving ARV among mothers; this conclusion was derived from an analysis of 108 HIV-infected mothers in China [60]. One research in Hong Kong is also in support of this point of view [61].

Attempts to compare the cost and benefits for testing late and untested HIV-infected women have been previously undertaken [37–39]. However, these analyses failed to account for receipt of remedies in labor and during the postnatal visits among untested HIV-infected women. The guideline in South Africa recommends all pregnant women who need triple therapy and breastfeeding to receive a FDC compatible regimen as a remedy [26], and FDC has been rolled out in South Africa since 2013 [62]. We found that those remedial treatments would avert 9.76% of pediatric HIV cases compared with lack of treatment.

Furthermore, since the differences between the promptly treated cohort and remedy cohort are obvious, our focus was to study the impacts of different feeding patterns and breastfeeding coverage between the two cohorts.

A.

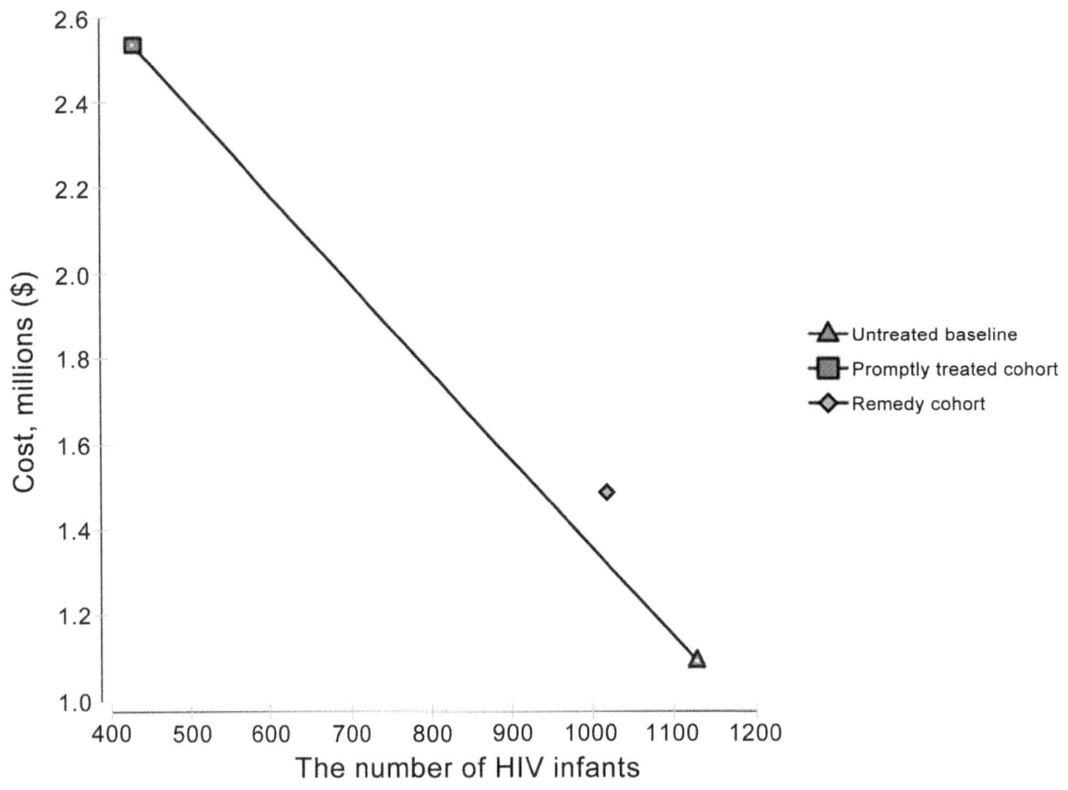
2.6
2.4
2.2
2.0
1.8
1.6
1.4
1.2
1.0
Cost, millions ($)
400 500 600 700 800 900 1000 1100 1200
The number of HIV infants
Untreated baseline
Promptly treated cohort
Remedy cohort

B.

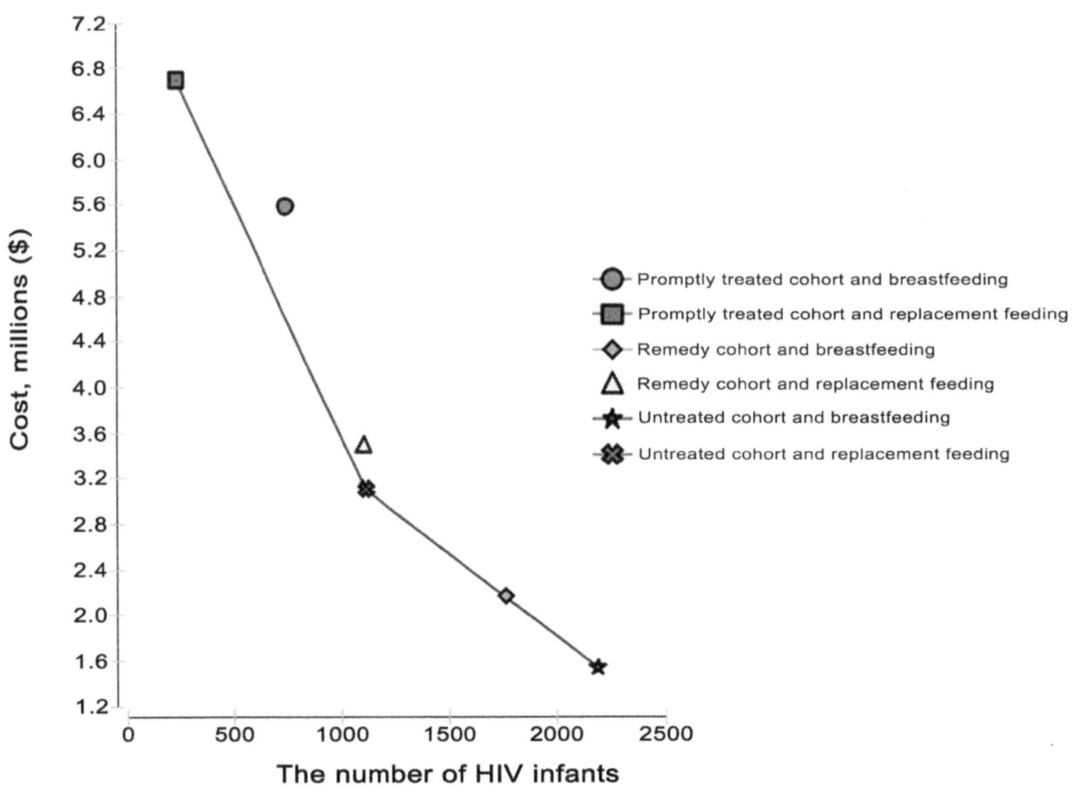
7.2
6.8
6.4
6.0
5.6
5.2
4.8
4.4
4.0
3.6
3.2
2.8
2.4
2.0
1.6
1.2
Cost, millions ($)
0 500 1000 1500 2000 2500
The number of HIV infants
Promptly treated cohort and breastfeeding
Promptly treated cohort and replacement feeding
Remedy cohort and breastfeeding
Remedy cohort and replacement feeding
Untreated cohort and breastfeeding
Untreated cohort and replacement feeding

Figure 3. The cost-effectiveness frontier of different strategy combinations. The cost-effectiveness frontier (solid line) includes strategies that maybe cost-effective if the incremental cost-effectiveness ratio is less than the accepted threshold. Strategies that are not on the frontier are dominated, meaning that they are not efficient use of resources. In figure 3.A, irrespective of the feeding patterns, remedial cohort is less cost-effective. In figure 3.B, mothers' prompt treatment and replacement feeding cohort is the most cost-effective intervention, followed by the promptly treated cohort being assigned to breastfeeding.

Our model is in good agreement with other studies [12,35,60] and demonstrates that formula feeding results in a substantial decrease in HIV transmission risk and is cost-effectiveness, but formula is sometimes unaffordable for most HIV infected women because of the resource-limited settings[14,40]. As our results show, although breastfeeding strategy is less cost-effective, we can't ignore the impact of willingness to pay. In sub-Saharan Africa, more deaths would be caused than saved by formula feeding [40]. Breast milk contains nutrients, agents and antibodies that protect the infant from the risk of childhood diseases such as diarrhoea. Without being breastfed, an infant runs the risk of becoming seriously ill with diseases other than HIV. Where treatment for them is limited or inaccessible, an infant's health can be compromised. Similarly, unsafe and unreliable replacement feeding when clean water and resources are unavailable can also be a danger to an infant's health [64]. Breastfeeding is therefore highly widespread in low- and middle-income countries.

One influential factor for MTCT is the coverage of exclusive breastfeeding. Coovadia et al. confirmed that exclusive breastfeeding from about ages of 6 weeks to 6 months carried an HIV transmission risk of about 4% in South Africa [63]. In our study, each time the rate of breastfeeding coverage in HIV-infected women reduced 5%, there were about 59 and 19 infants whose infections were prevented in the promptly treated cohort and remedy cohorts, respectively. In addition, severity of maternal HIV condition influences the breastfeeding coverage and infants' HIV status. Eighteen-month follow-up of an observational cohort in the Kesho Bora study [41] showed that mothers in less severe disease were more willing to breastfeed their children than mothers in serious condition. Maybe they felt too weak to breastfeed and they were more concerned about HIV transmission or ARV toxicity for their breastfed children. Other researches showed that mothers who chose to replacement feed were more likely to have CD4 counts less than 200 cells/mm^3 than those who chose exclusively breastfeeding. [30]This opinion was also supported in a South African study [65]. A reference showed a significant correlation between associated mothers'CD4 counts and infants' HIV status. they found that if the concentration of CD4 counts$\geq$350 cells/mm^3, the HR of infants infected HIV was 0.59 [80]. Delicio found that if the CD4 cell counts lower than 350 cells/mm^3, it would increase the risk of MTCT more than 12 times. [81]What's more, there was no relationship between gestational age and CD4 counts [82].

Early initiation of ART is important for achievement of an undetectable viral load well before delivery. Thus, women should be encouraged to plan pregnancies and attend antenatal care sufficiently early to diagnose HIV infection, assess the HIV stage, and initiate ART or antiretroviral prophylaxis promptly [16]. The latest WHO guidelines stated that lifelong ARV treatment should be provided for all pregnant women and breastfeeding women with HIV, known as Option B Plus [66]. Countries that do not have the resources to provide lifelong ARV should offer the mother ARV for her own health when she finishes breastfeeding, known as Option B. If the mother is not eligible, she may stop taking ARV one full week after cessation of breastfeeding in low- and middle-income countries. In the 22 priority countries of the Global Plan, there are more than half of them implementing the OPTION B regimen policy for preventing the mother-to-child transmission of HIV among pregnant women living with HIV in 2013 [2]. For example, in South Africa, OPTION B is the main regimen policy because of limited resources [2]. Although providing antiretroviral treatment until complete cessation of breastfeeding (Option B) has numerous advantages and has been preferable in our model, and despite the fact that South Africa recently announce a switch to Option B [63], the switch to Option B will present further challenges, such as operational issues, the cost of increasing the number of women on ART, adherence to lifelong ART, emergence of ARV resistance, and long-term side effects to the fetuses, infants, and mothers [67].

Several limitations of this study deserve mention. First, similar to any cost-effectiveness analysis [53,68,69], our study is limited in its inability to model perfectly the complexities of clinical medicine and accurately estimate probabilities and cost. Problems include the lack of empirical data on the effects of FDC [70–72] during postnatal intervention. We have used counseling cost but the cost of home visits, Non-Governmental Organization and community involvement was not included in our model. Further, the sensitivity and specificity of each HIV test were not incorporated into the decision tree.

Second, our model does not reflect the practices of elective cesarean section (ECS). ECS before labor has been introduced as an intervention for the PMTCT of HIV and significantly lowers the risk of mother-to-child transmission of HIV infection [73].However, most of the studies of ECS among HIV infected women were conducted exclusively in North America and Europe [74]. In developing countries, such as South Africa, the risks and benefits associated with ECS are seldom explored [74]. The European Mode of Delivery Collaboration Organization had found that the role of mode of delivery in the management of HIV infected women should be assessed in light of risks as well as benefits and the risk/benefits ratio depended upon the underlying rate of MTCT [74].

The ECS rate is lower in South Africa than that of some developed countries, such as 50.7% in France [75]. A multi-country study in Sub-Saharan Africa showed 1276 women underwent ECS, giving a frequency of 6.2% (range 4.1–16.8%) [74]. Further confirmation was also given by another two studies in South Africa, which showed that only 13.24% and 10.92% of HIV-infected mothers underwent ECS, respectively [16,30,32]. The low rates indicate that ECS may have not served as ubiquitous practices in South Africa. Thus, the effectiveness of ECS in South Africa is also unable to be evaluated due to inadequate parameters in our model.

Third, mixed feeding during the first several months of life which is not included in our model is a influencing factor of HIV transmission [76]. Mixed feeding infants are nearly 11 times (HR 10.87) more likely to acquire infection than the exclusively breastfed children [30]. However, some women in resource-limited settings are malnourished and their breast milk is not sufficient for their infants [77]. As a result, it is difficult to bring the exclusive breastfeeding into force in South Africa [40].

Table 3. Results and Outcomes of each cohorts of 10,000 HIV infected pregnant women.

Status	Feeding patterns	Incremental cost US($)	Infant HIV cases averted		Life years saved		Incremental cost-effectiveness
			Total	*Incremental cost (per, $)*	*Total*	*Incremental cost(per, $)*	
Baseline	-	-	-	-	-	-	-
(no intervention)							
Promptly treated cohort	-	2063.05	698	1439391.2	21009.8	68.51	Undominated[$]
Remedy cohort	-	3579.66	110	391806.75	3311	118.33	Extended dominated[&]
Untreated cohort	Breastfeed	-	-	-	-	-	-
Untreated cohort	Replacement feed	1461.19	1073	1568400	32297.3	48.56	Undominated
Promptly treated cohort	Replacement feed	4059.88	883	3584863.5	26578.3	134.88	Undominated
Remedy cohort	Breastfeed	1508.69	421	635167.86	12672.1	50.12	Extended dominated
Promptly treated cohort	Breastfeed	5826.72	360	2094217.3	10836	193.26	Extended dominated
Remedy cohort	Replacement feed	37296.63	11	383788.86	331.1	1159.13	Extended dominated

&: extended dominated, means exclude any interventions that have a higher ICER than more effective interventions.
$: undominated, strategies on the cost-effectiveness frontier, meaning that they are more cost-effective.

In addition, establishment of an intervention to reduce vertical transmission of HIV may have important secondary benefits [55], such as prevention of horizontal transmission, vigilant follow-up infant care to prevent opportunistic infections and etc [71]. These benefits have not been quantified in developing countries and hence are not included in the model.

It should be also noted that in this study, interventions for mothers and exposed infants were only evaluated from the moment when the treatment of the mother began until the end of first 18 months of life for the HIV-exposed infants, although the effectiveness associated with these interventions has been estimated for HIV-exposed infants. Meanwhile, the assumption that infants complied with exclusive breastfeeding from ages of 6 weeks to 6 months if their mothers intended to breastfeed may overestimate the results of exclusive breastfeeding. So we draw our conclusion carefully and do not extend the results throughout the whole period of breast milk exposure. The effectiveness of long-term interventions is unknown.

Another limitation in our study is that we extrapolated most assumptions from a limited number of relatively small-scale studies; thus, precise and reliable estimates of the effectiveness of large-scale prevention programs are needed.

Finally, our estimates of new HIV infections do not take into account dynamic spread at the population level or differences at risk populations, and many factors can cause variability in both the cost and effects of interventions.

Despite all these limitations, our model truly reflected the progress of MTCT. We assigned the HIV-infected pregnant women in South Africa as our target population and once pregnant, individuals were assigned different strategies (promptly treated or not). The CD4 counts were also taken into account as to reflect the severity of the HIV disease. Most of the confirmed interventions were included in our model in light of mothers' HIV-status and the corresponding diseases progress, such as the ART treatment, the Triple ARV prophylaxis and the feeding patterns. In addition, we took remedial preventions and the impacts of different feeding patterns into account. Our study should assist the governments of developing countries, such as South Africa, on strategic decision making regarding the health resource allocation.

Conclusions

In summary, our study demonstrates the cost-effectiveness of antenatal HIV testing and treatments, remedy treatments, and their combinations with different feeding patterns. Antenatal HIV testing and standard prompt treatments constitute a cost-effective strategy even in a resource-limited setting like South Africa. Compared with the promptly treated cohort, remedy during labor or the postnatal period is less cost-effective. Although we should pay more attention to the impact of willingness to pay and the advantages of breastfeeding in resource-limited setting can not be ignored, we still suggest choosing replacement feeding as far as possible. Hopefully, these data will enlighten public health policy decisions in South Africa regarding the implementation of remedial treatments and replacement feeding interventions.

Acknowledgments

The authors gratefully acknowledge X.J. and J. C. for assistance in model development, analyses, and manuscript preparation. Thank the teachers of Department of Epidemiology of School of Public Health of Tianjin Medical University for instruction and copyediting. We are also indebted to the Journal Prep Services Company and RLipkin (City University of New York, New York, USA) and He H.N. for their contributions.

Author Contributions

Conceived and designed the experiments: WY CL. Analyzed the data: WY CL. Wrote the paper: WY CL XF. Designed and revised the figures and tables in the manuscript: XL GZ. Data collection of this study: XF LF. Provided full discussion and revision: ZC JM.

References

1. World Health Organization (2013) Global update on HIV treatment 2013: results, impact and opportunities. Available:http://www.who.int/hiv/pub/progressreports/update2013/en/index.html. Accessed 21 August 2013.
2. World Health Organization (2012) Global report: UNAIDS Report on the global AIDS epidemic. Available:http://www.unaids.org/en/media/unaids/contentassets/documents/epidemiology/2012/gr2012/20121120_UNAIDS_Global_Report_2012_en.pdf. Accessed 15 August 2013.
3. Low A, Gavriilidis G, Larke N, Lajoie M-R, Drouin O, et al. (2013) Impact of antiretroviral on the incidence of opportunistic infections in resource-limited settings: a systematic review and meta-analysis. Available:http://www.who.int/hiv/events/2013/IAS_poster_ARVopport.pdf?ua = 1. Accessed 15 May 2013.
4. Diaz T, Chu SY, Conti L, Nahlen BL, Whyte B, et al. (1994) Health insurance coverage among persons with AIDS: Results from a multistate surveillance project. Am J Public Health 84: 1015–1018.
5. Bassett IV, Regan S, Chetty S, Giddy J, Uhler LM, et al. (2010) Who starts ART in Durban, South Africa? Not everyone who should. AIDS 24 Suppl 1: S37–S44.
6. Sabharwal CJ, Sepkowitz K, Mehta R, Shepard C, Bodach S, et al. (2011) Impact of accelerated progression to AIDS on public health monitoring of late HIV diagnosis. AIDS Patient Care STDS 25: 143–151.
7. Weis KE, Liese AD, Hussey J, Gibson JJ, Duffus WA (2010) Associations of rural residence with timing of HIV diagnosis and stage of disease at diagnosis, South Carolina 2001–2005. J Rural Health 26: 105–112.
8. Ziegler JB, Cooper DA, Johnson RO, Gold J (1985) Postnatal transmission of AIDS-associated retrovirus from mother to infant. Lancet 1: 896–898.
9. Read JS (2000) Preventing mother to child transmission of HIV: the role of caesarean section. Sex Transm Infect 76: 231–232.
10. Read JS (2003) Human milk, breastfeeding and transmission of human immunodeficiency virus type 1 in the United States. American Academy of Pediatrics Committee on Pediatric AIDS. Pediatrics 112: 1196–1205.
11. Horvath T, Madi BC, Iuppa IM, Kennedy GE, Rutherford G, et al. (2009) Interventions for preventing late postnatal mother-to-child transmission of HIV. Cochrane Database Syst Rev CD006734.
12. Nduati R, John G, Mbori-Ngacha D, Richardson B, Overbaugh J, et al. (2000) Effect of breastfeeding and formula feeding on transmission of HIV-1: a randomized clinical trial. JAMA 283: 1167–1174.
13. World Health Organization (2000) Effect of breastfeeding on infant and child mortality due to infectious diseases in less developed countries: a pooled analysis. WHO Collaborative Study Team on the Role of Breastfeeding on the Prevention of Infant Mortality. Lancet 355: 451–455.
14. Bositis CM, Gashongore I, Patel DM (2010) Updates to the World Health Organization's Recommendations for the Use of Antiretroviral Drugs for Treating Pregnant Women and Preventing HIV Infection in Infants. Med J Zambia 37: 111–117.
15. World Health Organization (2006) The role of the health sector in strengthening systems to support children's healthy development in communities affected by HIV/AIDS. Available: http://whqlibdoc.who.int/publications/2007/9789241595964_eng.pdf. Accessed 23 August 2013.
16. de Vincenzi I (2011) Triple antiretroviral compared with zidovudine and single-dose nevirapine prophylaxis during pregnancy and breastfeeding for prevention of mother-to-child transmission of HIV-1 (Kesho Bora study): a randomised controlled trial. Lancet Infect Dis 11: 171–180.
17. Gaillard P, Fowler MG, Dabis F, Coovadia H, Van Der Horst C, et al. (2004) Use of antiretroviral drugs to prevent HIV-1 transmission through breast-feeding: from animal studies to randomized clinical trials. J Acquir Immune Defic Syndr 35: 178–187.
18. Chasela CS, Hudgens MG, Jamieson DJ, Kayira D, Hosseinipour MC, et al. (2010) Maternal or infant antiretroviral drugs to reduce HIV-1 transmission. N Engl J Med 362: 2271–2281.
19. Shapiro RL, Hughes MD, Ogwu A, Kitch D, Lockman S, et al. (2010) Antiretroviral regimens in pregnancy and breast-feeding in Botswana. N Engl J Med 362: 2282–2294.
20. Kramer MS, Chalmers B, Hodnett ED, Sevkovskaya Z, Dzikovich I, et al. (2001) Promotion of Breastfeeding Intervention Trial (PROBIT): a randomized trial in the Republic of Belarus. JAMA 285: 413–420.
21. Wikipedia (15 May 2013) HIV/AIDS in South Africa. Available:http://en.wikipedia.org/wiki/HIV_in_South_Africa. Accessed 04 March 2014.
22. The South African Department of Health (2008) Report on the national hiv and syphilis prevalence survey south africa. Available: http://www.doh.gov.za/docs/antenatal-f.html. Accessed 12 March 2013.
23. The Joint United Nations Programme on HIV and AIDS (2008) 2008 Report On the Global AIDS Epidemic. Available:http://www.amarc.org/documents/manuals/JC1510_2008GlobalReport_en.pdf. Accessed 04 March 2013.
24. Mayosi BM, Lawn JE, van Niekerk A, Bradshaw D, Abdool Karim SS, et al. (2012) Health in South Africa: changes and challenges since 2009. Lancet 380: 2029–2043.
25. Health Department of Republic of South Africa (2010) Annual Report 2010–2011. Available: http://www.doh.gov.za/docs/reports/annual/2011/annual_report2010-11.pdf. Accessed 01 Nov 2013.
26. Health Department of Republic of South Africa (2012) South African antiretroviral treatment guideline2013. Available:http://www.doh.gov.za/docs/policy/2013/ART_Treatment_Guidelines_Final_25March2013.pdf. Accessed 30 August 2013.
27. World Health Organization (2012) Countdown to 2015 maternal,newborn&-child surval: building a future for women and children. Available:http://www.countdown2015mnch.org/documents/2012report/2012-complete-no-profiles.pdf. Accessed 09 August 2013.
28. The Joint United Nations Programme on HIV and AIDS (2012) Global Report: UNAIDS Report on the Global AIDS Epidemic 2012. Available:http://www.unaids.org/en/media/unaids/contentassets/documents/epidemiology/2012/gr2012/20121120_UNAIDS_Global_Report_2012_with_annexes_en.pdf. Accessed 11 August 2013.
29. The Joint United Nations Programme on HIV and AIDS (2012) World AIDS Day Report-Results. Available:http://www.unaids.org/en/media/unaids/contentassets/documents/epidemiology/2012/gr2012/jc2434_worldaidsday_results_en.pdf. Accessed 11 August 2013.
30. Coovadia HM, Rollins NC, Bland RM, Little K, Coutsoudis A, et al. (2007) Mother-to-child transmission of HIV-1 infection during exclusive breastfeeding in the first 6 months of life: an intervention cohort study. Lancet 369: 1107–16.
31. Kuhn L, Sinkala M, Kankasa C, Semrau K, Kasonde P, et al. (2007) High Uptake of Exclusive Breastfeeding and Reduced Early Post-Natal HIV Transmission. PLoS ONE 2(12): e1363.
32. Bland RM, Little KE, Coovadia HM, Coutsoudis A, Rollins NC, et al. (2008) Intervention to promote exclusive breast-feeding for the first 6 months of life in a high HIV prevalence area. AIDS 22(7) 883–891.
33. The Joint United Nations Programme on HIV and AIDS (2009) Overview of breastfeeding patterns, Available:http://www.childinfo.org/breastfeeding_overview.html. Accessed 13 May 2013.
34. Leshabari SC, Koniz-Booher P, Åstrøm AN, de Paoli MM, Moland KM (2006) Translating global recommendations on HIV and infant feeding to the local context: the development of culturally sensitive counselling tools in the Kilimanjaro Region, Tanzania. Implementation Science 1:(22).
35. Nagelkerke NJ, Jha P, de Vlas SJ, Korenromp EL, Moses S, et al. (2002) Modelling HIV/AIDS epidemics in Botswana and India: impact of interventions to prevent transmission. Bull World Health Organ 80: 89–96.
36. Grundmann N, Iliff P, Stringer J, Wilfert C (2011) Presumptive diagnosis of severe HIV infection to determine the need for antiretroviral therapy in children less than 18 months of age. Bull World Health Organ 89: 513–520.
37. Gibb DM, Ades AE, Gupta R, Sculpher MJ (1999) Costs and benefits to the mother of antenatal HIV testing: estimates from simulation modelling. AIDS 13: 1569–1576.
38. Mauskopf JA, Paul JE, Wichman DS, White AD, Tilson HH (1996) Economic impact of treatment of HIV-positive pregnant women and their newborns with zidovudine. Implications for HIV screening. JAMA 276: 132–138.
39. Ecker JL (1996) The cost-effectiveness of human immunodeficiency virus screening in pregnancy. Am J Obstet Gynecol 174: 716–721.
40. Soderlund N, Zwi K, Kinghorn A, Gray G (1999) Prevention of vertical transmission of HIV: analysis of cost-effectiveness of options available in South Africa. BMJ 318: 1650–1656.
41. Kesho Bora Study Group (2010) Eighteen-month follow-up of HIV-1-infected mothers and their children enrolled in the Kesho Bora study observational cohorts. J Acquir Immune Defic Syndr 54: 533–541.
42. Estill J, Egger M, Blaser N, Vizcaya LS, Garone D, et al. (2013) Cost-effectiveness of point-of-care viral load monitoring of antiretroviral therapy in resource-limited settings: mathematical modelling study. AIDS 27: 1483–1492.
43. Sturt AS, Dokubo EK, Sint TT (2010) Antiretroviral therapy (ART) for treating HIV infection in ART-eligible pregnant women. Cochrane Database Syst Rev: CD008440.
44. World Health Organization (2006) WHO HIV and Infant Feeding Technical Consultation Held on behalf of the Inter-agency Task Team (IATT) on Prevention of HIV Infections in Pregnant Women, Mothers and their Infants. Available: http://www.who.int/maternal_child_adolescent/documents/pdfs/who_hiv_infant_feeding_technical_consultation.pdf. Accessed 13 May 2013.
45. TreeAge Software Inc (2011) TreeAge Pro 2011 User's Manual. Available: http://installers.treeagesoftware.com/treeagepro/TP2012/TreeAgePro-2012-Manual.pdf. Accessed 21 June 2013.
46. Siegfried N, van der Merwe L, Brocklehurst P, Sint TT (2011) Antiretroviral for reducing the risk of mother-to-child transmission of HIV infection. Cochrane Database Syst Rev: CD003510.
47. The Petra Team (2002) Efficacy of three short-course regimens of zidovudine and lamivudine in preventing early and late transmission of HIV-1 from mother

to child in Tanzania, South Africa, and Uganda (Petra study): a randomised, double-blind, placebo-controlled trial. Lancet.359: 1178–1186.
48. Mosen DM, Horberg M, Roblin D, Gullion CM, Meenan R, et al. (2010) effect of once-daily FDC treatment era on initiation of cART. Dovepress.2: 19–26.
49. Mbori-Ngacha D, Nduati R, John G, Reilly M, Richardson B, et al. (2001) Morbidity and Mortality in Breastfed and Formula-Fed Infants of HIV-1–Infected Women A Randomized Clinical Trial. JAMA. 286(19): 2413–2420.
50. Index mundi (2014) World Facebook, South Africa Infant mortality rate. Available: http://www.indexmundi.com/south_africa/infant_mortality_rate.html. Accessed 20 April 2014.
51. Waning B, Kaplan W, King AC, Lawrence DA, Leufkens HG, et al. (2009) Global strategies to reduce the price of antiretroviral medicines: evidence from transactional databases. Bull World Health Organ 87: 520–528.
52. Kahn JG, Marseille E, Moore D, Bunnell R, Were W, et al. (2011) CD4 cell count and viral load monitoring in patients undergoing antiretroviral therapy in Uganda: cost-effectiveness study. BMJ 343: d6884.
53. Kim LH, Cohan DL, Sparks TN, Pilliod RA, Arinaitwe E, et al. (2013) The cost-effectiveness of repeat HIV testing during pregnancy in a resource-limited setting. J Acquir Immune Defic Syndr 63: 195–200.
54. Antiretroviral Therapy Cohort Collaboration (2008) Life expectancy of individuals on combination antiretroviral therapy in high-income countries: a collaborative analysis of 14 cohort studies. Lancet 372: 293–299.
55. Marseille E, Kahn JG, Mmiro F, Guay L, Musoke P, et al. (1999) Cost-effectiveness of single-dose nevirapine regimen for mothers and babies to decrease vertical HIV-1 transmission in sub-Saharan Africa. Lancet 354: 803–809.
56. Chin J (1991) The epidemiology and projected mortality of AIDS. Available: http://www.popline.org/node/317283. Accessed 20 April 2013.
57. McClamroch K, Behets F, Van Damme K, Rabenja LN, Myers E (2007) Cost-effectiveness of treatment strategies for cervical infection among women at high risk in Madagascar. Sex Transm Dis 34: 631–637.
58. Creese A, Floyd K, Alban A, Guinness L (2002) Cost-effectiveness of HIV/AIDS interventions in Africa: a systematic review of the evidence. Lancet 359: 1635–1643.
59. Westheimer EF, Urassa W, Msamanga G, Baylin A, Wei R, et al. (2004) Acceptance of HIV testing among pregnant women in Dar-es-Salaam, Tanzania. J Acquir Immune Defic Syndr 37: 1197 1205.
60. Li B, Zhao Q, Zhang X, Wu L, Chen T, et al. (2013) Effectiveness of a prevention of mother-to-child HIV transmission program in Guangdong province from 2007 to 2010. BMC Public Health 13: 591.
61. Lee PM, Wong KH (2007) Universal antenatal human immunodeficiency virus (HIV) testing programme is cost-effective despite a low HIV prevalence in Hong Kong. Hong Kong Med J 13: 199–207.
62. South Africa Government Services (2013) Department of Health starts rolling out fixed-dose combination antiretroviral. Available:http://www.services.gov.za/services/content/news/antiretrovirals/en_ZA. Accessed 08 April 2013.
63. Coovadia HM, Rollins NC, Bland RM, Little K, Coutsoudis A, et al. (2007) Mother-to-child transmission of HIV-1 infection during exclusive breastfeeding in the first 6 months of life: an intervention cohort study. Lancet 369: 1107–1116.
64. Avert (2012) HIV & AIDS in South Africa. Available: http://www.avert.org/hiv-aids-south-africa.htm. Accessed 22 April 2013.
65. World Health Organization (2010) Antiretroviral drugs for treating pregnant women and preventing HIV infections in infants: recommendations for a public health approach 2010 geneva switzerland. Available:http://whqlibdoc.who.int/publications/2010/9789241599818_eng.pdf.Acces -sed 25 August 2013.
66. World Health Organization (2013) Consolidated guidelines on the use of antiretroviral drugs for treating and preventing HIV infection:Recommendations for a public health approach. Available: http://apps.who.int/iris/bitstream/10665/85321/1/9789241505727_eng.pdf. Accessed 01 August 2013.
67. Moodley P, Parboosing R, Moodley D (2013) Reduction in perinatal HIV infections in KwaZulu-Natal, South Africa, in the era of more effective prevention of mother to child transmission interventions (2004–2012). J Acquir Immune Defic Syndr 63: 410–415.
68. McCabe CJ, Goldie SJ, Fisman DN (2010) The cost-effectiveness of directly observed highly-active antiretroviral therapy in the third trimester in HIV-infected pregnant women. PLoS One 5: e10154.
69. Liu X, Li C, Gong H, Cui Z, Fan L, et al. (2013) An economic evaluation for prevention of diabetes mellitus in a developing country: a modelling study. BMC Public Health 13: 729.
70. Jose R, Anton L, Pozniak, Joel E, Gallant, et al. (2008) Tenofovir Disoproxil Fumarate, Emtricitabine and Efavirenz Compared With Zidovudine/Lamivudine and Efavirenzin Treatment-Naive Patients 144-Week Analysis. J Acquir Immune Defic Syndr 47: 74–78.
71. Janssen N, Ndirangu J, Newell M-L, Bland RM (2010) Successful paediatric HIV treatment in rural primary care in Africa. Arch Dis Child 95: 414–421.
72. Gallant JE, Staszewski S, Pozniak AL, De Jesus E, Suleiman JMAH, et al. (2004) Efficacy and Safety of Tenofovir DF vs Stavudine in Combination Therapy in Antiretroviral-Naïve Patients A 3-Year Randomized Trial. JAMA 292: 191–201.
73. The European Mode of Delivery Collaboration (1999) Elective caesarean-section versus vaginal delivery in prevention of vertical HIV-1 transmission: a randomised clinical trial. Lancet 353: 1035–39.
74. Chu K, Cortier H, Maldonado F, Mashant T, Ford N, et al. (2012) Cesarean Section Rates and Indications in Sub-Saharan Africa:A Multi-Country Study from Medecins sans Frontieres. PLoS One 7(9):e44484.
75. Briand N, Jasseron C, Sibiude J, Azria E, Pollet J, et al. (2013) Cesarean section for HIV-infected women in the combination antiretroviral therapy era, 2000–2010. Am J Obstet Gynecol 209: 335.e1–12.
76. Becquet R, Ekouevi DK, Menan H, Amani-Bosse C, Becquet L, et al.(2008) Early mixed feeding and breastfeeding beyond 6 months increase the risk of postnatal HIV transmission: ANRS 1201/1202 Ditrame Plus, Abidjan, Côted'Ivoire. Preventive Medicine 47: 27–33.
77. International Treatment Preparedness Coalition (2009) Missing the Target: Failing Women, Failing Children:HIV, Vertical Transmission and Women's Health. Available:http://www.hivpolicy.org/Library/HPP001643.pdf. Accessed 29 August 2013.
78. Chatterjee A, Bosch RJ, Hunter DJ, Fataki MR, Msamanga GI, et al. (2007) Maternal disease stage and child undernutrition in relation to mortality among children born to HIV-infected women in Tanzania. J Acquir Immune Defic Syndr 46: 599–606.
79. United Nations Programme on HIV/AIDS (2008) Report on the global AIDS epidemic:Executive summary. Available:http://www.unaids.org/en/media/unaids/contentassets/dataimport/pub/globalreport/2008/jc1511_gr08_executivesummary_en.pdf. Accessed 20 August 2013.
80. Kovalchik SA (2012) Mother's CD4+ Count Moderates the Risk Associated with Higher Parity for Late Postnatal HIV-Free Survival of Breastfed Children: An Individual Patient Data Meta-Analysis of Randomized Controlled Trials. AIDS Behav 16: 79–85.
81. Delicio AM, Milanez H, Amaral E, Morais SS, Lajos GJ, et al. (2011) Mother-to-child transmission of human immunodeficiency virus in aten years period. Reprod Health 8: 35.
82. Temmerman M, Nagelkerke N, Bwayo J, Chomba EN, Ndinya-Achola J, et al. (1995) HIV-1 and immunological changes during pregnancy: a comparison between HIV-1-seropositive and HIV-1-seronegative women in Nairobi, Kenya. AIDS 9: 1057–1060.

6

Clinical Mentorship of Nurse Initiated Antiretroviral Therapy in Khayelitsha, South Africa: A Quality of Care Assessment

Ann Green[1*¤], Virginia de Azevedo[2], Gabriela Patten[3], Mary-Ann Davies[1], Mary Ibeto[3], Vivian Cox[3]

1 School of Public Health and Family Medicine, University of Cape Town, Cape Town, South Africa, **2** Department of Health, City of Cape Town, Cape Town, South Africa, **3** Médecins Sans Frontières Khayelitsha, Khayelitsha, South Africa

Abstract

Introduction: To combat the AIDS epidemic and increase HIV treatment access, the South African government implemented a nurse-based, doctor-supported model of care that decentralizes administration of antiretroviral treatment (ART) for HIV positive patients through nurse initiated and managed ART. Médecins Sans Frontières (MSF) implemented a mentorship programme to ensure successful task-shifting, subsequently assessing the quality of clinical care provided by nurses.

Methods: A before-after cross-sectional study was conducted on nurses completing the mentorship programme in Khayelitsha, South Africa, from February 2011-September 2012. Routine clinical data from 229 patient folders and 21 self-assessment questionnaires was collected to determine the number of patients initiated on ART by nurses; quality of ART management before-after mentorship; patient characteristics for doctor and nurse ART initiations; and nurse self-assessments after mentorship.

Results: Twenty one nurses were authorized by one nurse mentor with one part-time medical officer's support, resulting in nurses initiating 77% of ART eligible patients. Improvements in ART management were found for drawing required bloods (91% vs 99%, $p = 0.03$), assessing adherence (50% vs 78%, $p < 0.001$) and WHO staging (63% vs 91%, $p < 0.001$). Nurse ART initiation indicators were successfully completed at 95–100% for 11 of 16 indicators: clinical presentation; patient weight; baseline blood work (CD4, creatinine, haemoglobin); STI screening; WHO stage, correlating medical history; medications prescribed appropriately; ART start date; and documented return date. Doctors initiated more patients with TB/HIV co-infection and WHO Stage 3 and 4 disease than nurses. Nurse confidence improved for managing HIV-infected children and pregnant women, blood result interpretation and long-term side effects.

Conclusions: Implementation of a clinical mentorship programme in Khayelitsha led to nurse initiation of a majority of eligible patients, enabling medical officers to manage complex cases. As mentorship can increase clinical confidence and enhance professional development, it should be considered essential for universal ART access in resource limited settings.

Editor: Omar Sued, Fundacion Huesped, Argentina

Funding: These authors have no support or funding to report.

Competing Interests: The authors have declared that no competing interests exist.

* E-mail: annfordgreen@gmail.com

¤ Current address: Vanderbilt Institute for Global Health, Nashville, Tennessee, United States of America

Introduction

South Africa is one of the countries most severely affected by the AIDS pandemic, with an estimated 5.6 million people living with HIV & AIDS (PLWHA) and the largest antiretroviral treatment programme in the world [1]. Addressing the large numbers of patients requiring ART initiation and management has become a key priority. To increase the number of people that can access HIV care and management, the South African government implemented a task-shifting model in 2011 that certifies nurses for the administration of antiretroviral treatment (ART) for HIV positive patients [2]. Under this model of care, trained nurses initiate patients onto ART and continue management of their subsequent treatment. However, limitations to human resource capacity, infrastructure, drug supplies, and a lack of clinical mentorship for newly trained nurses have all contributed to inefficiencies in the system.

Task Shifting for ART Management and ART Initiation

As in South Africa, human resource constraints within a healthcare system often lead to some form of task-shifting, or re-distribution of health-related tasks to a cadre of lower level professionals [3]. A systematic review conducted in 2010 on task shifting for HIV care and treatment in Africa found that task shifting is an effective strategy for combating shortages in human resources for health in HIV care and treatment [4]. Specifically, the *Comprehensive International Programme of Research on AIDS* (CIPRA-

SA) and *Streamlining Tasks and Roles to Expand Treatment and Care for HIV* (STRETCH) randomized control trials conducted in South Africa found nurse monitored ART to be non-inferior to doctor monitored therapy [5][6][7]. Some doctor initiated patients, down-referred to a primary care facility managed by nurses, had twelve-month outcomes for stable ART patients that were as good as and, in some cases, better than those patients that were maintained under hospital-based ART care [8]. The time saving benefits of nurse initiated and managed ART (NIMART) [9] and proven high levels of nurse compliance with national treatment guidelines [10], support the notion that improved access to life-saving ART treatment in resource limited settings can be realized through shifting of tasks to medical assistants and nurses [11]. In fact, in 2008, the WHO released a new set of guidelines and recommendations on task shifting that assigned tasks related to ART initiation and management under the purview of nurses as well as doctors [3]. Despite this, there is still debate over whether nurse initiation of ART is sustainable and whether there are negative impacts on quality of care [12,13,14].

Most data on NIMART comes from trials rather than routine care settings, and, outside of the STRETCH trial, there is little research that explores the performance of NIMART graduates in the clinical management and initiation of ART and the quality of care provided. According to a recent study of initiation rates for NIMART graduates within seven South African provinces, of the 126 trained nurses that were sampled, only 72 (62%) nurses proceeded to actually initiating patients onto ART [15]. The South African Department of Health has since set a goal to have nurses initiating 85% of patients eligible for ART by 2016 [16]. Under this new model of care, clinical mentorship is a key factor in the process for NIMART graduates to independently initiate ART; however, there is little data on the effectiveness of clinical mentorship programs [17]. The objective of this study is to explore the quality of clinical care received by patients initiated or managed by nurses completing a clinical mentorship programme led by Médecins Sans Frontières (MSF) in Khayelitsha, South Africa.

The study had two main aims: to describe the characteristics of ART initiations done by nurse graduates of the MSF NIMART mentorship programme; to measure the quality of nurses' initiation and long-term clinical management of patients continuing ART in Khayelitsha City Health primary health care clinics.

Methods

Ethics Statement

Ethics approval for this study was provided by the University of Cape Town Human Research Ethics Committee, with permission to conduct the research also obtained from the Western Cape Provincial Research Committee, as well as the sub-district supervisor and facility manager for each selected clinic.

The basic principles of the South African Medical Research Council were upheld, which include autonomy, beneficence, non-maleficence and justice. Routine sources of data were used from each clinic, thus consent was not obtained from the individual patients or the nurse participants. The use of patient and nurse data without consent was approved by the ethics committees that approved this study, as both patient and nurse data was kept anonymous. The data collected is similar to the data reviewed during routine patient folder checks for quality control, and the nurses were aware of others accessing this information regarding their performance.

Study Overview

This was a before-after cross-sectional study involving patient folder reviews of clinic adult ART stationery and self-assessments completed by NIMART nurses before and after mentorship was undertaken. The study was conducted in the South African township of Khayelitsha, a sub-district with an estimated population of approximately 500,000 inhabitants, located on the outskirts of Cape Town in Western Cape Province, South Africa [18]. The healthcare needs of township residents are served through 8 primary health clinics, three community health centres and a recently developed district hospital. As of 2010, Khayelitsha's HIV burden is one of the largest in the country, with an antenatal HIV prevalence of 26% [19]. The high volume of patients requiring ART initiation and management highlights the need for task shifting in order to ensure access to care for all eligible patients. Following the South African government's 2009 mandate for universal ART access, the programme expanded rapidly with all 11 clinics providing access to ART by 2011.

Since February 2011, MSF has been implementing a NIMART training and mentorship program for nurses in Khayelitsha to become accredited to initiate ART [20]. As of December 31, 2013, 81 nurses have been or are being mentored through the MSF NIMART programme; 70 of which have been authorised to initiate ART independently. The mentorship programme follows the nurse-based, doctor-supported ART service model promoted by the Western Cape's Provincial HIV & AIDS, STI, and TB Directorate as depicted in Figure 1 [21]. The pre-requisites for NIMART authorization in the Western Cape of South Africa are: 1. Completion of a basic HIV course (from a list of approved courses that is adjusted as new courses become available); 2. Completion of PALSA Plus HIV training (a training on how to use South Africa's approved algorithmic tool for diagnosis and treatment of common opportunistic infections); 3. 40 hours of one-on-one mentorship.

This study focused on nurses completing the MSF NIMART mentorship programme and working in eight Khayelitsha facilities; a random sample of these nurses was chosen, with at least one nurse from each facility. Data from programme records was used to determine the number of nurses completing the NIMART mentorship program and receiving authorization to prescribe ART as well as the number and proportion of all patient ART initiations done by NIMART mentored nurses. Data was also collected through patient folder review to: 1) compare the quality of nurse ART management before and after NIMART training; 2) describe the quality of nurse ART initiations; and 3) compare patient characteristics for doctor and nurse ART initiations. Quality of ART initiation and management was assessed based on correct completion of standard clinical stationery components in use across all the study clinics. Data on patient characteristics included age, gender, weight, body mass index (BMI), creatinine and creatinine clearance, haemoglobin, alanine aminotransferase (ALT), tuberculosis (TB) status, pregnancy status, and WHO stage. Additionally, qualitative data comparing the level of nurse confidence before and after NIMART training was collected from a self-assessment survey that captured each nurse's perception of individual clinical confidence for a list of competencies on a level of 1-5 (1 = not very confident; 2 = somewhat confident; 3 = confident; 4 = very confident; 5 = confident if using manual).

The study period for reporting the number and proportion of NIMART nurse patient initiations and the number of nurses completing the NIMART mentorship programme spans from February 2011 to September 2012. The period for measuring quality of nurse ART management prior to mentorship was

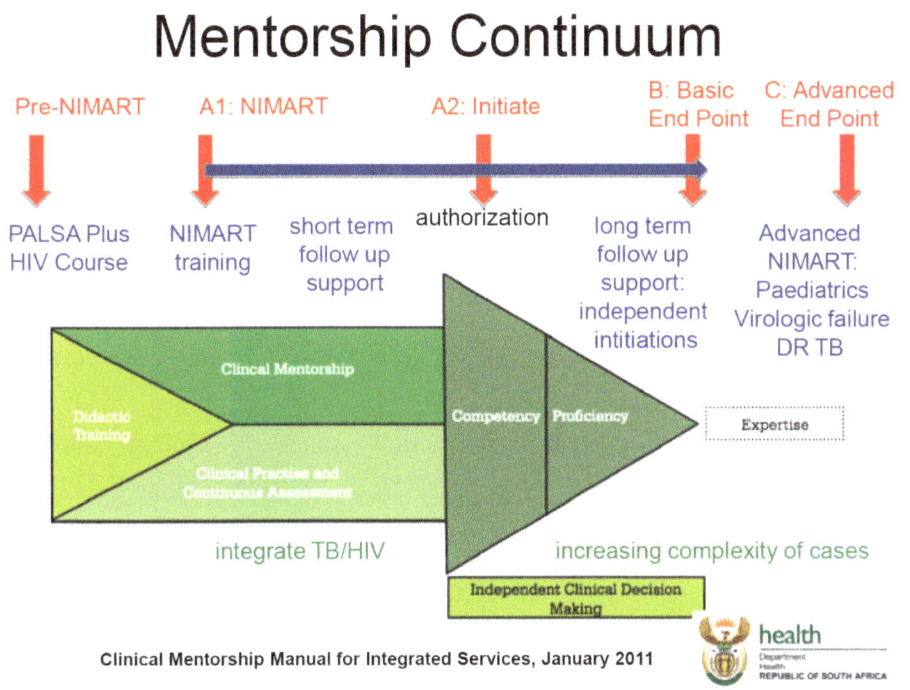

Figure 1. NIMART Clinical Mentorship Model for Integrated Services. Pre-NIMART: *PALSA Plus HIV course* training on use South Africa's approved algorithmic tool for diagnosis and treatment of common opportunistic infections; A1: *NIMART training* based on South African Ministry of Health guidelines; A2: *Authorization to initiate* is granted based on three required criteria: completion of basic HIV course, PALSA Plus HIV training, and 40 hours of one-on-one mentorship; B: *Basic End Point* is reached whereby the authorized nurses is conducting independent initiations; C: *Advanced End Point* is reached when skill level is expanded to include management of paediatric patients, virologic failure, and drug-resistant TB.

determined based on the nurse's authorization date, using data from February 2011 through the start date of each nurse's participation in the NIMART program, the "before period". The period for assessing ART management after mentorship was defined as the post-authorization date to September 2012, the "after period". For measuring the quality of nurse initiations and for collecting patient characteristics of nurse and doctor ART initiations, the study period was based on nurse authorization date through September 2012. The self-assessment questionnaires were completed on the start date of the NIMART mentorship programme. The same questionnaire was then repeated on the final date of the respective training.

For data on quality of nurse ART management, a nurse graduate was randomly selected from a list of each of the study clinics' mentored nurses. Patient folders were randomly sampled for the selected nurses, identifying ten folders for the before period and ten folders for the after period. Eighty patient folders in total were reviewed for the before and after periods, assessing quality of nurse ART management. An additional 80 folders were selected for assessing quality of nurse graduate ART initiation. The clinical stationery components chosen to assess quality of ART management and initiation included variables related to necessary laboratory testing, patient counselling, medication and side effect management, and adherence. To compare patient characteristics with those initiated on treatment by doctors, folders were randomly selected from a sampling frame of all doctor-led ART initiations at each clinic during the study period. All random selection was done using a random number generator programme (random.org) that includes a list randomizer function [22]. Figure 2 depicts a flow diagram for the sample selection process.

Programme data was summarized using appropriate descriptive statistics of frequency and percentage for categorical variables. The quality of nurse ART management and initiations were analysed by calculating the proportion of the chosen clinical stationery components correctly completed within the 10 folders reviewed for each nurse graduate and conducting chi-squared tests. Patient characteristics of both doctor and nurse ART initiations were analysed by calculating medians and inter-quartile ranges for continuous data and proportions for categorical data. Chi-squared tests were calculated where appropriate. Self-assessment data was summarized using descriptive statistics and rank sum tests. Where applicable the data was analysed using STATA statistical software version 12 [23].

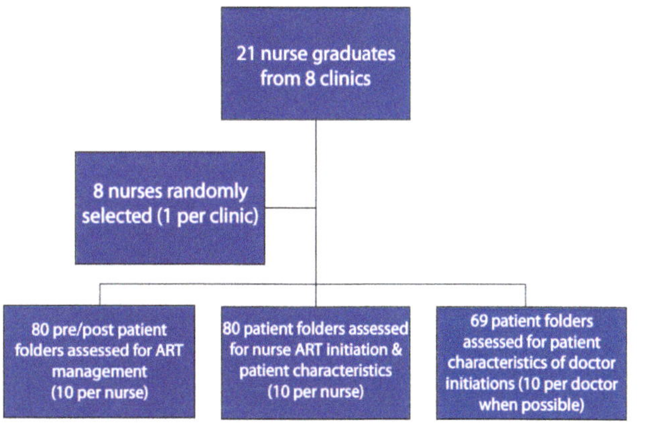

Figure 2. Sample selection flow diagram.

Results

There were 21 nurse graduates from the NIMART mentorship program during the study period. In the month of September 2012, 77% (173/223) of ART initiations in study clinics were done by nurse graduates. Three graduates resigned from their position during the study period. Twenty-one self-assessments were conducted before the NIMART mentorship program and again after completion of the program, two for each nurse graduate. Two nurses' before and after surveys for self-assessment analysis were excluded due to differing survey formats in the before and after period.

In terms of assessing the quality of nurse ART management following the NIMART mentorship program, there were significant improvements in the collection of required blood tests, patient HIV staging and nurse adherence assessment and documentation(Table 1). Of the 80 patient folders reviewed in each study period, one patient was referred to a doctor in the before period and two patients in the after period.

Analysis of nurse-managed ART initiation revealed that nurse graduates documented baseline CD4 count, calculated and entered patient HIV stage in accordance with patient medical history, and documented the ART initiation date and the prescribed medication 100% of the time(Table 2). In more than 90% of records reviewed, nurse graduates documented patient weight, past medical history, prior ART history and haemoglobin; screened for sexually transmitted infections; and documented a treatment plan and a return visit date. Pap smear data was only recorded in 14% of female records reviewed. Cotrimoxazole was prescribed in 76% of the patients requiring it.

Patients initiated on treatment by doctors had more advanced disease compared with those initiated by nurses(Table 3); median weight, BMI and haemoglobin levels were lower, and the median ALT was higher. A greater proportion of doctor-initiated patients had active TB and WHO Stage 3 or 4 disease.

Self-assessment data revealed a significant increase in nurse confidence level for nearly all clinical tasks measured, notably for management of children, body mass index calculation, creatinine clearance, prescribing with concurrent illness, recognition and management of side effects, pregnancy planning in HIV positive patients, and non-drug management and administration of post-exposure prophylaxis(Table 4).

Following the mentorship program nurses reported the lowest confidence scores in the following areas: cardiac failure, understanding of the ARV register, and procedures for lactate testing. Confidence did not significantly increase after mentoring in the following areas: TB screening, diagnosis and management in adults; cotrimoxazole prescription in adults; and management of the Department of Health first line regimen in adults. However, the confidence rates for these areas were moderately high (3–3.5) in the pre-test.

Discussion

This study found that a NIMART mentorship program successfully resulted in a majority of ART initiations conducted by nurses, which is an encouraging step toward reaching the South African National Strategic Plan's goal of 85% of eligible patients being initiated by nurses by 2016. The quality of ART management provided by nurses improved, as well as the nurses' confidence in their knowledge and management of HIV. The

Table 1. Quality of Nurse ART Management in Khayelitsha Clinics n = 80 patient clinical folders reviewed.

Indicator	Before	%	After	%	p-value
ART date recorded	80	100	79	98.8	0.316
Last viral load>400	4/54*	7.41	3/65*	4.6	0.519
Treatment plan documented for patients with viral load >400	2/4*	50	1/3*	33.3	0.659
Creatinine clearance recorded	13/74*	17.56	10/65*	15.4	0.73
Documented result of most recent bloods	74	92.5	75	93.8	0.755
Last required bloods drawn	73	91.25	79	98.8	**0.03**
TB screen done	63/76*	82.89	68/74*	91.9	0.098
STI screen done	71	88.75	75	93.8	0.263
Family planning offered	33/56*	58.93	37/55*	67.3	0.362
Pap smear recorded /referenced	4/60*	6.67	6/57*	10.5	0.455
Clinical presentation entered	80	100	80	100	
Problem list entered	33	41.25	36	45	0.632
Adherence assessed and documented	40	50	62	77.5	**<0.001**
Stage entered	50	62.5	73	91.3	**<0.001**
Stage correlates with known medical history	45	88	58	79.5	0.119
Treatment plan documented	58	72.5	66	82.5	0.13
Referred to doctor	1	1.25	2	2.5	0.56
Medication entered	80	100	80	100	
ARV dose entered correctly	64	80	64	80	
Cotrimoxazole prescribed	12	15	8	10	0.339
Should Cotrimoxazole have been prescribed	21	26.25	15	18.8	0.256

*Number of patients where particular indicator is applicable.

Table 2. Quality of Nurse ART Initiations in Khayelitsha Clinics n = 80.

	Number recorded	%
Patient weight documented	76	**95**
Patient BMI documented	60	75
Past medical history documented	73	91.3
Prior ART/history documented	73	91.3
If yes, was patient discussed with doctor	0	
Documented as 'No ART history'	33	41.3
Baseline CD4 documented	80	**100**
Creatinine documented	79	**98.8**
Creatinine clearance (CrCl) documented	43	53.8
IfCrCl<50, was patient discussed with doctor	0	
Not applicable	77	41.3
IfCrCl<50 and discussed by doctor, treatment documented	0	
Haemoglobin documented	78	**97.5**
Alanine aminotransferase (ALT) documented	70	87.5
IfALT>100, was patient referred to doctor	0	
ART initiation date recorded	80	**100**
TB screen done	61	76.3
On treatment	17	21.3
Investigation pending	1	1.3
STI screen done	76	**95**
Eligible for family planning	59	73.8
Family planning offered	42	71.2
Eligible for pap smear	59	73.8
Pap smear date recorded or referenced	8	13.6
Clinical presentation entered	80	**100**
Problem list entered	62	77.5
Stage entered	80	**100**
Stage correlates with known medical history	80	**100**
Treatment plan entered	74	92.5
Was patient seen or discussed with doctor in prior month	19	23.8
Medication entered	80	**100**
ARV dose entered correctly	66	82.5
Should Cotrimoxazole have been prescribed	41	51.3
Cotrimoxazole prescribed	30	37.5
Return date documented	79	**98.8**

quality of nurse initiation of patients onto ART following mentorship was satisfactory, allowing doctors to focus on patients with more advanced disease.

The study findings complement previous NIMART studies conducted in sub-Saharan Africa, whereby nurse ART management and initiation are recommended as effective strategies for addressing HIV care and treatment in low-resource settings. [4] However, this study has shown a higher percentage of nurse initiations than other studies. [15]

The MSF NIMART programme was conducted in line with the South African Ministry of Health (MoH) guidelines on NIMART mentorship with the intent to eventually hand over the programme. For this reason the results of the programme are seen as sustainable. MSF also supported the development of a Western Cape Provincial Trainer-of-NIMART Mentors course in 2011, and this course is now managed completely by the MoH without MSF involvement, producing +/− 20 new mentors a year.

Quality of Nurse ART Management

The nurse graduates successfully completed a number of ART management indicators both before and after the mentorship program, indicative of appropriate care of those on ART. The consistency in documentation is perhaps due to the fact that the nurses participating in the mentorship programme had significant prior experience in managing ART. Despite this, there are still some areas of concern in nurse management of ART, such as documentation of pap-smears for female patients. Consistent with other study findings [24], this is a topic to be included in future nurse mentorship programme content, especially given the high

Table 3. Patient Characteristics n = 80 n = 69.

	Nurse	Doctor	p-value
Age (median)	28 (IQR 24-35)	31 (IQR 24-39)	0.5654
Gender			0.352
Male	20 (25%)	22 (28%)	
Female	60 (75%)	47 (62%)	
Weight (median)	66 (IQR 61-78)	59 (IQR 52-70)	**<0.001**
Weight not recorded	3	0	
Infants	0	2	
BMI (median)	26 (IQR 23-31)	22 (IQR 19-26)	**0.0014**
Weight not recorded	3	0	
BMI not recorded	19	25	
Infants	0	2	
Creatinine (median)	62 (IQR 50-73)	66 (IQR 51-81)	0.2161
missing	1	2	
Creatinine clearance (median)	103 (IQR 80.5-125.5)	120 (IQR 71.5-154)	0.5926
missing	38	41	
Haemoglobin (median)	12 (IQR 11-13)	11 (IQR 9-13)	0.0463
missing	2	8	
Alanine aminotransferase (median)	18 (IQR 14-24)	26 (IQR 19-38)	**<0.001**
missing	11	6	
TB status			**<0.001**
On TB treatment	17	27	
Screen positive	0	0	
Screened negative	61	30	
Investigation Pending	1	1	
Not Screened	1	11	
Pregnant	3	1	0.453
WHO stage			**<0.001**
Stage 1	42	11	
Stage 2	11	13	
Stage 3	22	28	
Stage 4	5	12	
Missing Stage	0	5	

levels of cervical cancer throughout South Africa [25]. The absence of documented TB screening for all patients in an area with a high burden of TB-disease is also disconcerting, although improvements were observed after mentorship. Another concern is the low calculation rates of creatinine clearance (CrCl) for follow-up monitoring, although this may be attributed to the ART stationery in use not having a specific field to document the result. The ratio of Cotrimoxazole (Bactrim) being prescribed in patients that were eligible for it was also low. As this is an effective, affordable method for strengthening the immune system of HIV infected patients, it is imperative that the mentorship program place a strong focus on improving these rates moving forward.

Our results show that few patients were referred to doctors within the study clinics. This may result from the fact that the patients seen by nurses were characteristically not as ill, rather than nurse graduates not appropriately seeking professional guidance from doctors. The low level of doctors present within these clinics may contribute to the low levels of referrals. It is also possible that nurses consult a doctor or nurse for advice during the initiation process without documenting this advice in the patient folder.

Following completion of the NIMART mentorship program, there were improvements in indicators for drawing required bloods, assessing adherence and WHO staging. While the significant improvement in assessing adherence is encouraging (77.5%), there is still substantial room for improvement. Monitoring of patient adherence is crucial considering it is a key barrier to successfully keeping patients on treatment, and it will be important to continue focus on this area in future mentorship trainings.

Quality of Nurse ART Initiation

Overall, the high levels of completion for the majority of clinical indicators for ART initiation among nurse graduates suggest that such task shifting has been a success. While creatinine levels were consistently recorded at ART initiation, the calculation of creatinine clearance (CrCl) was often not included in the patient folder. Nurse graduates seem to pay more attention to creatinine

Table 4. Nurse Graduate Self-assessment n = 21 n = 21.

	Pre mean score	Post mean score	p-value
Section 1: Baseline Knowledge			
Modes of transmission - adults	3.3	3.8	0.0083
Modes of transmission - children	2.905	3.737	0.0060
Clinical course - adults	2.619	3.7	0.0016
Clinical course - children	2.278	3.5	0.0004
Signs and symptoms - adults	3.19	3.905	0.0014
Signs and symptoms - children	2.6	3.65	0.0043
Use of manuals –positive prevention& HIV	3.25	3.75	0.0247
Use of Department of Health stationery	2.8	3.789	0.0003
Core differences between adults & children	2.263	3.524	0.0013
Section 2: Before ARVs			
HIV counselling and testing - adults	3.25	3.85	0.0008
HIV counselling and testing - children	2.111	3.714	<0.0001
Diagnosis - adults	3	3.8	0.0003
Diagnosis - children	2	3.55	<0.0001
Staging - adults	3.3	3.905	0.0053
Staging - children	1.8	3.619	<0.0001
Body Mass Index calculation and management	3.2	3.952	<0.0001
Paediatric weight chart and management	1.789	3.474	<0.0001
TB screening - adults	3.476	3.857	0.1279
TB screening - children	2.476	3.476	0.0046
Pap smears and HIV	2.95	3.8	0.0007
Common opportunistic infections - adults	2.952	3.762	0.0013
Common opportunistic infections - children	2.1	3.381	0.0003
TB diagnosis and management - adults	3.05	3.571	0.0799
Drug side effects	2.905	3.824	0.0187
Cotrimoxazole use - adults	3.429	3.714	0.1654
Cotrimoxazole use - children	2.048	3.81	<0.0001
Section 3: Starting ARVs			
Eligibility criteria to start - adults	2.857	3.667	0.0029
Eligibility criteria to start - children	1.65	3.429	<0.0001
Fast-tracking criteria	2.762	3.75	0.0001
Blood result interpretation - adults	2.5	3.762	0.0003
Working withcreatinine clearance	2.1	3.905	<0.0001
Individual ART contra-indications	2.35	3.81	0.0004
Pre-start adherence counseling	2.55	3.7	0.0003
Department of Health1st line regimen - adults (ARVs, doses, side effects)	3	3.714	0.0870
Department of Health1st line regimen – children (ARVs, doses, side effects)	1.65	3.476	<0.0001
Prescribing w concurrent illnesses - TB, epilepsy, hypertension, diabetes	1.857	3.75	<0.0001
Normal course on ARVs	2.737	3.905	<0.0001
Side effects and their management:			
Skin, haematology, liver, kidney, psychiatric	2.143	3.6	0.0010
Recognition of side effects	2.667	3.429	0.0530
Understanding IRIS	2.35	3.571	0.0031
Long-term side effects	2.053	3.667	0.0002
Failing regimen - warning signs	2.4	3.667	0.0002
Diagnosis - clinical, immunological, virological	1.842	3.619	<0.0001
When to refer	2.333	3.857	<0.0001

Table 4. Cont.

	Pre	Post	
	mean score	mean score	p-value
Section 4: HIV & Pregnancy			
Family planning	3.095	3.762	0.0012
Wanting to fall pregnant	2.19	3.9	<0.0001
During pregnancy	2.571	3.7144	0.0005
After pregnancy - mother	2.35	3.762	0.0003
After pregnancy - child	2.1	3.5	0.0006
Section 5: Post-exposure Prophylaxis			
Non-drug management and administration	2.05	3.762	<0.0001
Drug regimen and indications	2.15	3.65	0.0006
Section 6: General			
Management of weight loss	2.7	3.571	0.0066
Routine clinical examination	2.438	3.667	0.0001
Cardiac failure	1.667	3.118	0.0005
Enlarged liver	1.81	3.313	0.0009
Neck stiffness	2.15	3.5	0.0009
Procedures for lactate testing	1.571	3.2	0.0001
Understanding the register	2.111	3.167	0.0186

clearance (CrCl) when initiating patients onto ART compared to when managing ART in patients already initiated. This may be due to a deeper sense of responsibility felt when personally initiating patients. Similar to nurse ART management results, further improvements are needed in rates of pap smears, prescription of Cotrimoxazole, and TB screening. There are low numbers of TB co-infected patients among those seen by nurse graduates, possibly due to the level of TB service integration at the study clinics.

Patient Characteristics between Doctor & Nurse Initiations

Our study findings indicate that doctors are initiating patients with more advanced disease than nurses, which is consistent with findings from some previous studies [4]. This suggests that nurses initiate patients with earlier stage disease, allowing doctors to concentrate their efforts on those with more advanced disease or more serious illness. This may affect the down referral of patients from doctors to nurses and may also impact the interpretation of patient outcomes when comparing nurse and doctor ART initiations.

Nurse Confidence

The NIMART mentorship program aimed to improve nurse confidence in HIV-related services for children, pregnant women, blood result interpretation and long-term side effects, suggesting a successful design of the training curriculum as these areas all showed significant improvements in nurse confidence level for the post-survey. It is important to note that these areas of greatest improvement in nurse confidence had the lowest confidence scores before training.

It is noted that some areas that did not see a significant increase in confidence level, such as TB screening and Cotrimoxazole prescription in adults, are in line with our findings in terms of areas needing improvement. The mean score for nurse confidence level in these areas was high in the pre-test (3.5, 3.4, respectively), possibly contributing to the lack of significant increase post-training. Certain areas, such as calculation of creatinine clearance (CrCl), had a highly significant improvement in nurse confidence level; however, that did not appear to translate into action. These factors will need to be taken into consideration for future mentorship trainings, being aware that confidence is not necessarily equal to competence and completion of routine practices.

Many clinical tasks related to paediatric HIV and treatment had low confidence scores on the pre-test and substantial improvement in the post-test; however, we did not specifically evaluate whether this resulted in more paediatric ART initiations. This is important as paediatric ART management has proven to be an especially challenging area in resource-limited settings, and the literature on task shifting of ART management for children is limited [15,26]. The implications for children's access to HIV treatment suggest that nurses in the study are now more confident, and potentially more competent, in handling paediatric HIV patients, improving quality of patient care and treatment. These results are a testament to the valuable role that mentorship can play in improving access to paediatric ART.

This research provides insightful feedback on the performance of NIMART graduates in the clinical management of ART and the quality of care provided. Generally the nurses report feeling empowered by the additional knowledge [27]. With the lack of a doctor's daily presence for many of the City of Cape Town clinics, this programme allows the nurse to manage stable patients without having to wait to discuss with a doctor. Doctor interactions are reserved for more complex patients, and most nurses seem happy with this distinction. The study was not designed as a comparison of quality of care between nurse and doctor; it did not investigate patient outcomes, nor did we look at the time to treatment initiation, all of which are important elements to consider when assessing appropriateness of task shifting to nurses for HIV care.

Limitations

The results of this study are limited by the fact that data were collected retrospectively from patient folders. The data may therefore be inaccurate if certain tasks were completed but not documented. The results therefore also rely on the clinical stationery in use at the time, as specific forms were not created for this study. Slight differences in the ART stationery existed between patient folders. Specifically, the TB symptom list for some folders included a checklist of boxes to aid completion of the register, which may have influenced documentation of TB symptoms. Not all study clinics had the same level of doctor involvement, potentially influencing the ability of nurses to refer sicker patients, and all study conclusions are based on one nurse mentor. The small number of nurses reviewed (8 of 21) may limit generalizability of results.

This study was restricted to adult ART initiations, and paediatric ART initiations were not included in the folder review. Western Cape NIMART nurses were not authorized to initiate ART on paediatric cases at the time of the study. The Western Cape NIMART guideline changed in 2014 to allow NIMART nurses to initiate paediatric ART following further mentorship and assessment.

While this study was not designed to assess whether this programme is reproducible in other settings, this model can be adapted as needed to suit any context. The basic HIV course is simply a training on the basics of HIV, and there is flexibility in how this is achieved, so long as the course covers the basics of what HIV is, modes of transmission, diagnosis and treatment. For the Western Cape model, the nurse does not have to have her PALSA Plus training completed before the 40 hours of mentorship starts and NIMART mentorship sessions can be used in place of some PALSA Plus sessions. Both the HIV course and PALSA Plus content could take place during the one-on-one mentorship for contexts were a specific HIV course or PALSA Plus guidelines were not available.

Conclusions

Implementation of a nurse-mentor driven NIMART mentorship programme led to competent nurse initiation of the majority of patients, enabling doctors to manage complex patient cases. Nurses improved their confidence in performing HIV related clinical tasks, nurses were initiating patients after mentorship and the quality of initiation and management was satisfactory. These results suggest that in regions where the HIV burden places large demands on health services, a nurse mentoring model could assist in ensuring system efficiency for task shifting.

Mentorship provides motivation for increased clinical confidence and improves the quality of clinical care provided by nurses in some areas, creating an opportunity for professional development through the provision of effective technical backup. Clinical mentorship should be considered an essential component of the public health approach to universal ART access in resource-limited settings. Further research is needed to determine whether NIMART mentorship for nurses improves linkage to and retention in ART care.

Acknowledgments

The authors would like to acknowledge research assistants, **Nikiwe Mkhosana** and **Nombulelo Raphahlelo**, of Médecins sans Frontières, Khayelitsha, as well as the dedicated staff at **Khayelitsha City of Cape Town clinics** who were involved in this study.

Author Contributions

Conceived and designed the experiments: AG GP MI VC. Performed the experiments: AG. Analyzed the data: AG GP VC. Wrote the paper: AG VdA GP MAD MI VC.

References

1. UNAIDS (2010)UNAIDS Report on the global AIDS epidemic 2010.WHO, Geneva.
2. South African National Department of Health (2011) Clinical Mentorship Manual for Integrated Services.
3. WHO (2008) Task shifting: rational redistribution of tasks among health workforce teams: global recommendations and guidelines. http://www.who.int/workforcealliance/knowledge/resources/taskshiftingguidelines/en/index.html.Accessed: 2012 March 24.
4. Callaghan M, Ford N, Schneider H (2010) A systematic review of task-shifting for HIV treatment and care in Africa. Human Resources for Health 8(8).
5. Sanne I, Orrell C, Fox MP, Conradie F, Ive P, et al. (2010) Nurse versus doctor management of HIV-infected patients receiving antiretroviral therapy (CIPRA-SA): a randomised non-inferiority trial. The Lancet 376(9734), pp. 33–40.
6. Fairall L, Bachmann MO, Lombard C, Timmerman V, Uebel K, et al. (2012) Task shifting of antiretroviral treatment from doctors to primary-care nurses in South Africa (STRETCH): a pragmatic, parallel, cluster-randomised trial. The Lancet 380(9845), pp. 889–898.
7. Kiweewa FM, Wabwire D, Nakibuuka J, Mubiru M, Bagenda D, et al. (2013) Noninferiority of a Task-Shifting HIV Care and Treatment Model Using Peer Counselors and Nurses Among Ugandan Women Initiated on ART: Evidence From a Randomized Trial. Journal of Acquired Immune Deficiency Syndromes 63(4).
8. Long L, Brennan A, Fox MP, Ndibongo B, Jaffray I, et al. (2011) Treatment outcomes and cost-effectiveness of shifting management of stable ART patients to nurses in South Africa: an observational cohort. PLoS Medicine 8(7), pp. e1001055.
9. Chung J (2008) Quantification of Physician-time Saved in a Task Shifting Pilot Program in Rwanda. Paper presented at the HIV/AIDS Implementers' Meeting. 3–7 June 2008. Kampala.
10. Shumbusho F, Van Griensven J, Lowrance D, Turate I, Weaver MA, et al. (2009) Task shifting for scale-up of HIV care: evaluation of nurse-centered antiretroviral treatment at rural health centres in Rwanda. PLoS Medicine 6(10), pp. e1000163.
11. Bemelmans M, Van Den Akker T, Ford N, Zachariah R, Harries A, et al. (2010) Providing universal access to antiretroviral therapy in Thyolo, Malawi through task shifting and decentralization of HIV/AIDS care. Tropical Medicine & International Health 15(12),pp. 1413–1420.
12. Naranbhai V, Karim QA, Naidoo K, Yende-Zuma N, Karim SSA (2012) Sustainability of task-shifting for antiretroviral treatment.The Lancet 380(9857), pp. 1907–1908.
13. Bachmann MO, Fairall L (2012) Sustainability of task-shifting for antiretroviral treatment–Authors' reply. The Lancet 380(9857), pp. 1908.
14. Kredo T, Bateganya M, Pienaar ED, Adeniyi FB (2012) Task shifting from doctors to non-doctors for initiation and maintenance of HIV/AIDS treatment. The Cochrane Library.
15. Cameron D, Gerber A, Mbatha M, Mutyabule J, Swart H (2012) Nurse-initiation and maintenance of patients on antiretroviral therapy: Are nurses in primary care clinics initiating ART after attending NIMART training. South African Medical Journal 102 (2), pp. 98–100.
16. South African National Department of Health (2011) National Strategic Plan for HIV and AIDS, STIs and TB, 2012–2016. Strategic Plan, South Africa.
17. Workneh G, Sherzer L, Kirk B, Draper H, Anabwani G, et al. (2013) Evaluation of the effectiveness of an outreach clinical mentoring programme in support of paediatric HIV care scale-up in Botswana. AIDS Care 25 (1), pp. 11–19.
18. Department of Social Services and Poverty Alleviation (2006) The Population Register Update: Khayelitsha 2005. Survey, Western Cape.
19. Médecins Sans Frontières (2011) Khayelitsha 2001–2011 ACTIVITY REPORT: 10 years of HIV/TB care at primary health care level. Activity report, Cape Town.
20. Médecins Sans Frontières (2012) Clinical Mentoring Toolkit. Available: http://msf.org.za/msf2012/publication/clinical-mentoring-toolkit.Accessed 2014 January 6.
21. Western Cape's HIV&AIDS, STI, TB Directorate (2012) Framework for Nurse Initiating and Management of Antiretroviral Therapy: Criteria of Mentors in NIMART. Circular, Cape Town.
22. Random.org website (2012) Available at: http://www.random.org/lists/.html.Accessed: 2012 November 19.

23. StataCorp (2011) Stata Statistical Software: Release 12. College Station, TX: StataCorp LP.
24. Bingham A, Bishop A, Coffey P, Winkler J, Bradley J, et al. (2003) Factors affecting utilization of cervical cancer prevention services in low-resource settings. Salud Pública de México 45, pp. 408–416.
25. International Agency for Research on Cancer (2010) GLOBOCAN 2008 Fast Stats: South African Republic. Available: http://globocan.iarc.fr/factsheet.asp [2012 October 11].
26. Penazzato M, Davies M A, Apollo T, Negussie E, Ford N (2013) Task shifting for the delivery of paediatric antiretroviral treatment: a systematic review. Journal of Acquired Immune Deficiency Syndromes doi: 10.1097/QAI.0000000000000024 [accessed 2013 December 17].
27. Stinson K, Giddy J, Cox V, Burton R, Ibeto M, et al (2014) Reflections on a decade of delivering PMTCT in Khayelitsha, South Africa. Southern African Journal of HIV Medicine, 15(1),pp. 30–32.

7

Increases in HIV Testing among Men Who Have Sex with Men — National HIV Behavioral Surveillance System, 20 U.S. Metropolitan Statistical Areas, 2008 and 2011

Laura A. Cooley*, Alexandra M. Oster, Charles E. Rose, Cyprian Wejnert, Binh C. Le, Gabriela Paz-Bailey for the NHBS Study Group¶

Division of HIV/AIDS Prevention, National Center for HIV, Viral Hepatitis, STD and TB Prevention, Centers for Disease Control and Prevention, Atlanta, Georgia, United States of America

Abstract

In 2011, 62% of estimated new HIV diagnoses in the United States were attributed to male-to-male sexual contact (men who have sex with men, MSM); 39% of these MSM were black or African American. HIV testing, recommended at least annually by CDC for sexually active MSM, is an essential first step in HIV care and treatment for HIV-positive individuals. A variety of HIV testing initiatives, designed to reach populations disproportionately affected by HIV, have been developed at both national and local levels. We assessed changes in HIV testing behavior among MSM participating in the National HIV Behavioral Surveillance System in 2008 and 2011. We compared the percentages tested in the previous 12 months in 2008 and 2011, overall and by race/ethnicity and age group. In unadjusted analyses, recent HIV testing increased from 63% in 2008 to 67% in 2011 overall ($P<0.001$), from 63% to 71% among black MSM ($P<0.001$), and from 63% to 75% among MSM of other/multiple races ($P<0.001$); testing did not increase significantly for white or Hispanic/Latino MSM. Multivariable model results indicated an overall increase in recent HIV testing (adjusted prevalence ratio [aPR] = 1.07, $P<0.001$). Increases were largest for black MSM (aPR = 1.12, $P<0.001$) and MSM of other/multiple races (aPR = 1.20, $P<0.001$). Among MSM aged 18–19 years, recent HIV testing was shown to increase significantly among black MSM (aPR = 1.20, $P=0.007$), but not among MSM of other racial/ethnic groups. Increases in recent HIV testing among populations most affected by HIV are encouraging, but despite these increases, improved testing coverage is needed to meet CDC recommendations.

Editor: Joan A Caylà, Public Health Agency of Barcelona, Spain

Funding: These authors have no support or funding to report. The National HIV Behavioral Surveillance System is funded by the Centers for Disease Control and Prevention (CDC). Study design and data collection are conducted by funded sites in accordance with a standardized protocol developed by CDC. Data analysis and preparation of the manuscript were conducted by CDC staff.

Competing Interests: The authors have declared that no competing interests exist.

* Email: LCooley@cdc.gov

¶ Membership of the NHBS Study Group is provided in the Acknowledgments.

Introduction

Approximately 1.1 million people in the United States are living with HIV [1], and an estimated 50,000 new infections occur each year [2]. Gay, bisexual, and other men who have sex with men (collectively referred to as MSM) and blacks or African Americans (hereafter referred to as blacks) continue to be disproportionately affected by HIV. While MSM represent only an estimated 4% of the male population in the United States [3], they accounted for approximately 79% of estimated new HIV diagnoses among adult and adolescent males and approximately 62% of estimated new HIV diagnoses overall in the United States in 2011 [4]. From 2008 to 2011, adult and adolescent MSM were the only group among whom the annual number of new HIV diagnoses increased [4]. Despite representing approximately 13% of the U.S. population [5], blacks accounted for 47% of estimated new HIV diagnoses in 2011 [4]. Considering the disproportionate burden of HIV among MSM and blacks, it is not surprising that the burden upon black MSM is also disproportionate; 39% percent of estimated new HIV diagnoses among MSM in 2011 occurred among black MSM [4]. Young black MSM are particularly affected. Though black MSM accounted for 39% of estimated new HIV diagnoses among MSM of all age groups in 2011, an estimated 58% of MSM aged 13–24 years diagnosed with HIV infection in 2011 were black [6].

Achieving awareness of HIV infection through testing is an essential first step to linking HIV-positive individuals to medical care and services, such as antiretroviral therapy, which can result in improved clinical outcomes [7]. Moreover, research has shown that once diagnosed with HIV, individuals reduce risk behaviors, which, in combination with viral suppression, can reduce the likelihood of transmitting HIV to others [8–10]. A recent analysis of U.S. HIV surveillance data estimated that of the adolescents and adults living with HIV infection at the end of 2010, 16% were living with undiagnosed infection [1]. Both the U.S. Department of Health and Human Services' *Healthy People 2020* and the National HIV/AIDS Strategy for the United States (NHAS) aim to reduce the percentage of persons living with undiagnosed HIV infection in the United States to 10% [11,12].

CDC currently recommends that individuals at increased risk for HIV infection, including sexually active MSM, should undergo HIV testing at least annually [13]. According to CDC's Sexually Transmitted Diseases (STDs) Treatment Guidelines, 2010, testing for STDs, including HIV, among MSM is indicated even more frequently (every three to six months) under certain circumstances, such as for MSM with multiple or anonymous partners, MSM having sex in conjunction with illicit drug use, or MSM whose sex partners participate in these activities [14]. Previous analyses suggest that more frequent HIV testing may be beneficial for all MSM, irrespective of self-reported risk behavior [15,16].

The importance of expanding HIV testing in populations disproportionately affected by HIV is described in NHAS [12]. Even before the release of NHAS in 2010, a variety of targeted testing initiatives were being developed at both national and local levels. CDC launched the Expanded HIV Testing Initiative (ETI) in 2007 to facilitate HIV diagnosis and linkage to medical care, focusing on the non-Hispanic black population. ETI was a three-year program intended to increase HIV testing in 25 U.S. jurisdictions; jurisdictions that received ETI funding were required to focus at least 80% of their activities on promoting opt-out HIV screening in high-morbidity clinical settings. With the remainder, they could support innovative methods to increase targeted HIV testing among high-risk populations (e.g., social networking approaches). For all persons newly diagnosed with HIV, jurisdictions had to ensure receipt of test results, linkage to medical care, and referral for partner services [17]. Jurisdictions were awarded between $510,000 and $6 million per year (for a total of $111 million), based proportionately on estimated 2005 AIDS diagnoses among blacks [18]. During 2007–2010, nearly 2.8 million tests were provided and more than 18,000 individuals were newly diagnosed with HIV. Sixty percent of these tests and 70% of the new diagnoses occurred among blacks [17]. A second ETI was funded in 2010 to expand routine testing services to reach a broader array of at-risk populations, including MSM (regardless of race or ethnicity) in 30 U.S. jurisdictions. A third initiative, intended to sustain progress made under the other two initiatives, was launched in 2012, extending eligibility to six additional jurisdictions [19].

Other testing initiatives arose during this time period, focused on populations likely overlapping with those targeted by CDC's ETIs. The Substance Abuse and Mental Health Services Administration (SAMHSA), for example, has funded multiple testing initiatives, including the Rapid HIV Testing Initiative (RHTI) during 2004–2007, designed to reduce HIV incidence among minority populations who may be at an even greater risk for acquiring or transmitting HIV associated with substance abuse and/or a mental health disorder [20]. In the private sector, the pharmaceutical company Gilead launched the HIV FOCUS program in 2010, to reduce the number of undiagnosed individuals through routine HIV screening in 10 cities heavily affected by HIV [21]. This list of initiatives, though far from an exhaustive review, helps illustrate the growing support for targeted testing throughout the public health community in the United States.

To describe HIV testing among MSM in the United States, we analyzed data from the National HIV Behavioral Surveillance System (NHBS). NHBS is a recurring cross-sectional survey designed to monitor selected sexual risk and drug-use behaviors, HIV testing experiences, use of prevention services, and HIV seroprevalence in three populations at high risk for HIV infection: MSM, injecting drug users, and heterosexual adults at increased risk of HIV infection [22]. Although previous analyses have examined differences in testing among various subpopulations of MSM [15,16,23,24], the purpose of this analysis was to understand changes in HIV testing over time. Accordingly, the objectives of this analysis were to describe recent HIV testing (during the 12 months before interview) among MSM in 20 U.S. metropolitan statistical areas (MSAs) in 2008 and 2011, by race/ethnicity and age group, and then to determine if recent HIV testing changed from 2008 to 2011 among MSM, overall and by race/ethnicity and age group.

Methods

National HIV Behavioral Surveillance System

NHBS data are collected in three-year rounds of annual rotating cycles which focus on one population per year; methods for NHBS have been described in detail elsewhere [22,23]. This analysis uses data from the MSM cycles of the second and third rounds of NHBS, conducted in 2008 and 2011 respectively. NHBS was conducted in 21 MSAs in 2008, and in 20 MSAs in 2011; the 20 MSAs common to both rounds were used in this analysis (Atlanta–Sandy Springs–Marietta, GA; Baltimore–Towson, MD; Boston–Cambridge–Quincy, MA–NH: Boston Quincy Division; Chicago–Joliet–Napierville, IL: Chicago–Joliet–Napierville Division; Dallas–Fort Worth–Arlington, TX: Dallas–Plano–Irving Division; Denver–Aurora–Broomfield, CO; Detroit–Warren–Livonia, MI: Detroit–Livonia–Dearborn Division; Houston–Sugar Land–Baytown, TX; Los Angeles–Long Beach–Santa Ana, CA: Los Angeles–Long Beach–Glendale Division; Miami–Ft. Lauderdale– Pompano Beach, FL: Miami Division; New Orleans–Metairie–Kenner, LA; New York–Northern New Jersey–Long Island, NY–NJ–PA: New York–White Plains–Wayne Division; New York–Northern New Jersey–Long Island, NY–NJ–PA: Nassau–Suffolk Division; New York–Northern New Jersey–Long Island, NY–NJ–PA: Newark–Union Division; Philadelphia–Camden– Wilmington, PA–NJ–DE–MD: Philadelphia Division; San Diego–Carlsbad–San Marcos, CA; San Francisco–Oakland–Fremont, CA: San Francisco–San Mateo–Redwood City Division; San Juan–Caguas–Guaynabo, PR; Seattle–Tacoma–Bellevue, WA: Seattle–Bellevue–Everett Division; and Washington–Arlington– Alexandria, DC–VA–MD–WV: Washington–Arlington–Alexandria Division). Together, these MSAs represented approximately 59% of the persons living with diagnosed HIV infection in large urban areas in 2010 [25].

Sampling, Eligibility, and Data Collection

NHBS staff recruited MSM using venue-based (or time-space) sampling (VBS). Because there is no accepted sampling frame for a hidden population like MSM, standard probability-based sampling methods are not possible [26,27]. VBS overcomes this limitation by sampling MSM where they congregate in the highest density, at known venues associated with the population [28]. Prior to recruitment, formative research was performed to identify appropriate venues, such as bars, clubs, social organizations, and street locations, that could be used for recruitment. In 2008, only venues at which 75% of men attending were MSM were eligible for inclusion. By 2011, venues had become more integrated by sexual orientation, thus this threshold was lowered to 50%. For each venue, days and times when MSM frequented these venues were also identified. From this list, venues and corresponding day/time periods were randomly selected for recruitment.

During recruitment, NHBS staff members systematically approached men for participation. For eligible men, informed consent was obtained, after which trained interviewers used a handheld computer to administer an anonymous, face-to-face interview. The standardized questionnaire, which lasted approximately 30 minutes, included questions regarding demographics, HIV-associated behaviors (including HIV testing history), and use of prevention and testing services. All participants, regardless of self-reported HIV infection status, were offered optional HIV testing, which was conducted after the interview in a private space. Participants received incentives for completing the interview and providing a specimen for HIV testing; the value varied by site, but $25 for the interview and an additional $25 for testing was typical.

Although our analysis criteria for both cycles were equivalent, eligibility criteria differed slightly for NHBS in 2008 versus 2011. For both surveys, individuals were considered eligible if they were born male and identified as male, were 18 years or older, had not previously completed any part of the current NHBS-MSM survey, resided in a participating MSA, were able to complete the survey in English or Spanish, and were capable of providing consent. In 2011, another requirement, reporting ever having had oral or anal sex with a man, was added [23].

Ethics Statement

Activities for NHBS were approved by local institutional review boards (IRBs) for each of the 20 participating MSAs. The project underwent a CDC review and approval process; because CDC staff were determined not to be directly engaged for the purposes of NHBS research, CDC IRB approval was not required [29,30]. All participants were explicitly assured during the recruitment process of the anonymous nature of the survey and the HIV testing. No personal identifiers were collected during enrollment, interview, or testing. All participants provided verbal informed consent to take part in the interview and to be tested for HIV. Verbal consent was documented electronically on the survey instrument by interviewers for all participants and on hard copy as required by local IRBs. Because data collection was anonymous, written consent was not possible and participant names or other personal identifiers were not linked to any NHBS instruments. All consent procedures, including verbal consent, were approved by local IRBs and CDC (see Table S1 for specific IRB information).

Analysis Inclusion Criteria

We restricted our analysis to men from the 20 MSAs that participated in both 2008 and 2011 who reported at least one male sex partner in the 12 months before interview and who provided answers to the questions regarding history of HIV testing. Of men who reported a positive HIV test result, we included only those who reported that their first positive test result occurred during the 12 months before interview.

Statistical Analysis

For 2008 and 2011, we compared the percentages of MSM who reported having a recent HIV test, stratified by race/ethnicity and age group. Next, we determined the percentages tested among each racial/ethnic group by age group. Bivariate analysis was performed using the chi-square test. All analyses were performed in SAS 9.3 (SAS Institute, Inc., Cary, NC).

Due to small sample sizes, we combined American Indian/Alaska Native, Asian, Native Hawaiian/other Pacific Islander, and multiple-race participants into one category for further analyses. Multiple-race participants accounted for less than 4% of the total sample both years. We conducted a hierarchical sensitivity analysis to assess the impact of testing among multiple-race blacks on single-race blacks and among multiple-race whites on single-race whites [31]. Specifically, we reclassified all multiple race blacks (including those who were biracial black/white) with the single-race blacks, and then, of the men who were left, we reclassified multiple race whites with the single-race whites. We reran the testing analysis and the results were unchanged. Because the results were similar either way, we left multiple-race blacks and whites with MSM of other/multiple races to be consistent with other NHBS publications.

To determine whether interview year was associated with recent HIV testing, we performed a multivariable analysis. Adjusted prevalence ratios (aPRs), *P*-values, and 95% confidence intervals (95% CIs) were estimated using a Poisson model with a robust standard error via the GENMOD procedure in SAS 9.3 [32]. Our main outcome was recent HIV testing (in the previous 12 months). To account for changes in the demographic composition of the sample and because demographic variables can be associated with HIV testing, the model was adjusted for race/ethnicity, age group, education, income, and MSA. From this model, we estimated the overall increase in recent HIV testing from 2008 to 2011. To explore whether temporal changes in recent HIV testing varied by race/ethnicity or age group, we then added interaction terms for race/ethnicity by interview year and age group by interview year. Next, to understand HIV testing among young MSM when stratified by race/ethnicity, we further expanded our model by adding a three-way interaction of race/ethnicity by age group by interview year, still using the overall sample.

Using the chi-square test, we examined the self-reported number of HIV tests in a two-year period to measure HIV testing frequency for men interviewed in 2008 and 2011. The percentage of men who tested twice in a two-year period was used as a proxy for annual testing; the percentage of men who were tested 3 or more times in two years was used to indicate testing more frequently than annually.

Results

Our analysis included 16,069 MSM (7,943 [49%] from 2008 and 8,126 [51%] from 2011), which includes 298 MSM (145 from 2008 and 153 from 2011) who reported a first positive test result less than 12 months before interview. Response rates for men approached to participate in NHBS in 2008 and 2011 have been described previously [23]. Sample characteristics for the men included in this analysis are presented by year in Table 1. In both years, the largest percentage of the sample was non-Hispanic white (42% in 2008 and 39% in 2011), followed by Hispanic/Latino (26% in 2008 and 27% in 2011), and then non-Hispanic black (24% in 2008 and 26% in 2011). The median age of the sample was 31 years in 2008 and 30 years in 2011.

Unadjusted prevalence of recent HIV testing in 2008 and 2011, as shown in Table 2, demonstrates an increase from 63% in 2008 to 67% in 2011 overall ($P<0.001$), from 63% to 71% among black MSM ($P<0.001$), and from 63% to 75% ($P<0.001$) among MSM of other/multiple races. Increases were not statistically significant for Hispanic/Latino MSM (from 63% to 65%, $P=0.2$) or white MSM (from 64% to 66%, $P=0.2$). Multivariable analyses demonstrate an overall adjusted increase in recent HIV testing (aPR = 1.07, $P<0.001$). This increase varied significantly by race/ethnicity ($P<0.001$ for the interaction term). Consistent with the unadjusted results, the adjusted increases in testing were significant for black MSM (aPR = 1.12, $P<0.001$) and MSM of other/multiple races (aPR = 1.20, $P<0.001$) (Table 2).

Table 1. Sample characteristics by year among men who have sex with men — National HIV Behavioral Surveillance System, 20 U.S. cities, 2008 and 2011.

	2008		2011	
	No.	(%)	No.	(%)
Total	7943		8126	
Race/Ethnicity*				
American Indian/Alaska Native	42	(1)	63	(1)
Asian/Native Hawaiian/Other Pacific Islanders	257	(3)	255	(3)
Black/African American	1926	(24)	2130	(26)
Hispanic/Latino	2037	(26)	2171	(27)
White	3361	(42)	3198	(39)
Multiple races	314	(4)	289	(4)
Age group (years)				
18–19	445	(6)	357	(4)
20–24	1509	(19)	1894	(23)
25–29	1561	(20)	1612	(20)
30–39	2194	(28)	1901	(23)
≥40	2234	(28)	2362	(29)
Education				
< High School	509	(6)	434	(5)
High School diploma or GED	1839	(23)	1961	(24)
Some college or technical degree	2537	(32)	2729	(34)
College degree or postgraduate education	3057	(38)	3002	(37)
Annual Household Income				
≤$19,999	2288	(29)	2484	(31)
$20,000–$39,000	2018	(25)	1983	(24)
$40,000–$74,999	1949	(25)	1958	(24)
≥$75,000	1563	(20)	1565	(19)

Percentages may not add to 100, due to rounding or missing values.
*Hispanics/Latinos can be of any race; categories are mutually exclusive.

The increase in recent testing did not vary overall by age group ($P = 0.4$ for the interaction term). Nevertheless, knowing that young MSM, and particularly young black MSM, are disproportionately affected by HIV, we investigated further, using the three-way interaction of race/ethnicity by age group by interview year to clarify differences in recent HIV testing by race/ethnicity among the youngest MSM. Although adjusted increases in recent HIV testing (Table 2) were not significant for young MSM aged 18–19 years (aPR = 1.05, $P = 0.3$), black MSM aged 18–19 years experienced significant increases in recent HIV testing (aPR = 1.20, $P = 0.007$), while MSM aged 18–19 years of other racial/ethnic groups did not (Table 3).

As shown in Figure 1, the distribution of HIV testing frequency among MSM during the 2 years before interview changed from 2008 to 2011 ($P<0.001$). The percentage of men who tested one time or less in the 2 years before interview (less than annually) decreased from 40% in 2008 to 34% in 2011. The percentage who tested twice in two years (annually) was similar (23% to 22%), while the percentage of men who tested three or more times in two years (more than annually) increased from 37% to 44%.

Discussion

In this analysis of NHBS data from 20 U.S. MSAs, we found that recent HIV testing increased among MSM from 2008 to 2011. Increases were more substantial among certain racial/ethnic groups, specifically black MSM. Increases were also substantial for MSM of other/multiple races, however, these men accounted for a small percentage of the total sample. Although we did not see significant increases in recent HIV testing among the youngest MSM overall, we did see significant increases among young black MSM, a subpopulation particularly affected by HIV. These differential increases might reflect an effect of testing initiatives focused on populations disproportionately affected by HIV.

Even in 2011, only 67% of the MSM participating in NHBS had been tested for HIV during the previous 12 months. According to NHBS data from 2008, the main reasons for not undergoing recent HIV testing included a perception of being at low risk for HIV infection, followed by a fear of testing positive, followed by a lack of time [22]; results for 2011 were similar (unpublished NHBS data). Data from another survey suggest that recent HIV testing may be even lower in different populations, for instance, MSM from smaller cities or rural areas. The National Survey of Family Growth (NSFG) estimates that only 39% of sexually active MSM interviewed during 2006–2010 had been

Table 2. HIV testing in previous 12 months among men who have sex with men — National HIV Behavioral Surveillance System, 20 U.S. cities, 2008 and 2011.

	2008		2011			aPR		
	No. Tested	(%)	No. Tested	(%)	*P*-value*	2011 vs 2008	(95% CI)	*P*-value†
Interview year§	5026	(63)	5478	(67)	**<0.001**	**1.07**	**(1.05,1.09)**	**<0.001**
Race/Ethnicity by interview year¶**								
Black/African American	1213	(63)	1510	(71)	**<0.001**	**1.12**	**(1.07,1.17)**	**<0.001**
Hispanic/Latino	1275	(63)	1402	(65)	0.2	1.02	(0.98,1.08)	0.3
White	2146	(64)	2096	(66)	0.2	1.03	(0.98,1.07)	0.2
Other/multiple races	387	(63)	456	(75)	**<0.001**	**1.20**	**(1.11,1.30)**	**<0.001**
Age group by interview year¶								
18–19	288	(65)	238	(67)	0.6	1.05	(0.95,1.17)	0.3
20–24	1045	(69)	1364	(72)	0.08	**1.06**	**(1.02,1.11)**	**0.008**
25–29	1066	(68)	1180	(73)	**0.002**	**1.10**	**(1.05,1.15)**	**<0.001**
30–39	1425	(65)	1322	(70)	**0.002**	**1.10**	**(1.05,1.15)**	**<0.001**
≥40	1202	(54)	1374	(58)	**0.003**	**1.14**	**(1.08,1.20)**	**<0.001**

aPR = Adjusted Prevalence Ratio and CI = Confidence Interval.
*Unadjusted *P*-value.
†Adjusted *P*-value.
§Adjusted for race/ethnicity, age group, education, income, and MSA; aPR presented for interview year.
¶Adjusted for race/ethnicity, age group, education, income, MSA, race/ethnicity by interview year, and age group by interview year; aPR presented for the interaction terms, race/ethnicity by interview year and age group by interview year.
**Hispanics/Latinos can be of any race; categories are mutually exclusive.

Table 3. HIV testing in previous 12 months, stratified by race/ethnicity and age group, among men who have sex with men — National HIV Behavioral Surveillance System, 20 U.S. cities, 2008 and 2011.

	2008		2011					
	No. Tested	(%)	No. Tested	(%)	*P*-value*	aPR† 2011 vs 2008	(95% CI)	*P*-value†
Race/Ethnicity§ by age group by interview year								
Black/African American								
18–19	137	(65)	129	(77)	**0.009**	**1.20**	**(1.05,1.38)**	**0.007**
20–24	361	(71)	508	(76)	**0.03**	1.07	(0.999,1.15)	0.055
25–29	247	(66)	323	(75)	**0.006**	**1.12**	**(1.03,1.23)**	**0.01**
30–39	282	(62)	296	(73)	**<0.001**	**1.16**	**(1.06,1.27)**	**0.002**
≥40	186	(49)	254	(55)	0.1	1.12	(0.98,1.27)	0.09
Hispanic/Latino								
18–19	95	(66)	72	(55)	0.06	0.87	(0.72,1.06)	0.2
20–24	277	(64)	401	(68)	0.1	1.08	(0.98,1.18)	0.1
25–29	284	(66)	302	(67)	0.9	0.98	(0.89,1.07)	0.7
30–39	389	(66)	376	(69)	0.4	1.04	(0.96,1.13)	0.3
≥40	230	(52)	251	(56)	0.2	1.08	(0.96,1.22)	0.2
White								
18–19	39	(63)	23	(58)	0.6	0.87	(0.62,1.21)	0.4
20–24	312	(71)	328	(69)	0.5	0.98	(0.90,1.07)	0.7
25–29	429	(72)	432	(74)	0.3	1.05	(0.98,1.12)	0.2
30–39	642	(66)	531	(68)	0.4	1.03	(0.97,1.10)	0.3
≥40	724	(56)	782	(59)	0.1	**1.07**	**(1.003,1.14)**	**0.04**
Other/multiple races								
18–19	17	(61)	13	(72)	0.4	1.21	(0.78,1.88)	0.4
20–24	93	(75)	125	(78)	0.5	1.04	(0.91,1.19)	0.5
25–29	105	(65)	119	(83)	**<0.001**	**1.32**	**(1.15,1.51)**	**<0.001**
30–39	111	(63)	113	(70)	0.1	1.12	(0.96,1.30)	0.1
≥40	61	(50)	86	(69)	**0.002**	**1.44**	**(1.17,1.79)**	**<0.001**

aPR = Adjusted Prevalence Ratio and CI = Confidence Interval.
*Unadjusted *P*-value.
†Adjusted for race/ethnicity, age group, education, income, MSA, race/ethnicity by interview year, age group by interview year, race/ethnicity by age group, and race/ethnicity by age group by interview year; aPR presented for the three-way interaction term, race/ethnicity by age group by interview year.
§Hispanics/Latinos can be of any race; categories are mutually exclusive.

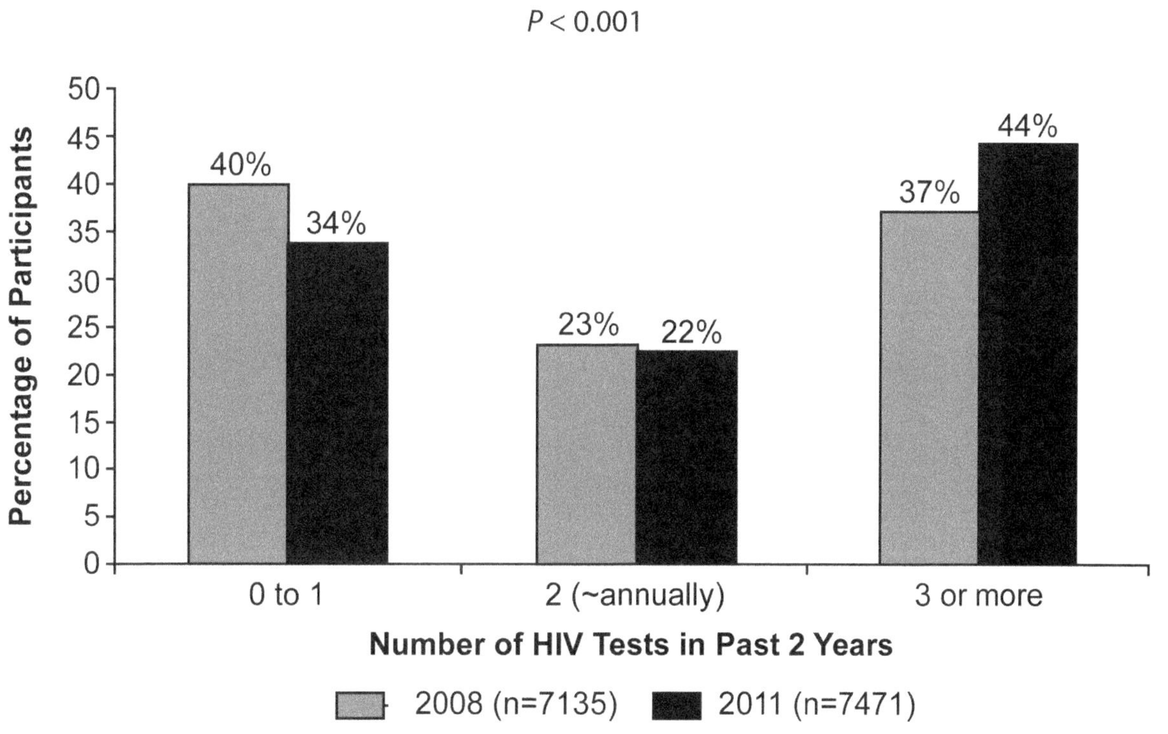

Figure 1. Number of HIV tests in a two-year period among MSM in 2008 and 2011. During the interview, NHBS participants were asked to report their HIV testing frequency in the two years before interview. Testing twice in a two-year period was used as a proxy for annual testing. The distribution of HIV testing frequency among MSM during the 2 years before interview, shown here, changed from 2008 to 2011 ($P<0.001$). The percentage of men who tested one time or less in the 2 years before interview (less than annually) decreased from 40% in 2008 to 34% in 2011. The percentage who tested twice in two years (annually) was similar (23% to 22%), while the percentage of men who tested three or more times in two years (more than annually) increased from 37% to 44%.

tested for HIV in the previous 12 months [33]. Although differences in the geographic areas, sampling methods, and mode of interview administration between NSFG and NHBS limit the comparability of the results, the basic message is the same; measures of recent HIV testing among MSM suggest that CDC recommendations for HIV testing frequency among MSM—that all sexually active MSM undergo HIV testing at least annually—have not yet been met. Although increases in recent HIV testing were observed in our analysis, there is more work to be done to increase HIV testing among populations most affected by HIV. HIV testing continues to play a critical role in the fight against HIV [7–10], and additional HIV testing efforts might benefit the MSM population.

Of MSM participating in NHBS who had tested for HIV in the previous 12 months, 5% were HIV-positive but unaware of their infection in 2011 [16], while 7% were in 2008 [15]. Furthermore, of the participants in both 2008 and 2011 who were found to be HIV-positive but unaware of their infection, approximately one third had been tested for HIV during the past six months [15,16]. These data suggest that, at least among sexually active MSM, annual testing may not be sufficient. In populations with a high HIV burden, more frequent HIV testing may be indicated. In our analysis, we found that the percentage of MSM who tested at least three times during the two years before interview increased, perhaps an early sign that at least some MSM are undergoing HIV testing more frequently.

A recently published analysis of 2008 and 2011 NHBS data showed that HIV prevalence among MSM participating in NHBS was stable from 2008 to 2011, however, awareness of infection among HIV-positive MSM increased during that time period [23]. Increased testing, among other factors such as reduced HIV stigma, may be contributing to the increase in awareness of HIV infection [34]. HIV surveillance data show that the annual number of HIV diagnoses among MSM continues to increase [4]. Increased testing, in addition to other factors such as increased incidence [2], may help explain this increase in diagnoses. Additional analyses are needed to examine this hypothesis and relationship.

This analysis is subject to several limitations. First, because the data were collected in 20 large MSAs with high HIV burden and most men were recruited from bars or dance clubs, study findings may be generalizable only to MSM who attend venues in large urban areas. Recruiting participants at venues, as is done with VBS, may result in selection bias; these data are not weighted to account for bias. Furthermore, the venue inclusion criteria changed from 2008 to 2011. Next, because date of most recent HIV test was self-reported, social desirability and recall biases may affect estimates. Finally, this study is cross-sectional and cannot be linked to any particular testing initiative, including CDC's ETI, thus causality cannot be established. Seventeen of the 20 NHBS sites were among the original 25 ETI jurisdictions, but despite the considerable overlap, NHBS was not designed to evaluate ETI.

Conclusions

As theorized in national strategic initiatives, achieving increased awareness of HIV infection through HIV testing is an important step towards reducing new HIV infections by leading to linkage to and engagement in HIV care, viral suppression, and behavioral change [7–10]. We found that recent HIV testing increased from

2008 to 2011 among black MSM, including young black MSM, which are populations disproportionately affected by HIV. HIV testing initiatives focused on populations most affected by HIV might be having a positive effect. While the finding of increased HIV testing among certain populations is encouraging, our analysis demonstrates that improved coverage of HIV testing is needed to meet CDC recommendations.

Supporting Information

Table S1 National HIV Behavioral Surveillance System (NHBS): Local institutional review boards (IRBs) by Metropolitan Statistical Area (MSA).

Acknowledgments

We would like to thank all of the NHBS 2008 and 2011 participants.

We would also like to thank members of the NHBS Study Group: Atlanta, GA: Jennifer Taussig, Robert Gern, Tamika Hoyte, Laura Salazar, Jianglan White, Jeff Todd, Greg Bautista; Baltimore, MD: Colin Flynn, Frangiscos Sifakis, Danielle German; Boston, MA: Debbie Isenberg, Maura Driscoll, Elizabeth Hurwitz, Miminos, Rose Doherty, Chris Wittke; Chicago, IL: Nikhil Prachand, Nanette Benbow; Dallas, TX: Sharon Melville, Praveen Pannala, Richard Yeager, Aaron Sayegh, Jim Dyer, Shane Sheu, Alicia Novoa; Denver, CO: Mark Thrun, Alia Al-Tayyib, Ralph Wilmoth; Detroit, MI: Emily Higgins, Vivian Griffin, Eve Mokotoff, Karen MacMaster; Houston, TX: Marcia Wolverton, Jan Risser, Hafeez Rehman, Paige Padgett; Los Angeles, CA: Trista Bingham, Ekow Kwa Sey; Miami, FL: Marlene LaLota, Lisa Metsch, David Forrest, Dano Beck, Gabriel Cardenas; Nassau-Suffolk, NY: Chris Nemeth, Bridget J. Anderson, Carol-Ann Watson, Lou Smith; New Orleans, LA: William T. Robinson, DeAnn Gruber, Narquis Barak; New York City, NY: Chris Murrill, Alan Neaigus, Samuel Jenness, Holly Hagan, Kathleen H. Reilly, Travis Wendel; Newark, NJ: Helene Cross, Barbara Bolden, Sally D'Errico, Afework Wogayehu, Henry Godette; Philadelphia, PA: Kathleen A. Brady, Althea Kirkland, Andrea Sifferman; San Diego, CA: Vanessa Miguelino-Keasling, Al Velasco, Veronica Tovar; San Francisco, CA: H. Fisher Raymond; San Juan, PR: Sandra Miranda De Leo'n, Yadira Rolo'n- Colo'n, Melissa Marzan; Seattle, WA: Maria Courogen, Tom Jaenicke, Hanne Thiede, Richard Burt; Washington, DC: Yujiang Jia,Jenevieve Opoku, Marie Sansone, Tiffany West, Manya Magnus, Irene Kuo; Behavioral Surveillance Team.

The findings and conclusions in this paper are those of the authors and do not necessarily represent the official position of the Centers for Disease Control and Prevention.

Author Contributions

Conceived and designed the experiments: LAC AMO CW GPB. Analyzed the data: LAC AMO CER CW BCL GPB. Contributed to the writing of the manuscript: LAC AMO CW GPB.

References

1. Centers for Disease Control and Prevention (2013) Monitoring Selected National HIV Prevention and Care Objectives by Using HIV Surveillance Data—United States and 6 Dependent Areas—2011. HIV Surveillance Supplemental Report. 18 (No.5). http://www.cdc.gov/hiv/library/reports/surveillance/. Accessed 2013 Nov 15.
2. Centers for Disease Control and Prevention (2012) Estimated HIV incidence in the United States, 2007–2010. HIV Surveillance Supplemental Report. 17(No.4). http://www.cdc.gov/hiv/topics/surveillance/resources/reports/#supplemental. Accessed 2013 Nov 15.
3. Purcell DW, Johnson CH, Lansky A, Prejean J, Stein R, et al. (2012) Estimating the population size of men who have sex with men in the United States to obtain HIV and syphilis rates. Open AIDS J 6: 98–107.
4. Centers for Disease Control and Prevention (2013) HIV Surveillance Report, 2011, vol 23. http://www.cdc.gov/hiv/topics/surveillance/resources/reports/. Accessed 2013 Nov 15.
5. U.S. Census Bureau (2010) Profile of General Population and Housing Characteristics: 2010. http://www.census.gov/. Accessed 2013 Aug 29.
6. Centers for Disease Control and Prevention HIV Surveillance Slide Set: HIV Surveillance in Men Who Have Sex with Men (MSM). http://www.cdc.gov/hiv/library/slideSets/index.html. Accessed 2014 Jan 13.
7. Castel AD, Greenberg AE, Befus M, Willis S, Samala R, et al. (2013) Temporal association between expanded HIV testing and improvements in population-based HIV/AIDS clinical outcomes, District of Columbia. AIDS Care 26: 785–789.
8. Weinhardt LS, Carey MP, Johnson BT, Bickham NL (1999) Effects of HIV counseling and testing on sexual risk behavior: a meta-analytic review of published research, 1985–1997. Am J Public Health 89: 1397–1405.
9. Marks G, Crepaz N, Senterfitt JW, Janssen RS (2005) Meta-analysis of high-risk sexual behavior in persons aware and unaware they are infected with HIV in the United States: implications for HIV prevention programs. J Acquir Immune Defic Syndr 39: 446–453.
10. Marks G, Crepaz N, Janssen RS (2006) Estimating sexual transmission of HIV from persons aware and unaware that they are infected with the virus in the USA. AIDS 20: 1447–1450.
11. U.S. Department of Health and Human Services (2010) Healthy People 2020. http://www.healthypeople.gov/2020/topicsobjectives2020/overview.aspx?topicid = 22 Accessed 2013 Nov 20.
12. Office of National AIDS Policy (2010) National HIV/AIDS Strategy. http://www.whitehouse.gov/sites/default/files/uploads/NHAS.pdf. Accessed 2013 Nov 9.
13. Branson BM, Handsfield HH, Lampe MA, Janssen RS, Taylor AW, et al. (2006) Revised recommendations for HIV testing of adults, adolescents, and pregnant women in health-care settings. MMWR Recomm Rep 55: 1–17; quiz CE11-14.
14. Workowski KA, Berman S (2010) Sexually transmitted diseases treatment guidelines, 2010. MMWR Recomm Rep 59: 1–110.
15. Centers for Disease Control and Prevention (2011) HIV testing among men who have sex with men—21 cities, United States, 2008. MMWR Morb Mortal Wkly Rep 60: 694–699.
16. Centers for Disease Control and Prevention (2013) HIV Testing and Risk Behaviors Among Gay, Bisexual, and Other Men Who Have Sex with Men - United States. MMWR Morb Mortal Wkly Rep 62: 958–962.
17. Centers for Disease Control and Prevention (2011) Results of the Expanded HIV Testing Initiative—25 jurisdictions, United States, 2007–2010. MMWR Morb Mortal Wkly Rep 60: 805–810.
18. Centers for Disease Control and Prevention (2007) Funding Opportunity Announcement CDC-PS07-768. http://www.cdc.gov/od/pgo/funding/PS07-768.htm. Accessed 2014 May 19.
19. Centers for Disease Control and Prevention (2012) Expanded Testing Initiative Overview. http://www.cdc.gov/hiv/resources/factsheets/PDF/HIV-ETP.pdf. Accessed: 2014 May 6.
20. Substance Abuse & Mental Health Services Administration (2004) SAMHSA's Rapid HIV Testing Initiative (RHTI). http://www.samhsa.gov/hivhep/rhti_factsheet02.aspx. Accessed 2013 Nov 20.
21. Gilead (2012) Gilead's HIV Focus Program. http://www.gilead.com/responsibility/hiv-focus-program. Accessed 11/20/2013.
22. Finlayson TJ, Le B, Smith A, Bowles K, Cribbin M, et al. (2011) HIV risk, prevention, and testing behaviors among men who have sex with men—National HIV Behavioral Surveillance System, 21 U.S. cities, United States, 2008. MMWR Surveill Summ 60: 1–34.
23. Wejnert C, Le B, Rose CE, Oster AM, Smith AJ, et al. (2013) HIV Infection and Awareness among Men Who Have Sex with Men-20 Cities, United States, 2008 and 2011. PLOS ONE 8: e76878.
24. Oster AM, Russell K, Wiegand RE, Valverde E, Forrest DW, et al. (2013) HIV infection and testing among Latino men who have sex with men in the United States: the role of location of birth and other social determinants. PLoS One 8: e73779.
25. Centers for Disease Control and Prevention (2013) Diagnosed HIV Infection among Adults and Adolescents in Metropolitan Statistical Areas—United States and Puerto Rico, 2011. HIV Surveillance Supplemental Report. 18 (No.8). http://www.cdc.gov/hiv/library/reports/surveillance/index.html. Accessed 2013 Nov 15.
26. Semaan S, Heckathorn DD, Des Jarlais DC, Garfein RS (2010) Ethical considerations in surveys employing respondent-driven sampling. Am J Public Health 100: 582–583; author reply 583–584.
27. Semaan S, Lauby J, Liebman J (2002) Street and network sampling in evaluation studies of HIV risk-reduction interventions. AIDS Rev 4: 213–223.
28. MacKellar DA, Gallagher KM, Finlayson T, Sanchez T, Lansky A, et al. (2007) Surveillance of HIV risk and prevention behaviors of men who have sex with men—a national application of venue-based, time-space sampling. Public Health Rep 122 Suppl 1: 39–47.
29. Centers for Disease Control and Prevention (1999) Guidelines for defining public health research and public health non-research. Atlanta, GA.
30. Code of Federal Regulations (1991) Protection of human subjects. 45 CFR 46.
31. Office of Management and Budget (2000) Provisional Guidance on the Implementation of the 1997 Standards for Federal Data on Race and Ethnicity, Appendix C: The Bridge Report: Tabulation Options for Trend Analysis.

http://www.whitehouse.gov/omb/inforeg_statpolicy#dr. Accessed 2014 Jun 20.

32. Barros AJ, Hirakata VN (2003) Alternatives for logistic regression in cross-sectional studies: an empirical comparison of models that directly estimate the prevalence ratio. BMC Med Res Methodol 3: 21.
33. Chandra A BV, Copen CE, Balaji A, Dinenno E (2012) HIV Testing in the U.S household population aged 15–44: data from the National Survey of Family Growth, 2006–2010. http://www.cdc.gov/nchs/data/nhsr/nhsr058.pdf. Accessed 2013 Sept 19.
34. Herek GM, Capitanio JP, Widaman KF (2002) HIV-related stigma and knowledge in the United States: prevalence and trends, 1991–1999. Am J Public Health 92: 371–377.

8

Sociodemographic Factors and Prejudice toward HIV and Hepatitis B/C Status in a Working-Age Population: Results from a National, Cross-Sectional Study in Japan

Hisashi Eguchi[1], Koji Wada[2]*, Derek R. Smith[3]

1 Department of Public Health, Kitasato University School of Medicine, Sagamihara, Kanagawa, Japan, **2** National Center for Global Health and Medicine, Tokyo, Japan, **3** School of Health Sciences, Faculty of Health, University of Newcastle, Ourimbah, Australia

Abstract

Background: In many countries, HIV, hepatitis B virus (HBV), and hepatitis C virus (HCV) infected individuals may face discrimination and mistreatment from coworkers. Effective interventions to reduce workplace discrimination are therefore needed to protect these vulnerable populations. The current study investigated potential associations between sociodemographic factors and prejudice toward HIV and HBV/HCV infected colleagues within a Japanese working population.

Methods: An online anonymous, nationwide internet survey was administered to a cross-section of approximately 3,000 individuals in Japan. The survey comprised 14 questions focusing on demographics (five items), basic HIV or HBV/HCV knowledge (eight items), and potential prejudice toward HIV or HBV/HCV infected colleagues (one item). The sociodemographic characteristics evaluated were sex, age, educational level, employment status, and individual income; with multiple logistic regression used for the analysis.

Results: In total, 3,055 individuals were recruited for the HIV related survey and 3,129 for the HBV/HCV related survey. Older age was significantly and positively associated with prejudice toward HIV infected colleagues ($p<0.01$) and negatively associated with prejudice toward HBV/HCV infected colleagues ($p<0.01$). Statistically significant associations were not observed between other sociodemographic characteristics and potential prejudice toward HIV and HBV/HCV infected coworkers.

Conclusion: Overall, this study suggests that age may be associated with prejudice toward HIV and HBV/HCV infected colleagues among the working age population of Japan. As such, policy makers should consider the age of participants when formulating efforts to reduce prejudice toward HIV and HBV/HCV infected workers.

Editor: Ratna B. Ray, Saint Louis University, United States of America

Funding: This study was funded by the Health Labour Sciences Research Grant of the Ministry of Health, Labour, and Welfare (H23-practical-Hepatitis-general-005). The funders had no role in the study design, data collection and analysis, decision to publish, or manuscript preparation.

Competing Interests: The authors have declared that no competing interests exist.

* E-mail: kwada-sgy@umin.ac.jp

Introduction

Research suggests that individuals diagnosed with HIV or HBV/HCV may face abuse, discrimination, and unfair treatment from coworkers [1] [2]. Furthermore, employers are often reluctant to hire people diagnosed with HIV, and may even dismiss a newly-diagnosed employee [3]. As a result, seropositive workers often avoid disclosing their infection status to employers in order to avoid prejudice and disadvantage [4] [5].

HBV/HCV infection initially entered the general Japanese population through blood transfusions, acupuncture, tattooing, and skin injury [6]. The spread of HCV infection was caused primarily by viral-contaminated blood products; and approximately 10,000 cases of infection occurred in individuals who received these products up to 1988 [7]. In recent years, the horizontal incidence of HBV/HCV infection in Japan has decreased steadily from 1.43% to 0.10% in men, and from 0.95% to 0.03% in women; although HBV carriers are most numerous in the 50–59 year age group, and the estimated number of HCV carriers is highest in individuals older than 50 years [8].

Intervention programs intended to improve the general population's knowledge of HIV and HBV/HCV and reduce stigma have often been inconsistent [9]. Older age independently predicted a stronger discriminatory attitude in a study from Hong Kong [10] for example, while it decreased the likelihood of receiving HIV screening in a previous study from the United States (US) [11]. Cultural values and social-cognitive factors are also known to affect HBV screening intention [12].

To the authors' knowledge, no studies have yet explored the association between sociodemographic factors and prejudice toward HIV and HBV/HCV infected colleagues in Japanese working populations. As such, the current study was undertaken to examine associations between sociodemographic factors and prejudice toward HIV and HBV/HCV infected colleagues in this large demographic. We hypothesized that sociodemographic factors may effect prejudice toward HIV and HBV/HCV infected colleagues.

Methods

Participants and conduct of the survey

This study comprised a HIV related survey and a HBV/HCV related survey. Around 3,000 individuals of working age (between 20 and 69 years of age), without sex or age bias, were randomly extracted from the registry of an Internet research company (among a randomly selected group of 7,937 persons from a total of 1.60 million registrants), and a survey of this population was then carried out via the Internet in September 2011. A random number generator was used to select participants, with the study population itself comprising of individuals who were interested in participating a survey with financial incentives for responding. The web survey company contacted selected registrants to respond to the survey and ceased recruitment when the total number of participants reached the target number. Sample size calculation was based on an expected percentage of having prejudiced toward HIV and HBV/HCV infected colleagues of 40% with an expected confidence interval precision of ± 5% [13]. The minimum sample size required was 248 participants. Participants were recruited in clusters, targeting 300 individuals for each sex in each age group. The survey consisted of 14 questions on each participant's sociodemographic characteristics (five items), basic knowledge of factors affecting HIV or HBV/HCV (eight items), and potential prejudice toward HIV or HBV/HCV infected colleagues. The sociodemographic characteristics investigated were sex, age, educational level, employment status, and individual income.

Participant characteristics

Age was stratified into five groups: 20–29, 30–39, 40–49, 50–59, and 60–69 years. Educational level was divided into four categories as follows: lower than or equal to high school graduation; technical college or junior college; higher than university; and others. Employment status was classified into five groups: manager, regular employee, non-regular employee, others, and student. The other employment status included: unemployment, agriculture, fishery, forestry, and self-employed business owners. Annual individual income was classified in three equal groups as follows: low, <1 million yen (<12,500 US$); middle, 1–3 million yen (12,500–24,999 US$); and high, >3 million yen (≥ 25,000 US$) (with an exchange rate of 1 US$ equaling around 80 Japanese yen at the time).

HIV or HBV/HCV knowledge and prejudice toward infected colleagues

Eight questions were developed based on previous studies, with responses measured on a two-point scale (0 = No, I did not know, or 1 = Yes, I knew). Cronbach's alpha was 0.82 for the HIV related survey and 0.92 for the HBV/HCV related survey. The sum of each item was calculated, with the higher score suggesting greater knowledge on HIV and HBV/HCV. Prejudice toward HIV and HBV/HCV infected individuals was determined based on the response to the following question: "If I found that people with whom I work were infected with HIV or HBV/HCV, I think I would look at him/her to be a homosexual, someone who engaged in sexual relationships with an unspecified number of people, or a drug addict."

Participant responses toward HIV infected individuals were initially measured on a five-point scale (1 = I think so; 2 = I think so, to a degree; 3 = I do not really think so; 4 = I do not think so at all; and 5 = not sure), and then further dichotomized into a two-point scale (1 = I think so and I think so to a degree; and 0 = I do not really think so and I do not think so at all). The "Not sure" (5) response on the initial five-point scale (n = 230) was omitted during analysis to allow for a direct comparison between results from the HIV and the HBV/HCV related surveys. Responses to the HBV/HCV related survey were initially measured on a four-point scale (1 = I think so; 2 = I think so to a degree; 3 = I do not really think so; and 4 = I do not think so at all), and then further dichotomized into a two-point scale (1 = I think so and I think so to a degree; and 0 = I do not really think so and I do not think so at all).

Statistical analysis

Multiple logistic regression analyses were used to investigate the associations between each sociodemographic factors and prejudice toward HIV and HBV/HCV infected colleagues. Given that the outcome of interest was not rare, we subsequently applied Zhang's formula of adjustment when calculating the results [14]. Statistical analysis was performed using SPSS version 17.0 (IBM, Chicago, IL, USA). A two-tailed p value of 0.05 was considered significant, unless otherwise indicated.

Ethics

The study aims and protocol were approved by the institutional ethics committee of Kitasato University School of Medicine in 2011. Participants were informed in advance that their participation was strictly voluntary and that all information provided would remain confidential. Individuals who consented to participate in the survey were able to access a designated website upon verification of their personal information, after which time they could then complete the survey online. Participants had the option to not respond to any part of the questionnaire at any time, and also the option to discontinue the survey at any point. Consent was implied based on voluntary participation according to the ethics code for public health research in Japan [15].

Results

The survey was sent to 7,937 individuals and closed after each stratum of gender and age group reached its target sample size. Recruitment was terminated when the number of participants reached 3,055 in the HIV related survey and 3,129 in the HBV/HCV related survey. Each of the five age groups (20–29, 30–39, 40–49, 50–59, and 60–69 years old) contained approximately 20% of the total participants. Participant characteristics are summarized in Table 1. Educational level distribution was significantly different between participants of the HIV and HBV/HCV related surveys ($p<0.01$). Mean HIV knowledge score was higher than the mean HBV/HCV knowledge score ($p<0.01$). Participants answering, "strongly agree" and "agree" about prejudice toward infected colleagues constituted 39.8% and 23.7% of total participants in the HIV and HBV/HCV related surveys, respectively.

Table 2 summarizes the associations between sociodemographic factors and prejudice toward infected colleagues. The age and educational level distributions were significantly different in the HIV related survey ($p<0.01$, 0.03 respectively). The HIV knowledge score of "strongly agree" and "agree" respondents was also lower than that observed among the "disagree and strongly disagree" respondents ($p<0.01$). Sex, age, employment status, and individual income distributions were significantly different in the HBV/HCV related survey ($p<0.01$, 0.01, 0.01, and 0.04, respectively). The HBV/HCV knowledge score of "strongly agree" and "agree" respondents was lower than

Table 1. Participant characteristics.

	HIV		HBV/HCV		p
	n = 3,055	(%)	n = 3,129	(%)	
Sex					
Male	1,532	(50.1)	1,549	(49.5)	0.61
Female	1,523	(49.9)	1,580	(50.5)	
Age (yr)					
20–29	607	(19.9)	618	(19.8)	1.00
30–39	611	(20.0)	628	(20.1)	
40–49	612	(20.0)	627	(20.0)	
50–59	616	(20.2)	632	(20.2)	
60–69	609	(19.9)	624	(19.9)	
Educational level					
Junior high school or high school	878	(28.7)	693	(22.1)	<0.01
Technical college or junior college	767	(25.1)	572	(18.3)	
University and graduate school	1,368	(44.8)	1,084	(34.6)	
Others	42	(1.4)	780	(24.9)	
Employment status					
Manager	244	(8.0)	231	(7.4)	0.78
Regular employee	852	(27.9)	845	(27.0)	
Non-regular employee	522	(17.1)	540	(17.3)	
Undergraduate student	201	(6.6)	211	(6.7)	
Others	1236	(40.5)	1302	(41.6)	
Individual income					
Low (<1 million yen/year)	1,210	(39.6)	1,236	(39.5)	0.07
Middle (1–3 million yen/year)	1,052	(34.4)	1,149	(36.7)	
High (>3 million yen/year)	793	(26.0)	744	(23.8)	
Having prejudiced opinions about infected colleagues					
Strongly agree and agree	1,215	(39.8)	742	(23.7)	-
Disagree and strongly disagree	1,610	(52.7)	2,387	(76.3)	
Not sure	230	(7.5)	-	-	
	Mean	SD	Mean	SD	
Knowledge score (0–8)	6.64	1.91	5.33	2.94	<0.01

observed in the "disagree" and "strongly disagree" respondents ($p<0.01$).

Logistic regression analyses revealed that older age was significantly associated with increased prejudice toward HIV infected colleagues ($p<0.01$) and decreased prejudice toward HBV/HCV infected colleagues ($p<0.01$), after adjusting for other sociodemographic factors and basic knowledge (Table 3). Sex, educational level, employment status, and individual income were not significantly associated with prejudice toward HIV or HBV/HCV infected colleagues.

Discussion

In the current study we investigated associations between sociodemographic factors and prejudice toward HIV and HBV/HCV infected colleagues among the Japanese working age demographic for what appears to be the first time. Our findings suggest that older age was independently associated with increased prejudice toward HIV infected colleagues and decreased prejudice toward HBV/HCV infected colleagues, after controlling for other sociodemographic factors and knowledge level. No other associations between other sociodemographic factors and these attitudes were elucidated in the current study. These results suggest that health promotion authorities should carefully consider the target population age when implementing interventions to reduce prejudice toward HIV and HBV/HCV infected colleagues in the workplace in Japan, as elsewhere.

It is reasonable to hypothesize that age reflects an individual's historical background, and therefore, may play an important contextual role in their reaction toward HIV. Our current findings are consistent with previous research which found that older age was independently associated with increased prejudice toward HIV infected colleagues [10] [16]. Individuals older than 40 years of age experienced the so-called 'AIDS panic' of January of 1987, which was caused by media reports of a Japanese woman in Kobe who had been diagnosed with AIDS, and died soon after the initial report. It has been suggested that this particular panic rose from a societal concern that the government was unable to prevent HIV from entering Japan [17]. From this the resulting panic sharply increased negative information about HIV in the Japanese mass

Table 2. Statistical associations between socio-demographic factors and prejudiced attitudes towards infected colleagues.

	Prejudiced toward infected HIV colleagues (n = 3,055)							Prejudice toward infected HBV/HCV colleagues (n = 3,129)				
	Strongly agree and agree	**(%)**	**Disagree and strongly disagree**	**(%)**	**Not sure**	**(%)**	**p**	**Strongly agree and agree**	**(%)**	**Disagree and strongly disagree**	**(%)**	**p**
Sex												
Male	629	(41.1)	790	(51.6)	113	(7.4)	0.35	409	(26.4)	1140	(73.6)	<0.01
Female	586	(38.5)	820	(53.8)	117	(7.7)		333	(21.1)	1247	(78.9)	
Age												
20–29	209	(34.4)	343	(56.5)	55	(9.1)	<0.01	174	(28.2)	444	(71.8)	0.01
30–39	226	(37.0)	342	(56.0)	43	(7.0)		160	(25.5)	468	(74.5)	
40–49	238	(38.9)	323	(52.8)	51	(8.3)		142	(22.6)	485	(77.4)	
50–59	258	(41.9)	320	(51.9)	38	(6.2)		125	(19.8)	507	(80.2)	
60–69	284	(46.6)	282	(46.3)	43	(7.1)		141	(22.6)	483	(77.4)	
Educational level												
Junior high school or high school	347	(39.5)	451	(51.4)	80	(9.1)	0.03	150	(21.6)	543	(78.4)	0.52
Technical college or junior college	304	(39.6)	410	(53.5)	53	(6.9)		139	(24.3)	433	(75.7)	
University and graduate school	551	(40.3)	728	(53.2)	89	(6.5)		267	(24.6)	817	(75.4)	
Others	13	(31.0)	21	(50.0)	8	(19.0)		186	(23.8)	594	(76.2)	
Employment status												
Manager	101	(41.4)	130	(53.3)	13	(5.3)	0.06	59	(25.5)	172	(74.5)	<0.01
Regular employee	344	(40.4)	445	(52.2)	63	(7.4)		240	(28.4)	605	(71.6)	
Non-regular employee	195	(37.4)	287	(55.0)	40	(7.7)		107	(19.8)	433	(80.2)	
Others	516	(41.7)	626	(50.6)	94	(7.6)		283	(25.1)	1019	(74.9)	
Student	59	(29.4)	122	(60.7)	20	(10.0)		53	(21.7)	158	(78.3)	
Individual income (JPY)												
Low (<1 million yen/year)	465	(38.4)	640	(52.9)	105	(8.7)	0.20	264	(21.4)	972	(78.6)	0.04
Middle (1–3 million yen/year)	415	(39.4)	565	(53.7)	72	(6.8)		285	(24.8)	864	(75.2)	
High (>3 million yen/year)	335	(42.2)	405	(51.1)	53	(6.7)		193	(25.9)	551	(74.1)	
	Mean	SD	Mean	SD	Mean	SD	p	Mean	SD	Mean	SD	p
Knowledge score (0–8)	6.46	(1.85)	6.92	(1.71)	5.66	(2.89)	<0.01	4.76	(3.09)	5.51	(2.87)	<0.01

Table 3. Univariable and multivariable analyses of association between sociao-demographic factors and the prejudiced attitudes toward HBV/HCV or HIV infected colleagues.

	Prejudiced toward infected HIV colleagues (n = 2,825)				Prejudice toward infected HBV/HCV colleagues (n = 3,129)			
	Univariable model[a]		Multivarible model[b]		Univariable model[a]		Multivarible model[b]	
	OR (95% CI)	p	OR (95% CI)	p	OR (95% CI)	p	OR (95% CI)	p
Sex								
Male	ref		ref		ref		ref	
Female	0.94 (0.85–1.02)	0.16	0.93 (0.83–1.05)	0.25	0.79 (0.68–0.90)	<0.01	0.87 (0.73–1.03)	0.14
Age								
20–29	ref		ref		ref		ref	
30–39	1.05 (0.91–1.20)	0.51	0.99 (0.83–1.15)	0.85	0.90 (0.74–1.09)	0.29	0.80 (0.63–1.00)	0.06
40–49	1.11 (0.97–1.25)	0.12	1.04 (0.88–1.20)	0.65	0.79 (0.64–0.97)	0.03	0.70 (0.54–0.90)	0.01
50–59	1.16 (1.02–1.29)	0.02	1.08 (0.93–1.24)	0.31	0.68 (0.54–0.85)	0.00	0.61 (0.46–0.81)	0.00
60–69	1.24 (1.13–1.35)	<0.01	1.16 (1.01–1.30)	0.03	0.79 (0.64–0.97)	0.03	0.70 (0.52–0.92)	0.02
Test for linear trend[d]	p<0.01		p<0.01		p<0.01		p<0.01	
Educational level								
Junior high school or high school	ref		ref		ref		ref	
Technical college or junior college	0.98 (0.86–1.10)	0.72	1.02 (0.90–1.14)	0.34	1.12 (0.92–1.34)	0.26	1.16 (0.95–1.40)	0.13
University and graduate school	0.99 (0.89–1.09)	0.86	1.05 (0.94–1.17)	0.64	1.13 (0.96–1.33)	0.15	1.17 (0.98–1.37)	0.08
Others	0.87 (0.52–1.31)	0.55	0.90 (0.53–1.36)	0.85	1.10 (0.91–1.31)	0.32	1.12 (0.93–1.34)	0.24
Test for linear trend[d]	p = 0.79		p = 0.60		p = 0.31		p = 0.21	
Employment status								
Manager	ref		ref		ref		ref	
Regular employee	1.00 (0.83–1.17)	0.97	1.07 (0.90–1.25)	0.44	1.11 (0.87–1.37)	0.39	1.04 (0.80–1.33)	0.74
Non-regular employee	0.92 (0.75–1.11)	0.41	1.01 (0.80–1.24)	0.94	0.76 (0.56–1.03)	0.08	0.78 (0.53–1.10)	0.15
Others	0.71 (0.51–0.95)	0.02	0.79 (0.53–1.11)	0.18	0.98 (0.70–1.33)	0.92	0.88 (0.56–1.32)	0.57
Student	1.03 (0.88–1.19)	0.68	1.07 (0.88–1.26)	0.51	0.84 (0.64–1.09)	0.20	0.88 (0.63–1.20)	0.46
Individual income (JPY)								
Low (<1 million yen/year)	ref		ref		ref		ref	
Middle (1–3 million yen/year)	1.01 (0.90–1.11)	0.90	0.93 (0.81–1.06)	0.31	1.15 (1.00–1.32)	0.05	1.11 (0.92–1.32)	0.24
High (>3 million yen/year)	1.07 (0.97–1.17)	0.18	0.98 (0.82–1.14)	0.77	1.20 (1.03–1.38)	0.02	1.04 (0.81–1.31)	0.65
Test for linear trend[d]	p = 0.20		p = 0.79		p = 0.01		p = 0.31	
Knowledge score	0.87 (0.83–0.90)	<0.01	0.87 (0.84–0.91)	<0.01	0.92 (0.90–0.95)	<0.01	0.93 (0.90–0.96)	<0.01

[a]Each factor was entered into the univariable model separately.
[b]All factors were entered into the multivariable model simultaneously.
[c]ref: Reference category OR: odds ratio.
[d]Test for linear trends were performed by modelling the group scores of age, educational level and individual income as one variable.

media [18]. Once disseminated, this biased information led to discrimination against HIV infected people. As such, this unfortunate historical episode illustrates the need to consider the age of the target population to effectively reduce discrimination toward HIV infected colleagues in the workplace.

Older people in Japan may have different attitudes towards HBV/HCV infection, resulting from different initial exposure to HBV/HCV related information, when compared with younger people. The current study revealed that older age was independently associated with decreased prejudice toward HBV/HCV infected colleagues. It is worth noting that HCV hepatitis, when caused by HCV-contaminated fibrinogen concentrate, is termed Yakugai-hepatitis in Japan; where the characters Yakugai mean "health hazards due to pharmaceuticals" [7]. Until 1988, approximately 10,000 individuals who had received HCV-contaminated fibrinogen concentrate were diagnosed with HCV infection in Japan [7]. As a result, it is reasonable to assume that Yakugai-hepatitis positive individuals in Japan are more commonly perceived as victims, at least by the older generation. Since 1988, blood donated at Japanese blood centers has been screened for HBV, and HBV vaccinations have also been administered to infants born to HBV infected mothers. By contrast, most acute hepatitis B cases in contemporary Japanese society result from sexual transmission between young people [19] [20] [21]. Younger people in Japan may therefore perceive HBV infection as the responsibility of the individual and something that is acquired through immoral behavior. Thus, any intervention to decrease prejudice toward HBV/HCV infected colleagues will clearly need to consider the age of the target population in its design.

The mean HIV knowledge score in the current study was higher than that observed for HBV/HCV, which is consistent with previous research [22]. Since establishing government resources for medical and public health support of HIV infected people in Japan, the stigma surrounding HIV has diminished significantly over time [22]. Increased knowledge of HIV or HBV/HCV has previously been shown to reduce prejudice toward infected colleagues [23] [24]. Lessons may therefore, be learned from successful HIV public health interventions to improve the knowledge about HBV/HCV. Japanese public health centres/municipal health centres represent an existing on-the-ground resource for community health promotion [25] and may therefore be well-placed to serve an increasing workplace role in this regard.

Sex, educational level, employment status, and individual income were not independently associated with prejudice toward infected colleagues in the present study. This is somewhat different to other research from Western and African regions which demonstrated strong associations between sociodemographic factors, stigma, and discrimination against people living with HIV [26] [27] [28]. Cultural values and social-cognitive factors are related to health beliefs [12], and these are known to influence the perceptions of blood-borne diseases in other parts of Asia, such as China [29]. In a Japanese setting, at least in the current study, the effect of sociodemographic factors on prejudice toward HIV or HBV/HCV infected colleagues may be limited.

Although it appears to have been the first of its kind, there are several potential limitations to the current study. Firstly, 230 respondents who answered "not sure" on having prejudiced opinions about infected colleagues were omitted from the analysis, as previously described. The distribution of sex, age, employment status, individual income and having prejudiced opinions about infected colleagues among this omitted group was not significantly different from the remaining respondents. However, the proportion of "junior high school or high school" and "others" in the educational level category were found to be higher, while the proportion of "technical college or junior college" and "university and graduate school" were lower among the omitted group. Their knowledge score was also lower among the omitted group. As a result, the potential effect of excluding this particular group on the overall results may still be considered. Secondly, our study population presumably had internet access in order to complete the survey, and therefore may be more aware of HIV and HBV/HCV through access to online information [30]. Our results may therefore not be generalized to individuals without internet access, or in other countries and settings. Thirdly, our study population were higher educated and with lower income than the general Japanese working population; with only 25% of respondents having completed junior high or high school compared with 46% among the general Japanese working population [31] and 40% of respondents having an income of less than 1 million yen compared with 8.6% of that [32]. Fourthly, we could not be entirely certain about individuals who stated their educational category as 'others,' given that this could include college and/or high school drop-outs or simply participants who did not want to answer the question. Finally, although HBV and HCV are distinct diseases with different characteristics, different modes of transmission, and have different therapeutic options and goals; we did not measure prejudiced toward these diseases separately.

Conclusion

Overall, this study suggests that age may be associated with prejudice toward HIV and HBV/HCV infected colleagues among the working age population of Japan. As such, policy makers should carefully consider the age of participants when formulating efforts to reduce prejudice toward HIV and HBV/HCV infected workers.

Author Contributions

Conceived and designed the experiments: HE KW. Performed the experiments: KW. Analyzed the data: HE. Contributed reagents/materials/analysis tools: HE KW DS. Wrote the paper: HE KW DS.

References

1. Gifford SM, O'Brien ML, Smith A, Temple-Smith M, StoovÉ M, et al. (2005) Australian men's experiences of living with hepatitis C virus: Results from a cross-sectional survey. J Gastroenterol Hepatol 20: 79–86.
2. Dray-Spira R, Gueguen A, Lert F, Group* tVS (2008) Disease severity, self-reported experience of workplace discrimination and employment loss during the course of chronic HIV disease: differences according to gender and education. Occup Environ Med 65: 112–119.
3. Lim VK, Teo TS, Teo AC, Tan KT (1999) HIV and youths in Singapore—knowledge, attitudes and willingness to work with HIV-infected persons. Singapore Med J 40: 410–415.
4. Narai R, Oyama T, Ogawa M, Yamaguchi T, Kinaga T, et al. (2007) HBV- and HCV- infected workers in the Japanese workplace. J Occup Health 49: 9–16.
5. McGoldrick C (2012) HIV and employment. Occ Med (London) 62: 242–253.
6. Yoshizawa H (2002) Hepatocellular carcinoma associated with hepatitis C virus infection in Japan: projection to other countries in the foreseeable future. Oncology 62 Suppl 1: 8–17.
7. Yasunaga H (2007) Risk of authoritarianism: fibrinogen-transmitted hepatitis C in Japan. The Lancet 370: 2063–2067.
8. Tanaka J, Kumagai J, Katayama K, Komiya Y, Mizui M, et al. (2004) Sex- and age-specific carriers of hepatitis B and C viruses in Japan estimated by the prevalence in the 3,485,648 first-time blood donors during 1995–2000. Intervirology 47: 32–40.
9. Corrigan PW, Penn DL (1999) Lessons from social psychology on discrediting psychiatric stigma. Am Psychol 54: 765–776.
10. Lau JT, Tsui HY (2005) Discriminatory attitudes towards people living with HIV/AIDS and associated factors: a population based study in the Chinese general population. Sex Transm Infect 81: 113–119.

11. Fortenberry JD, McFarlane M, Bleakley A, Bull S, Fishbein M, et al. (2002) Relationships of stigma and shame to gonorrhea and HIV screening. Am J Public Health 92: 378–381.
12. Veen YJJ, Empelen P, Looman CWN, Richardus JH (2013) Social-Cognitive and Socio-Cultural Predictors of Hepatitis B Virus-Screening in Turkish Migrants, the Netherlands. J Immigr Minor Health: Aug 4. [Epub ahead of print].
13. Cabinet office (2000) Opinion poll about AIDS. [Online]. Cabinet office website. Available: http://www8.cao.go.jp/survey/h12/h12-aids/ (in Japanese). Accessed 2014 April 11.
14. Zhang J, Yu KF (1998) What's the relative risk? A method of correcting the odds ratio in cohort studies of common outcomes. JAMA 280: 1690–1691.
15. Ministry of Education C, Sports Science and Technology & Ministry of Health, Labour and Welfare (2002) Ethical Guidelines for Epidemiological Research. [Online]. Ministry of Health, Labour and Welfare website. Available http://www.mhlw.go.jp/seisakunitsuite/bunya/hokabunya/kenkyujigyou/i-kenkyu/dl/02-02.pdf (in Japanese). Accessed 2014 April 11.
16. Bermingham S, Kippax S (1998) HIV-related discrimination: a survey of New South Wales general practitioners. Aust N Z J Public Health 22: 92–97.
17. Ikegami C (1997) HIV prevention and community-based organizations in Japan. J Acquir Immune Defic Syndr Hum Retrovirol 14 Suppl 2: S51–57.
18. Hirata S, Watanabe M, Katsuno S (1995) AIDS in the Japanse Mass Media: Content Analysis of Articles about AIDS from 1982 to 1992 in the Japanese Newspaper. Jpn J Health and Human Ecology 61: 2–15.
19. Kubo N, Furusyo N, Sawayama Y, Otaguro S, Nabeshima S, et al. (2003) A patient in whom only hepatitis B virus (HBV) was thought to have been contracted, by kissing, from a same-sex partner coinfected with HBV and human immunodeficiency virus-1. J Infect Chemother 9: 260–264.
20. Yamada N, Yotsuyanagi H, Koitabashi Y, Nagase Y, Okuse C, et al. (2008) Epidemiology and clinical features of acute hepatitis B in Japan_Analysis with an emphasis on genotype A HBV_. Kanzo 49: 553–559.
21. Sako A, Yasunaga H, Horiguchi H, Hashimoto H, Masaki N, et al. (2011) Acute hepatitis B in Japan: Incidence, clinical practices and health policy. Hepatol Res 41: 39–45.
22. Krauskopf K, McGinn TG, Federman AD, Halm EA, Leventhal H, et al. (2011) HIV and HCV health beliefs in an inner-city community. J Viral Hepat 18: 785–791.
23. Wang G, Wada K, Hoshi K, Sasaki N, Ezoe S, et al. (2013) Association of knowledge of HIV and other factors with individuals' attitudes toward HIV infection: a national cross-sectional survey among the Japanese non-medical working population. PLoS One 8: e68495.
24. Eguchi H, Wada K (2013) Knowledge of HBV and HCV and individuals' attitudes toward HBV- and HCV-infected colleagues: a national cross-sectional study among a working population in Japan. PLoS One 8: e76921.
25. Smith DR (2009) Public health centres in contemporary Japan. Public health 123: 196–197.
26. Feyissa GT, Abebe L, Girma E, Woldie M (2012) Stigma and discrimination against people living with HIV by healthcare providers, Southwest Ethiopia. BMC Public Health 12: 522.
27. Akena D, Musisi S, Joska J, Stein DJ (2012) The association between aids related stigma and major depressive disorder among HIV-positive individuals in Uganda. PLoS One 7: e48671.
28. Nyamathi A, Ekstrand M, Zolt-Gilburne J, Ganguly K, Sinha S, et al. (2013) Correlates of Stigma among Rural Indian Women Living with HIV/AIDS. AIDS Behav 17: 329–339.
29. Smith DR, Ning W (2010) Emerging workplace issues for Chinese health care workers in the new millennium: HIV/AIDS. Work 37: 297–300.
30. Kontos EZ, Emmons KM, Puleo E, Viswanath K (2012) Contribution of communication inequalities to disparities in human papillomavirus vaccine awareness and knowledge. Am J Public Health 102: 1911–1920.
31. The Organization for Economic Co-operation and Development (OECD) (2013) Education at a Glance 2013.
32. National Tax Agency (2013) Salary for private sector employee actual condition statistical research 2012.

Beneficial Effect of Isoniazid Preventive Therapy and Antiretroviral Therapy on the Incidence of Tuberculosis in People Living with HIV in Ethiopia

Kesetebirhan Delele Yirdaw[1]*, Degu Jerene[1], Zewdu Gashu[1], M. E. Edginton[2], Ajay M. V. Kumar[3], Yohannes Letamo[4], Beniam Feleke[5], Alula M. Teklu[6], Solomon Zewdu[7], Bill Weiss[7], Andrea Ruff[7]

1 Clinical Department, Johns Hopkins University TSEHAI Project, Addis Ababa, Ethiopia, **2** Center for Operational Research, International Union against Tuberculosis and Lung Disease, Paris, France, **3** International Union against Tuberculosis and Lung Disease, South-East Asia Regional Office, New Delhi, India, **4** Health Research and Technology Transfer Support Process, Southern Nations Nationalities and People's Region Health Bureau, Hawassa, Southern Nations Nationalities and People's Region, Ethiopia, **5** Care and treatment branch, TB/HIV unit, Centers for Disease Control and Prevention, Addis Ababa, Ethiopia, **6** PCM Department, Johns Hopkins University TSEHAI Project, Addis Ababa, Ethiopia, **7** Bloomberg School of Public Health, Johns Hopkins University, Baltimore, Maryland, United States of America

Abstract

Background: IPT with or without concomitant administration of ART is a proven intervention to prevent tuberculosis among PLHIV. However, there are few data on the routine implementation of this intervention and its effectiveness in settings with limited resources.

Objectives: To measure the level of uptake and effectiveness of IPT in reducing tuberculosis incidence in a cohort of PLHIV enrolled into HIV care between 2007 and 2010 in five hospitals in southern Ethiopia.

Methods: A retrospective cohort analysis of electronic patient database was done. The independent effects of no intervention, "IPT-only," "IPT-before-ART," "IPT-and-ART started simultaneously," "ART-only," and "IPT-after-ART" on TB incidence were measured. Cox-proportional hazards regression was used to assess association of treatment categories with TB incidence.

Results: Of 7,097 patients, 867 were excluded because they were transferred-in; a further 823 (12%) were excluded from the study because they were either identified to have TB through screening (292 patients) or were on TB treatment (531). Among the remaining 5,407 patients observed, IPT had been initiated for 39% of eligible patients. Children, male sex, advanced disease, and those in Pre-ART were less likely to be initiated on IPT. The overall TB incidence was 2.6 per 100 person-years. As compared to those with no intervention, use of "IPT-only" (aHR = 0.36, 95% CI = 0.19–0.66) and "ART-only" (aHR = 0.32, 95% CI = 0.24–0.43) were associated with significant reduction in TB incidence rate. Combining ART and IPT had a more profound effect. Starting IPT-before-ART (aHR = 0.18, 95% CI = 0.08–0.42) or simultaneously with ART (aHR = 0.20, 95% CI = 0.10–0.42) provided further reduction of TB at ~80%.

Conclusions: IPT was found to be effective in reducing TB incidence, independently and with concomitant ART, under programme conditions in resource-limited settings. The level of IPT provision and effectiveness in reducing TB was encouraging in the study setting. Scaling up and strengthening IPT service in addition to ART can have beneficial effect in reducing TB burden among PLHIV in settings with high TB/HIV burden.

Editor: Emma S. McBryde, Royal Melbourne Hospital, Australia

Funding: Funding for the course was from an anonymous donor and the Department for International Development, UK. The funders had no role in study design, data collection and analysis, decision to publish, or preparation of the manuscript.

Competing Interests: The authors have declared that no competing interests exist.

* Email: kcgp2005@yahoo.com

Introduction

The TB/HIV syndemic is a global public health challenge accounting for nearly 25% of all HIV-associated deaths [1]. Of 8.7 million estimated incident tuberculosis (TB) cases in 2011, about 13% were among people living with HIV (PLHIV) [1]. The African region, with 80% of the estimated HIV-infected TB cases, bears the brunt of the epidemic [1]. Ethiopia has the dual distinction of being a high TB burden country with incidence of 277 TB cases per 100,000 people per year [2] as well as a high HIV burden country with adult (15–49) HIV prevalence of 1.5% [3]. The prevalence of HIV among TB patients was estimated at 8% [1].

To reduce the burden of TB among PLHIV, the World Health Organization (WHO) recommends Intensified Case Finding (ICF), Isoniazid Preventive Therapy (IPT), Infection control, and early initiation of antiretroviral therapy (ART) [4]. Of these, ART is the most potent and widely implemented TB preventive intervention among PLHIV [4]. Although anti-retroviral drugs lower the risk of TB through immune reconstitution, the risk remains much higher than in HIV-uninfected individuals despite achievement of good CD4 cell recovery, emphasizing the need to implement other preventive interventions such as IPT. Observational studies done in Brazil and South Africa have shown that the combined effect of ART and IPT in preventing TB among PLHIV is significantly higher compared to using only ART [5–7]. Despite strong recommendations globally, the uptake of IPT has been limited due to difficulties in excluding active TB, added pill burden for patients, side effects, poor adherence to IPT, and concerns about development of drug resistance. In a review done by the WHO guidelines group, adherence for IPT ranged from 34–98% [4].

One study in Ethiopia demonstrated the effectiveness of IPT in reducing TB burden among PLHIV [8]. But, there is no published evidence on uptake and completion rates of IPT among PLHIV in Ethiopia, or its effectiveness in reducing TB incidence in combination with ART, when implemented under routine programmatic settings. There are also uncertainties regarding timing of IPT initiation in relation to ART. The WHO has identified these issues as priority areas for operational research [4]. In this study, we assessed the uptake and effectiveness of IPT in reducing TB incidence, when used alone or in combination with ART and the effect of timing of initiation of IPT in relation to initiation of ART in a population of PLHIV in Southern Ethiopia.

Methods

Ethics Considerations

Approval was obtained from the National Research Ethics Review Committee of Ethiopia. Furthermore, the original data collection for the pre-existing, de-identified/de-linked datasets used for this study was given a non-research determination and subsequent approval for secondary analysis by IRBs of Centers for Disease Control and Prevention (CDC) and Johns Hopkins University School of Public Health (JHSPH). Additional approval was obtained from the Ethics Advisory Group of the International Union against Tuberculosis and Lung Disease (IUATLD). Informed consent was not obtained since data was de-identified/de-linked before analysis.

Study Design and Setting

This is a cohort study based on a secondary analysis of an electronic database of patients under care at five HIV/ART clinics in the Southern Nations, Nationalities and People's Region (SNNPR).The SNNPR, south of the Ethiopian capital Addis Ababa, has a population of about 17 million [9]. According to the latest Demographic and Health Survey of Ethiopia, the HIV prevalence for the region was estimated at 0.9% in 2011 [3]. Health services in the region are provided by 14 governmental, six non- government hospitals and 180 health centers. All public hospitals have provided ART and IPT for eligible patients based on the national ART and TB/HIV guidelines since 2005 and 2008 respectively. Eligibility for ART was based on the following criteria: all WHO stage 4 clients, WHO stage 3 clients with CD4≤ 350 and WHO stage 1 or 2 with CD4≤200. In the absence of CD4 testing, WHO stages 3 and 4 were eligible for ART. The first line ARV regimens used were according to national and international guidelines [10].

At each visit all HIV infected clients were screened for TB, using WHO recommended symptom-based screening, and symptomatic patients were evaluated by diagnostic tests (sputum smear microscopy, chest radiography, clinical evaluation) and with treatment provided where indicated [11]. Clients screening negative for TB and without contraindications were eligible to start IPT at any time. Tuberculin skin test (TST) was not done for patients before IPT initiation. IPT was provided for a period of 6 months at a dosage of 300 mg/day for adults and 5–10 mg/kg/day for children [11]. Patients collected their drugs every month until the treatment course was completed. Patients on IPT were monitored monthly for development of active TB, adherence to treatment and adverse drug reactions. All patient details were documented by trained and supervised health care workers, standardized to maintain accuracy [10,12] and all services were provided free to the patients.

Study Period and Population

The sampling frame constituted all 20 hospitals in SNNP region. All PLHIV newly enrolled in chronic HIV care in five randomly selected hospitals of SNNP region of Ethiopia between September 2007 and August 2010 constituted the study population. All cases of prevalent TB (TB cases already on treatment at the time of enrolment into HIV care and those diagnosed within one month of enrolment) were excluded from the cohort.

Variables and Source of Data

The primary outcome variable was 'incident TB', defined as any new TB case that was diagnosed after one month of enrolment into HIV care. The primary exposures of interest were initiation of IPT and/or ART. We extracted data on these and other key covariates from the existing electronic database which included baseline WHO clinical stage, baseline CD4 count, age, sex, history of cotrimoxazole use, IPT completion and duration of ART intake. The data correspond to data on national forms for care of patients with HIV. The data were collected to support clinical decision-making and reporting to the government. All patients enrolling in HIV care at the clinic were registered in the database. Demographic information and other key milestones, like date of enrollment to care, date of ART initiation, date of IPT initiation, date of patient visit, and date of tuberculosis treatment initiation were recorded for each patient.

Data Analysis

Epi Info statistical software Version 3.4 (United States Centers for Disease Control and Prevention, Atlanta, GA) and MS Access 2007 were used to clean and analyze the data. Person-time incidence rates, incidence rate ratios and hazard ratios were calculated using Stata statistical software Version 12. Person-time at risk of TB was accrued from the date of enrolment in chronic care until death, transfer to other facility, loss to follow-up (LTFU), appearance of incident TB, or last visit. Any patient over four weeks late for a scheduled appointment who failed to return to the ART programme and could not be located by "case managers" was classified as LTFU. The following two variables were treated as time-updated variables: IPT intake, with patients accruing person time in IPT groups after time of IPT initiation; ART intake, with patients accruing person time in ART groups after time of ART initiation. Based on this, patients were divided into six exposure categories to assess the combined effect of IPT intake, and ART treatment. 'No intervention' period when neither IPT nor ART were initiated; 'IPT only' period when IPT was the only treatment received; 'ART only' period when ART was the only treatment received; 'IPT before ART' period when ART was taken after IPT initiation; 'IPT & ART simultaneously' when IPT was initiated within two weeks of ART initiation; and 'IPT after ART' period when IPT was taken after ART initiation'. A more elaborate pictorial description of this time splitting process is found in figure S1. Similar procedure was followed to assess the overall effect of IPT completion and duration of ART treatment.

Missing values for baseline CD4 (22%) and WHO stage (10%) were calculated by multiple imputation methods using multivariate normal (mvn) regression. Twenty five data sets were generated. Site, year of enrolment, sex, age, cotrimoxazole use, ART status, INH use, and incident TB were used as regular variables to impute them. Survival methods were used to assess the relationship of independent variables listed above to incident TB. Participants were censored from the risk set after the first new TB diagnosis - multiple outcomes were not allowed. We fit a multivariable Cox proportional hazards regression model. Stratification was used to correct for effect of within-group correlation at site level on the relationship between independent and dependent variables. We constructed the model using stepwise techniques, adding one independent variable at a time to the model. The decision rule for addition of a variable to the model was if significance was less than 0.05, and the rule for removal was at significance more than 0.1. *P* values for risk ratios were calculated using chi-square test.

A secondary analysis was done taking the definition of incident TB as that occurring two months after enrolment. Finally, sensitivity analysis was done to assess if baseline characteristic of patients not on follow-up differed from those on follow-up and to see the effect of IPT on TB incidence, assuming 25% of randomly selected patients who were lost to follow-up or dead developed TB at time of censoring. The final dataset and program codes to generate the results of the study are presented as supporting information S1.

Results

Baseline Characteristics

Of the 7097 patients, 867 were excluded because they were transferred in; a further 823 (12%) were excluded from the study because they were either identified to have TB through screening (292 patients) or were on TB treatment (531). Thus, there were 5407 patients studied. (Figure 1)

Median age was 30 years (range, 0.16–82) and the median follow-up duration was two years with inter-quartile range (IQR) of 0.2–4 years. Most of the patients were adults more than 14 years of age (91%) and the proportion of females was 57%. (Table 1) Among patients on ART, patients with higher baseline CD4 count, and WHO disease stage 1 or 2 were more likely to have active follow-up at the end of the study (data not shown). Median baseline CD4 count was lowest for the 'ART only' group (152/mm^3) followed by 'IPT after ART' (160/mm^3), and 'IPT and ART Simultaneously' (187/mm^3). Higher baseline CD4 counts were recorded for the 'IPT only' group (375/mm^3) followed by 'IPT before ART' groups (242/mm^3) and 'no intervention' group (216/mm^3).

IPT Initiation and Completion

IPT was initiated for 2131 (39%) patients, and 44% of them initiated IPT during Pre-ART care (Tables 1 and 2). Adults, women, those having CD4 count more than 100, those with earlier WHO disease stage and those having initiated ART were more likely to receive IPT. There was documented completion of IPT in 24% of those who started treatment. There were no statistically significant associations between IPT completion and other covariates.

Incident Tuberculosis

There were 295 incident TB cases in this study cohort during 11,290 person-years (PY) of observation, making the overall TB incidence rate 2.6 per 100 PY of follow-up (95% CI: 2.3–2.9) (Table 3). The TB incidence rate in those who took IPT was 0.7 per 100 PY and 6.1 per 100 PY for those who did not (IRR: 0.11; 95% CI: 0.08–0.15 before controlling for effect of ART). This protective effect of IPT intake persisted whether IPT completion was documented or not.

The first six months on ART represented the period with the highest risk (TB incidence 8.0 per 100 PY; 95% CI: 6.0–10), followed by Pre-ART period (TB incidence 3.9 per 100 PY; 95% CI: 3.3–4.6). After the first 6 months it decreased progressively with increase in length of time on ART. TB incidence was higher among 'ART only' and 'No intervention' treatment categories as compared to 'IPT only', 'IPT before ART', 'IPT & ART simultaneously' or 'IPT after ART'. Patients who took IPT and were eventually started on ART or those who started both simultaneously had lower risk of developing TB as compared to those who took ART only. The combined effect of IPT and ART when started at the same time reduced TB incidence by 57% (IRR: 0.43; 95%CI 0.18–0.86) as compared to those who took ART only (Table 3).

Cox Proportional Hazards Modeling

During bivariable analysis, male sex, cotrimoxazole use, advanced disease stage, and having a lower CD4 count were associated with increased relative hazard for developing TB (Table 3). On the other hand, being on IPT (irrespective of completion status), and taking ART for longer duration were each associated with lower relative hazard of developing TB. After controlling for sex, WHO stage, baseline CD4, and cotrimoxazole use, ART intake was protective against TB, and more so with greater duration of ART as compared to those not on ART. In bivariable analysis, all treatment categories showed protective effect but it was higher for 'IPT only' (HR 0.24, 95% CI 0.13–0.44), 'IPT before ART' (0.25, 95% CI 0.11–0.59), 'IPT & ART simultaneously' (HR 0.36; 95% CI 0.17–0.74) and 'IPT after ART' (HR 0.19, 95% CI 0.11–0.34). After controlling for sex, WHO stage, baseline CD4, and cotrimoxazole use, the 'ART only' group (aHR 0.32, 95% CI 0.24–0.43) had higher protective effect as well.

In the 'IPT after ART' group, TB incidence in the first six months after ART initiation was 0.2 per 100 PY as compared to those who were started on ART only which was at 6.2 per 100 PY. The median time for IPT initiation for the 'IPT after ART' group was nine months (IQR-3 months to 1.6 years).

Hazard ratios were calculated taking the definition of incident TB to be new TB disease diagnosed after two months from enrolment and the results were similar to those of the original analysis. Sensitivity analysis was also done taking those started on ART and assuming 25% of those lost to follow-up or dead developed TB. IPT was still protective of TB (Table 4). The percentages of patients lost to follow-up or dead among 'IPT before ART', 'ART only', 'IPT and ART simultaneously', and 'IPT after ART' treatment groups were 9%, 39%, 17%, and 9% respectively. The overall lost or death among ART patients was 24%.

Discussion

Over a third of PLHIV received IPT and its use was associated with 65% reduction in tuberculosis occurrence in patients who had not yet started ART. On the other hand, using only ART was associated with 68% reduction in TB incidence. The effect of ART use was directly proportional to the duration of treatment. Despite that, TB incidence among patients on ART for more than three

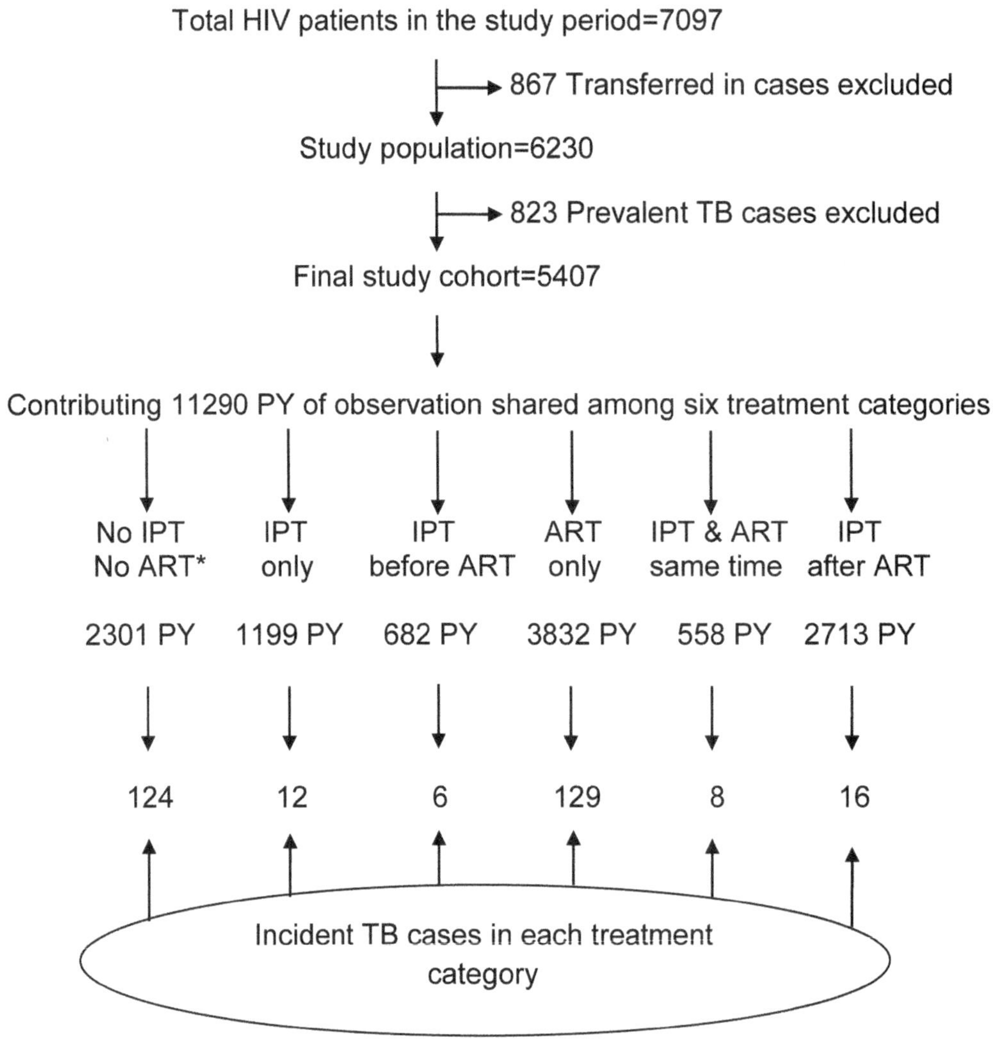

Figure 1. Cohort profile of study population, SNNP region, Ethiopia, September 2007 to August 2010. Of 7,097 patients enrolled in chronic HIV care, 5,407 were eligible for analysis contributing a total of 11,290 PY of follow-up. These were further classified into six treatment categories based on the combination of treatment received, IPT and/or ART, as well as the timing of IPT initiation with respect to ART. There were 295 incident TB cases diagnosed in the study period. IPT-Isoniazid Preventive Therapy; ART-antiretroviral therapy; TB-Tuberculosis; HIV-Human Immunodeficiency virus; PY-person year. * 'No IPT NO ART' group is equivalent to no intervention group.

and a half years remained about four times as high as the current estimate for the general population of Ethiopia which is 240 per 100,000 per year [2]. Combining IPT and ART resulted in further reduction in TB incidence, reaffirming the synergistic role of the two interventions. Timing of IPT initiation relative to ART initiation did not make any difference in reduction of TB incidence. Taking IPT before starting ART was associated with 82% reduction in TB incidence while starting IPT & ART simultaneously resulted in 80% reduction. TB incidence was much higher during the first six months of ART suggesting a possibility of TB immune reconstitution inflammatory syndrome (IRIS) which occurs in the face of very low CD4 count [13]. In the study cohort, 40% of TB cases diagnosed in this period had CD4 below 100, supporting the aforementioned premise.

The protective effect of ART and IPT was similar to what was previously reported in Ethiopia [8,14].The protective effect obtained from combining ART and IPT including the beneficial effect of starting IPT before ART is well documented in the studies done in South Africa and Brazil [5,6]. Significant TB incidence reduction among patients who started IPT and ART simultaneously was a new finding.

The protective effect of initiating IPT after starting ART, which was at 92%, should not be confused with this being the best option to prevent TB in the first six months. This group of patients was actually low risk for TB to begin with. TB incidence for this group prior to IPT initiation but after ART was 0.2 per 100 PY as compared to those who took ART only at 6.2 per 100 PY. Patients in the 'IPT after ART' group survived initial treatment period without experiencing TB and thus were likely to have been healthier overall. So, a policy offering IPT after ART initiation and after the risky period of TB has passed allows those at risk for it to develop TB disease and would benefit only the minority who were not at risk for TB in the first place. What would be rational is to initiate IPT before ART if possible or simultaneously with ART. This would benefit all patients but particularly those at risk for TB IRIS in the first six months. Of course, IPT should be offered if for some reason it was not initiated during these periods because it would further decrease TB.

Table 1. Characteristics of HIV infected patients in chronic HIV care in SNNP region, Ethiopia, September 2007 to August 2010.

Category	Sub-category	Number (%)
Age (years)	<15	475 (9)
	15–50	4683 (87)
	>50	249 (5)
Sex	Female	3095 (57)
	Male	2312 (43)
WHO Stage	Stage 1 & 2	3182 (59)
	Stage 3 & 4	2225 (41)
CPT initiation	Yes	3926 (73)
	No	1481 (27)
Baseline CD4 (count/mm^3)	<100	1002 (19)
	100–199	1545 (29)
	200–349	1590 (29)
	≥350	1270 (23)
IPT intake	Yes	2131 (39)
	No	3276 (61)
Timing of IPT initiation*	Before ART initiation	939 (44)
	After ART initiation	1192 (56)
ART initiation	Yes	3183 (59)
	No	2224 (41)

*among those who initiated IPT (n = 2131); IPT-Isoniazid Preventive Therapy; ART-antiretroviral therapy; CPT-Cotrimoxazole Preventive Therapy; WHO-World Health Organization; HIV-Human Immunodeficiency virus.

TST-positive patients benefit the most from IPT as compared to those who are TST- negative [4]. In studies where TST status was not determined results were mixed with some showing protective effect and others not [4]. Ethiopia is a high TB burden country with TST positivity among the general population reaching up to 66% [4,15]. In this study TST status was not determined, yet the

Table 2. Characteristics of HIV infected patients in Chronic HIV care who took IPT in SNNP region, Ethiopia, September 2007 to August 2010.

Category	Sub-category	Total	Took IPT, n (%)	RR (95% CI)	*P* value
Total		5407	2131 (39)		
Age (years)	<15	475	125 (26)	1.0	
	15–50	4683	1898 (41)	**1.54 (1.34–1.77)**	**<0.001**
	>50	249	108 (43)	**1.65 (1.34–2.03)**	**<0.001**
Sex	Female	3095	1279 (41)	1.0	
	Male	2312	852 (37)	**0.89 (0.83–0.95)**	**<0.001**
WHO Stage	Stage 1 and 2	3182	1318 (41)	1.0	
	Stage 3 and 4	2225	813 (37)	**0.88 (0.82–0.94)**	**<0.001**
CPT initiation	Yes	3926	1751 (45)	1.0	
	No	1481	380 (26)	**0.58 (0.52–0.63)**	**<0.001**
Baseline CD4 (count/mm^3)	<100	1002	345 (34)	1.0	
	100–199	1545	635 (41)	**1.19 (1.08–1.33)**	**0.001**
	200–349	1590	638 (40)	**1.17 (1.05–1.29)**	**0.004**
	≥350	1270	513 (40)	**1.17 (1.05–1.31)**	**0.004**
ART initiation	Yes	3183	1606 (50)	**1.0**	
	No	2224	525 (24)	**0.47 (0.43–0.51)**	**<0.001**

IPT-Isoniazid Preventive Therapy; ART-antiretroviral therapy; CPT-Cotrimoxazole Preventive Therapy; WHO-World Health Organization; HIV-Human Immunodeficiency virus.

Table 3. Incidence rate of TB among HIV infected patients in Chronic HIV care in SNNP region, Ethiopia, September 2007 to August 2010.

Category	Sub-category	Incident TB cases	Peron-years	Incidence rate per 100 person-years	Unadjusted HR (95% CI)	Adjusted HR (95% CI)
Total		295	11290	2.6		
Age (years)	<15	23	1099	2.1	1	
	15–49	253	9624	2.6	1.24 (0.81–1.91)	
	>49	19	568	3.3	1.61 (0.87–2.95)	
Sex	Female	139	6705	2.1	1	1
	Male	156	4585	3.4	**1.57 (1.25–1.97)**	**1.42 (1.13–1.79)**
CPT status	No	16	1546	1.0	1	
	Yes	279	9745	2.9	**3.16 (1.90–5.23)**	**2.15 (1.25–3.69)**
WHO Stage	Stage 1 or 2	74	6468	1.1	1	1
	Stage 3 or 4	221	4822	4.6	**4.05 (3.11–5.28)**	**3.80 (2.87–5,04)**
Baseline CD4	<100	93	2017	4.6	1	1
	100–199	82	3537	2.3	**0.54 (0.40–0.73)**	**0.70 (0.52–0.95)**
	201–349	84	3343	2.5	**0.59 (0.44–0.80)**	**0.59 (0.43–0.81)**
	>349	36	2394	1.5	**0.32 (0.22–0.47)**	**0.36 (0.23–0.56)**
IPT Intake & completion*	No IPT	244	3969	6.1	1	1
	IPT Completion	16	1975	0.8	**0.14 (0.08–0.23)**	**0.15 (0.09–0.26)**
	IPT non-completion	35	5347	0.7	**0.12 (0.08–0.17)**	**0.13 (0.09–0.19)**
Duration on ART*	No ART	136	3505	3.9	1	1
	0–5 months	76	952	8.0	0.90 (0.65–1.25)	**0.38 (0.27–0.54)**
	6–24 months	45	2868	1.6	0.76 (0.49–1.19)	**0.30 (0.19–0.48)**
	25–42 months	25	2519	1.0	**0.43 (0.23–0.82)**	**0.15 (0.08–0.28)**
	>42 months	13	1445	0.9	**0.37 (0.14–0.95)**	**0.10 (0.04–0.27)**
IPT and/or ART*	No intervention	124	2306	5.4	1	1
	IPT only	12	1199	1.0	**0.24 (0.13–0.44)**	**0.36 (0.19–0.66)**
	IPT before ART	6	682	0.9	**0.25 (0.11–0.59)**	**0.18 (0.08–0.42)**
	ART only	129	3832	3.4	**0.74 (0.58–0.96)**	**0.32 (0.24–0.43)**
	IPT & ART Simultaneously	8	558	1.4	**0.36 (0.17–0.74)**	**0.20 (0.10–0.42)**
	IPT after ART	16	2713	0.6	**0.19 (0.11–0.34)**	**0.08 (0.05–0.15)**

*Controlled for sex, WHO stage, baseline CD4, and Cotrimoxazole status; HR-Hazard Ratio; CI- Confidence Interval; IPT-Isoniazid Preventive Therapy; ART-antiretroviral therapy; CPT-Cotrimoxazole Preventive Therapy; WHO-World Health Organization; HIV-Human Immunodeficiency virus.

Table 4. Sensitivity analysis for effectiveness of IPT with or without ART using Cox proportional hazards model among patients on ART assuming those who were lost to follow-up and dead developed TB in SNNP region, Ethiopia, September 2007 to August 2010.

Category	Sub-category	Incident TB+lost+dead	Person-years	Incidence rate per 100 person-years	Unadjusted HR (95% CI)	Adjusted HR (95% CI)
IPT and/or ART*	No intervention	93	1018	9.1	1	1
	IPT only	9	370	2.4	**0.36 (0.18–0.71)**	**0.40 (0.20–0.80)**
	IPT before ART	15	682	2.2	**0.42 (0.24–0.74)**	**0.45 (0.25–0.80)**
	ART only	266	3832	6.9	0.93 (0.73–1.19)	**0.69 (0.53–0.89)**
	IPT & ART Simultaneously	14	558	2.5	**0.39 (0.22–0.70)**	**0.35 (0.20–0.62)**
	IPT after ART	41	2713	1.5	**0.30 (0.20–0.46)**	**0.22 (0.15–0.34)**

*Controlled for sex, WHO stage, cotrimoxazole use, and baseline CD4; HR-Hazard Ratio; CI- Confidence Interval; IPT-Isoniazid Preventive Therapy; ART-antiretroviral therapy; WHO-World Health Organization; HIV-Human Immunodeficiency virus.

protective effect of IPT was comparable to those studies with positive TST status [4].

Patients ever started on cotrimoxazole were found to be at higher risk for TB. This is not surprising, considering that those with advanced immune-suppression who were eligible for it would have also been at risk for TB [4,11].The association persisted even after controlling for other potential confounding variables.

This study has implications for policy and practice. We now have additional data on the effectiveness of IPT in preventing TB in routine care setting. A simple modeling indicates that, tripling the IPT coverage in two year time in the study region from the current level following the recommended IPT initiation would reduce the number of TB patients among PLHIV in care by 27% than if no more patients were initiated on IPT after this (Text S1). This should help convince health workers, patients, and policy makers in quickly addressing the IPT implementation challenges to harness its benefit [16]. The potential benefit of initiating IPT before ART or simultaneously with ART if coupled with effective implementation of TB screening could reduce TB burden in the first six months of ART intake. The IPT coverage in this cohort of HIV infected patients is over twice the national average of 18% for HIV infected patients in chronic care in Ethiopia [1,17,18] but the coverage rate was slightly lower in children. This suggests the need to look for and address additional underlying factors that lead to lower IPT use rate in the pediatric population in particular and the PLHIV in general. A study done in South Africa indicates that lack of knowledge and experience among providers about TB screening and IPT use as well as lack of awareness of benefits of IPT among patients contributed to low IPT use [19]. IPT use for those with advanced HIV disease was found to be lower as comparable to those with less advanced disease. But since the risk for TB is higher in this group, IPT use should have been relatively higher as well. Initiating more patients as such could be challenging due to higher rates of symptomatic patients in this group and the difficulty faced by health care workers in excluding active TB. Late presentation of patients to chronic HIV care adds to this burden [16]. This is another reminder for the need to have feasible, improved, and less expensive diagnostic methods in such settings.

There are several points that make the finding of this study important. The study showed the level to which IPT intervention was scaled up and the resultant effectiveness on reduction of TB risk. The study was done in routine clinical care setting in a low-income country and this will add to the limited evidence of IPT effectiveness under such conditions. A previous study done in Ethiopia on factors affecting occurrence of TB showed IPT use prevented TB (adjusted odds ratio 0.35). Similar assessments were done in Brazil and South Africa and comparable results were documented in the effectiveness of IPT with ART while IPT coverage (10 and 13% respectively) and effectiveness of 'IPT only' (43 and 13% respectively) were much lower than the findings from our study [5,6]. In a different study in Tanzania, IPT was not found to be effective at all [20]. Our study presents new evidence on the effect of timing of IPT initiation with respect to ART. There are ongoing clinical trials looking into this which will clear uncertainties [21].

Although coverage of IPT for this cohort of HIV infected patients was lower than the expected, it was more than twice the prior estimate for the national average of 18% among HIV infected patients in chronic care [1,17,18]. The coverage is even higher for patients ever started on ART. It was also better than reported coverage in other African countries such as Mozambique (<1%); but lower than that of South Africa where it was 46% in 2011 [22,23]. The relatively better IPT coverage rate in this cohort could be attributed to the technical support provided by JHU TSEHAI, a PEPFAR-supported program, which involved monthly site-level mentoring, training health care providers, IPT-focused update sessions, and improved data capturing system.

Long-term ART was associated with greater reduction of risk of TB in this study. The result is comparable to a study done in South Africa that found that TB risk decreased significantly with long-term ART treatment although it remained at four times the risk to the general population [7]. Findings of higher TB incidence in the early months of ART in this study were similar to findings from a large multinational cohort study in six sub-Saharan African countries with TB incidence in the first three months being 13 per 100 PY, a bit higher than TB incidence in Pre-ART period at 10.5 per 100 PY [24].

Our findings should be interpreted cautiously because of some important limitations. Missing data and incomplete documentation were the major limitations for some variables. Missing data for baseline CD4 and WHO stage were accounted for by imputation. IPT completion was documented in 24% of the records only, which did not allow for thorough comparison on the effect of IPT by adherence rate. Being on ART was associated with higher completion of IPT in Brazil [24], for example, but this was not demonstrated in the present study. Also, because of the limited number of variables in the database, we were not able to include variables such as anemia and body-mass index in our analyses. TB diagnosis was presumptive or was based on sputum and chest x-ray results in most cases, which might have led to over or under estimation of the actual number of TB cases. Patients who were lost to follow-up or died had lower CD4 counts and more advanced WHO disease stage putting them at greater risk for TB as compared to those active in follow-up. Hence, TB incidence was likely to be a bit higher in this study population.

The strengths of this study include that it was adequately powered to study the relationship between the effect of ART used alone and with IPT in reducing TB because of large sample size and adequate number of events. Since all study records were included the potential for selection bias was reduced.

Conclusions

This study indicates that IPT intake in addition to ART could be beneficial in reducing risk of TB among PLHIV in high TB and HIV setting in resource-limited countries. The most benefit would be harnessed if IPT was initiated before or at the same time with ART. The gap in IPT coverage should be addressed urgently and in particular children less than 14 years with HIV that represent a group at significant risk for TB must be prioritized. Further studies are needed to assess the level of adherence, and barriers to IPT provision.

Supporting Information

Figure S1 Splitting of subjects according to time-updated. Coding of time updated variables: ART = 0 means ART not received; ART = 1 means ART received; IPT = 0 means IPT not received; IPT = 1 means IPT received; Subject 1 received no intervention for nine years for which reason value of both ART and IPT was set to '0' for the whole duration. Subject 2 received no intervention for the first three years but after that IPT was received and stayed in care for seven years. So the value of IPT was updated to '1' in the period where IPT was received. Subject 3 received no intervention for the first three years but after that ART was received and stayed in care for six years. So the value of ART was updated to '1' in the period where ART was received. Subject 4 received no intervention for the first four years, took IPT for three years followed by initiation of ART. In the period ART was initiated, this subjected was exposed for the effects of both ART and IPT for three years but with the effect of IPT coming first. So the value of IPT was updated to '1' in the period where IPT only was received, then after ART initiation, both values of ART and IPT was made to be '1'. Subject 5 experienced the same chain of events as in Subject 4, except ART initiation preceded IPT initiation. Subject 6 received no intervention for the first five years followed by initiation of both ART and IPT at the same time and stayed in care for five years. For this reason, value of ART and IPT was updated to '1' at the same time. Subjects 2–5 contributed person-time of follow-up to more than one treatment category.

Text S1 Estimated effect of IPT scale-up on incidence of TB/HIV co-infection.

Supporting Information S1 Dataset and program codes.

Acknowledgments

This research was supported through an operational research course, which was jointly developed and run by the Centre for Operational Research, International Union against Tuberculosis and Lung Disease, France, The Union South-East Asia Regional Office and the Operational Research Unit (LUXOR), Medecins sans Frontieres, Brussels-Luxembourg. Additional support for running the course was provided by the Center for International Health, University of Bergen, Norway. Collection of the original programmatic data was undertaken by JHU-TSEHAI with CDC/PEPFAR (U2GPS000858). The Sothern Nations Nationalities and People's regional health bureau facilitated the study.

DISCLAIMER

The findings and conclusions in this paper are those of the authors and do not necessarily represent the views of their organizations or funding agencies.

Author Contributions

Conceived and designed the experiments: KDY ZG DJ. Performed the experiments: KDY DJ ZG MEE AMVK YL BF AMT SZ BW AR. Analyzed the data: KDY. Contributed reagents/materials/analysis tools: KDY DJ ZG MEE AMVK YL BF AMT SZ BW AR. Wrote the paper: KDY DJ ZG MEE AMVK YL BF AMT SZ BW AR.

References

1. World Health Organisation (2013) Global Tuberculosis Report 2013. Geneva, Switzerland.
2. Federal Ministry of Health Ethiopian Health and Nutrition Research Institute (2011) First Ethiopian national population based TB prevalence survey. Ethiopia.
3. Ethiopian Statistical Agency (2011) Demographic and health survey.
4. World Health Organisation (2011) Guideline for Intensified TB case-findings and isoniazid Preventive Therapy for HIV positive patients in resource constrained settings. Geneva, Switzerland.
5. Golub JE, Pronyk P, Mohapi L, Thsabangu N, Moshabela M, et al. (2009) Isoniazid preventive therapy, HAART and tuberculosis risk in HIV-infected adults in South Africa: a prospective cohort. AIDS 23: 631–636.
6. Golub JE, Saraceni V, Cavalcante SC, Pacheco AG, Moulton LH, et al. (2007) The impact of antiretroviral therapy and isoniazid preventive therapy on tuberculosis incidence in HIV-infected patients in Rio de Janeiro, Brazil. AIDS 21: 1441–1448.
7. Gupta A, Wood R, Kaplan R, Bekker L-G, Lawn SD (2012) Tuberculosis incidence rates during 8 years of follow-up of an antiretroviral treatment cohort in South Africa: comparison with rates in the community. PLoS One 7: e34156.
8. Kibret KT, Yalew AW, Belaineh BG, Asres MM (2013) Determinant factors associated with occurrence of tuberculosis among adult people living with HIV after antiretroviral treatment initiation in Addis Ababa, Ethiopia: a case control study. PLoS One 8: e64488.
9. Ethiopian Population Census Commission (2008) Summary and Statistical Report of the 2007 Population and Housing Census.
10. Federal HIV/AIDS Prevention and Control Office & Federal Ministry of Health (2008) Guideline for Antiretroviral Therapy, Ethiopia.
11. Federal Ministry of Health (2012) Guidelines for clinical and programmatic management of TB, Leprosy and TB/HIV in Ethiopia. Addis Ababa, Ethiopia.
12. Federal Ministry of Health (2010) Health management information system (HMIS) participants' handout & instruments. Ethiopia.
13. World Health Organisation (2010) Treatment of tuberculosis guideline 4th edition. 2010. Geneva, Switzerland.
14. Jerene D, Næss A, Lindtjørn B (2006) Antiretroviral therapy at a district hospital in Ethiopia prevents death and tuberculosis in a cohort of HIV patients. AIDS Research and Therapy 3: 10.
15. Tegbaru B, Wolday D, Messele T, Legesse M, Mekonnen Y, et al. (2006) Tuberculin skin test conversion and reactivity rates among adults with and without human immunodeficiency virus in urban settings in Ethiopia. Clinical and Vaccine immunology 13: 784–789.
16. Getahun H, Granich R, Sculier D, Gunneberg C, Blanc L, et al. (2010) Implementation of isoniazid preventive therapy for people living with HIV worldwide: barriers and solutions. AIDS 24: S57–65.
17. Federal Ministry of Health (2004) National TB/HIV Surveillance Progress Report and Findings. Ethiopia.
18. Federal HIV/AIDS Prevention and Control Office & Federal Ministry of Health (2012) Country Progress Report on HIV/AIDS Response. Ethiopia.
19. Lester R, Hamilton R, Charalambous S, Dwadwa T, Chandler C, et al. (2010) Barriers to implementation of isoniazid preventive therapy in HIV clinics: a qualitative study. AIDS 24.
20. Kabali C, von Reyn C, Brooks D, Waddell R, Mtei L, et al. (2011) Completion of isoniazid preventive therapy and survival in HIV-infected, TST-positive adults in Tanzania. The International Journal of Tuberculosis and Lung Disease 15: 1515–1522.
21. Granich R, Gupta S, B Suthar A, Smyth C, Hoos D, et al. (2011) Antiretroviral therapy in prevention of HIV and TB: update on current research efforts. Current HIV research 9: 446–469.
22. Auld AF, Mbofana F, Shiraishi RW, Alfredo C, Sanchez M, et al. (2013) Incidence and Determinants of Tuberculosis among Adults Initiating Antiretroviral Therapy–Mozambique, 2004–2008. PloS one 8: e54665.
23. Chehab JC, Vilakazi-Nhlapo AK, Vranken P, Peters A, Klausner JD (2013) Current Integration of Tuberculosis (TB) and HIV Services in South Africa, 2011. PloS one 8: e57791.
24. Durovni B, Cavalcante SC, Saraceni V, Vellozo V, Israel G, et al. (2010) The implementation of isoniazid preventive therapy in HIV clinics: the experience from the TB/HIV in Rio (THRio) study. AIDS (London, England) 24: S49.

10

The Sensitivity and Specificity of Using a Computer Aided Diagnosis Program for Automatically Scoring Chest X-Rays of Presumptive TB Patients Compared with Xpert MTB/RIF in Lusaka Zambia

Monde Muyoyeta[1]*, Pragnya Maduskar[2], Maureen Moyo[1], Nkatya Kasese[1], Deborah Milimo[1], Rosanna Spooner[1], Nathan Kapata[3], Laurens Hogeweg[2], Bram van Ginneken[2], Helen Ayles[1,4]

1 Department of medicine, School of Medicine, University of Zambia, ZAMBART Project, Lusaka, Zambia, **2** Diagnostic Image Analysis Group, Radboud University Medical Center, Nijmegen, The Netherlands, **3** National TB program, Ministry of Health, Lusaka, Zambia, **4** Clinical research department, Faculty of Infectious and Tropical Diseases, London School of Hygiene and Tropical Medicine, London, United Kingdom

Abstract

Objective: To determine the sensitivity and specificity of a Computer Aided Diagnosis (CAD) program for scoring chest x-rays (CXRs) of presumptive tuberculosis (TB) patients compared to Xpert MTB/RIF (Xpert).

Method: Consecutive presumptive TB patients with a cough of any duration were offered digital CXR, and opt out HIV testing. CXRs were electronically scored as normal (CAD score $\leq$60) or abnormal (CAD score>60) using a CAD program. All patients regardless of CAD score were requested to submit a spot sputum sample for testing with Xpert and a spot and morning sample for testing with LED Fluorescence Microscopy-(FM).

Results: Of 350 patients with evaluable data, 291 (83.1%) had an abnormal CXR score by CAD. The sensitivity, specificity, positive predictive value (PPV) and negative predictive value (NPV) of CXR compared to Xpert were 100% (95%CI 96.2–100), 23.2% (95%CI 18.2–28.9), 33.0% (95%CI 27.6–38.7) and 100% (95% 93.9–100), respectively. The area under the receiver operator curve (AUC) for CAD was 0.71 (95%CI 0.66–0.77). CXR abnormality correlated with smear grade ($r = 0.30$, $p < 0.0001$) and with Xpert C_T($r = 0.37$, $p < 0.0001$).

Conclusions: To our knowledge this is the first time that a CAD program for TB has been successfully tested in a real world setting. The study shows that the CAD program had high sensitivity but low specificity and PPV. The use of CAD with digital CXR has the potential to increase the use and availability of chest radiography in screening for TB where trained human resources are scarce.

Editor: Robert J. Wilkinson, Institute of Infectious Diseases and Molecular Medicine, South Africa

Funding: Funding sources: T9-370-114 World Health Organization through the stop TB partnership-TB REACH wave 2 grant. http://www.stoptb.org,/global/awards/tbreach/grantees2.asp, Sub grant- Delft Imaging systems-CAD4TBII, http://www.delftimagingsystems.com/tb-solutions/cad4tb. The funders had no role in study design, data collection and analysis, decision to publish, or preparation of the manuscript.

Competing Interests: The authors have declared that no competing interests exist.

* E-mail: monde@zambart.org.zm

Introduction

Recently there has been renewed interest in the role of chest x-ray (CXR) in the diagnosis of tuberculosis (TB), especially with advances that have been made with digital technology [1,2]. Particularly, there has been an increasing interest in developing computer aided diagnostic systems for detection of TB [3–5]. The advances in digital technology have made CXR cheaper, easier to use because films and chemicals are no longer needed and more reliable because automatic exposure control largely avoids unreadable images and also makes it possible to score CXRs digitally using computer aided diagnosis (CAD) [6–8]. In high burden TB and HIV settings, the use of CXR in TB diagnosis has been limited by the scarcity of personnel that can interpret CXR correctly but also by the large work load required to read CXRs manually [3]. Digital scoring of CXR therefore has the potential to increase the use of CXR in these settings as it does not have these limitations.

Studies have shown high variability in human scoring of CXRs with wide ranges of sensitivity and specificity [9–15]. Furthermore, inter-reader and intra-reader agreement also vary widely, although the use of standard classification systems for CXR scoring has improved agreement [10–12,16–18]. On the other hand, CAD systems have the potential to reduce inter-reader and intra-reader variability and also the potential to reduce detection errors [19,20]. Additionally, CAD is trained on digital CXR images and performance might vary with the quality of the scanned films.

The resurgence of TB has seen renewed interest and progress in new technologies for diagnosis of TB such as the molecular based tool, the Xpert MTB/RIF (Xpert) [21–23]. Whilst Xpert has been shown to have high sensitivity and high specificity [24–28], its extensive use in resource constrained settings is partly limited by its high cost [23,29]. It has been suggested that extensive use of Xpert in these settings can be achieved by using Xpert in conjunction with other screening tests [29]. Chest radiography can be used as a pre-screening tool for TB with other more sensitive but expensive tests such as Xpert [9,29]. In this way, the cost of diagnosis can be minimized through pre-selecting patients so that only those who are most likely to benefit from an expensive but sensitive tool have access, thus improving cost effectiveness.

As part of a TB REACH Xpert implementation evaluation project we conducted a prospective study to evaluate the use of a CAD program to digitally score CXRs of presumptive TB patients as a pre-screening test to access Xpert or Fluorescence microscopy (FM) diagnosis. In this paper, we report the sensitivity and specificity of a CAD program compared to Xpert and describe the relationship between CAD score and TB detection by Xpert, smear microscopy and clinical TB diagnosis. We also describe the association between patients presenting symptoms and bacillary load with the degree of CXR abnormality.

Ethics statement

The study had ethical approval from the University of Zambia Ethics committee. The requirement to obtain individual written informed consent was waived for presumptive TB patients being screened as part of the case finding activities, as this was part of routine health care and all modalities of TB diagnosis included are currently recommended as best practice.

Methods

Study setting and study population

The study was conducted in a primary health care facility in Lusaka, Zambia. The health facility is located in peri-urban Lusaka, and offers services to a population with a high burden for TB and HIV [30]. The facility notifies over 2,000/100,000 population TB patients yearly, although a low proportion of these cases are microbiologically confirmed.

The study population comprised individuals from the catchment population of the primary health care facility that presented to the health facility and met the definition of a presumptive TB patient. A presumptive TB patient was defined as any patient of any age who presented with a cough of any duration with or without other symptoms of TB and was able to submit a sputum sample. Data presented in this study was collected between June and July 2013 from consecutive patients presenting during the study period.

Study design and study procedures

This was a cross sectional prospective study. Enhanced case finding activities were conducted in the community with the aim of raising awareness around tuberculosis; symptoms of TB, the link between TB and HIV, and the importance of seeking care early. Patients with a cough of any duration were encouraged to visit the clinic to be assessed for TB. An open access point was established at the health facility to streamline the diagnostic process. The open access point allowed patients to present directly to the TB services without queuing up in the general outpatient clinic before being investigated for TB, thus bypassing a known barrier to TB diagnosis of busy overburdened clinics. A presumptive TB patient register was maintained at the open access point. Patients that presented to the open access point were registered by allocation of a presumptive TB patient number; socio-demographic data, and history of presenting symptoms were collected in line with requirements for clinical management of presumptive TB patients. After registration, a CXR request form and HIV counseling and testing request form with the presumptive TB patient number were printed only for patients that met the definition of a presumptive TB patient. Patients that did not meet the definition of a presumptive TB patient were directed to see a clinician for assessment and management of their symptoms. Presumptive TB patients were directed to the CXR unit (Odelca-DR, Delft Imaging Systems, The Netherlands) located within the same premises. After the CXR was done, patients were directed to the HIV counseling and testing unit where opt out HIV testing was offered in accordance with the current local guidelines for patient management.

Procedure for automatic scoring of CXR

At the CXR unit, patients were registered by scanning in the presumptive TB patient number that had been allocated at the point of registration. The CXRs were scored by a software system (CAD4TB, version 1.08, Diagnostic Image Analysis Group, The Netherlands) [4] developed for automatic detection of abnormalities suggestive of pulmonary tuberculosis. The CAD4TB software had been trained with labeled samples to distinguish between normal and abnormal CXRs. For this purpose, 945 consecutive digital CXRs (514 abnormal, 431 normal) acquired at two sites with a high TB prevalence in Sub-Saharan Africa, located in Lusaka, Zambia, and Cape Town, South Africa, were used as the training database. The CAD4TB abnormality score was calculated by combining the output of two detection systems, a textural abnormality detection and a shape abnormality detection system. These detection systems analyze the abnormalities in the unobscured lung fields which were segmented automatically as described by van Ginneken et al. [31]. The textural abnormality system was trained with various descriptive features calculated from normal and abnormal circular patches in the image to train a *k*-nearest neighbor classifier [32] (*k*-NN) to differentiate between a normal/abnormal patch in the image. These descriptive features included moments of intensity distributions of Gaussian derivative filtered images [33] and the patch position relative to the segmented lung fields. All patches in the lung fields were classified using the trained classifier to assign a probability of being abnormal. A textural abnormality score was calculated by fusing the probabilistic labels of all the patches. The shape abnormality detection system was included in the software to handle the CXR images where the lung fields were not accurately segmented. This can occur if the CXR contains substantial parenchymal abnormalities or large amounts of pleural fluid [34]. Therefore, a shape model as mentioned in [4] was constructed using lung shapes of normal CXRs in the training dataset, which was utilized to compute a shape abnormality score between 0 and 100. A high shape abnormality score reflects a very abnormal image.

The two abnormality scores computed from the above described detection systems were used as image descriptive features to train a *k*-NN classifier to estimate the combined abnormality score for a new CXR image. The combined abnormality score is in the range of 0 to 100, where a higher score is indicative of more severe abnormalities present on the CXR image.

Using previously collected CXR data from the same population, an appropriate threshold for the CAD score was determined. The area under the receiver operating (ROC) curve on a test set of 969 CXRs (458 normal, 511 abnormal) using a radiological reference

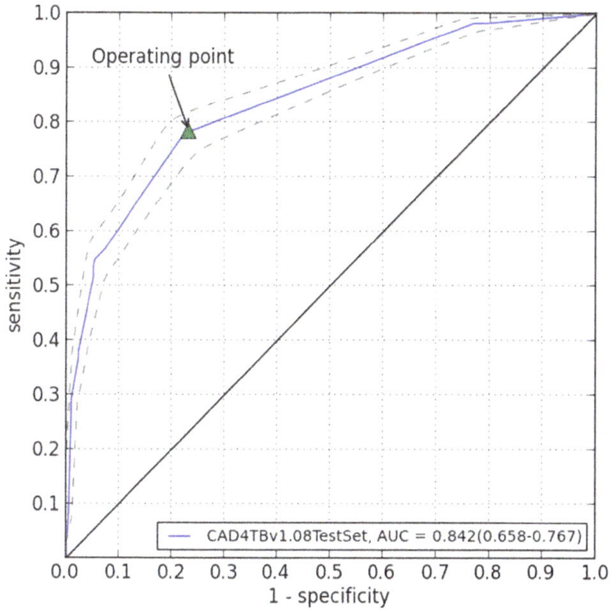

Figure 1. ROC on a test set of 969 CXRs.

standard is shown in Figure 1. A threshold of 61 was chosen based on the shown ROC curve at the operating point where 78% sensitivity and 77% specificity was achieved. For this study, a CAD score of 61 and greater was considered abnormal whilst a CAD score less than or equal to 60 was considered to be normal.

Procedure for sputum testing and TB diagnosis

Xpert MTB/RIF (Cepheid, Inc., Sunnyvale, CA, USA) (Xpert) instruments and LED fluorescent microscopy (FM) were placed in the laboratory at the primary health care facility described above. All patients were requested to submit two spot sputum samples; one spot sample was tested with Xpert whilst the other was tested with FM. For FM testing, a further morning sample was also requested in line with the National TB Program (NTP) guidelines for testing with sputum smear microscopy. FM and Xpert testing were done according to the standard operating procedures [35,36]. Briefly, GeneXpert lysate was added to the sputum sample using 2X the volume of the sample, the mixture was incubated for a maximum of 15 minutes with intermittent vortexing. After the incubation 2 mls of the sample were added to the Xpert cartridge and loaded into the Xpert instrument within 30 minutes. Any leftover samples were stored at 4 degrees for a maximum of 12 hours. Slides were prepared and stained using Auramine "O" stain at the primary health care facility and for blinding purposes, the slides were read by a centrally located team who were not aware of the Xpert results. Smears were graded positive for: 10 to 19 AFB were seen in 100 microscopic fields (scored as scanty positive), when 20 to 99 AFB were seen in 100 fields (scored as 1+), when 1 to 10 AFB were seen per field in at least 50 fields (scored as 2+), and when more than 10 AFB were seen per field in at 20 fields (scored as 3+). Patients that were not TB detected by either FM or Xpert underwent a clinical review of

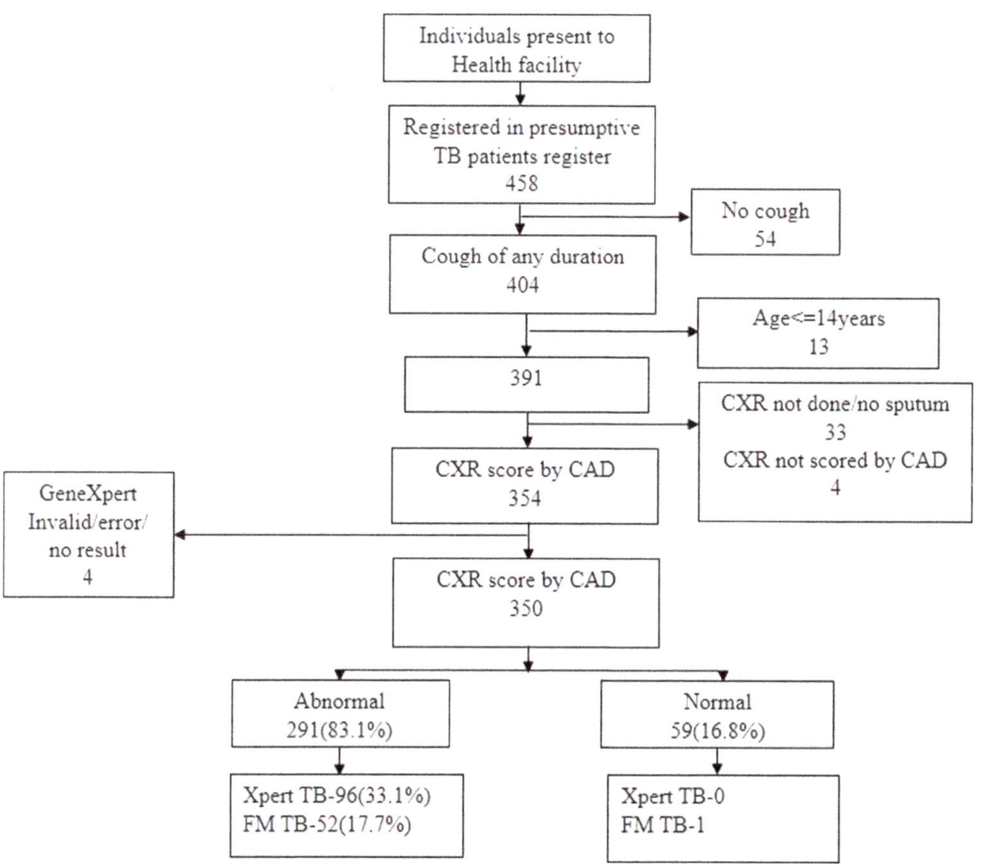

Figure 2. Patient flow.

Table 1. Baseline characteristics of presumptive TB patients with abnormal and Normal Chest x-ray.

	All	Abnormal CXR	Normal CXR	p-Value
	350(%)	291(%)	59(%)	
Gender				0.007
Male	215(61.4)	187(64.3)	27(45.8)	
Female	135(38.6)	103(35.4)	32(54.2)	
Mean age(SD)	36.5(11.6)	36.2(11.4)	37.7(12.4)	0.369
Cough duration				0.912
<2week	93(26.7)	76(26.1)	17(28.8)	0.691
2-8 weeks	226(64.6)	189(64.9)	37(62.7)	0.771
>8 weeks	31(8.9)	26(8.9)	5(8.5)	0.444
Previous TB				0.269
No	272(77.7)	223(76.6)	49(83.0)	
Yes	78(22.3)	68(23.4)	10(16.9)	
HIV status				0.018
Negative	148(42.3)	115(39.5)	33(55.9)	
Positive	190(54.3)	166(57.0)	24(40.7)	
Unknown status	12(3.4)	10(3.4)	2(3.4)	
Fever				0.053
No	74(21.1)	56(19.2)	18(30.5)	
Yes	276(78.9)	235(80.8)	41(69.5)	
Weight loss				<0.0001
No	173(49.3)	131(45.0)	42(71.2)	
Yes	177(50.7)	160(55.0)	17(28.8)	
Chest pains				0.565
No	29(8.3)	23(7.9)	6(10.2)	
Yes	321(91.7)	268(92.1)	53(89.8)	
Shortness of breath				<0.0001
No	246(70.3)	192(66.0)	54(91.5)	
Yes	104(29.7)	99(34.0)	5(8.5)	
Night sweats				0.025
No	111(31.7)	85(29.2)	26(44.1)	
Yes	239(68.3)	206(70.8)	33(55.9)	
Smear result				
Negative	298(85.1)	240(82.5)	58(98.3)	<0.0001
Scanty positive	8(2.3)	8(2.7)	0	0.225
1+	12(3.4)	12(4.1)	0	0.105
2+	17(4.9)	16(5.5)	1(1.7)	0.160
3+	15(4.3)	15(5.1)	0	0.059
Xpert Ct				
No TB detected	254(72.6)	195(67.0)	59(100.0)	<0.0001
>28(very low TB)	16(4.6)	16(5.5)	0	0.049
22-28(low TB)	20(5.7)	20(6.9)	0	0.022
16-22(medium TB)	36(10.3)	36(12.4)	0	0.001
<16(high TB)	24(6.9)	24(8.2)	0	0.010

symptoms, as well as physical examination by a clinician. The clinician also reviewed the CXR independent of the CAD score to decide whether or not to commence TB treatment.

Definition of TB diagnosis

A diagnosis of TB in this study was defined as bacteriologically confirmed TB or clinical TB. Bacteriologically confirmed TB was defined as Xpert TB detected or FM positive (AFB positive) whereas clinical TB was defined as TB treatment commenced on

Table 2. Sensitivity, specificity of CXR compared to GeneXpert MTB/RIF.

Compared to gold standard-Xpert TB Detected				
	Sensitivity (%)	**Specificity%**	**PPV**	**NPV**
	(95%CI)	**(95%CI)**	**(95%CI)**	**(95%CI)**
CXR regardless of smear status N = 350				
All*	96/96 (100%)	59/254 (23.2%)	96/291(33.0%)	59/59 (100%)
	(96.2–100)	(18.2–28.9)	(27.6–38.7)	(93.9–100)
HIV positive	57/57 (100%)	24/133 (18.0%)	57/166 (34.3%)	24/24 (100%)
	(93.7–100)	(11.9–25.6)	(27.2–42.1)	(85.7–100)
HIV negative	35/35 (100%)	33/113 (29.2%)	35/115 (30.4%)	33/33 (100%)
	(90.0–100)	(21.0–38.5)	(22.2–39.7)	(89.4–100)
Smear microscopy negative followed by CXR N = 298				
All*	45/45 (100%)	58/253 (22.9%)	45/240 (18.7%)	58/58 (100%)
	(92.1–100)	(17.9–28.6)	(14.0–24.3)	(93.8–100)
HIV positive	34/34 (100%)	24/133 (18.0%)	34/143 (23.8%)	24/24 (100%)
	(89.7–100)	(11.9–25.6)	(17.1–31.6)	(85.7–100)
HIV negative	10/10 (100%)	32/112 (28.6%)	10/90 (11.1%)	32/32 (100%)
	(69.1–100)	(20.4–37.9)	(5.4–19.5)	(89.1–100)

*includes Unknown HIV status.

patients without bacteriologically confirmed TB but clinician decided to commence TB treatment based on symptoms, CXR and physical examination.

Data Analysis

All data analysis were conducted using STATA Statistical Software (Stata Corporation Version 11. College Station, TX, USA). The performance of the CAD system was evaluated using the area under the receiver operating characteristic (ROC) curve. The ROC curve with 95% confidence interval was constructed using bootstrapping [37]. Initially a descriptive data analysis was done to describe the population that participated in the study. Patient characteristics were compared between patients with an abnormal CXR score and those with a normal CXR score. Significance testing was done using the chi-squared test and the t-test for categorical and continuous variables, respectively. The sensitivity, specificity, positive predictive value (PPV) and negative predictive value (NPV) for the CAD program were determined against Xpert TB detected. The sensitivity, specificity, PPV and NPV were initially calculated (with respective 95% confidence intervals) for the CAD program regardless of smear microscopy status. Then assuming that only patients with a smear negative result would proceed to Xpert testing, CAD program performance was also assessed restricted to patients that were smear negative. Further the sensitivity and specificity of CAD at different CAD thresholds was determined. A ROC curve comparing CAD to Xpert was constructed using Xpert TB as the reference standard. Further data analysis was performed to determine the correlation between CAD score and bacillary load using smear grade and Xpert C_T for microscopy and Xpert respectively. To perform this analysis, Pearson's correlation coefficient was determined with respective p-values and 95% confidence intervals. Logistic regression analysis was performed to determine the association between selected patient characteristics and symptoms with abnormal CXR. To perform this analysis, CAD score as the outcome variable was grouped to form a binary score of $\leq$60 and >60. In univariable analysis, statistical significance was considered to be a p value of $\leq$0.05 and for inclusion in the final multivariable analysis, only variables with a p value of $\leq$0.25 were included.

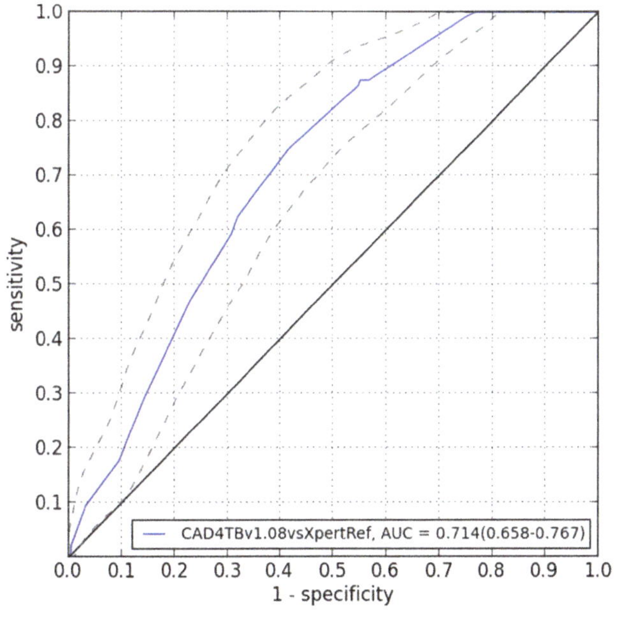

Figure 3. ROC curve comparing CAD score to Xpert TB as the reference standard.

Results

Among all patients that presented to the open access point during the study period, 404/458 (88.2%) met the definition of a

Table 3. Sensitivity and specificity at different CAD score thresholds with Xpert TB as the reference standard.

Sensitivity	1-specificity	CAD Threshold
0	0	99
0.01	0.00	99
0.02	0.00	97
0.09	0.03	95
0.16	0.08	94
0.18	0.09	93
0.29	0.14	92
0.47	0.23	91
0.59	0.31	88
0.60	0.31	86
0.63	0.32	84
0.75	0.42	82
0.86	0.55	81
0.88	0.55	76
0.88	0.56	74
0.88	0.57	72
0.99	0.75	69
1.00	0.77	61
1.00	0.98	60
1.00	1.00	56

presumptive TB patient (figure 2). Amongst these, 13 were aged less than 15 years and were not included in the analysis. 33 patients did not have a CXR or were unable to provide a sputum sample for testing, 4 did not have a CAD reading for their CXR and 4 had an invalid Xpert result giving 350 presumptive TB patients with full data available (See figure 2). Among these 350 patients 291 (83.1%) had a CXR scored as abnormal (CAD>60) and the rest were scored as normal (CAD≤60). Among 291 patients with abnormal CAD score, Xpert detected TB in 96 (33.0%) and FM detected TB in 52 (17.9%) all of whom were also detected using Xpert. Among those with normal CXR, Xpert did not detect any TB, whilst 1 patient was FM positive (1.7%).

There were 215 (61.4%) males and 135 (38.6%) females in the study population. The mean age of study participants was 36.5 (SD 11.6). The majority of patients had a cough of duration 2–8 weeks; 226 (64.6%). HIV positive individuals made up 54.3% of the study population. The proportion of patients with an abnormal CXR was higher among HIV positive patients ($p = 0.018$), those with fever ($p = 0.053$), weight loss ($p < 0.0001$), shortness of breath ($p < 0.0001$) and night sweats ($p = 0.025$) (Table 1).

The sensitivity, specificity, PPV and NPV of CAD compared to Xpert were 100% (95%CI 96.2–100), 23.2% (95%CI 18.2–28.9), 33.0% (95%CI 27.6–38.7) and 100% (95% 93.9–100), respectively. The specificity of CAD among HIV positive individuals was lower than among negative individuals; 18.0% compared to 29.2% ($p = 0.039$). If CXRs were only done in those with a negative smear result, the performance of the CAD program did not change and was similar to when all individuals were considered (see Table 2).

Using Xpert as the reference standard, the area under the ROC curve for CAD was 0.71 (95%CI 0.66–0.77) (See figure 3). The sensitivity of CAD at different CAD threshold is shown in table 3.

Comparing CAD score and bacillary load, the correlation coefficient for smear grade compared to CAD score was $r = 0.30$(95%CI 0.29–0.31) $p < 0.0001$, and for Xpert C_T, $r = 0.37$(95%CI 0.36–0.38) $p < 0.0001$.

Patient characteristics associated with abnormal chest x-ray were male gender adjusted odds ratio (aOR) 2.33(95%CI 1.27–4.26); HIV positive status aOR 1.89 (95%CI 1.02–3.50); and reporting the symptom shortness of breath aOR 4.20 (1.55–11.39) (table 4)

Overall, 97 (27.7%) patients had a confirmed diagnosis of TB by either FM or Xpert. Among patients without a confirmed diagnosis, clinical TB diagnosis was made in 71 out of 253 (28.1%) patients (results not shown).

Discussion

To our knowledge this is the first prospective study to report the use and performance of a computer aided diagnosis system for detection of TB in a real world setting. In this high HIV prevalence setting, the CAD program performed well in both HIV positive and HIV negative patients.

The sensitivity and NPV of CAD was high, and this finding is similar to what has been shown by other studies that have assessed CXR performance for diagnosis of TB [9,11,29]. The difference in this study is that we assessed automatic reading of CXR whereas other works assessed CXR using human readers. Similarly, the low specificity observed in this study is similar to findings by Theron et al. who also found that specificity of CXR alone was below 30% [29] though this study assessed human scorers.

These findings demonstrate the potential role automatic CXR scoring has especially where qualified human resources are scarce. In a previous study performed in the same setting on a similar population, using the same CAD program, we observed that

Table 4. Univariable and multivariable odds ratios showing patient characteristics associated with abnormal CAD score (61–100).

	CAD score ≥61 N = 291(%)	Unadjusted OR	95%CI	Adjusted OR	95%CI
Gender					
Female	103 (35.4)	1.00		1.00	
Male	188 (64.6)	2.16	1.23–3.81	2.33	1.27–4.36
Age group					
15–24	30 (10.3)	1.00			
25–34	112 (38.5)	0.93	0.32–2.69		
≥35	145 (49.8)	0.73	0.26–2.03		
Missing	4 (1.4)	-			
Cough duration					
<2week	76 (26.6)	1.00	-		
2–8 weeks	189 (64.9)	1.14	0.61–2.15		
>8 weeks	26 (8.9)	1.16	0.39–3.47		
Previous TB					
No	223 (76.6)	1.00			
Yes	68 (24.8)	1.50	0.72–3.10		
HIV status					
Negative	115 (39.5)	1.00	-	1.00	
Positive	166 (57.0)	1.98	1.11–3.53	1.89	1.02–3.50
Unknown status	10				
Fever					
No	56 (19.2)	1.00	-		
Yes	235 (80.8)	1.84	0.98–3.44		
Weight loss					
No	131 (45.0)	1.00	-	1.00	
Yes	160 (55.0)	3.02	1.64–5.55	1.72	0.88–3.36
Chest pains					
No	23 (7.9)	1.00	-		
Yes	268 (92.1)	1.32	0.51–3.39		
Shortness of breath					
No	192 (66.0)	1.00	-	1.00	
Yes	99 (34.0)	5.57	2.16–14.37	4.20	1.55–11.39
Night sweats					
No	85 (29.2)	1.00	-		
Yes	206 (70.8)	1.91	1.08–3.39		
Number of symptoms					
1	3 (1.0)	1.00			
2	21 (7.2)	2.10	0.63–12.31		
3	43 (14.8)	2.87	0.52–15.77		
4	97 (33.30	5.39	1.01–28.84		
5 or more	127 (43.6)	9.77	1.79–53.42		

automatic scoring was similar to that by human readers [20]. The CAD program used in this study meets the criteria for a good screening test. Initial screening tests should have a very high sensitivity so that true positive cases will not be missed. In this study, the sensitivity of CAD compared to Xpert was 100% and expectedly the PPV was low. As shown in table 3, a higher threshold for CAD can be chosen at minimal loss of sensitivity, i.e. at a threshold of 76, 88% sensitivity and 45% specificity (much higher than reported in this study) can be achieved. This is applicable in a setting where a higher throughput is required per day, for example, where access to Xpert machines is limited.

HIV infection was significantly associated with abnormal CXR though the specificity of CAD was significantly lower in this group compared to HIV negative individuals. These findings are expected because it is known from literature that HIV positive individuals tend to present with atypical nonspecific CXR changes which can be due to a myriad number of opportunistic infections that can mimic TB in clinical presentation [38–41].

The AUROC for CAD of 0.71 was significantly greater than 0.5 suggesting that the ability by CAD to discriminate between patients with TB and those without TB was more than a chance occurrence. CAD seemed able to discern changes synonymous with TB to a certain degree. CAD's ability to discern changes likely due to TB are also observed through the finding that bacillary load was linearly correlated to the degree of CXR abnormality though this linear association was weak as indicated by the finding of correlation coefficients that were between the values 0.5 and −0.5.

The association between abnormal CXR and some symptoms of TB suggests that CAD performance could possibly be improved by adding symptoms. A regression model can be built that takes into account the CAD score and symptoms to estimate the likelihood of having TB and this could result in improved specificity of CAD. Different abnormal CAD score thresholds could be set depending on individual patients' clinical presentation. Validation of these findings is required with larger studies performed in various settings.

Still 56% among those with highly abnormal CXR did not have TB detected by Xpert. Patients that were Xpert or FM negative underwent clinical assessment which included review of CXR and symptoms as well as physical examination by a clinician to decide whether or not to start TB treatment. Clinical diagnosis of TB was made in 28.1% of these cases and several reasons can be advanced for this finding. Firstly, the CAD system will also score CXR changes due to pneumonia as highly abnormal. Secondly, it is well known that the sensitivity of Xpert among smear negative patients ranges from 60–80% [25,26,28] and in this study, only 15% of the participants were smear positive. Finally, the sensitivity of Xpert can be marginally improved when more than one sputum specimen is examined for each patient [29]. However in this study only one sample was tested per patient, and this may have limited the sensitivity of the Xpert test.

The findings in this study suggest that CAD score can be used to pre-screen patients prior to using Xpert or FM testing. Individuals with a low CAD score ≤60 are very unlikely to have TB and therefore could be offered antibiotics and follow up. In situations where resources are limited and Xpert is not available to all patients suspected of having TB then its use could be targeted by CAD score.

The major limitation of this study was that we used Xpert as the gold standard for determining the sensitivity and specificity of CAD as opposed to using mycobacterial culture. However, single Xpert test has been shown to have a sensitivity of ~98% in smear positive samples and ~75% in smear negative samples [28,42]. Despite the acknowledged limitation, this study still provides useful information on the performance of CAD, especially when used in a high burden setting area where use of such technology is likely to have the most impact. Further studies are required to validate use of CAD as well as to ascertain the cost effectiveness of using CAD to prescreen patients.

Conclusion

The advances that have been made with digital technology have made it possible to score chest radiographs automatically using computer aided diagnosis software programs. This prospective study is the first to demonstrate that CAD has the ability to discriminate CXR as normal or abnormal and that its ability to discriminate between patients with TB and those without TB was more than a chance occurrence. There is potential for roll-out of digital x-ray technology with CAD programs, especially in high burden settings where human resources are scarce. In such situations, CAD and CXR can be used as a pre-screening tool before applying more expensive diagnostic tests but cost effectiveness of such strategies would have to be ascertained. These findings need to be validated with larger studies, using mycobacterial culture as a gold standard.

Acknowledgments

Ab Schaap is acknowledged for his technical assistance on databases and Frank Vijn (Delft Imaging) for the technical assistance with the digital X-ray Unit. Timothy Manja and Mapopa Njovu, the study radiographer and study clinician are acknowledged for their role in data collection, reviewing CXRs and patient management. The authors would like to acknowledge project staff members for their role of data collection.

Author Contributions

Conceived and designed the experiments: HA M. Muyoyeta M. Moyo. Performed the experiments: M. Muyoyeta M. Moyo N. Kasese DM RS. Analyzed the data: M. Muyoyeta PM. Contributed reagents/materials/analysis tools: PM LH BG N. Kasese DM M. Muyoyeta N. Kapata HA. Wrote the paper: HA M. Muyoyeta N. Kapata M. Moyo N. Kasese DM RS PM LH BG. Designed CAD software: BG LH PM.

References

1. Iademarco MF, O'Grady J, Lonnroth K (2012) Chest radiography for tuberculosis screening is back on the agenda. Int J Tuberc Lung Dis 16: 1421–1422.
2. Toman K, Frieden T (2004) Toman's tuberculosis: case detection, treatment and monitoring: questions and answers; TFrieden T, editor. Geneva: World Health Organisation.
3. Jaeger S, Karargyris A, Candemir S, Siegelman J, Folio L, et al. (2013) Automatic screening for tuberculosis in chest radiographs: a survey. Quant Imaging Med Surg 3: 89–99.
4. Hogeweg L, Mol C, de Jong PA, Dawson R, Ayles H, et al. (2010) Fusion of local and global detection systems to detect tuberculosis in chest radiographs. Med Image Comput Comput Assist Interv 13: 650–657.
5. Jaeger S, Karargyris A, Candemir S, Folio L, Siegelman J, et al. (2013) Automatic Tuberculosis Screening Using Chest Radiographs. IEEE Trans Med Imaging.
6. Kurihara Y, Yoshida S, Geshi H, Kubo Y, Kitazoe Y (2001) Economic analysis of a filmless system based on the hospital information system. Stud Health Technol Inform 84: 1166–1170.
7. Muto H, Tani Y, Suzuki S, Yokooka Y, Abe T, et al. (2011) Filmless versus film-based systems in radiographic examination costs: an activity-based costing method. BMC Health Serv Res 11: 246.
8. Naul LG, Sincleair ST (2001) Radiology goes filmless. What does this mean for primary care physicians? Postgrad Med 109: 107–110, 113.
9. Story A, Aldridge RW, Abubakar I, Stagg HR, Lipman M, et al. (2012) Active case finding for pulmonary tuberculosis using mobile digital chest radiography: an observational study. Int J Tuberc Lung Dis 16: 1461–1467.
10. Balabanova Y, Coker R, Fedorin I, Zakharova S, Plavinskij S, et al. (2005) Variability in interpretation of chest radiographs among Russian clinicians and implications for screening programmes: observational study. Bmj 331: 379–382.
11. Hoog AH, Meme HK, van Deutekom H, Mithika AM, Olunga C, et al. (2011) High sensitivity of chest radiograph reading by clinical officers in a tuberculosis prevalence survey. Int J Tuberc Lung Dis 15: 1308–1314.
12. Dawson R, Masuka P, Edwards DJ, Bateman ED, Bekker LG, et al. (2010) Chest radiograph reading and recording system: evaluation for tuberculosis screening in patients with advanced HIV. Int J Tuberc Lung Dis 14: 52–58.
13. Shah S, Demissie M, Lambert L, Ahmed J, Leulseged S, et al. (2009) Intensified tuberculosis case finding among HIV-Infected persons from a voluntary counseling and testing center in Addis Ababa, Ethiopia. J Acquir Immune Defic Syndr 50: 537–545.
14. van Cleeff MR, Kivihya-Ndugga LE, Meme H, Odhiambo JA, Klatser PR (2005) The role and performance of chest X-ray for the diagnosis of tuberculosis: a cost-effectiveness analysis in Nairobi, Kenya. BMC Infect Dis 5: 111.
15. Lewis JJ, Charalambous S, Day JH, Fielding KL, Grant AD, et al. (2009) HIV infection does not affect active case finding of tuberculosis in South African gold miners. Am J Respir Crit Care Med 180: 1271–1278.
16. Nyboe J (1968) Results of the international study on x-ray classification. Bull Int Union Tuberc 41: 115–124.

17. Shaw NJ, Hendry M, Eden OB (1990) Inter-observer variation in interpretation of chest X-rays. Scott Med J 35: 140–141.
18. Graham S, Das GK, Hidvegi RJ, Hanson R, Kosiuk J, et al. (2002) Chest radiograph abnormalities associated with tuberculosis: reproducibility and yield of active cases. Int J Tuberc Lung Dis 6: 137–142.
19. Jaeger S, Karargyris A, Antani S, Thoma G (2012) Detecting tuberculosis in radiographs using combined lung masks. Conf Proc IEEE Eng Med Biol Soc 2012: 4978–4981.
20. Maduskar P, Muyoyeta M, Ayles H, Hogeweg L, Peters-Bax L, et al. (2013) Detection of tuberculosis using digital chest radiography: automated reading vs. interpretation by clinical officers. Int J Tuberc Lung Dis 17: 1613–1620.
21. World Health Organisation (2011) Rapid implementation of the Xpert MTB/RIF diagnostic test: Technical and operational 'How- to'. Practical considerations (WHO/HTM/TB/2011.2).
22. Small PM, Pai M (2010) Tuberculosis diagnosis—time for a game change. N Engl J Med 363: 1070–1071.
23. Pai M, Palamountain KM (2012) New tuberculosis technologies: challenges for retooling and scale-up. Int J Tuberc Lung Dis 16: 1281–1290.
24. Ntinginya EN, Squire SB, Millington KA, Mtafya B, Saathoff E, et al. (2012) Performance of the Xpert(R) MTB/RIF assay in an active case-finding strategy: a pilot study from Tanzania [Short communication]. Int J Tuberc Lung Dis 16: 1468–1470.
25. O'Grady J, Bates M, Chilukutu L, Mzyece J, Cheelo B, et al. (2012) Evaluation of the Xpert MTB/RIF Assay at a Tertiary Care Referral Hospital in a Setting Where Tuberculosis and HIV Infection Are Highly Endemic. Clin Infect Dis 55: 1171–1178.
26. Theron G, Peter J, van Zyl-Smit R, Mishra H, Streicher E, et al. (2011) Evaluation of the Xpert(R) MTB/RIF Assay for the Diagnosis of Pulmonary Tuberculosis in a High HIV Prevalence Setting. Am J Respir Crit Care Med.
27. Sekadde MP, Wobudeya E, Joloba ML, Ssengooba W, Kisembo H, et al. (2013) Evaluation of the Xpert MTB/RIF test for the diagnosis of childhood pulmonary tuberculosis in Uganda: a cross-sectional diagnostic study. BMC Infect Dis 13: 133.
28. Boehme CC, Nicol MP, Nabeta P, Michael JS, Gotuzzo E, et al. (2011) Feasibility, diagnostic accuracy, and effectiveness of decentralised use of the Xpert MTB/RIF test for diagnosis of tuberculosis and multidrug resistance: a multicentre implementation study. Lancet 377: 1495–1505.
29. Theron G, Pooran A, Peter J, van Zyl-Smit R, Kumar Mishra H, et al. (2012) Do adjunct tuberculosis tests, when combined with Xpert MTB/RIF, improve accuracy and the cost of diagnosis in a resource-poor setting? Eur Respir J 40: 161–168.
30. Zachery D, Schaap A, Muyoyeta M, Mulenga D, Brown J, et al. (2012) Changes in tuberculosis notifications and treatment delay in Zambia when introducing a digital X-ray service. Public Health Action 2: 56–60.
31. van Ginneken B, Stegmann MB, Loog M (2006) Segmentation of anatomical structures in chest radiographs using supervised methods: a comparative study on a public database. Med Image Anal 10: 19–40.
32. Duda RO, Hart PE, Stork DG (2001) Pattern Classification. New York: John Wiley and Sons.
33. Arzhaeva Y, Tax DMJ, van Ginneken B (2009) Dissimilarity-based calssification in the absence of local ground truth: apllication to diagnostic interpretation of chest radiographs. Pattern Recognition 42: 1768–1776.
34. Seghers D, Loeckx D, Maes F, Vandermeulen D, Suetens P (2007) Minimal shape and intensity cost path segmentation. IEEE Trans Med Imaging 26: 1115–1129.
35. Cepheid (2009) Xpert MTB/RIF:Two-hour detection of MTB and resistance to rifampicin. Cepheid. pp. 3–4.
36. Rieder HL, van Deun A, Kam KM, Kim SJ, Chonde TM, et al. (2007) Priorities for Tuberculosis Bacteriology Services in Low-Income Countries; Union) IUATaLDT, 68 Boulevard Saint-Michel P, France, editors: International Union Against Tuberculosisand Lung Disease (The Union).
37. Efron B (1979) "Bootstrap methods: another look at jackknife" The annals of Statistics.
38. Barnes PF, Bloch AB, Davidson PT, Snider DE Jr. (1991) Tuberculosis in patients with human immunodeficiency virus infection. N Engl J Med 324: 1644–1650.
39. Chamie G, Luetkemeyer A, Walusimbi-Nanteza M, Okwera A, Whalen CC, et al. (2010) Significant variation in presentation of pulmonary tuberculosis across a high resolution of CD4 strata. Int J Tuberc Lung Dis 14: 1295–1302.
40. Pepper T, Joseph P, Mwenya C, McKee GS, Haushalter A, et al. (2008) Normal chest radiography in pulmonary tuberculosis: implications for obtaining respiratory specimen cultures. Int J Tuberc Lung Dis 12: 397–403.
41. Pitchenik AE, Rubinson HA (1985) The radiographic appearance of tuberculosis in patients with the acquired immune deficiency syndrome (AIDS) and pre-AIDS. Am Rev Respir Dis 131: 393–396.
42. Boehme CC, Nabeta P, Hillemann D, Nicol MP, Shenai S, et al. (2010) Rapid molecular detection of tuberculosis and rifampin resistance. N Engl J Med 363: 1005–1015.

11

Attitudes of People in the UK with HIV Who Are Antiretroviral (ART) Naïve to Starting ART at High CD4 Counts for Potential Health Benefit or to Prevent HIV Transmission

Alison J. Rodger[1]*, Andrew Phillips[1], Andrew Speakman[1], Richard Gilson[1], Martin Fisher[2], Ed Wilkins[3], Jane Anderson[4], Margaret Johnson[5], Rebecca O'Connell[6], Simon Collins[7], Jonathan Elford[8], Lorraine Sherr[1], Fiona C. Lampe[1] and for the ASTRA (Antiretrovirals, Sexual Transmission Risk and Attitudes) Study Group¶

1 University College London, London, United Kingdom, **2** Brighton and Sussex University Hospitals NHS Trust, Brighton, United Kingdom, **3** Pennine Acute Hospitals NHS Trust, Manchester, United Kingdom, **4** Homerton University Hospital NHS Foundation Trust, London, United Kingdom, **5** Royal Free NHS London Foundation Trust, London, United Kingdom, **6** Newham University NHS Hospital Trust, London, United Kingdom, **7** HIV i-Base, London, United Kingdom, **8** City University London, London, United Kingdom

Abstract

Objective: To assess if a strategy of early ART to prevent HIV transmission is acceptable to ART naïve people with HIV with high CD4 counts.

Design: ASTRA is a UK multicentre, cross sectional study of 3258 HIV outpatients in 2011/12. A self-completed questionnaire collected sociodemographic, behavioral and health data, and attitudes to ART; CD4 count was recorded from clinical records.

Methods: ART naïve participants with CD4 $\geq$350 cells/μL (n = 281) were asked to agree/disagree/undecided with the statements (i) I would want to start treatment now if this would slightly reduce my risk of getting a serious illness, and (ii) I would want to start treatment now if this would make me less infectious to a sexual partner, even if there was no benefit to my own health.

Results: Participants were 85% MSM, 76% white, 11% women. Of 281 participants, 49.5% and 45.2% agreed they would start ART for reasons (i) and (ii) respectively; 62.6% agreed with either (i) or (ii); 12.5% agreed with neither; 24.9% were uncertain. Factors independently associated ($p<0.1$) with agreement to (i) were: lower CD4, more recent HIV diagnosis, physical symptoms, not being depressed, greater financial hardship, and with agreement to (ii) were: being heterosexual, more recent HIV diagnosis, being sexually active.

Conclusions: A strategy of starting ART at high CD4 counts is likely to be acceptable to the majority of HIV-diagnosed individuals. Almost half with CD4 >350 would start ART to reduce infectiousness, even if treatment did not benefit their own health. However a significant minority would not like to start ART either for modest health benefit or to reduce infectivity. Any change in approach to ART initiation must take account of individual preferences. Transmission models of potential benefit of early ART should consider that ART uptake may be lower than that seen with low CD4 counts.

Editor: Scarlett L. Bellamy, University of Pennsylvania School of Medicine, United States of America

Funding: The ASTRA study presents independent research funded by the National Institute for Health Research (NIHR) under its Programme Grants for Applied Research funding scheme(RP-PG-0608-10142). The views expressed in this presentation are those of the authors and not necessarily those of the NHS, the NIHR or the Department of Health. The funders had no role in study design, data collection and analysis, decision to publish, or preparation of the manuscript.

Competing Interests: The authors have declared that no competing interests exist.

* E-mail: alison.rodger@ucl.ac.uk

¶ Membership of the ASTRA Study Group is provided in the Acknowledgments.

Introduction

Untreated HIV-infection causes progressive CD4 depletion and increasing risk of AIDS-defining illnesses and death. It is uncontroversial that antiretroviral treatment (ART) should be started before immunosuppression is advanced and the risk of serious illness becomes significant. However there is no clear consensus regarding precisely when (at what CD4 count) an HIV-infected person should start ART. In the current (2012) European AIDs Clinical Society guidelines, commencement of ART is recommended with a CD4 count below 350 cells/μL [1]. With asymptomatic HIV infection and a CD4 count between 350–500 cells/μL it is recommended that ART be considered, but deferred at counts >500 cells/μL [1]. Similar recommendations on CD4 thresholds are made by the UK 2012 guidelines [2]. In July 2012, WHO guidelines, which are influential for treatment programmes in developing countries, recommended starting ART at a threshold of 500 CD4 cells/μL [3]. In contrast, in 2012 the U.S. Guideline Committee, the DHHS [4], and the IAS-USA [5], recommended that ART be initiated in all people with HIV, regardless of CD4 count. Recommendations to start at CD4 counts above 350 cells/μL are based on evidence from observational studies and trials with deferral strategies to start below 250 cells/μL, and remain controversial [6].

Randomized Control Trial (RCT) evidence of the clinical effectiveness of starting ART (at higher CD4 counts) is currently being evaluated in the START trial [7], an international trial that has almost fully recruited 4600 participants and also in the TEMPRANO trial [8] - now fully recruited with 1600 participants in Côte D'Ivoire. In START, HIV-infected individuals with CD4 count >500 cells/μL are randomized to immediate ART initiation or deferral until CD4 count has declined to 350 cells/μL. The results of TEMPRANO are expected in 2015 and START in 2016. However, even if clinical benefit were shown in randomized evaluation, the absolute risk reduction of ill health associated with early ART is likely to be modest, given the low risk of serious illness with CD4 counts >350 cells/μL [9].

However, the potential individual clinical benefit of earlier treatment is not the only factor under consideration in the debate regarding when people diagnosed with HIV should start ART. There is increasing interest in a policy of early ART to reduce HIV transmission. Observational studies report that people on ART with a suppressed viral load have markedly reduced infectiousness [10–12]. The HPTN 052 RCT prospectively evaluated the effect of ART on prevention of HIV transmission to HIV negative heterosexual partners. This study reported 96% reduction of transmissions in serodifferent couples (CD4 count 350–550 cells/μL at entry) assigned to the early ART arm [13] compared to those where ART was differed to CD4 count <250 cells/μL. The results of this landmark trial in 2011 dramatically increased interest in the use of ART for prevention. UK, European, WHO and American guidelines now recommend explaining to all HIV positive individuals that there is a beneficial effect of ART on infectiousness and that ART be offered to anyone who wants to take it to reduce transmission risk [2,4,14,15].

The question arises as to whether a policy of ART for all people diagnosed with HIV should be adopted, even in the absence of evidence of significant individual health benefit.

There remain unanswered questions prior to widespread roll out of ART for prevention of transmission for people with higher CD4 counts. Issues include the durability of the prevention effect and, especially in a non-trial setting, the lack of precise transmission risk estimates for sex without the use of condoms (particularly for anal sex), long term adherence and tolerability of treatment, and the potential for transmission of resistant strains. In addition there are issues in resource-restrained environments with insufficient roll out of ART to those under 350 cells/μL [16]. One of the most significant unknowns, however, is the extent to which a policy of early ART would be acceptable to people with HIV, particularly if there was little or no individual health benefit to starting therapy at higher CD4 counts.

The aim of this study was to use data from the ASTRA (Antiretroviral, Sexual Transmission Risk and Attitudes) UK multi-centre questionnaire study of outpatients with HIV, to investigate attitudes to earlier ART (i) for modest potential health benefit, and (ii) to reduce infectiousness, among ART-naïve HIV diagnosed individuals with CD4 count ≥350cells/μL.

Methods

Ethics statement

Ethical approval for the ASTRA study was obtained via the National Research Ethics Service (10/H0720/70).

ASTRA was a cross-sectional self-administered questionnaire study in 3258 outpatients recruited from February 2011 to December 2012 at eight UK outpatient HIV clinics. The overall response rate was 64%. The questionnaire collected information on demographic, social, lifestyle, HIV and health-related factors, in addition to beliefs about sexual transmission risk, and attitudes to early ART (for participants who were ART naïve only). Most recent CD4 count and viral load were recorded from clinical records for all participants. In addition, 2983 (92%) of the 3258 participants gave consent for linkage of their questionnaire data with routine clinical information from their HIV clinic records. The full methods for the ASTRA study are published elsewhere [17].

Of 3258 participants, 3202 gave information on ART status of which 364 (11.4%) reported that they had never taken ART. Of these 364, a further 6 participants were excluded as linked clinical data recorded ART use at the time of the questionnaire. Of the remaining 358 participants 281 had a CD4 cell count of ≥ 350cells/μL (according to CD4 count recorded in the study log) and are included in this analysis (8.6% of the total ASTRA sample).

Participants who were ART naïve were asked the extent to which they agreed with the following statements: (i) I would want to start treatment now if this would slightly reduce my risk of getting a serious illness; (ii) I would want to start treatment now if this would make me less infectious to a sexual partner, even if there was no benefit to my own health

Response options were: strongly agree; tend to agree; undecided or no opinion; tend to disagree; strongly disagree. Factors associated with agreement ('strongly agree' or 'tend to agree', versus all other responses) to statements (i) (starting for modest health benefit) and (ii) (starting to reduce infectiousness) were assessed.

Factors considered were demographic and social factors [age group, gender/sexuality, ethnicity, country of birth, employment status, education, financial hardship, current partner, children, social support (assessed by a modified version of the Duke UNC Functional Social Support Questionnaire [18]); HIV-related factors [time since HIV diagnosis, latest CD4 count]; health-related factors [hepatitis C diagnosis ever, recent diagnosed sexually transmitted infection; depressive symptoms ('major depressive disorder' according to PHQ-9 [19]; moderate or high physical symptom distress (assessed by a modified version of the Memorial Symptoms Assessment Scale Short-Form [20]); lifestyle factors [smoking status, alcohol use (assessed by modified WHO AUDIT-C questionnaire) and alcohol dependency (assessed by CAGE questionnaire [21], recent recreational drug use]; recent sexual activity; ART optimism (agreement with the statement 'better HIV treatment means people are less worried about infecting others').

Chi-squared tests and chi-squared tests for trend were used to assess the univariable associations of the above factors with agreement to attitude questions (i) and (ii). Logistic regression analysis was used to produce unadjusted odds ratios with 95%

confidence intervals, and to assess multivariable associations. The final multivariable models were developed as follows: first all factors with p≤0.1 in univariable associations were included in an intermediate model; next each of the other factors was added to the intermediate model individually, and retained if p≤0.1. Results are presented as adjusted odds ratios (OR) with 95% confidence intervals. Likelihood ratio tests were used to produce p-values. ART optimism variables were not considered as potential factors to be included in the multivariable model as they were considered too similar to the outcomes of interest (attitudes to early ART).

Results

Overall, 281 ART naïve participants were included in this analysis (Table 1). Of these 85.0% were MSM, 3.9% heterosexual men and 11.0% women. The mean age was 39.5 years (range 20 to 71 years). Ethnicity was 76.2% white, 8.5% Black African and 15.3% other ethnicity. CD4 count was 350–499 mm^3, 500–699 mm^3 and ≥700 mm^3 in 35.2%, 38.1% and 26.7% respectively. Overall 74.4% were in employment and 46.3% university educated. In terms of sufficient money to cover basic needs, less than half (44.8%) reported always having sufficient money to cover basic needs. Half (50.5%) had a stable partner of whom 47.2% were also HIV positive. In terms of health behaviours; 43.4% were current smokers, 24.2% had hazardous or harmful drinking on CAGE screen and 53.0% had used recreational drugs in the previous 3 months.

Figure 1 shows attitudes to starting early ART. A quarter (25.3%) of participants strongly agreed that they would want to start ART now to slightly reduce risk of serious illness, while a similar number (24.2%) tended to agree with this statement. A further quarter (25.3%) was undecided, and the remaining quarter disagreed (tend to disagree 16%, strongly disagree: 9.3%). A similar pattern of response was apparent for wanting to start ART now to reduce infectiousness even if there was no health benefit, although the proportions who were undecided was somewhat higher (30.2%).

Combining the 'strongly' and 'tend to' responses, the percentages of participants agreeing that they would want to start ART now to: (i) slightly reduce risk of serious illness was 49.5% (139/281) and (ii) to reduce infectiousness even if there was no health benefit was 45.2% (127/281). Overall, 32.0% (90/281) of participants agreed with both statements (i) and (ii), 30.6% (86/291) agreed with one of the two statements, 12.5% (35/281) disagreed with both statements, and 24.9% (70/281) were uncertain.

Table 1 shows the unadjusted associations of agreement with statements (i) and (ii) with other factors (demographic, socio-economic, health-related, lifestyle, sexual activity and ART optimism). In unadjusted analysis, 'wanting to start ART for modest health benefit' was associated with being heterosexual compared to MSM (p = 0.080), greater levels of financial hardship (p = 0.004, test for trend), low levels of social support (p = 0.017, trend), having a lower CD4 count (p = 0.09, trend), shorter length of time since HIV diagnosis (p = 0.019, trend), having moderate or high physical symptom distress scores (p = 0.016) and agreeing that ART meant people were less worried about infecting others (p = 0.005). Univariable associations with starting ART for (ii) to reduce infectiousness even if there was no health benefit were being heterosexual compared to MSM (p = 0.092), shorter length of time since HIV diagnosis (p = 0.001, trend), being sexually active in the past 3 months (p = 0.056) and agreeing that ART meant people were less worried about infecting others (p<0.001). Among participants who were sexually active, there was no evidence that the proportion wanting to start to reduce infectiousness differed between those having condom-protected compared to condom-less sex (Table 1).

Table 2 and 3 show factors included in the final multivariable models for agreement with statements (i) and (ii). The ART optimism variable was not included in these models. Factors that remained independently associated (p<0.1) with wanting to start ART for (i) modest health benefit were: having a lower CD4 count; a more recent HIV diagnosis; financial hardship; presence of moderate or high physical symptom distress. In addition, absence of major depressive disorder by PHQ-9 was significantly associated with wanting to start ART for health benefit once the other factors were included in the model. Factors independently associated (p≤0.1) with (ii) wanting to start ART to reduce infectiousness even if there was no health benefit were: having a more recent HIV diagnosis; being heterosexual compared to MSM; being currently sexually active.

Discussion

This is the first study to our knowledge to assess the acceptability of ART at high CD4 counts to reduce the risk of transmission to others in people with HIV in a general clinic setting. We found that almost one half (45%) of HIV-diagnosed individuals not on ART with CD4 ≥350cells/μL reported that they would want to start early ART to reduce infectiousness, even with no health benefit and that half (50%) would want to start for modest health benefit i.e. a small reduction in risk of serious illness. Overall, 62.6% would want to start ART for either or both reasons, 12.5% indicated they would not want to start for either reason, while 24.9% were uncertain. People who had lived longer with HIV were much less likely to want to start ART for either reason, and those with higher CD4 counts were less likely to want to start for modest health benefit.

There is now overwhelming evidence of the reduction in infectiousness through heterosexual sex when the HIV positive partner is on ART with a suppressed VL, although evidence for reduction in infectiousness through anal sex is still lacking [22]. It is therefore entirely appropriate that this should be explained to all people with HIV and ART offered to those who wish to take it to reduce infectiousness; a stance reflected in current guidelines in this area [1,3,4,14]. It is, however, a different matter to advance a general recommendation of ART for all those with diagnosed HIV to prevent transmission as a public health measure. Indeed a key factor in determining in the acceptability and therefore the success of such a strategy of 'ART for prevention of HIV transmission' must be the willingness of people who are HIV positive to voluntarily take ART at higher CD4 counts for what may be a minimal absolute reduction in personal risk of adverse clinical outcomes

It is also important to consider the generalizability of 'when to start' RCTs which may show modest health gain. The success of ART is highly dependent on readiness to start and motivation to adhere to treatment. Trial participants are a selected group who necessarily must agree in principle to randomisation to early treatment, and may well have a preference for early ART, or high motivation to adhere to ART. The promise of a slight health gain may not universally be viewed by people who are HIV positive as a sufficient incentive to start ART at high CD4 counts and individual preferences and concerns need to be taken into account.

We found that those with high CD4 counts (>700 cells/μL) were much less likely to want to start ART for a small reduction in the risk of serious illness, most likely reflecting their perception of

Table 1. Association of factors with (i) wanting to start ART for modest health benefit* and (ii) wanting to start ART to reduce infectiousness* among 281 ART naïve people with CD4≥350/cells/μL.

		N	n (%) who agree with (i) would start for modest health benefit	P value	n (%) who agree with (ii) Would start to reduce infectiousness	P value
TOTAL		281	139 (49.5)		127 (45.2)	
Gender/Sexuality group	MSM	239	113 (47.3)	0.080	103 (43.1)	0.092
	Heterosexual men and women	42	26 (61.9)		24 (57.1)	
Ethnicity	White	214	101 (47.2)	0.17	94 (43.9)	0.44
	Black African/other ethnicity	67	38 (56.7)		33 (49.3)	
Born in UK?	Yes	170	80 (47.1)	0.48	77 (45.3)	0.82
	No	107	55 (51.4)		47 (43.9)	
Age group (Years)	≤30	44	19 (43.2)	0.64	21 (47.7)	0.88
	30–50	196	100 (51.0)		90 (45.9)	
	>50	31	15 (48.4)		13 (41.9)	
Employment	Employed	209	98 (46.9)	0.14	93 (44.5)	0.69
	Other	72	41 (56.9)		34 (47.2)	
Education	Uni education	130	65 (50.0)	0.78	62 (47.7)	0.42
	Other	147	71 (48.3)		63 (42.9)	
'Money to cover basic needs?' (financial hardship)	Yes, always	126	50 (39.7)	0.004 trend	53 (42.1)	0.22 trend
	Yes, mostly	82	44 (53.7)		38 (46.3)	
	Yes, sometimes	43	24 (55.8)		18 (41.9)	
	No	27	18 (66.7)		16 (59.2)	
Stable partner	Yes, HIV +ve	67	33 (49.3)	0.19	25 (37.3)	0.30
	Yes, HIV −ve	75	31 (41.3)		37 (49.3)	
	No partner	138	75 (54.3)		65 (47.1)	
Have children	Yes	43	26 (60.5)	0.12	22 (51.2)	0.41
	No	237	113 (47.7)		105 (44.3)	
Social support group (measure of supportive relationships, modified Duke UNC FSSQ)	1: High	79	31 (39.2)	0.017 trend	31 (39.2)	0.76 trend
	2–4	171	89 (52.0)		85 (49.7)	
	5: Low	27	17 (63.0)		9 (33.3)	
Time since HIV diagnosis	≤3 months	30	17 (56.7)	0.019 trend	14 (46.7)	0.001 trend
	3 months–2 years	91	52 (57.1)		53 (58.2)	
	2–5 years	79	36 (45.6)		38 (48.1)	
	>5 years	78	31 (39.7)		21 (26.9)	
CD4 count/cells/μL from clinic records	350–499	99	54 (54.5)	0.090 trend	43 (43.4)	0.46 trend
	500–699	107	54 (50.5)		47 (43.9)	
	≥700	75	31 (41.3)		37 (49.3)	
Smoking status	Current	122	60 (49.2)	0.92	53 (43.4)	0.61
	Ex	68	35 (51.5)		29 (42.6)	
	Never	91	44 (48.4)		45 (49.5)	
Heavy drinking# (modified WHO AUDIT-C)	No	247	124 (50.2)	0.51	108 (43.7)	0.18
	Yes	34	15 (44.1)		19 (55.9)	
Alcohol misuse (by CAGE)	No	213	105 (49.3)	0.92	93 (43.7)	0.36
	Yes	68	34 (50.0)		34 (50.0)	
Recreational drug past 3 months	No	132	62 (47.0)	0.43	56 (42.4)	0.38
	Yes	149	77 (51.7)		71 (47.7)	
Major depression symptoms (by PHQ-9)	No	239	121 (50.6)	0.35	108 (45.2)	0.99

Table 1. Cont.

		N	n (%) who agree with (i) would start for modest health benefit	P value	n (%) who agree with (ii) Would start to reduce infectiousness	P value
	Yes	42	18 (42.9)		19 (45.2)	
Moderate/high physical symptom distress$ (modified MSAS-SF questionnaire)	No	239	111 (46.4)	0.016	109 (45.6)	0.74
	Yes	42	28 (66.7)		18 (42.9)	
Hepatitis C diagnosis ever	No	254	127 (50.0)	0.58	118 (46.5)	0.19
	Yes	27	12 (44.4)		9 (33.3)	
STI in past 3 months	No	237	115 (48.5)	0.46	106 (44.7)	0.71
	Yes	44	24 (54.5)		21 (47.7)	
Sexually active (vaginal/anal sex) in past 3 months	No	61	28 (45.9)	0.53	21 (34.4)	0.056
	Yes	220	111 (50.5)		106 (48.2)	
Sexual activity category in past 3 months:	No vaginal/anal sex status partner(s)	61	28 (45.9)	0.36	21 (34.4)	0.20
	Condom-protected sex only	86	49 (57.0)		45 (52.3)	
	Condom-less sex HIV+ve partners only	75	33 (44.0)		34 (45.3)	
	Condom-less sex HIV-ve or unknown status partner(s)	51	24 (47.1)		23 (45.1)	
Agree ART mean people less worried infecting others (ART optimism)	Yes	100	61 (61.0)	0.005	60 (60.0)	<0.001
	No/unsure	175	76 (43.4)		64 (35.6)	

* tend to agree or strongly agree combined, versus undecided/tend to disagree/strongly disagree combined.
P values by chi-squared tests, and chi-squared tests for trend.
#usual alcohol intake of at least 5 units 4 or more times a week, or at least 10 units 2–3 times a week.
$score of 10 or more, based on total distress score for 19 physical symptoms, each scored 0 (symptom not present or no distress) to 4 (distressed very much by symptom).

their current low risk of such health problems. We also found a strong association with financial hardship. People experiencing greater levels of financial hardship were considerably more likely to want to start ART for modest health benefit perhaps indicating the vulnerability of their situation and the unwillingness to consider even a small health risk due to the potential impact on an already precarious financial situation. We also found that those who scored higher for physical symptom distress were more likely to wish to start ART for modest health benefit, which may indicate optimism about the potential health benefits of ART, or that they perceive that their current symptoms may be due to uncontrolled HIV infection. Conversely participants who met criteria for major

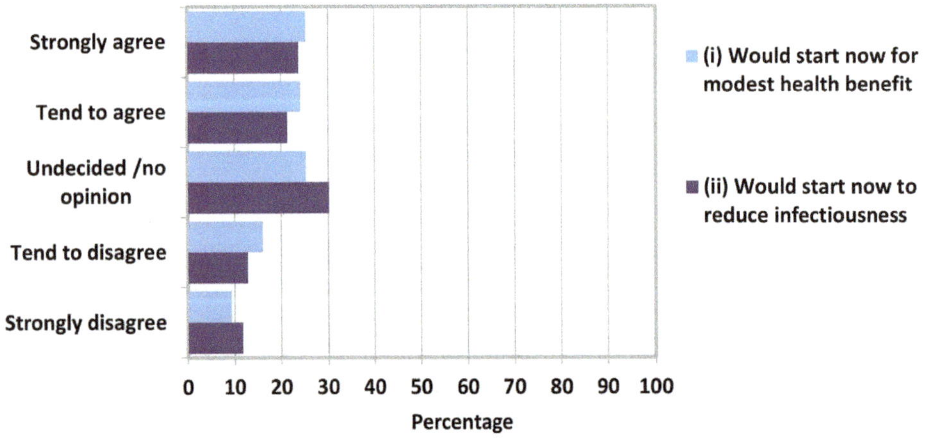

Figure 1. Attitudes to early ART among 281 ART naïve individuals with CD4 ≥350cells/µL.

Table 2. Independent association of factors with (i) wanting to start ART for modest health benefit* in ART naïve people with CD4≥350/cells/μL.

		N	n (%) who agree*	P value	Unadjusted odds ratio (95% CI)	Adjusted odds ratio (95% CI) # (N = 275)	P value for adjusted model#
TOTAL		281	139 (49.5)				
'Money to cover basic needs?'(financial hardship)	Yes, always	126	50 (39.7)	0.004 trend	1	1	0.007 trend
	Yes, mostly	82	44 (53.7)		1.8 (1.0, 3.1)	1.8 (1.0, 3.3)	
	Yes, sometimes	43	24 (55.8)		1.9 (1.0, 3.9)	2.2 (1.0, 4.7)	
	No	27	18 (66.7)		3.0 (1.3, 7.3)	2.8 (1.1, 7.5)	
Time since HIV diagnosis	≤3 months	30	17 (56.7)	0.019 trend	1.0 (0.4, 2.3)	0.8 (0.3, 2.0)	0.038 trend
	3 months–2 years	91	52 (57.1)		1	1	
	2–5 years	79	36 (45.6)		0.6 (0.3, 1.2)	0.6 (0.3, 1.1)	
	>5 years	78	31 (39.7)		0.5 (0.3, 0.9)	0.4 (0.2, 0.8)	
CD4 count cells/μL	350–499	99	54 (54.5)	0.090 trend	1	1	0.044 trend
	500–699	107	54 (50.5)		0.8 (0.5, 1.5)	0.8 (0.4, 1.4)	
	≥700	75	31 (41.3)		0.6 (0.3, 1.1)	0.5 (0.3, 1.0)	
Major depression (PHQ-9 MDD)	No	239	121 (50.6)	0.35	1	1	0.019
	Yes	42	18 (42.9)		0.7 (0.4, 1.4)	0.4 (0.2, 0.9)	
Moderate/high physical symptom distress$ (modified MSAS questionnaire)	No	239	111 (46.4)	0.016	1	1	0.046
	Yes	42	28 (66.7)		2.3 (1.2, 4.6)	2.3 (1.0, 5.1)	

*tend to agree or strongly agree combined, versus undecided/tend to disagree/strongly disagree combined.
#using logistic regression analysis; p values by likelihood ratio test.
$score of 10 or more, based on total distress score for 19 physical symptoms, each scored 0 (symptom not present or no distress) to 4 (distressed very much by symptom).

Table 3. Independent association of factors with (ii) wanting to start ART to reduce infectiousness* among 281 ART people who were ART naïve with CD4≥350cells/μL.

		N	n (%) who agree*	P value	Unadjusted odds ratio (95% CI)	Adjusted odds ratio (95% CI): # (N = 278)	P value for adjusted model#
TOTAL		281	127 (45.2)				
Gender/sexuality	MSM	239	103 (43.1)	0.092	1	1	0.058
	Heterosexual men and women	42	24 (57.1)		1.8 (0.9, 3.4)	2.0 (1.0, 4.1)	
Time since HIV diagnosis	≤3 months	30	14 (46.7)	0.001 trend	0.6 (0.2, 1.4)	0.6 (0.2, 1.5)	0.001 trend
	3 months–2 years	91	53 (58.2)		1	1	
	2–5 years	79	38 (48.1)		0.7 (0.4, 1.2)	0.7 (0.3, 1.3)	
	>5 years	78	21 (26.9)		0.3 (0.1, 0.5)	0.2 (0.1, 0.5)	
Sexually active in past 3 months	No	61	21 (34.4)	0.056	1	1	0.025
	Yes	220	106 (48.2)		1.8 (1.0, 3.2)	2.0 (1.1, 3.9)	

* tend to agree or strongly agree combined, versus undecided/tend to disagree/strongly disagree combined;
#using logistic regression analysis; p values by likelihood ratio test.

depressive symptoms were less likely to wish to start ART for health benefit, perhaps indicating a reduced interest or concern in their health, or lack of motivation to take regular medication or a negative low mood meant that positive health or future benefits did not resonate as important in their life choices.

People who had lived longer with diagnosed HIV were less likely to want to start immediate ART, either for reasons of health or reduced infectivity. Individuals who have lived longer with untreated HIV and potentially through an era where early treatment was not on the agenda and there was a great awareness of drug toxicities, may perceive their current health status as good without being on ART. The association with time since HIV diagnosis was particularly strong for not wanting to start to reduce infectiousness. Individuals with longstanding infections have had years to assess issues of infectiousness and potentially adapt sexual practices and other risks, so may be less interested in ART to reduce infectiousness. Conversely individuals diagnosed recently have been diagnosed in an era where early ART is very much on the agenda, new treatments are safe and tolerable, and ART may be generally more favourably perceived.

Modelling work to assess the impact of ART on population transmission has considered issues such as adherence to ART and sexual risk behaviour change on ART, but the potential lower uptake of ART has not generally been considered, presumably partly due to lack of data on the acceptability of taking ART to individuals with high CD4 counts [23]. Our results are consistent with the view that uptake and adherence might well be somewhat lower if ART is initiated in people where there is not a clear and immediate personal health risk.

One potential limitation of our study is that the study was conducted only in UK HIV outpatients, and the majority of participants were MSM. Results may not be generalizable to other settings, in particular to resource-limited settings. We had limited power to assess differences according to gender/transmission group. Our data suggested demographic variation in likelihood of wanting to start immediate ART, with some evidence that heterosexual men and women were more likely to want to start than MSM. However confidence intervals for this estimate were wide. In addition, the views we are reporting were expressed in 2011/12 and we should consider that attitudes to early ART to prevent transmission might change rapidly as the publicity around treatment for prevention gains momentum. Likewise, results from ongoing randomized trials could cause a further shift in views. In addition, in this large quantitative study we were not able to explore in depth motivations for responses to the questions regarding early ART. Further qualitative research in this area would be beneficial.

The only other data that we are aware of in this area is from the HPTN 052 trial itself, which was conducted, largely in heterosexual couples in 9 countries [13]. After the HPTN 052 study results of 96% reduction in HIV transmission in the early treatment arm were made public, ART was offered to all HIV positive participants in the delayed arm. However, even with the knowledge that ART had a dramatic effect on risk of transmission, 20% of participants in the deferred ART group - who had agreed at study entry to possible randomisation to initiate ART at higher CD4 count - chose not to initiate ART [24]. This indicates that even in this highly select study population a significant proportion of people feel reluctance to initiate ART primarily to prevent transmission.

In conclusion, a strategy of starting ART at high CD4 counts is likely to be acceptable to the majority of HIV-diagnosed individuals. Nearly two thirds of ART naïve respondents with CD4>350/mm^3 said they would start immediate ART either for modest health benefit or to reduce infectiousness and almost one half would start to reduce infectiousness even if there were no health benefits. Nonetheless, our results suggest that any change in ART initiation must carefully consider individual needs and preferences. It is unlikely to be universally acceptable to initiate ART at a high CD4 count, even if modest health benefits become established in randomized trials. This information on potential uptake of earlier ART should be incorporated into transmission models of the potential population benefit of early ART.

Acknowledgments

We wish to acknowledge all ASTRA study participants and the ASTRA clinic teams and study team as follows:

- Mortimer Market Centre: Richard Gilson; Simon Edwards; Lewis Haddow; Simon Gilson; Christina Broussard; Robert Pralat; Sonali Wayal
- Royal Free Hospital: Alison Rodger; Jeff McDonnell; Margaret Johnson; Aderonke Adebiyi
- Royal Sussex County Hospital Brighton: Martin Fisher; Nicky Perry; Alex Pollard; Serge Fedele; Louise Kerr; Lisa Heald; Wendy Hadley; Kerry Hobbs; Julia Williams; Elaney Youssef; Celia Richardson; Sean Groth
- North Manchester General Hospital: Ed Wilkins; Yvonne Clowes; Jennifer Cullie; Cynthia Murphy; Christina Martin; Valerie George; Andrew Thompson
- Homerton University Hospital: Jane Anderson; Sifiso Mguni; Damilola Awosika; Rosalind Scourse
- Eastbourne Sexual Health Clinic: Kazeem Aderogba; Caron Osborne; Sue Cross; Jacqueline Whinney; Martin Jones
- Newham University Hospital: Dr Rebecca O'Connell; Cheryl Tawana
- Whipps Cross University Hospital: Monica Lascar; Zandile Maseko, Gemma Townsend, Vera Theodore, Jas Sagoo.
- Marina Daskalopoulou
- ASTRA advisory group: Lorraine Sherr; Graham Hart; Simon Collins; Anne Johnson; Anna-Maria Geretti; Bill Burman; Alec Miners; Jonathan Elford

Author Contributions

Conceived and designed the experiments: AR AP FL. Performed the experiments: RG MF EW JA AR MJ RO'C. Analyzed the data: FL. Wrote the paper: AR. Contributed to the study design: AS RG MJ SC JE LS. Contributed to interpretation of the data: AS RG MJ SC JE LS. Contributed to writing of the paper: AS RG MJ SC JE LS.

References

1. http://europeanaidsclinicalsociety.org/images/stories/EACS-Pdf/EacsGuidelines-v6.1-2edition.pdf. Accessed 2013 Nov 14.
2. Williams I, Churchill D, Anderson J, Boffito M, Bower M, et al. (2012) British HIV Association Guidelines for the Treatment of HIV-1-positive adults with antiretroviral therapy 2012. HIV Med 13 (Suppl 2):1–85.
3. Hirnschall G, Harries AD, Easterbrook PJ, Doherty MC, Ball A, et al. (2013) The next generation of the World Health Organization's global antiretroviral guidance. J Int AIDS 30;16:18757
4. US Department of Health and Human Services. Guidelines for the use of antiretroviral agents in HIV-1-infected adults and adolescents. Available: http://aidsinfo.nih.gov/guidelines. Accessed 2013 Nov 14.
5. Thompson MA, Aberg JA, Hoy JF, Telenti A, Benson C, et al. (2012) Antiretroviral treatment of adult HIV infection. 2012 Recommendations of the International Antiviral Society – USA Panel. JAMA 308:387–402.
6. Sabin C, Cooper D, Collins S, Schechter M (2013) Rating evidence in treatment guidelines: a case example of when to initiate combination antiretroviral therapy (cART) in HIV-positive asymptomatic persons. AIDS 27(12):1839–46
7. Babiker AG, Emery S, Fätkenheuer G, Gordin FM, Grund B, et al for the INSIGHT START Study Group (2013) Considerations in the rationale, design and methods of the Strategic Timing of Anti-Retroviral Treatment (START) study. Clin Trials 10 (1 Suppl):S5–S36.
8. Early Antiretroviral Treatment and/or Early Isoniazid Prophylaxis Against Tuberculosis in HIV-infected Adults (ANRS 12136 TEMPRANO). ClinicalTrials.gov Identifier: NCT00495651
9. Lodwick RK, Sabin CA, Porter K, Ledergerber B, van Sighem A, et al. (2010) Death rates in HIV-positive antiretroviral-naive patients with CD4 count greater than 350 cells per microL in Europe and North America: a pooled cohort observational study. Lancet 376 (9738):340–5.
10. Quinn TC, Wawer MD, Sewankambo N, Serwadda D, Li C, et al. (2000) Viral load and heterosexual transmission of HIV type 1. N Engl J Med 342:921–929.
11. Donnell D, Baeten JM, Kiarie J, Thomas KK, Stevens W, et al. (2010) Heterosexual HIV-1 transmission after initiation of antiretroviral therapy: a prospective cohort analysis. Lancet 375:2092–2098.
12. Attia S, Egger M, Müller M, Zwahlen M, Low N (2009) Sexual transmission of HIV according to viral load and antiretroviral therapy: systematic review and meta-analysis. AIDS 23:1397–1404.
13. Cohen MS, Chen YQ, McCauley M, Gamble T, Hosseinipour MC, et al. (2011) Prevention of HIV-1 infection with early antiretroviral therapy. N Engl J Med 365:493–505.
14. World Health Organization. Guidance on Couples HIV Testing and Counseling, including antiretroviral therapy for treatment and prevention in serodiscordant couples. Recommendations for a public health approach. 2012. Available: http://www.who.int/hiv/pub/guidelines/9789241501972/en/. Accessed 2013 Nov 14.
15. Department of Health. BHIVA and EAGA position statement on the use of antiretroviral therapy to reduce HIV transmission. Available: https://www.gov.uk/government/publications/bhiva-and-eaga-position-statement-on-the-use-of-antiretroviral-therapy-to-reduce-hiv-transmission. Accessed 2013 Nov 14.
16. Coutsoudis A, Goga A, Desmond C, Barron P, Black V, et al. (2013) Is Option B+ the best choice? Lancet 381(9863):269–71
17. Speakman A, Rodger A, Phillips AN, Gilson R, Johnson M, et al. (2013) The 'Antiretrovirals, Sexual Transmission Risk and Attitudes' (ASTRA) Study. Design, methods and participant characteristics. PLoS One 8(10):e77230
18. Broadhead WE, Gehlbach SH, De Gruy FV, Kaplan BH (1988) The Duke-UNC Functional Social Support Questionnaire. Measurement of social support in family medicine patients. Med Care 26: 709–723. Available: http://www.jstor.org/stable/3765493. doi:10.1097/00005650-198807000-00006. PubMed: 3393031.
19. Kroenke K, Spitzer RL, Williams JB (2001) The PHQ-9: validity of a brief depression severity measure. Joun Gen Intern Med 16 (9): 606–613.
20. Chang VT, Hwang SS, Feuerman M, Kasimis BS, Thaler HT (2000) The memorial symptom assessment scale short form (MSAS-SF). Cancer 89: 1162–1171.
21. Mayfield D, McLeod G, Hall P (1974) The CAGE questionnaire: validation of a new alcoholism screening instrument. The American Journal of Psychiatry 131: 1121–1123.
22. Rodger AJ, Bruun T, Vernazza P, Collins S, Estrada V, et al. (2013) Further research needed to support a policy of antiretroviral therapy as an HIV prevention initiative. Antivir Ther 18(3):285–7
23. Granich RM, Gilks CF, Dye C, De Cock KM, Williams BG (2009) Universal voluntary HIV testing with immediate antiretroviral therapy as a strategy for elimination of HIV transmission: a mathematical model. Lancet. 373(9657):48–57.
24. T. Gamble M, McCauley J, Talley P, Dusara P, Maliwichi M, et al. for the HPTN 052 Study Team. Acceptance of ART in the Delay Arm after Notification of Interim Study Results: Data from HPTN 052. Poster #550, 20th CROI, Atlanta, March 3rd to 6th, 2013.

12

Multi-Level Factors Affecting Entry into and Engagement in the HIV Continuum of Care in Iringa, Tanzania

Erica H. Layer[1]*, Caitlin E. Kennedy[2], Sarah W. Beckham[2], Jessie K. Mbwambo[3], Samuel Likindikoki[3], Wendy W. Davis[4], Deanna L. Kerrigan[1], Heena Brahmbhatt[5], the LTC Tanzania Collaborative Study Team¶

1 Department of Health, Behavior and Society, Johns Hopkins Bloomberg School of Public Health, Baltimore, Maryland, United States of America, **2** Department of International Health, Johns Hopkins Bloomberg School of Public Health, Baltimore, Maryland, United States of America, **3** Department of Psychiatry, Muhimbili University of Health and Allied Sciences, Dar es Salaam, Tanzania, **4** Department of Epidemiology, Johns Hopkins Bloomberg School of Public Health, Baltimore, Maryland, United States of America, **5** Department of Population, Family and Reproductive Health, Johns Hopkins Bloomberg School of Public Health, Baltimore, Maryland, United States of America

Abstract

Progression through the HIV continuum of care, from HIV testing to lifelong retention in antiretroviral therapy (ART) care and treatment programs, is critical to the success of HIV treatment and prevention efforts. However, significant losses occur at each stage of the continuum and little is known about contextual factors contributing to disengagement at these stages. This study sought to explore multi-level barriers and facilitators influencing entry into and engagement in the continuum of care in Iringa, Tanzania. We used a mixed-methods study design including facility-based assessments and interviews with providers and clients of HIV testing and treatment services; interviews, focus group discussions and observations with community-based providers and clients of HIV care and support services; and longitudinal interviews with men and women living with HIV to understand their trajectories in care. Data were analyzed using narrative analysis to identify key themes across levels and stages in the continuum of care. Participants identified multiple compounding barriers to progression through the continuum of care at the individual, facility, community and structural levels. Key barriers included the reluctance to engage in HIV services while healthy, rigid clinic policies, disrespectful treatment from service providers, stock-outs of supplies, stigma and discrimination, alternate healing systems, distance to health facilities and poverty. Social support from family, friends or support groups, home-based care providers, income generating opportunities and community mobilization activities facilitated engagement throughout the HIV continuum. Findings highlight the complex, multi-dimensional dynamics that individuals experience throughout the continuum of care and underscore the importance of a holistic and multi-level perspective to understand this process. Addressing barriers at each level is important to promoting increased engagement throughout the continuum.

Editor: Michael H. Chung, University of Washington, United States of America

Funding: This work was supported by USAID | Project SEARCH, Task Order No. 2, funded by the US Agency for International Development under Contract No. GHH-I-00-07-00032-00, beginning 30 September 2008, and supported by the President's Emergency Plan for AIDS Relief. Publication of this article was funded in part by the Open Access Promotion Fund of the Johns Hopkins University Libraries. The funders had no role in study design, data collection and analysis, decision to publish, or preparation of the manuscript.

Competing Interests: The authors have declared that no competing interests exist.

* Email: erica.layer@gmail.com

¶ Membership of the LTC Tanzania Collaborative Study Team is provided in the Acknowledgments.

Introduction

In the past decade, the scale-up of antiretroviral therapy (ART) has led to an unprecedented number of people living with HIV (PLHIV) on treatment, resulting in decreased HIV-related morbidity, mortality and onward transmission [1,2]. Despite these considerable gains, ART coverage remains low. In 2012, treatment coverage in low and middle income countries was estimated at 61% of all eligible individuals under the 2010 World Health Organization (WHO) HIV treatment guidelines. However, under new WHO treatment guidelines, which recommend ART initiation at $\leq$500 cells/mm^3, this ART coverage represents only 34% of the people eligible in 2013 [3,4] and considerable obstacles to universal treatment access remain.

Successful ART programs depend on the progression of PLHIV through a number of stages. This continuum of care, also referred to as a cascade of care or HIV care pathway, includes HIV testing and counseling (HTC), linkage to care (defined here as the initial engagement with the health system to receive HIV care and treatment services following an HIV diagnosis), eligibility assessment and clinical staging or CD4 testing, pre-ART care, ART initiation and lifelong ART adherence and retention in care. Considerable losses along each stage of this continuum have been well documented, especially in the pre-ART initiation [5–7] and

Table 1. Summary of data collection across methods.

Facility-based data collection				
	Client IDIs	**Provider IDIs**	**Direct observations**	**Facility checklists**
HTC (n = 4)	23	7	4	4
CTC (n = 4)	24	8	4	4
PMTCT (n = 4)	24	7	4	4
VMMC (n = 1)	4	4	3	0
Total	**75**	**26**	**15**	**12**

Community-based data collection				
	Client IDIs	**Provider/key informant IDIs**	**Direct observations**	**Focus group discussions**
Support groups (n = 5)	30	10	5	5
Spiritual healers (n = 2)	12	4	1	0
Traditional healers (n = 12)	0	12	2	0
Government liaison (n = 4)	0	4	0	0
Total	**42**	**30**	**8**	**5**

Longitudinal interview participants					
	Men		**Women**		**Total**
	ART	**No ART**	**ART**	**No ART**	
Urban	6	7	10	8	**31**
Rural	7	4	4	2	**17**
Total	**13**	**11**	**14**	**10**	**48**

HTC: HIV testing and counseling; CTC: Care and treatment center; PMTCT: Prevention of mother-to-child transmission; VMMC: Voluntary medical male circumcision; IDIs: In-depth interviews; ART: Anti-retroviral therapy.

retention stages [8]. However, factors contributing to suboptimal progression at each stage of the continuum are poorly understood. A systematic review of factors affecting linkages to ART in sub-Saharan Africa found that key barriers to engagement included transport costs and distance to health facilities, stigma and fear of disclosure and limited human resources [9]. MacPherson et al. reported that socio-cultural norms, support networks and limited human resources and laboratory capacity affected progression throughout the continuum in Malawi [10].

The Iringa region of Tanzania is located 500 kilometers (km) southwest of Dar es Salaam and has a population of approximately 900,000 people. The Tanzam Highway, a conduit between Dar es Salaam and Northern Zambia, cuts through Iringa, which is also home to large tea and timber plantations, leading to high rates of mobility which potentially contribute to HIV risk. Most people in Iringa are involved in small-scale agriculture [11]. A majority of the population lives more than 2 km from the nearest health facility, while over one third of rural residents live greater than 5 km away [12]. Iringa has the second highest HIV prevalence (9.1%) in the country [12]. It is estimated that only 68.6% of women and 52.7% of men in Iringa have ever been tested for HIV and received their results (26.0% and 28.2% in the past year, respectively) [12]. Thus, many individuals are unaware of their HIV serostatus and miss the opportunity for linkage to care and treatment services. Consistent with findings across sub-Saharan Africa, findings from other regions of Tanzania indicate that a substantial portion of individuals who receive a positive HIV diagnosis are not referred for subsequent care, and among those who *are* referred, many fail to register for services and clinical staging [13,14]. Country-level estimates suggest that less than one third of those eligible for ART based on WHO 2013 guidelines are receiving it [3].

While there is considerable need to improve access to and retention in HIV services in Iringa and elsewhere, little is known about barriers or facilitators to linkages throughout the HIV continuum of care. In this study, we examined multi-level barriers and facilitators influencing entry into and engagement in the continuum of care in Iringa, Tanzania.

Methods

Between March and November 2013 we used a mixed-methods approach to examine individual, facility and community level factors affecting linkages to HIV care and treatment.

Facility-based data collection

At the facility level, we conducted assessments of a sample of HIV testing and treatment services, including HTC sites (n = 4), care and treatment centers (CTC) (n = 4), prevention of mother to child transmission (PMTCT) services (n = 4) and voluntary medical male circumcision (VMMC) outreach sites (n = 1). Facilities were purposively sampled throughout Iringa region to ensure diversity in urban/rural location and facility size. At each facility, we completed a structured facility checklist to gather basic operational information, a direct observation to collect information on the flow of clientele through each facility, provider-client interactions, client-client interactions, wait times, and the general ambience. In addition, convenience sampling was used to identify providers (n = 26) and HIV-infected clients (n = 75) at facilities who participated in qualitative in-depth interviews (IDIs). Facility-based data collection is summarized in Table 1.

Community-based data collection

In addition to facility-based data, we visited community-based providers of HIV care and support services, including support groups (n = 5), traditional healers (n = 12) and spiritual/religious healers (n = 2) sampled from urban and rural areas throughout Iringa region. In-depth qualitative interviews were conducted with providers (n = 52) and clients (n = 42) of these services who were conveniently sampled at these locations. IDIs were conducted with government representatives who had worked with traditional healers in the region (n = 4). We also conducted direct observations at community-based facilities. Finally, focus group discussions (FGD) were organized with existing support groups for PLHIV (n = 5) (Table 1).

Cohort of PLHIV

To further explore the social context and dynamics of barriers and facilitators of engagement in care, we conducted longitudinal interviews with 48 PLHIV followed prospectively at three time points over the course of six months. Participants were stratified by gender, ART status and urban/rural location (Table 1).

Data analysis

All data were collected by trained Tanzanian research assistants. Interviews and focus groups were recorded, transcribed, and translated into English. Analysis of qualitative data was conducted through a multi-stage process using a narrative and case study approach. First, each individual interview with providers and clients was summarized and re-written in brief narrative form, with particular attention to structured categories of interest related to linkages within the continuum of care. Second, for each facility, these individual narrative summaries from both client and provider interviews were brought together with data from the facility checklist and observations to develop a case summary report for that facility. In this way, the analysis brought together a variety of perspectives on individual-level, provider-level, and facility-level barriers and facilitators to engagement in HIV services for a particular setting. Similar methodology was employed for the longitudinal interviews that also sought to document the story or trajectory of each participant through the continuum of care and key factors linked to continuity or breakages in progression. Key themes were identified across these narratives and developed into a conceptual framework summarizing findings across levels and steps in the continuum of care.

Ethics Statement

All participants provided oral informed consent prior to data collection. Written consent was not obtained because the authors felt that asking individuals to disclose their full names by providing written consent would decrease participants' anonymity. Participants received 10,000 Tanzanian Shillings (~USD6) at the end of each interview or FGD for their time and transport. Ethical approval, including the decision to obtain oral informed consent, was obtained from Muhimbili University of Health and Allied Sciences, the Tanzania National Institute for Medical Research and Johns Hopkins Bloomberg School of Public Health.

Results

We present factors influencing engagement at each stage of the continuum of HIV care and treatment, including HTC, linkage to care, clinical staging, pre-ART care, ART and cross-cutting issues. At each stage in the HIV care continuum, we identified barriers and facilitators at the individual, facility, community, and structural levels, presented in a multi-level continuum of care framework (Figure 1). Representative quotes from key themes are summarized in Table 2. In the cohort of PLHIV, data collectors made multiple attempts to contact cohort participants for follow-up interviews. If the participant could not be reached after three separate attempts (including phone calls and visits to the participant's home of record), the participant was designated as lost to follow up. Seven participants (3 females, 4 males) were lost to follow up during the second round of data collection and two participants (both male) were lost to follow up for the third round of data collection, for an overall retention rate of 81%.

HIV testing and counseling

HTC is available in Iringa through a mix of client-initiated and provider-initiated services. Client-initiated voluntary counseling and testing services are offered through both static and mobile services. Provider-initiated testing and counseling (PITC) should be routinely practiced in all health facilities. In addition, PITC services are offered routinely with VMMC and antenatal care (ANC) services.

Study participants described a perception that HIV is characterized by severe illness and that infected individuals would be visibly sick. Participants described a strong reluctance to test while healthy and said that individuals often distrust positive test results if they are not sick and therefore often seek multiple HIV tests to confirm positive results. Fear of the stress of an HIV-positive test result and internalized stigma were additional individual-level barriers to HTC, especially among asymptomatic individuals (Table 2, quote 1.1).

A majority of our participants received HTC only after being sick for extended periods of time. Medical care was sought at multiple health facilities for recurring illnesses but HTC was rarely recommended during these visits. Despite the government policy of PITC, this service was not routinely offered to participants in our study and providers missed critical cases among these clients (Table 2, quote 1.2.1).

Persistent stock-outs of HIV test kits, which were common throughout Iringa region for the duration of this study, prevented access to HTC services. Service providers noted that they routinely turned clients away, while clients explained that the stock-out had caused many people to give up on HIV testing completely (Table 2, quote 1.3.1).

In addition, women in our study were often denied antenatal care (ANC) services unless they brought their male partners to the first ANC visit for couples HIV testing. During a direct observation of a PMTCT facility, a data collector noted a poster on the wall that stated (in Swahili), "It is required for a pregnant woman to come with her husband/partner on her first [ANC] visit. You will not be served without following this." Multiple women in our study reported being denied ANC services because they were not accompanied by a male partner, and participants shared stories of friends who delayed ANC services or avoided them altogether (Table 2, quote 1.4.1 and 1.4.2). While Tanzania national guidelines do not support this practice, they do encourage increased male participation and recommend that ANC providers promote "couple/partner HIV/STI testing and counseling for all young women" [15]. Service providers interviewed for this study

Table 2. Selected themes and quotes from study participants.

LTC Stage	Theme	Quote
1. HTC	1.1 Fear of testing	1.1.1 "People are intimidated by the idea of testing– whether positive or negative–they are afraid. They don't go for testing if they are not sick. They have a belief that knowing your HIV status is the end of your life. They think that you will die immediately after knowing your status." –HTC client, M, 36
	1.2 Inadequate PITC	1.2.1 "I was treated at a dispensary at home and they failed to diagnose me. They referred me to a hospital. I was treated more than twice [without being advised to test for HIV], and then I decided by myself to check my health [get an HIV test]." –HTC client, F, 47
	1.3 HIV test kit stock-out	1.3.1 "We are losing so many clients. It's very disgusting for someone who leaves his house knowing he is going to the hospital for services. [He thinks] "I am going to get [HTC] services." And then when he gets there, he finds there are no services. It's not only here; this is the problem for all places in this district. I think it's also in all places in Tanzania … So that's a big problem. We face some difficulties in delivering HCT services." –HTC provider, F, 55
	1.4 Denying pregnant women ANC/PMTCT services until partner attends	1.4.1 "When women go to the [ANC] clinic, they are asked to bring their husbands. They don't get other services until they bring their husbands. So the husbands are motivated because they tell themselves that their partner won't get the services unless they bring them to the clinic and they can't stay without those services. That's how they get tested [for HIV]." -PMTCT Provider, F, 41; 1.4.2 "I already knew that when you go to the ANC clinic for the first time, you must go with a man - your partner. But he was not present; whenever I made a phone call to him he would say, "I will come" or "I will make arrangements." Time was passing and even when I came for the first time, the nurse sent me back … The nurse told me, "Go to advise your husband [to come with you to the clinic] so that we can help you." -PMTCT client, F, 31
	1.5 Visiting traditional healers	1.5.1 "I took my wife to a traditional healer. I thought she was bewitched. I thought she was bewitched because she was being treated [at the hospital] but did not heal. What will he tell you? He will tell you that he has the medicine and that the patient has been bewitched. He cannot tell you that she has HIV. They want her to suffer and most of them are liars … There isn't one [who would advise a client to go to a hospital]." –Cohort participant, M, 30
	1.6 Belief that ART is efficacious	1.6.1 "I came here [for HTC] voluntarily. I decided to check on my HIV status because a lot of people who get tested get [ART] services and are doing well. I decided to come here for testing so that I will start taking [ART] medications before my health deteriorates. If they find that I am HIV infected, I know I will comply well with the treatment regimen and there will be few side effects … Your health will be at stake if you wait for a fever before you get tested." –HTC client, F, 30
	1.7 PLHIV testimonials	1.7.1 "We help people to realize that HIV is not such a scary disease … There are a lot of people who are going for testing right now due to our influence. Some come here for advice. They go for HIV testing and are initiated on ART. They are doing well now because of us. They were so afraid of HIV testing before the group was established. I decided to disclose my status in public to save others. Some people who have symptoms come to me for advice. I tell them about everything that they have to do so that they are started on medications." –Support group member, F, 34
2. Linkage to care	2.1 Feeling healthy at diagnosis	2.1.1 "I saw that my body was good and I didn't have any problem. I was not sick so I decided to stay strong like that without following up on anything." –Cohort participant, F, 28
	2.2 Separately located services	2.2.1 "[It's challenging when a client] has tested in centers that do not have other services. You give the client a referral letter to go to another place. When he reaches a certain place [CTC] and starts hesitating, he will stop. But if he tested here, he would be escorted to the CTC by the VCT service provider." –CTC provider, F, 38
	2.3 Challenges during initial linkage	2.3.1 "When I reached [the doctor's room at the CTC] they told me that I should go back to the reception. When I saw that man [from reception] he was so strict. He said 'I told you to go there [to the doctor].' But I said, 'They told me that I should come back here [to reception].' But he insisted that I should go up. Then I went back upstairs again. When I reached there, they asked what is wrong with me. I told them, 'I was sent to bring you this note [referral letter from HTC]. I totally don't understand the process in this place.' Then they said since the doctor is not around I should leave and come back on Tuesday." –HTC client, M, 33; 2.3.2 "I would expect that when you come here [to the CTC] for the first time, providers should explain what you are supposed to do. But here they are so rude and say, "We have already told you to do this and this" when they haven't told you anything. So it happens that you don't understand what to do because they fail to explain, and if you make a little mistake then they start to yell at you, and so it happens that you start answering them rudely." -HTC client, M, 36
3. Clinical staging and CD4 testing	3.1 Ineffective systems for CD4 testing	3.1.1 "It was troublesome; we used to wake up at 6 am to get [CD4] testing. When you reach there, you find a long line of people and the machine takes only 50 patients, so when you reach 50 it was finished. The others [who did not get tested] had to leave; I had to go there for about a week. I managed to get tested in the second week … You have to wake up about 4 or 5 in the morning so that you can be early; when you are later than that you get turned away." –CTC client, F, 45
4. Pre-ART care	4.1 Cotrimoxazole stock-outs	4.1.1 "Frankly speaking there is not enough [cotrimoxazole]. Most of the time they are disturbing us so much. And for some people who are starting [pre-ART care], when they are coming for the first month, they are told to go and buy them [cotrimoxazole], and in the next month they are told to go and buy them, and in the next month they are told to go and buy them. Now it reaches a point when he sees that he would be better off to go and buy them rather than coming here [to the CTC]; he is wasting his time." -Client, M, 45

Table 2. Cont.

LTC Stage	Theme	Quote
5. ART initiation, adherence and retention	5.1 HIV as a "normal" disease	5.1.1 "During the beginning when we were getting this [CTC] service there used to be very few people. So I felt very bad when I was told that I had the infection … later on I felt normal as they [CTC providers] continued giving me this medication [ART], so as the number of people kept on increasing, I kept on encouraging myself that it is better if I continue using the medication. Initially I felt so weak, I felt like my fellows were somehow stigmatizing me. But after the number of people kept on increasing then I felt like it is just a normal thing and since then I have been feeling good." -Client, M, 47
	5.2 Disrespectful treatment by service providers	5.2.1 "When I reached there [CTC] they said, 'How many are late?' We raised our hands. They said, 'Every day we tell you to come early. When is your time?' One of us raised our hand and said, 'At 8 AM.' The provider said, 'Why are you coming at 9 and we have so much work to do? …Today you will get service at 12.' And surely we were seen at 12. They left, I don't know where, maybe to drink tea, until we got tired, that is when they came back and gave us services." -Cohort participant, F, 42; 5.2.2 "I was on the waiting bench. That's where they weigh us before we enter into the doctor's room. That's when a nurse said, 'You are wearing tight pants and the way you are seated is seductive and you have even applied eye liner. Who are you trying to attract? You just want to hurt others [i.e. infect others].' That was so painful … I stopped attending those services [at the regional hospital] because of the statements used in there. I just stayed home because I had already lost hope because of the statements used by some nurses over there. There were very good services until one nurse spoke to me in a very bad way that made me feel worthless, maybe because of the way I am. So I felt really sad. My heart doesn't feel like going back there because I feel sad every time I see her." –CTC client, F, 31
	5.3 Spiritual healing	5.3.1 "PLHIV can go for the [ART] medications, but we know that it is prayers that sets them free from their problems, not medication. I can say that the medications have their own position but it's very minor, prayers are the main deal." – Spiritual healer, F, 38
	5.4 Support groups	5.4.1 "Disclosing your status makes you strong in such a way that you can't be shaken by any enemy who will try to speak against your status. First and foremost I have my freedom, I don't have bitterness. I have peace of mind wherever I go; it's because of this group."-Support group member, F, 34
	5.5 Home based care providers	5.5.1 "It is easy [to follow up with clients who miss appointments] currently because of these HBCs. We just look where [the patient] comes from and then we just use the HBC from there. [The HBC] tries to follow [the patient], sometimes someone may die and we don't have the information. So [the HBC] will give us the information … If [the patient] just decided not to come, then [the HBC] will also tell us, but currently, by using the HBCs, a majority [of patients] have returned back to the service." -Provider, F, 43
6. Cross-cutting	6.1 Not receiving services	6.1.1 "The ones who are missing CTC services are so many because of the distance. Someone comes, yet he is being told that maybe [cotrimoxazole] is not in stock, you see. And most of them are told to go and buy. Then he comes in the next month then they are telling him, 'You have not had your CD4 checked so we cannot change the medications for you [i.e. initiate ART], so you are supposed to go and buy [cotrimoxazole] again.' So that situation is what leads to that [dropping out of services]. First, he is looking at the distance and he is wasting his time. On the day that he comes, he has to prepare the whole day for not working. So when he prepares that day and then he sees that he doesn't get that service, he sees that it is not a productive work going there [to the CTC]." -Client, M, 45
	6.2 Stigma and discrimination	6.2.1 "I felt that I was discriminated against by my relatives. My relatives did not even contribute a cent to help me nor did they escort me [to the hospital]. And it is not that my relatives do not have the means, they are people who are able to. I was really discriminated [against]. Even my neighbors, my in-laws would even ban their children from coming to my home. They would say, 'You better not eat anything there.' One time, my sister-in-law got sick when she was pregnant, but she said, 'I will try, better I hire someone [else] to take care of me. Because my sister-in-law has AIDS, she might infect me.' Therefore I felt bad." –Client, F, 39
	6.3 Service provider burnout	6.3.1 "We are losing hope because we do this hard job with no motivation of any kind. The work is very hard. You just receive people's problems and you are supposed to help them, but there is nothing that you are going to gain, so it really breaks our hearts … The work is very hard but the government cannot help us … There are other times that our fellows [other service providers] have no plans to help patients who are admitted in the ward who need that service. He might be sick in bed, but he is not attended … If there were incentives then someone would work wholeheartedly." – CTC provider, F, 55

explained that they required women to bring their partners in order to increase male involvement, which appears to be a misrepresentation of national guidelines, with the unintended negative consequence of discouraging single women from seeking care.

Traditional healers offered an alternative to the formal health system and some individuals attended these services after multiple failed attempts to determine the cause of their illness. Clients of traditional healers were rarely advised to test for HIV and noted they were always told that they were bewitched and in need of traditional medicine, preventing further engagement with the health system (Table 2, quote 1.5.1).

Several factors facilitated HTC, including the perception that ART is highly efficacious, often as a result of witnessing health

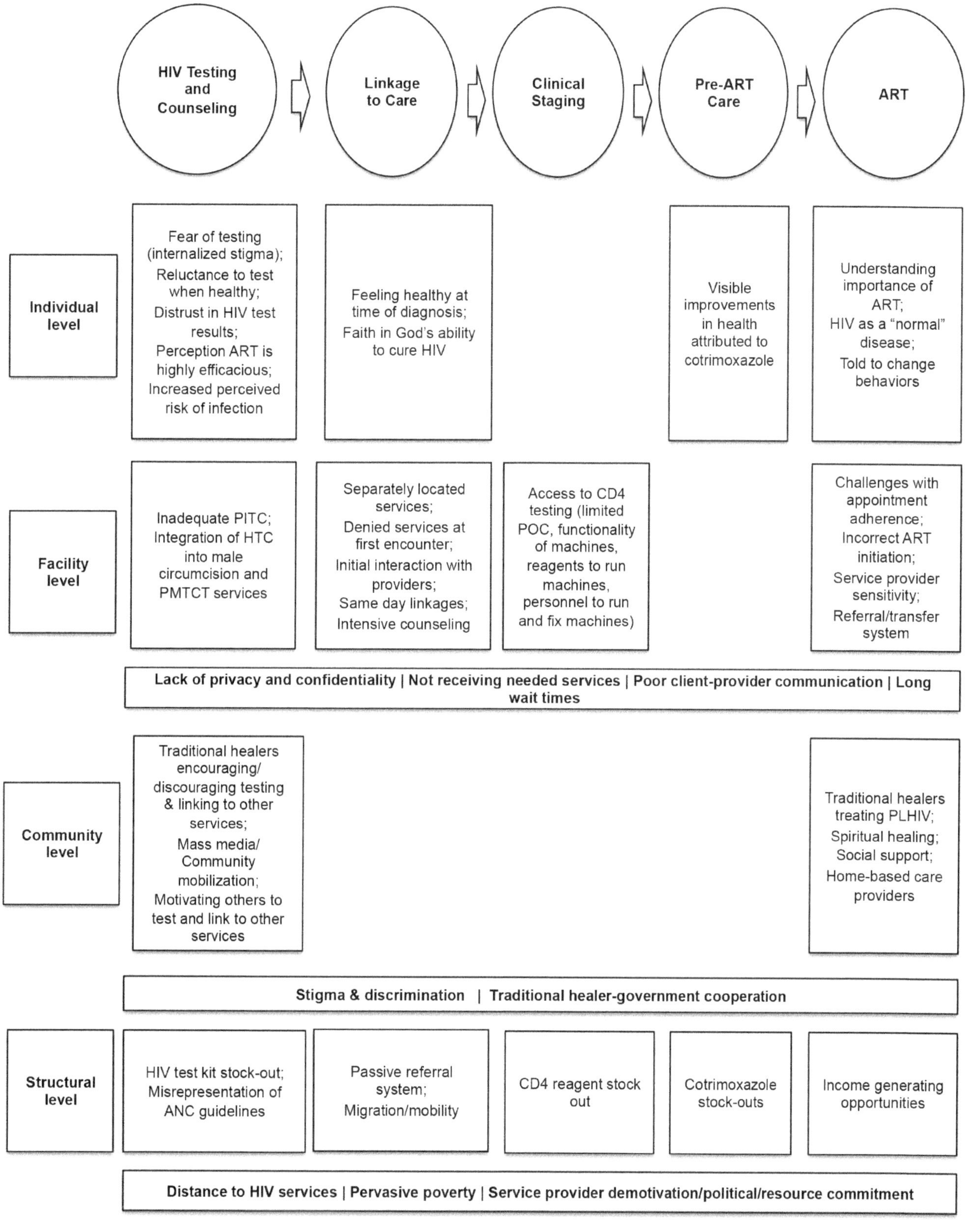

Figure 1. Barriers and facilitators influencing entry into and engagement in the continuum of care.

improvements when a friend or relative initiated ART; increased perceived risk of infection resulting from an AIDS-related death of a spouse or family member; or having multiple sexual partners (Table 2, quote 1.6.1). Mass media promoting HTC, mobile HIV testing services, community mobilization and PLHIV testimonials were additional facilitating factors (Table 2, quote 1.7.1).

Access to and linkage to care

Following HTC, all additional HIV services in Iringa are provided at CTCs. The linkage to care phase includes the process of a newly diagnosed HIV-infected individual successfully progressing from an HTC facility to a CTC for assessment of ART eligibility.

One key facilitator prompting linkage to care was severe illness at the time of HIV diagnosis. These clients expressed relief in determining the cause of their illness and were happy to immediately link to a CTC in order to initiate treatment. In contrast, participants widely acknowledged that asymptomatic individuals were much less likely to link to a CTC because they either did not believe the HIV test results or did not see the point in receiving care (Table 2, quote 2.1.1). Several clients of spiritual healing services also delayed linking to care because they had faith that God would either cure them or stop disease progression.

Co-located HTC and CTC services facilitated linkages to care. Participants agreed that linking a person to a CTC on the same day increased that person's chance of continuing to receive HIV services, especially when a service provider personally escorted the client. However, many HTC facilities were stand-alone, so clients were given a referral card and told to travel to the nearest CTC on their own which was noted as a key point at which individuals drop out of services (Table 2, quote 2.2.1). In addition, providers had no way to follow up with patients to ensure successful linkage to treatment and care services because no active tracking systems existed in the facilities we assessed.

Clients often encountered challenges during their initial visit and were told to leave and return on another day due to restricted opening hours, limited capacity for enrollment and shortages of providers (Table 2, quote 2.3.1). Some participants also expressed frustration at the way they were treated by CTC providers during their initial visit (Table 2, quote 2.3.2).

Clinical Staging and CD4 testing

After successfully linking to HIV care and treatment services, clients undergo clinical and/or laboratory staging to determine whether they are eligible for either pre-ART or ART care. In Iringa, this process most commonly involved a medical evaluation and CD4 testing. According to national guidelines, ART initiation is recommended for individuals with WHO stage 3 and 4 clinical criteria, regardless of CD4 cell count, and for adults and adolescents with a CD4 count <350 cells/mm3, regardless of clinical symptoms [15].

While government guidelines allow for ART initiation in individuals based on clinical evaluation, all participants in our study reported being required to receive CD4 testing before ART initiation. This process was a major challenge for most CTC clients in this study. From the results of the facility checklist, we found that of the four CTC facilities visited, only one had a working CD4 machine, while two had machines that were either broken or lacked reagents. Clients were required to get a referral letter from their original CTC, travel long distances, were often turned away and test results were commonly lost, forcing clients to repeat the process multiple times (Table 2, quote 3.1.1). Because of these inconveniences, participants said that many PLHIV lose hope and drop out of HIV services at this stage.

Pre-ART care

Following staging, PLHIV who are not yet eligible for ART engage in pre-ART care services until they are eligible to initiate ART. This stage in the continuum of care should include regular clinical assessments for ART eligibility and consistent HIV care. According to Tanzanian guidelines, individuals in this stage of the continuum of care should receive cotrimoxazole prophylaxis, a combination of antibiotics used to treat a range of opportunistic infections associated with HIV [15]. Clients are expected to return to the CTC monthly for monitoring and to receive cotrimoxazole, free of charge, and should receive CD4 testing every six months until eligible for ART initiation.

Many ART-ineligible clients who were enrolled in pre-ART care viewed receiving cotrimoxazole as the main benefit of attending monthly appointments. In fact, several clients attributed dramatic improvements in their health to this medication. Unfortunately, chronic stock-outs were common; six out of 11 facilities reported cotrimoxazole stock-outs at the time of the facility checklist and study participants were often told to purchase the medication from a private pharmacy. Participants listed this as a significant factor for drop out of pre-ART care services (Table 2, quote 4.1.1).

ART initiation, adherence and retention

The next stage in the continuum of care is ART initiation. Current Tanzanian national guidelines recommend ART for individuals with CD4 counts of ≤350 cells/mm3 or those with severe or advanced clinical disease. After initiating ART, PLHIV are counseled to adhere to daily ART regimens and should return for regular clinic appointments for assessment, counseling and medication refills.

Many ART clients reported high levels of ART adherence due to health improvements experienced after ART initiation. Additionally, clients were motivated to continue attending CTC services because seeing other PLHIV made them feel that they were "not alone" and helped them to see HIV as a "normal" disease (Table 2, quote 5.1.1).

There were potential provider-level factors that acted as barriers to ART initiation and adherence. Several cohort participants reported that they were told by their doctors to discontinue ART when they became healthy. Participants also noted that they were not initiated on ART, even after their clinical symptoms indicated ART initiation or when their CD4 count was well below 200. However, these situations were reported by only a few study participants and were not supported by observations or interviews with providers, so the generalizability of these findings is not known.

One of the most significant barriers to retention in CTC services was disrespectful and abusive treatment by service providers. Almost all participants in this study encountered negative experiences where they were shouted at, "scolded" or "punished" by one or more providers. Often, negative interactions occurred when a client disobeyed rules set by providers, most commonly arriving late or missing an appointment (Table 2, quote 5.2.1). When clients returned to the CTC on a day other than their assigned clinic day, they were often either denied services completely or forced to wait until the end of the day as punishment or "correction" for their behavior. Harsh and disrespectful treatment was the most common reason for CTC clients to disengage from care (Table 2, quote 5.2.2).

Visiting traditional and spiritual healers were common alternate pathways to care. While most traditional healers said that they were unable to treat HIV, several noted that they routinely diagnosed, treated and cured PLHIV. In addition, *all* spiritual healers expressed faith in God's ability to cure HIV and encouraged their clients to trust in God's healing powers, and one spiritual healer explained that prayers helped PLHIV more than ART (Table 2, quote 5.3.1). A majority of alternate healers said that while they did not discourage clients from attending HIV services, they generally did not actively encourage attendance at HIV services, and several participants knew of people who were encouraged to stop taking ART while participating in spiritual healing services. Most clients of traditional and spiritual healers in this study attended alternate healing services in parallel with CTC services. These individuals were aware of the importance of ART for their survival, but had hope that they might be cured through alternate healing systems, so continued to attend both services. Clients of spiritual healers also discussed the support they received from other PLHIV during healing services as a reason for continued attendance.

Support groups for PLHIV were identified throughout Iringa region. These groups were generally initiated and managed by PLHIV in the community and members attended regular meetings. Each group visited in this study also had an economic strengthening component through income generating activities or savings programs. Members of PLHIV support groups benefitted in many ways which facilitated their involvement in CTC services, including through social support and income generating opportunities. Most group members said they were no longer "embarrassed" of being HIV-positive and did not feel ashamed to attend CTC services because they knew that they were not alone (Table 2, quote 5.4.1). Clients of HIV services who were not members of support groups expressed their desire for more opportunities for support and income generating activities but were not aware of organized groups in the area.

Home based care providers (HBCs), community volunteers who serve as a link between the health system and community by visiting PLHIV in their homes and following up after missed appointments, were present in two CTC facilities in this study. In these facilities, HBCs were mentioned as a very effective system for following up with patients who did not attend their CTC visits since they lived and worked at the village level. Service providers at the only CTC facility with HBCs said that they rarely lost clients to follow-up due to the strong support provided by HBCs (Table 2, quote 5.5.1).

Cross-cutting themes

In addition to the themes presented above which correspond to a specific stage within the continuum of care, several cross-cutting themes were identified which influenced engagement in HIV services at all stages.

Participants described frustration after traveling long distances for care only to be turned away if they arrived outside of clinic hours, if providers were too busy to serve them, if there were stock-outs of HIV test kits and cotrimoxazole or when they encountered challenges accessing CD4 testing services (Table 2, quote 6.1.1). Poor communication between providers and clients limited clients' abilities to fully understand their situation, which led to misunderstanding important concepts such as what CD4 levels mean, the difference between cotrimoxazole and ART, and the importance of lifelong ART adherence. Finally, long wait times and severe crowding, especially at CTC facilities, caused frustration and led some PLHIV to disengage from care.

Stigma, discrimination and internalized stigma were very common themes throughout this study which impeded individuals' ability to access and participate in HIV services. Participants commonly reported that people avoided HTC due to fear of discrimination they would face if others discovered their HIV status, and many CTCs had waiting areas or queues that were outside, making the patients visible to all other hospital attendees or even people passing by. Some CTC clients traveled long distances to avoid seeing people that they knew at CTC facilities in their communities, while others discussed the "humiliation" they were forced to endure every time they attended CTC services. Many clients of HIV services also shared experiences of being discriminated against in their communities (Table 2, quote 6.2.1). Because of the real and perceived social stigma, many participants had not disclosed their HIV status to anyone outside of their immediate family, and many had not disclosed to their spouses due to fear of violence or abandonment.

Service providers discussed challenges they faced which ultimately led to burn out and lower quality care, including severe shortages of staff, lack of incentives and inadequate training. Doctors were often assigned to multiple departments while providers mentioned that they turned clients away from HTC or CTC services if they came towards the end of the day, since they were too exhausted to see more clients (Table 2, quote 6.3.1).

Individual trajectories

While the results presented above highlight specific factors which affect an individual's decision to engage in HIV services, these single barriers and facilitators do not capture the complexity of participant experiences, which often involve multiple competing priorities and challenges. To illustrate this complexity, we present three case studies from participants in the longitudinal cohort to contextualize the themes within a person's life trajectory. All names are pseudonyms.

Emmanuel: Disengagement following poor quality care. In 2011, Emmanuel's wife was pregnant. She told him that it was mandatory for men to accompany their wives to ANC services for HIV testing; if he did not attend, his wife would not receive services. Emmanuel hesitantly agreed to accompany his wife. At this visit, he was diagnosed with HIV even though he felt healthy and had no visible signs of illness.

His wife encouraged him to pursue further HIV care services, so he immediately travelled to the nearest CTC which was more than two hours away via public transportation. However, he became frustrated with the poor quality of care and long distances and disengaged from HIV services after only four visits.

Emmanuel's decision to disengage from care was a culmination of several factors, including inadequate services, being told repeatedly to return on a different day, and the cost associated with each trip. During his visits, he noted that he was not provided with any education or medication. He explained, "I gave them my [CTC] card and they would tell me to come back the next month. I would go the next month, again they would write for me [to come back the next month], without getting any medication." Similarly, he tried four times to receive his CD4 test results but was denied every time and told to return on another day. Emmanuel explained that he could not justify wasting his time and money on CTC visits when the quality of services was so low and he was in good health, so he disengaged from care and never returned.

Linda: Internalized stigma. In 2005, Linda was diagnosed with HIV after being chronically ill for several years. Before her HIV diagnosis, Linda had frequent fevers, chest pain and tuberculosis. Even after completing tuberculosis treatment, she continued to experience recurrent illness but had never been advised to test for HIV by health providers. After ruling out all other possible problems, Linda decided to receive HTC.

After receiving her HIV-positive diagnosis, Linda was shocked and contemplated suicide. She recalled, "I wished to take ten tablets at once so that I would die. That's what I was thinking."

However, several service providers supported her and convinced her to accept her diagnosis and engage in HIV care and treatment services.

Linda did not disclose her HIV status to her husband or her children for one year due to fear of abandonment and discrimination. She believed that people perceived HIV to be a disease brought about by casual sex, and thought that PLHIV were viewed as "hooligans" or "prostitutes." Linda found this particularly challenging because she was an older woman and felt that she was being harshly judged by people in her community.

Linda's decision to receive treatment was challenging and complex. When she arrived for services, extremely long lines, poor ventilation, and waiting for long periods in public where others could identify her as HIV-positive made her feel humiliated. Despite these challenges, Linda continued to engage in HIV services, which is due in large part to her participation in a support group for PLHIV. The group helped her to cope with the challenges she faced while waiting for CTC services and made her understand the importance of ART adherence for her survival.

Furaha: Verbal abuse from service providers. Furaha was diagnosed with HIV in 2007 after suffering from recurrent illnesses for more than one year. She was relieved when she received her HIV diagnosis because she finally discovered what was bothering her and felt happy that she could get relief. She said that her health improved dramatically after ART initiation and she attended CTC services regularly for five years. In 2012 however, she disengaged from care due to missing one CTC appointment because she was working away from home. When she returned on another date, she was scolded and yelled at by the providers who refused to give her ART. She tried to return several weeks later but was still denied services as a punishment for missing one appointment and did not want to continue to face service providers who treated her so poorly.

During the period that she was disengaged from care, Furaha purchased cotrimoxazole from the pharmacy and "borrowed" ART from her friends who were engaged in CTC services. She expressed concern and anxiety about not being able to adhere to ART and said, "I have to go back because I don't want to die. I have to take the medications to stay alive ...I pray that they accept me without scolding".

During the course of this study, Furaha was successfully able to re-engage in care. The doctor "warned" her not to repeat missing appointments, but agreed to allow her to resume ART, but only after repeating three weeks of ART training.

Discussion

Understanding factors which motivate and prevent PLHIV from engaging in and adhering to care at each step along the continuum is critical to successful HIV treatment and prevention efforts. Our findings are consistent with previous studies assessing barriers and facilitators throughout various stages of the HIV care continuum [9,10,16–19]. While many of the barriers presented here have been looked at independently as factors associated with negative care outcomes, few if any studies have looked holistically at all of these multiple levels and types of factors influencing the full continuum of care in a given setting. This study highlights the complex interplay of these factors and the need to provide comprehensive solutions which address the multiple challenges to providing HIV treatment and care services.

An individual's health was a strong influencing factor in progression through the continuum of care. Those who were visibly sick and had ruled out other causes of disease were most likely to seek HTC services, accept their diagnosis and immediately link to care and treatment. Further, these individuals were also the most likely to see dramatic improvements in their health after initiating cotrimoxazole and/or ART, and therefore viewed these medications as important for sustained health. In contrast, healthy participants in our study expressed reluctance to receive HTC and were more likely to delay linking to care or disengage from care and treatment services, which is consistent with other findings throughout sub-Saharan Africa [20–23]. When faced with additional barriers to care such as long distances, high transport costs, stigma and risk of verbal abuse from providers, these individuals often chose not to engage in care because the perceived need for medical care was outweighed by multiple barriers and competing priorities. As treatment guidelines evolve to recommend ART initiation at higher CD4 counts, more people will initiate ART before a noticeable decline in health. Identifying these individuals and ensuring successful progression through the continuum of care is critical, but will be challenging. Fully implementing the policy of universal and routine PITC services in all health facilities to normalize HTC, and behavior change communication strategies to promote earlier testing and engagement in care, could change the current social norms around HIV testing and promote earlier uptake of HIV services.

Persistent stock-out of supplies, including HIV test kits, CD4 reagents and cotrimoxazole were common throughout Iringa region during this study. In addition to causing frustration and demotivation among service providers and clients, these stock-outs decreased trust in the health system, promoted disengagement from care and led to poor health outcomes. HTC providers noted that they routinely turned clients away during frequent HIV test kit stock-outs and believed that these people would give up and not return at a later date. In addition, lack of timely CD4 counts due to broken machines or missing reagents led to an inability to determine ART eligibility and has been shown delay ART initiation [10,24,25]. Provision of free cotrimoxazole, which was described by our study participants as the most important element of pre-ART care, has been shown to double retention in pre-ART care services [26]. Unfortunately, this benefit was undermined by chronic cotrimoxazole stock-outs which led to deep dissatisfaction and reduced clients' perceived need to attend monthly visits. Participants in our study who did not believe they would receive required services were less likely to invest in the time, money and effort needed to attend visits to health facilities. Stock-outs of HIV-related medication and supplies have been documented in other African settings [27–30] and these findings highlight the need to strengthen supply chain management systems. In addition, point of care CD4 testing, which provides immediate results for use in patient care, could eliminate many of the logistical and operational barriers to CD4 testing noted in this study [31–33].

Provider attitudes and treatment of clients were significant barriers to retention in care and the main reason for disengagement from CTC services among clients of ART care. Many study participants endured verbal abuse and disrespectful treatment by providers at CTC facilities because accepting this mistreatment was the only way to receive ART. However, several clients disengaged from care when they could no longer handle being degraded, ridiculed and punished, even though they knew their health would suffer as a consequence. These findings point to a clear need to improve provider-client interactions as a means of reducing disengagement from care. Physical and verbal abuse against patients has been reported in a variety of health settings throughout sub-Saharan Africa [34–37]. In a study in South Africa, Jewkes et al. described providers' abusive treatment as "a complex interplay of concerns including organizational issues, professional insecurities, perceived need to assert 'control' over the environment and sanctioning of the use of coercive and punitive measures to do so, and an underpinning ideology of patient inferiority" [38]. They explained that violence was allowed to become commonplace due to lack of accountability and limited action taken by managers against service providers who abuse patients, which appears consistent with our findings. Service providers in our study discussed burnout and demotivation as a result of staff shortages, unrealistic workloads and lack of supervision and training. Health-system level changes to increase human resources, provide incentives, ensure adequate support systems and provide ongoing training and supervision are needed to increase service provider motivation and improve client-provider interactions.

Consistent with other studies, our findings suggest that HIV-related stigma and discrimination are key barriers to engagement in HIV services throughout the continuum, leading to suboptimal levels of HTC [39], disclosure [40], retention in care [41] and ART adherence [42,43]. Negative health outcomes resulting from HIV-related stigma have been well documented [44–48] and our findings highlight the need for stigma-reduction strategies to accompany HIV prevention and treatment efforts. While effective interventions to reduce community-level stigma and damaging social norms are not well-defined [49], there is general consensus that that four basic approaches are effective in reducing stigmatizing attitudes among individuals and groups, including information, skills-building, counselling and PLHIV testimonials [50,51].

Community-level approaches to HIV service delivery could be one strategy to reduce barriers at multiple levels identified in our study. A growing body of evidence suggests that novel strategies to bring HIV services to the community level through task shifting, such as home-based HIV testing [52–55] and home-based ART initiation [56] and delivery [57–61] are effective, feasible and acceptable [62]. In addition, positive side effects of home-based ART delivery programs include increased community-level social support and decreased discrimination [61,63], and clients of these services reported saving time and money due to reduced clinic visits [64]. These novel community-based strategies would require significant political commitment and operational research to tailor programs to the local context, but may have the potential to strengthen all stages of the HIV care continuum by improving identification of HIV-infected individuals, simplifying linkages to care, improving retention in ART care programs, and reducing structural-level barriers such as distance, cost and stigma and discrimination.

Finally, leveraging and expanding services and opportunities identified in this study which facilitate engagement in care, including PLHIV support groups, income generating opportunities, HBC providers and government engagement with alternate healing systems, could strengthen linkages to care and help to reduce the impact of additional barriers to engagement and retention in care in this setting.

Strengths of this study include the diversity of respondents and data collection methods which provided multiple perspectives on factors affecting the continuum of care in Iringa. In addition, the longitudinal nature of the qualitative cohort allowed us to gain an in-depth understanding of the complexity of PLHIV's experiences as they moved through the continuum of care. At the facility level, our interviews with clients of HIV services and service providers, direct observations and facility checklists allowed us to triangulate findings. In addition, interviews and focus group discussions with members of support groups, traditional healers and spiritual healers add a unique dimension and understanding to community-level influence throughout the continuum of care.

Despite these strengths, the study has several limitations. First, HIV test kit stock-outs limited our ability to interview newly diagnosed clients, especially those who chose not to link to further care and treatment services, which could have provided valuable insight into barriers at this stage. Another limitation was our inability to recruit HIV-infected clients of traditional healers. Traditional healers universally noted that PLHIV do not disclose their status, and they therefore were not aware of any HIV-positive clients. While we would have liked to understand the perspective of this group, we were able to capture experiences from longitudinal cohort participants who had visited traditional healers themselves or knew of people who had.

Conclusion

This study presents a multi-level framework for understanding barriers and facilitators to linkages to care in Iringa, Tanzania. Our findings highlight the complex, multi-dimensional dynamics that individuals experience throughout the continuum of care and underscore the importance of taking a holistic and multi-level perspective to understand this process. Interventions to address single barriers identified in this study are insufficient; our findings illustrate how multiple barriers interact and influence decisions about engagement in care. Addressing barriers at multiple levels is needed to promote increased engagement and retention in care.

Acknowledgments

We would like to thank all of the study participants who contributed to this study. We appreciate the support and contributions from the many individuals who have contributed in a wide variety of ways to this study and the Research to Prevention (R2P) project, especially Charlene Brown, Vincent Wong, Alison Cheng, and Sarah Sandison.

The LTC Tanzania Collaborative Study Team includes Jacob Ntogwisangu, Ard Mwampashi, Catherine Shembilu, David Gitagno, Lilian Mgeni, Maureen Peter, Editha Laizer and Emmanuel Massawe, all from Muhimbili University of Health and Allied Sciences.

Author Contributions

Conceived and designed the experiments: CEK JKM SL DLK HB. Performed the experiments: EHL SWB JKM SL. Analyzed the data: EHL CEK SWB WD DLK HB. Contributed reagents/materials/analysis tools: EHL CEK SWB JKM SL DLK HB WD. Contributed to the writing of the manuscript: EHL CEK SWB JKM SL WD DLK HB.

References

1. Joint United Nations Programme on HIV/AIDS (UNAIDS) (2013) Getting to zero: HIV in eastern and southern Africa. 2013 report on the HIV epidemic in eastern and southern Africa. Available: http://www.unicef.org/esaro/Getting-to-Zero-2013.pdf. Accessed 10 January 2014.
2. Cohen MS, Chen YQ, McCauley M, Gamble T, Hosseinipour MC, et al. (2011) Prevention of HIV-1 infection with early antiretroviral therapy. New England journal of medicine 365: 493–505.
3. Joint United Nations Programme on HIV/AIDS (UNAIDS) (2013) UNAIDS report on the global AIDS epidemic 2013. Available: http://www.unaids.org/en/media/unaids/contentassets/documents/epidemiology/2013/gr2013/unaids_global_report_2013_en.pdf. Accessed 9 January 2014.
4. World Health Organization (2013) Consolidated guidelines on the use of antiretroviral drugs for treating and preventing HIV infection. Available: http://apps.who.int/iris/bitstream/10665/85321/1/9789241505727_eng.pdf. Accessed 10 January 2014.
5. Rosen S, Fox MP (2011) Retention in HIV care between testing and treatment in sub-Saharan Africa: a systematic review. PLoS medicine 8: e1001056.

6. Kranzer K, Govindasamy D, Ford N, Johnston V, Lawn SD (2012) Quantifying and addressing losses along the continuum of care for people living with HIV infection in sub-Saharan Africa: a systematic review. J Int AIDS Soc 15: 17383.
7. Mugglin C, Estill J, Wandeler G, Bender N, Egger M, et al. (2012) Loss to programme between HIV diagnosis and initiation of antiretroviral therapy in sub-Saharan Africa: systematic review and meta-analysis. Trop Med Int Health 17: 1509–1520.
8. Fox MP, Rosen S (2010) Patient retention in antiretroviral therapy programs up to three years on treatment in sub-Saharan Africa, 2007–2009: systematic review. Trop Med Int Health 15 Suppl 1: 1–15.
9. Govindasamy D, Ford N, Kranzer K (2012) Risk factors, barriers and facilitators for linkage to antiretroviral therapy care: a systematic review. AIDS 26: 2059–2067.
10. MacPherson P, MacPherson EE, Mwale D, Bertel Squire S, Makombe SD, et al. (2012) Barriers and facilitators to linkage to ART in primary care: a qualitative study of patients and providers in Blantyre, Malawi. J Int AIDS Soc 15: 18020.
11. CIA: The World Factbook. Available: https://www.cia.gov/library/publications/the-world-factbook/geos/tz.html. Accessed 10 June 2014.
12. Tanzania Commission for AIDS (TACAIDS), Zanzibar AIDS Commission (ZAC), National Bureau of, Statistics (NBS) OotCGSO, and Macro International Inc. (2013) Tanzania HIV/AIDS and Malaria Indicator Survey 2011–12. Dar es Salaam, Tanzania.
13. Mshana GH, Wamoyi J, Busza J, Zaba B, Changalucha J, et al. (2006) Barriers to accessing antiretroviral therapy in Kisesa, Tanzania: a qualitative study of early rural referrals to the national program. AIDS Patient Care & STDs 20: 649–657.
14. Ferguson L, Grant AD, Watson-Jones D, Kahawita T, Ong'ech JO, et al. (2012) Linking women who test HIV-positive in pregnancy-related services to long-term HIV care and treatment services: a systematic review. Tropical Medicine & International Health 17: 564–580.
15. Tanzania Ministry of Health and Social Welfare, National AIDS Control Program (2012) National Guidelines for the Management of HIV/AIDS. Dar es Salaam, Tanzania. Available: www.nacp.go.tz/site/download/nationalguideline42012.pdf. Accessed: 15 December 2013.
16. Musheke M, Ntalasha H, Gari S, McKenzie O, Bond V, et al. (2013) A systematic review of qualitative findings on factors enabling and deterring uptake of HIV testing in Sub-Saharan Africa. BMC Public Health 13: 220.
17. Bogart LM, Chetty S, Giddy J, Sypek A, Sticklor L, et al. (2013) Barriers to care among people living with HIV in South Africa: contrasts between patient and healthcare provider perspectives. AIDS Care 25: 843–853.
18. Roura M, Busza J, Wringe A, Mbata D, Urassa M, et al. (2009) Barriers to sustaining antiretroviral treatment in Kisesa, Tanzania: a follow-up study to understand attrition from the antiretroviral program. AIDS patient care and STDs 23: 203–210.
19. Tomori C, Kennedy CE, Brahmbhatt H, Wagman JA, Mbwambo JK, et al. (2013) Barriers and facilitators of retention in HIV care and treatment services in Iringa, Tanzania: the importance of socioeconomic and sociocultural factors. AIDS Care.
20. Feldacker C, Johnson D, Hosseinipour M, Phiri S, Tweya H (2012) Who Starts? Factors Associated with Starting Antiretroviral Therapy among Eligible Patients in Two, Public HIV Clinics in Lilongwe, Malawi. PloS one 7: e50871.
21. Topp SM, Li MS, Chipukuma JM, Chiko MM, Matongo E, et al. (2012) Does provider-initiated counselling and testing (PITC) strengthen early diagnosis and treatment initiation? Results from an analysis of an urban cohort of HIV-positive patients in Lusaka, Zambia. J Int AIDS Soc 15: 17352.
22. Lessells RJ, Mutevedzi PC, Cooke GS, Newell M-L (2011) Retention in HIV care for individuals not yet eligible for antiretroviral therapy: rural KwaZulu-Natal, South Africa. Journal of acquired immune deficiency syndromes (1999) 56: e79.
23. Tayler-Smith K, Zachariah R, Massaquoi M, Manzi M, Pasulani O, et al. (2010) Unacceptable attrition among WHO stages 1 and 2 patients in a hospital-based setting in rural Malawi: can we retain such patients within the general health system? Trans R Soc Trop Med Hyg 104: 313–319.
24. Bassett IV, Wang B, Chetty S, Mazibuko M, Bearnot B, et al. (2009) Loss to care and death before antiretroviral therapy in Durban, South Africa. Journal of acquired immune deficiency syndromes (1999) 51: 135.
25. Govindasamy D, van Schaik N, Kranzer K, Wood R, Mathews C, et al. (2011) Linkage to HIV care from a mobile testing unit in South Africa by different CD4 count strata. JAIDS Journal of Acquired Immune Deficiency Syndromes 58: 344–352.
26. Kohler PK, Chung MH, McGrath CJ, Benki-Nugent SF, Thiga JW, et al. (2011) Implementation of free cotrimoxazole prophylaxis improves clinic retention among antiretroviral therapy-ineligible clients in Kenya. AIDS 25: 1657–1661.
27. Muhamadi L, Nsabagasani X, Tumwesigye MN, Wabwire-Mangen F, Ekström A-M, et al. (2010) Inadequate pre-antiretroviral care, stock-out of antiretroviral drugs and stigma: Policy challenges/bottlenecks to the new WHO recommendations for earlier initiation of antiretroviral therapy (CD<350 cells/μL) in eastern Uganda. Health policy 97: 187–194.
28. Schouten EJ, Jahn A, Ben-Smith A, Makombe SD, Harries AD, et al. (2011) Antiretroviral drug supply challenges in the era of scaling up ART in Malawi. Journal of the International AIDS Society 14: S4.
29. Harding R, Simms V, Penfold S, Downing J, Powell RA, et al. (2013) Availability of essential drugs for managing HIV-related pain and symptoms within 120 PEPFAR-funded health facilities in East Africa: A cross-sectional survey with onsite verification. Palliative medicine: 0269216313498637.
30. Pasquet A, Messou E, Gabillard D, Minga A, Depoulosky A, et al. (2010) Impact of drug stock-outs on death and retention to care among HIV-infected patients on combination antiretroviral therapy in Abidjan, Côte d'Ivoire. PloS one 5: e13414.
31. Jani IV, Sitoe NE, Alfai ER, Chongo PL, Quevedo JI, et al. (2011) Effect of point-of-care CD4 cell count tests on retention of patients and rates of antiretroviral therapy initiation in primary health clinics: an observational cohort study. The Lancet 378: 1572–1579.
32. Faal M, Naidoo N, Glencross DK, Venter WD, Osih R (2011) Providing immediate CD4 count results at HIV testing improves ART initiation. JAIDS Journal of Acquired Immune Deficiency Syndromes 58: e54–e59.
33. Wynberg E, Cooke G, Shroufi A, Reid SD, Ford N (2014) Impact of point-of-care CD4 testing on linkage to HIV care: a systematic review. J Int AIDS Soc 17: 18809.
34. Yakong VN, Rush KL, Bassett-Smith J, Bottorff JL, Robinson C (2010) Women's experiences of seeking reproductive health care in rural Ghana: challenges for maternal health service utilization. J Adv Nurs 66: 2431–2441.
35. d'Oliveira AFPL, Diniz SG, Schraiber LB (2002) Violence against women in health-care institutions: an emerging problem. The Lancet 359: 1681–1685.
36. Manongi RN, Nasuwa FR, Mwangi R, Reyburn H, Poulsen A, et al. (2009) Conflicting priorities: evaluation of an intervention to improve nurse-parent relationships on a Tanzanian paediatric ward. Hum Resour Health 7: 50.
37. Campbell C, Scott K, Madanhire C, Nyamukapa C, Gregson S (2011) A 'good hospital': nurse and patient perceptions of good clinical care for HIV-positive people on antiretroviral treatment in rural Zimbabwe–a mixed-methods qualitative study. Int J Nurs Stud 48: 175–183.
38. Jewkes R, Abrahams N, Mvo Z (1998) Why do nurses abuse patients? Reflections from South African obstetric services. Social science & medicine 47: 1781–1795.
39. Turan JM, Bukusi EA, Onono M, Holzemer WL, Miller S, et al. (2011) HIV/AIDS stigma and refusal of HIV testing among pregnant women in rural Kenya: results from the MAMAS Study. AIDS Behav 15: 1111–1120.
40. Tsai AC, Bangsberg DR, Katz IT, Haberer JE, Conrad Muzoora MBChB M, et al. (2013) Internalized stigma, social distance, and disclosure of HIV seropositivity in rural Uganda. Annals of Behavioral Medicine: 1–10.
41. Naar-King S, Bradford J, Coleman S, Green-Jones M, Cabral H, et al. (2007) Retention in care of persons newly diagnosed with HIV: outcomes of the Outreach Initiative. AIDS patient care and STDs 21: S-40–S-48.
42. Rintamaki LS, Davis TC, Skripkauskas S, Bennett CL, Wolf MS (2006) Social stigma concerns and HIV medication adherence. AIDS Patient Care & STDs 20: 359–368.
43. Rao D, Kekwaletswe T, Hosek S, Martinez J, Rodriguez F (2007) Stigma and social barriers to medication adherence with urban youth living with HIV. AIDS care 19: 28–33.
44. Mahajan AP, Sayles JN, Patel VA, Remien RH, Ortiz D, et al. (2008) Stigma in the HIV/AIDS epidemic: a review of the literature and recommendations for the way forward. AIDS (London, England) 22: S67.
45. Prachakul W, Grant JS, Keltner NL (2007) Relationships among functional social support, HIV-related stigma, social problem solving, and depressive symptoms in people living with HIV: a pilot study. Journal of the Association of Nurses in AIDS Care 18: 67–76.
46. Sayles JN, Ryan GW, Silver JS, Sarkisian CA, Cunningham WE (2007) Experiences of social stigma and implications for healthcare among a diverse population of HIV positive adults. Journal of Urban Health 84: 814–828.
47. Vanable PA, Carey MP, Blair DC, Littlewood RA (2006) Impact of HIV-related stigma on health behaviors and psychological adjustment among HIV-positive men and women. AIDS and Behavior 10: 473–482.
48. Bogart LM, Cowgill BO, Kennedy D, Ryan G, Murphy DA, et al. (2008) HIV-related stigma among people with HIV and their families: a qualitative analysis. AIDS and Behavior 12: 244–254.
49. Stangl AL, Lloyd JK, Brady LM, Holland CE, Baral S (2013) A systematic review of interventions to reduce HIV-related stigma and discrimination from 2002 to 2013: how far have we come? J Int AIDS Soc 16: 18734.
50. Brown L, Macintyre K, Trujillo L (2003) Interventions to reduce HIV/AIDS stigma: What have we learned? AIDS Education and Prevention 15: 49–69.
51. Sengupta S, Banks B, Jonas D, Miles MS, Smith GC (2011) HIV interventions to reduce HIV/AIDS stigma: a systematic review. AIDS Behav 15: 1075–1087.
52. Were WA, Mermin JH, Wamai N, Awor AC, Bechange S, et al. (2006) Undiagnosed HIV infection and couple HIV discordance among household members of HIV-infected people receiving antiretroviral therapy in Uganda. JAIDS Journal of Acquired Immune Deficiency Syndromes 43: 91–95.
53. Kimaiyo S, Were M, Shen C, Ndege S, Braitstein P, et al. (2010) Home-based HIV counseling and testing in western Kenya. East African Med J 87: 100–108.
54. Lugada E, Levin J, Abang B, Mermin J, Mugalanzi E, et al. (2010) Comparison of home and clinic-based HIV testing among household members of persons taking antiretroviral therapy in Uganda: results from a randomized trial. JAIDS Journal of Acquired Immune Deficiency Syndromes 55: 245–252.
55. Tumwebaze H, Tumwesigye E, Baeten JM, Kurth AE, Revall J, et al. (2012) Household-based HIV counseling and testing as a platform for referral to HIV care and medical male circumcision in Uganda: a pilot evaluation. PLoS One 7: e51620.

56. MacPherson P, Lalloo D, Choko A (2013) Home assessment and initiation of ART following HIV self-testing: a cluster-randomized trial to improve linkage to ART in Blantyre, Malawi.
57. Weidle PJ, Wamai N, Solberg P, Liechty C, Sendagala S, et al. (2006) Adherence to antiretroviral therapy in a home-based AIDS care programme in rural Uganda. The Lancet 368: 1587–1594.
58. Mermin J, Were W, Ekwaru JP, Moore D, Downing R, et al. (2008) Mortality in HIV-infected Ugandan adults receiving antiretroviral treatment and survival of their HIV-uninfected children: a prospective cohort study. The Lancet 371: 752–759.
59. Mpiima D, Birungu J, Alwedo S, C L (2012) Successful community interventions to improve retention and reduce loss to follow up of patients taking antiretroviral therapy – The AIDS Support Organization (TASO).
60. Kipp W, Konde-Lule J, Saunders LD, Alibhai A, Houston S, et al. (2010) Results of a community-based antiretroviral treatment program for HIV-1 infection in western Uganda. Current HIV research 8: 179–185.
61. Wools-Kaloustian KK, Sidle JE, Selke HM, Vedanthan R, Kemboi EK, et al. (2009) A model for extending antiretroviral care beyond the rural health centre. Journal of the International AIDS Society 12: 22.
62. Suthar AB, Ford N, Bachanas PJ, Wong VJ, Rajan JS, et al. (2013) Towards universal voluntary HIV testing and counselling: a systematic review and meta-analysis of community-based approaches. PLoS medicine 10: e1001496.
63. Apondi R, Bunnell R, Awor A, Wamai N, Bikaako-Kajura W, et al. (2007) Home-based antiretroviral care is associated with positive social outcomes in a prospective cohort in Uganda. JAIDS Journal of Acquired Immune Deficiency Syndromes 44: 71–76.
64. Jaffar S, Amuron B, Foster S, Birungi J, Levin J, et al. (2010) Rates of virological failure in patients treated in a home-based versus a facility-based HIV-care model in Jinja, southeast Uganda: a cluster-randomised equivalence trial. The Lancet 374: 2080–2089.

13

Incidence of and Risk Factors Associated with Pulmonary and Extra-Pulmonary Tuberculosis in Saudi Arabia (2010–2011)

Ziad Ahmed Memish[1,2]*, Elija Afolabi Bamgboye[1,3], Naila Abuljadayel[1], Hanan Smadi[1], Mohamed Salamh Abouzeid[1], Rafat Faisal Al Hakeem[1]

1 Public Health Directorate, Ministry of Health, Riyadh, Kingdom of Saudi Arabia, **2** College of Medicine, Alfaisal University, Riyadh, Kingdom of Saudi Arabia, **3** Department of Epidemiology and Medical Statistics, University of Ibadan, Ibadan, Nigeria

Abstract

Setting: National Tuberculosis Program, Department of Public Health, Ministry of Health, Kingdom of Saudi Arabia (KSA).

Objective: To summarize data on the incidence of tuberculosis and associated risk factors for cases reported during 2010–2011.

Design: Retrospective analysis of routinely collected data through an established national disease notification system of the Ministry of Health in KSA.

Results: The estimated incidence of all forms of tuberculosis fell from 15.8/100000 (95% CI: 15.3/100,000–16.3/100,000) in 2010 to 13.8/100,000 (95% CI: 13.4/100,000–14.2/100,000) in 2011. Saudis experienced a decrease from 11.8/100,000 (95% CI: 11.3/100,000 to 12.3/100,000) in 2010 to 9.9/100,000 (95% CI: 9.5/100,000–10.4/100,000) in 2011 while the incidence in non-Saudis declined from 24.7/100,000 (95% CI: 23.6/100,000 to 25.7/100,000) in 2010 to 22.5/100,000 (95% CI: 21.5/100,000 to 23.4/100,000) in 2011. The proportion of Extra Pulmonary TB (EPTB) which increased minimally from 30% in 2010 to 32% in 2011 was higher than global figures and strongly associated with age, sex, nationality and occupation.

Conclusion: The current estimated incidence of about 14/100,000 in 2011 is less than half its estimated value of 44/100000 in 1990. Without prejudice to any under-reporting, the KSA appeared to be on the course for TB elimination by 2050 having reached the first milestone set by WHO. The proportion of EPTB remains higher than global figure and age, sex, nationality and occupation were significant independent predictors of EPTB.

Editor: Angelo A. Izzo, Colorado State University, United States of America

Funding: The authors have no support or funding to report.

Competing Interests: The authors have declared that no competing interests exist.

* E-mail: zmemish@yahoo.com

Introduction

With an estimated 8.5–9.2 million cases and 1.2–1.5 million deaths in 2010, tuberculosis (TB) is the second leading cause of death after HIV from any single agent and continues to be a major global public health concern. [1] The target set by the STOP TB Partnership, WHO and Millennium Development Goals is to reduce the prevalence of TB to half of its value in 1990 by 2015. KSA has made tremendous efforts towards the world plan to eliminate TB. The incidence of new TB cases in KSA of 22/100,000 in 2009 and this compared favorably with the situation in developed countries, and much lower than the overall incidence of 174/100,000 reported in the WHO EMRO region in the same year is noteworthy. [1–3] Interestingly, the WHO has signified of its intention to make KSA a model country in the worldwide elimination of TB. [4] Therefore, the current study examines the reported cases of TB in 2010 and 2011 with special interest in its epidemiology that may assist the National Tuberculosis Program (NTP) in KSA revise their policies to achieve their goal of elimination.

Methodology

KSA has a well-established national infectious diseases notification system whereby all the different health affairs (13 provinces and 7 districts) and report all notifiable diseases to the central registry at the Ministry of Health. It is mandatory to notify the health authority of any case of TB diagnosed from any of the health institutions to the Regional Directorate of Health Affairs. The data on TB for 2010 to 2011 for new cases were retrieved and analyzed retrospectively using SPSS (version 15.0). [5] Data for the denominator of the incidence rate (population of KSA) were derived from Saudi Arabia Statistical Health Statistics 2010 and 2011. The binary logistic regression model was fitted to the data with type of TB as dependent variable and age, sex, nationality and occupation as independent variables. This binary logistic analysis technique was used to assess the association between risk factors (predictors) and the probability of TB patient being pulmonary (PTB) or extra-pulmonary (EPTB) at 5% significance level. The forward selection procedure was used to fit the variables and the results of the Hosmer-Lesmeshow tests revealed that the model fit was adequate. [5].

Results

Incidence Rate of Tuberculosis

Table 1 showed 70% of the 4,293 new TB patients notified in 2010 as well as the 3,872 cases in 2011 (a 10% decline) were PTB and the remaining 30%, EPTB. The commonest diagnosis of EPTB were lymphadenitis (45%), central nervous system (7%), gastrointestinal (5%), and renal TB (0.7%) while about 31% were not defined with respect to site of disease as presented in Table 2. Given that the total population of the KSA in 2010 was 27,136,977, the overall estimated incidence rate of TB was 15.8/100,000 (95% CI: 15.3/100,000–16.3/100,000). The estimated population of Saudi Arabia in 2011 was 28,016,602 at a growth rate of 3.19% per annum. Thus the estimated incidence of TB in 2011 was 13.8 per 100,000 population (95% CI: 13.4/100,000–14.2/100,000) a decline of about 13% from the rate in 2010.

The non-Saudis in 2010 with a population of 8,429,401 constituted 31.06% of the total population of the KSA. And the incidence rates of TB estimated separately for Saudis and non-Saudis were 11.8/100,000 (95%CI: 11.31/100,000 to 12.29/100,000) and 24.7/100,000 (95%CI: 23.6/100,000 to 25.7/100,000) respectively. The difference in the incidence rates between the Saudis and non- Saudis was statistically significant, $P<0.001$. The incidence rates declined in 2011 to give 9.92/100,000 (95% CI: 9.48/100,000–10.36/100,000) for Saudis and 22.49/100,000 (95% CI: 21.49/100,000 to 23.4/100,000) for non-Saudis respectively.

Smear Analysis

The proportion of all new TB patients in 2010 and 2911 that were smear-positive was higher among non-Saudis than the Saudis $P<0.05$. However, a lower proportion was smear negative in 2010, lower among non-Saudis (11%) compared to Saudis (15%). The proportion of EPTB patients slightly increased from 30% in 2010 to 32% in 2011. The increase was more noticeable among the non-Saudis than the Saudis as shown in Table 3. In each year, about 13% of PTB patients were smear negative while about 2% of the patients did not have result of smear analysis.

HIV Prevalence among New TB Patients

Table 4, Panel 1 showed a total of 77 and 66 new TB patients were also HIV positive in 2010 and 2011 respectively, giving a prevalence of 1.8% (95% CI: 1.4%–2.2% and 1.7% (95% CI: 1.3%–2.1%) respectively among new TB patients. The TB patients from the Africanregion has the highest proportion of HIV positives with an overall prevalence of 8% among new TB patients followed by patients from the Eastern Mediterranean region (WHO EMRO) which accounted for about 24% giving a prevalence of 2.5% over the two years of study but slightly higher in 2010. There were no HIV patients from countries in the European region and neither TB nor HIV were from the Americas and 1.2% of the new TB patients who are Saudi Arabia citizens were positive for HIV increasing from 1.1% in 2010 to 1.4% in 2011.

The proportion of new TB cases positive for HIV were higher in Jeddah (3.8%) and Asser (3.2%) than the national average (1.8%) and other health regions of Saudi Arabia.

Province/District (Health Affairs)

The distribution of the new TB cases according to the Health Affairs (13 provinces and 7 districts) classification within the KSA is shown in Table 4. More than 60% of the TB patients were from Jeddah and Riyadh and another 15% from the Eastern health affair and holy Mecca. The remaining 25% were located in the remaining nine health affairs of the Kingdom with Jazan contributing about 7%. Also, about a third of non-Saudi TB patients were from Jeddah, higher than the 23% of Saudis but an almost equal proportion (30%) of Saudi and Non- Saudi were from Riyadh. A higher proportion (77% and above) of TB patients from Mecca, Jeddah, Jazan, and Eastern health affair were of the pulmonary type, much higher than the proportion of patients from Riyadh (62%). Riyadh, the capital of KSA which contributed about 32% of all new TB patients in 2010 accounted for more than 40% of EPTB. This pattern was sustained in 2011 even though a majority of the health affairs reported lesser cases. The Eastern health affair appeared to be the notable area with an increased frequency of new TB patients in 2011.

Risk Factors Associated with Extra-pulmonary Tuberculosis

The overall mean age of patients with PTB (36.4 years, SD = 17.0 years) appeared similar to patients with EPTB (35.0 years, SD = 16.4 years) as shown in Table 5. But the difference was statistically significant, $P<0.05$. The mean age of 35.6 years, (SD = 16.8 years) for patients in 2010 was also statistically significantly lower than the mean of 36.4 years (SD = 16.8 years) for patients in 2011 ($P<0.05$).

The proportion of female EPTB patients was higher than their PTB counterparts, $P<0.01$. The association between patient occupation and type of TB was also statistically significant, $P<0.01$. Housewives and workers sharing the same household environment had more proportions with EPTB than those who were self-employed. About 71% of the non-Saudis had pulmonary TB, slightly higher than their Saudi counterparts $P<0.01$.

Table 1. The distribution of new TB cases by Pulmonary and Extra-Pulmonary among Saudis and Non-Saudis (2010–2011).

Nationality	2010		Total 2010	2011		Total 2011
	Pulmonary (%)	Extra-Pulmonary		Pulmonary (%)	Extra-Pulmonary	
Non-Saudi Arabia	1503(72.3)	575(27.7)	2078(48.4)	1366(69.8)	591(30.2)	1957(50.5)
Saudi	1485(67.0)	730(33.0)	2215(51.6)	1275(66.6)	640(33.4)	1915(49.5)
TOTAL	2988(69.6)	1305(30.4)	4293(100.0)	2641(68.2)	1231(31.8)	3872(100)

Table 2. The sites of new Extra-Pulmonary Tuberculosis patients in Saudi Arabia by nationality 2010–2011.

Type	2010		Total	2011		Total
	Saudi	Non-Saudi		Saudi	Non-Saudi	
BONE	64 (8.8)	36 (6.3)	100 (7.7)	74(11.6)	35 (5.9)	109 (8.9)
GASTROINTESTINAL	46 (6.3)	21 (3.7)	67(5.1)	41 (6.4)	29 (4.9)	70 (5.7)
LYMPHATIC	320(43.8)	270(47.0)	590(45.2)	278(43.4)	260(44.0)	538(43.7)
MILIARY	19 (2.6)	13 (2.3)	32 (2.5)	15 (2.3)	15 (2.5)	30 (2.4)
NERVOUS	57(7.8)	40 (7.0)	97 (7.4)	45 (7.0)	39 (6.6)	84 (6.8)
RENAL	6(0.8)	3 (0.5)	9 (0.7)	3 (0.5)	4 (0.7)	7 (0.6)
OTHERS	218(29.9)	192(33.4)	410(31.4)	184(28.8)	209(35.4)	393(31.9)
TOTAL	**730**	**575**	**1305**	**640**	**591**	**1231**

The odds ratios for each of the variables age, sex, nationality and occupation and their 95% confidence limits from the logistic regression analysis presented in Table 6 revealed them as significant predictors of the probability of a TB patient being of the Extra Pulmonary type $P<0.01$. Younger TB patients were more likely to be EPTB than older patients. For example a TB patient less than 5 years of age was almost 5 times more likely to have EPTB than was a patient 65 years and above. Similarly, females and non-Saudis were more likely to be diagnosed with EPTB. Also, TB patients with semi-skilled jobs were statistically significantly less likely to have EPTB compared to students which was the reference category.

Discussion and Conclusion

The overall incidence rate of TB in Saudi Arabia observed in this study was estimated at about 16 and 14 per 100,000 populations for 2010 and 2011 respectively. According to the World Health Organization report published in 2011, [2] the incidence of TB was reported as 18 per 100,000 people in KSA. Available reports have shown that the incidence of 16 per 100,000 observed in 2010 appeared similar to what it was since 200. [3] But the decline in 2011 may be a cumulative effect of the gains in the control mechanism to eliminate TB in the Kingdom. The estimated incidence rate of TB in 1990 was 44 per 100,000 and the current estimate which has remained stable for three years is about half the incidence in 1990. If one recognizes that one of the targets set to achieve the objective of WHO for TB elimination was to reduce its incidence rate to half of its value in 1990 by 2015, one could safely conclude that Saudi Arabia is on track. Although, there could be some reservations that the TB data source in KSA might suffer from under reporting and consider effect seriously the interpretation of this study. But one should also realize that while the likelihood of under-reporting of TB cases cannot be wished away, there is also the fear of over-reporting because of lack of central system for the reporting a case. The NTP in KSA has integrated the care of TB into the health care system and all hospitals under the Ministry of Health, the special hospitals for the armed forces such as the National Guard, the military hospital, the security forces, other private hospitals, and health care centers all provide care and support for TB patients. But each of these hospitals report new TB patients directly to the Ministry of Health database, someone might receive care in one hospital where he has been registered as a new patient only to present in another hospital as a new patient. Perhaps the over reporting may offset the under reporting, but this study recommends an assessment of the completeness of registration of tuberculosis in the Kingdom in a separate study. But one may infer from this study that a significant progress in implementing the STOP strategy of TB in line with international recommendations has been made in KSA and a good evidence of a high-level political support and utilization of available resources. [4] The economic fortunes of Saudi Arabia with a stable GDP per capita around 20,300 dollars over the years and remarkable investment of about 7% of her annual budget usually allocated to health care services. [6] This is expected to facilitate the dream of eliminating TB to less than 1/100.000 by the year 2050. [7].

The observed proportion of EPTB in this study is an increase over the figures in 1997 when EPTB accounted for 28.2% of all reported TB cases [8] and the findings in 1991 when the

Table 3. The distribution of smear positives, negative and EPTB in new tuberculosis patients in Saudi Arabia by nationality and year.

Smear Analysis	2010		Total	2011		Total
	Saudi	Non-Saudi		Saudi	Non-Saudi	
Positive	1079(48.7)	1222(58.8)	2301(53.6)	913(47.7)	1142(58.3)	2055(53.1)
Negative	332(15.0)	237(11.4)	569(13.3)	319(16.7)	206(10.5)	525(13.6)
EPTB	730(33.0)	575(27.7)	1305(30.4)	640(33.4)	591(30.2)	1231(31.8)
Not done	77(3.5)	46(2.7)	118(2.7)	44(2.2)	21(1.1)	65(1.7)
TOTAL	**2215**	**2078**	**4293**	**1915**	**1957**	**3872**

Table 4. The distribution of new tuberculosis patients in Saudi Arabia Province/District (Health Affairs) by type 2010–2011.

District	2010		Total	2011		Total
	Pulmonary	Extra-Pulmonary		Pulmonary	Extra-Pulmonary	
Aseer	97 (3.0)	52 (3.9)	149 (3.3)	83 (3.0)	51(4.1)	134 (3.3)
Albaha	29 (0.9)	6 (0.4)	35 (0.8)	30 (1.1)	17(1.4)	47 (1.2)
Bishan	14 (0.4)	7 (0.5)	21(0.5)	8 (0.3)	5 (0.4)	13 (0.3)
Eastern	159 (5.0)	40 (3.0)	199 (4.4)	191 (6.8)	21 (1.7)	212 (5.7)
Hafr El-Baten	28 (0.9)	18 (1.3)	46 (1.0)	22 (0.8)	8 (0.6)	30 (0.7)
Hail	16 (0.5)	8 (0.6)	24 (0.5)	13 (0.5)	5 (0.4)	18 (0.4)
Hassa	71 (2.2)	79 (5.9)	150 (3.3)	42 (1.5)	60 (4.8)	102 (2.5)
Jizan	219 (6.8)	59 (4.4)	278 (6.1)	179 (6.4)	56 (4.5)	235 (5.8)
Jeddah	978(30.5)	257 (19.2)	1235 (27.2)	883 (31.5)	303(24.3)	1186 (29.3)
Al-Joof	16 (0.5)	22 (1.6)	38 (0.8)	14 (0.5)	6 (0.5)	20 (0.5)
Medinah	149 (4.6)	42 (3.1)	191 (4.2)	150 (5.4)	49 (3.9)	199 (4.9)
Makkah	243 (7.6)	43 (3.2)	286 (6.3)	179 (6.4)	40 (3.2)	219 (5.4)
Najran	25 (0.8)	27 (2.0)	52 (1.1)	33 (1.2)	23 (1.8)	56 (1.4)
Nothern	18 (0.6)	9 (0.7)	27 (0.6)	13 (0.5)	15 (1.2)	28 (0.7)
Qaseem	81 (2.5)	58 (4.3)	139 (3.1)	100 (3.6)	43 (3.4)	143 (3.5)
Qounfoda	24 (0.7)	10 (0.7)	34 (0.7)	23 (0.8)	8 (0.6)	31 (0.8)
Qurayat	6 (0.2)	5 (0.4)	11 (0.2)	7 (0.2)	0 (0.0)	7 (0.2)
Riyadh	912(28.4)	541 (40.4)	1453 (32.0)	700 (25.0)	489 (39.2)	1189 (29.3)
Tabouk	49 (1.5)	26 (1.9)	75 (1.6)	55 (2.0)	20 (1.6)	75 (1.9)
Taif	74 (2.3)	30 (2.2)	104 (2.3)	78 (2.8)	30 (2.4)	108 (2.7)

proportion was only 11.7%. [9] The seemingly low prevalence of HIV in Saudi Arabia has defeated a link with HIV as a possible explanation. [10] It is generally known that HIV and Mycobacterium tuberculosis have a synergistic interaction and each propagates the progression of the other so that increasing HIV prevalence can show up as more cases of EPTB. [11] Therefore the increase in EPTB might probably be due to the availability of better diagnostic facilities and better reporting system, leading to the identification of more cases. Also, that the proportion of EPTB increased among non Saudis is consistent with previous reports that foreigners could change the epidemiology of TB as reported in Germany, Denmark and USA. [12–14].

The result of the logistic regression analysis that showed persons less than 15 years of age were likely to have EPTB than was a person 65 years and above was similar to an earlier study which reported the preponderance of EPTB in the younger age group. [9] Young age as an independent risk factor for EPTB observed in this study has also been reported in earlier studies from Nepal, USA and Europe. [15–17] The usual explanation has been the possibility of a higher probability of reactivation at an extra-pulmonary site at younger ages after primary infection in the lungs. That a higher proportion of PTB was found at higher ages as observed in this study may also suggest a higher likelihood of reactivation of TB in the lungs at older ages. This is more likely the effect of decreased local immunity in the lungs in the elderly. A large pool of latent tuberculosis have been reported in an earlier nationwide community study in Saudi Arabia. [18] And this is more likely to be the source of possible reactivation taken place in older ages. [19].

The significance of people in semi- skilled jobs less likely to have EPTB compared to students could also be attributed to age as the students were more likely to be younger and childhood TB is usually a reflection of new infections. That females were more likely to be diagnosed with EPTB than males was consistent with results of previous studies by Al-Otaibi [9] who reported a higher proportion of EPTB among females and others. [12,14,20] No clear explanation have been offered other than a suggestion of possible roles of endocrine factors.

Also the fact that non-Saudis had a significantly excess odds of EPTB compared to Saudis is not new as other studies have found that non -Saudis tended to have EPTB more than PTB. [9,21] The pre-employment screening at entry, which prominently targets PTB could have missed out a number of EPTB which later show up for treatment. The most common site EPTB observed in this study was lymph nodes, which was similar to other previous studies from KSA, Nepal and Turkey, [15,22,23] which have reported that lymph nodes accounted for nearly half the cases of EPTB. Other forms of EPTB were TB of the bone, gastro and CNS which is consistent with other studies from Saudi Arabia. [1,21] The fact that more than 60% of patients TB patients were received from Jeddah and Riyadh health affairs is not surprising because the foreigners work in the major cities of the country. Riyadh, which contributed about 32% of all new tuberculosis patients in 2010 accounted for more than 40% of EPTB. This again can be explained as a fall out that the foreigners were more likely to be based in the capital city, [6] and a study from the USA reported higher rates in cities. [24] The observed 54% smear-positive among new TB patients in this study is consistent with what was observed in KSA in previous years but higher than global values. [1,21] However, the non-Saudis (59%) have maintained their higher values than Saudis (49%). These values were higher than values in the Eastern Mediterranean region. One

Table 5. The distribution of new tuberculosis patients in Saudi Arabia by type and selected demographic characteristics 2010–2011.

		2010		Total 2010	2011		Total 2011
		Pulmonary (%)	Extra-Pulmonary		Pulmonary (%)	Extra-Pulmonary	
Age group	0–4	15(0.5)	24(1.8)	39(0.9)	10(0.4)	20(1.6)	30(0.8)
	5–14	80(2.7)	62(4.8)	142(3.3)	60(2.3)	52(4.2)	112(2.9)
	15–24	731(24.5)	249(19.1)	980(22.8)	561(21.2)	233(18.9)	794(20.5)
	25–34	923(30.9)	421(32.3)	1344(31.3)	804(30.4)	420(34.1)	1224(31.6)
	35–44	426(14.3)	244(18.7)	670(15.6)	435(16.5)	204(16.6)	639(16.5)
	45–54	348(11.6)	136(10.4)	484(11.3)	344(13.0)	124(10.1)	468(12.1)
	≥65	242(8.1)	91(7.0)	333(7.8)	221(8.4)	87(7.1)	308(8.0)
Sex	Female	1113(37.2)	567(43.4)	1680(39.1)	1006(38.1)	525(42.6)	1531(39.5)
	Male	1875(62.8)	738(56.6)	2613(60.9)	1635(61.9)	706(57.4)	2341(60.5)
Occupation	Skilled workers	174(5.8)	74(5.7)	248(5.8)	172(6.5)	72(5.8)	244(6.3)
	Semi-skilled (Vocational training)	222(7.4)	73(5.6)	295(6.9)	258(9.8)	70(5.7)	328(8.5)
	Unskilled workers	365(12,2)	132(10.1)	497(11.6)	355(13.4)	179(14.5)	534(13.8)
	Housewives and workers	882(29.5)	454(34.8)	1336(31.1)	789(29.9)	405(32.9)	1194(30.8)
	Self-employed	1107(37.0)	464(35.6)	1571(35.6)	844(32.0)	381(31.0)	1225(31.6)
	Students	238(8.0)	108(8.3)	346(8.1)	223(8.4)	124(10.1)	347(9.0)
Nationality	Eastern Mediterranean	508(17.0)	158(12.1)	666(15.5)	484(18.3)	199(16.2)	683(17.6)
(WHO Regions)	South East Asia(SEAR)	572(19.1)	302(23.1)	874(20.4)	508(19.2)	256(20.8)	764(19.7)
	Western Pacific Region(WPR)	109(3.6)	47(3.6)	156(3.6)	127(4.8)	58(4.7)	185(4.8)
	African Region(AR)	286(9.6)	59(4.5)	345(8.0)	222(8.4)	72(5.8)	294(7.6)
	European Region(EUR)	19(0.6)	8(0.6)	27(0.6)	20(0.8)	2(0.2)	22(0.6)
	Others not Indicated	9(0.3)	1(0.1)	10(0.2)	5(0.2)	4(0.3)	9(0.2)
	The Americas	0	0	0	0	0	0
	Saudi Arabia	1485(49.7)	730(55.9)	2215(51.6)	1275(48.3)	640(52.0)	1915(49.5)
	Western Pacific Region(WPR)	109(3.6)	47(3.6)	156(3.6)	127(4.8)	58(4.7)	185(4.8)
TOTAL		**2988**	**1305**	**4293**	**2641**	**1231**	**3872**

Table 6. Logistic regression predicting extra-pulmonary tuberculosis from occupation, age, nationality, and sex.

Variable		Odds ratio	95% CI OR	P value
Occupation	Skilled	0.96	0.72–1.27	0.748
	Semi-skilled	0.73	0.55–0.98	0.034
	Unskilled	1.13	0.87–1.47	0.349
	House-jobs	1.02	0.82–1.27	0.848
	Self-employed	0.96	0.78–1.18	0.663
	Student (ref)	1		
Age	0–4	4.69	2.77–7.96	<0.001
	5–14	2.07	1.49–2.88	<0.001
	15–24	1.03	0.83–1.28	0.768
	25–34	1.43	1.17–1.75	<0.001
	35–44	1.55	1.25–1.92	<0.001
	45–54	1.11	0.88–1.39	0.386
	55–64	1.10	0.86–1.41	0.462
	65+(ref)	1		
Nationality	Non Saudi	1.33	1.19–1.49	<0.001
	Saudi(ref)	1		
Sex	Female	1.21	1.08–1.36	0.001
	Male(ref)	1		

cannot readily explain this differential. Also the overall proportion of smear negative (13%) which was lower among non-Saudis (11%) and higher among Saudis (15%) were generally lower than global values. [1].

The results of our study corroborate similar studies that found a decrease in the overall TB incidence. The current estimate of the incidence rate of TB of about 14/100000 is less than half its value of 44/100000 in 1990. Without prejudice to any under-reporting of cases, the KSA appeared to have reached the first milestone set by WHO for TB eradication by 2050. The proportion with EPTB among new TB patients remains higher than global figures and suggested younger age, non-Saudis, female gender and semi-skilled occupation may be its significant independent risk factors for EPTB relative to PTB in KSA. Based on our results TB control programs might target young, female, and non-Saudi populations for early diagnosis of EPTB. The Kingdom needs more attention on the role of HIV among the TB patients.

Acknowledgments

The authors are grateful to Dr. Pai Madhukar, Department of Epidemiology & Biostatistics, McGill University, Montreal, Canada for his critical review and intellectual scientific contributions to improve the manuscript.

Author Contributions

Conceived and designed the experiments: ZAM RFA NA. Performed the experiments: NA MA. Analyzed the data: EAB. Contributed reagents/materials/analysis tools: ZAM RFA NA. Wrote the paper: ZAM EAB NA HS.

References

1. World Health Organization (2011) WHO Report. Global Tuberculosis Control.
2. World Health Organization (2011) WHO report. Saudi Arabia tuberculosis profile, Geneva: World Health Organization.
3. Waness A, Abu El-Sameed Y, Mahboub B, Noshi M, Al Jahdali H, et al. (2011) Respiratory disorders in the Middle East: a review. Respirology; 16: 755–766.
4. WHO, EMRO website. Stop Tuberculosis: Saudi Arabia to become a model for TB elimination. Available: www.emro.who.int/tuberculosis/.../worldtuberculosis-day-2011-campaign. Accessed 2013 May 13.
5. IBM (1968) Statistical Package for Social Scientist (SPSS). Version 15, IBM Corporation,
6. Saudi Arabia, Health Statistical Year Book (2011) 103–117.
7. Al-Kahtani NH, Al-Jeffri MH (2003) Manual of the National TB Control Program. Ministry of Health, Saudi Arabia.
8. Index mundi website. Saudi Arabia-incidence of tuberculosis. Available: http://www.indexmundi.com/facts/saudi-arabia indexmundi. Accessed 2012 Aug 24.
9. AL-Otaibi F, ElHazmi MM (2010) Extra-pulmonary tuberculosis in Saudi Arabia. Indian J. Pathol Microbiol; 53(2) 227–31.
10. Alothman AF, Mohajer K, Balkhy H, BMC Proceedings (2011) Prevalence of HIV-infection in Saudi Arabia; 5 (Suppl 6) p:252 doi:10,1186/1753-6561-5-S6-P252).
11. Jaryal A, Raina R, Sarkar M, Sharma A (2011) Manifestations of tuberculosisin HIV/AIDS patients and its relationship with CD4 count. Lung India (serial online, cited 2013 14 May); 28; 263–6.
12. World Health Organization (1994) Report on the technical consultation meeting on Tuberculosis in the Eastern Mediterranean Region, Cairo, Egypt, WHO-EM/TUB/184-E/L.
13. García-Rodríguez JF, Álvarez-Díaz H, Lorenzo-García MV, Mariño-Callejo A, Fernández-Rial Á, et al. (2011) Extrapulmonary tuberculosis: epidemiology and risk factors. Enferm Infecc Microbiol Clin. Aug-Sep; 29(7): 502–9.
14. Lin JN, Lai CH, Chen YH, Lee SS, Tsai SS, et al. (2009) Risk factors for extra-pulmonary tuberculosis compared to pulmonary tuberculosis. Int J Tuberc Lung Dis; 13(5): 620–5.
15. Ministry of Health (1997) Tuberculosis. Annual Health Report. Riyadh (KSA): Ministry of Health; p.46–9.
16. Fiske CT, Griffin MR, Erin H, Warkentin J, Lisa K, et al. (2010) Black race, sex, and extrapulmonary tuberculosis risk: an observational study BMC Infectious Diseases 10: 16 Available: http://www.biomedcentral.com/1471-2334/10/16.
17. Al-Kassimi FA, Abdullah AK, al-Hajjaj MS, al-Orainey IO, Bamgboye EA, et al. (1993) Nationwide community survey oftuberculosis in Saudi Arabia. Tuber Lung Dis; 74: 254–60.
18. Dubrow EL (1976) Reactivation of tuberculosis: A problem of aging. J. Am Geriatr Soc; 24: 481–7.
19. Gunal S, Yang Z, Agarwal M, Koroglu M, Anci ZK, et al. (2011) Demographic and microbial characteristics of extrapulmonary tuberculosis cases diagnosed in Malatya,Turkey, 2001–2007 BMC Public Health 11: 154 Available: http://www.biomedcentral.com/1471-2458/11/154.

20. Peto HM, Pratt RH, Harrington TA, LoBue PA, Armstrong LR (2009) Epidemiology of extrapulmonary tuberculosis in the United States, 1993–2006. Clin Infect Dis; 49(9): 1350–7.
21. Abouzeid MS, Zumia AI, Felemban S, Alotaibi B, O'Grady J, et al. (2010) Tuberculosis in Saudis and Non-Saudis in the Kingdom of Saudi Arabia- A10 Year Retrospective Study (2000–2009). PLos ONE 7(6): e39478. Doi:1371/journal.pone.0039478.
22. Gonzalez OY, Adams G, Teeter LD, Bui TT, Musser JM, et al. (2003) Extra-pulmonary manifestations in a large metropolitan area with a low incidence of tuberculosis. Int J Tuberc Lung Dis; 7(12): 1178–85.
23. Cailhol J, Decludt B, Che D (2005) Socio-demographic factors that contribute to the development of extrapulmonary tuberculosis were identified. J Clin Epidemiol; 58: 1066–71.
24. Oren E, Winston CA, Pratt R, Robison VA, Narita M (2011) Epidemiology of urban tuberculosis in the United States, 2000–2007. Am J Public Health; 101: 1256–63.

Trends in AIDS-Defining Opportunistic Illnesses Incidence over 25 Years in Rio de Janeiro, Brazil

Lara Coelho*, **Sandra Wagner Cardoso, Rodrigo Teixeira Amancio, Ronaldo Ismério Moreira, Dayse Pereira Campos, Valdiléa Gonçalves Veloso, Beatriz Grinsztejn, Paula Mendes Luz**

Instituto de Pesquisa Clínica Evandro Chagas, Fundação Oswaldo Cruz, Rio de Janeiro, Brasil

Abstract

Objectives: To assess the temporal trends in incidence of AIDS-defining opportunistic illnesses in an urban cohort of a middle-income country.

Methods: HIV infected patients aged ≥18 years at cohort entry were included in this analysis. We calculated incidence rates per 1000 persons-years of observation for the first opportunistic illness presented after cohort enrollment, from 1987 to 2012. Trends for overall and specific opportunistic illnesses were tested and incidence rate ratios for the most recent calendar period were calculated as the ratio between the incidence rate observed in the most recent period of the study (2009–2012) and the incidence rate observed in first period of the study (1987–1990).

Results: Overall, 3378 patients were included in this analysis; of which 1119 (33%) patients presented an opportunistic illness during follow up. Incidence rates of all opportunistic illnesses decreased over time, and the overall opportunistic illness incidence rates fell from 295.4/1000 persons-years in 1987–1990 to 34.6/1000 persons-years in 2009–2012. Tuberculosis, esophageal candidiasis, cerebral toxoplasmosis and *Pneumocystis jirovecii* pneumonia were the most incident opportunistic illnesses in the cohort. Tuberculosis had the highest incidence rate in the study period. The peak in tuberculosis incidence occurred in 1991–1993 (80.8/1000 persons-years). Cerebral toxoplasmosis was the third most incident opportunistic illness in the study, with a peak of incidence of 43.6/1000 persons-year in 1987–1990.

Conclusions: All opportunistic illnesses incidence rates decreased over the years but they still occur in an unacceptable frequency. Tuberculosis co-infection among HIV-infected persists as an important challenge for health care professionals and policy makers in our setting. Impressively high rates of cerebral toxoplasmosis were found suggesting that its incidence among HIV-infected is linked to the high prevalence of *Toxoplasma gondii* infection in the general population.

Editor: Mark Wainberg, McGill University AIDS Centre, Canada

Funding: BG and PML acknowledge funding from the National Council of Technological and Scientific Development (CNPq) and the Research Funding Agency of the State of Rio de Janeiro (FAPERJ). The funders had no role in study design, data collection and analysis, decision to publish, or preparation of the manuscript.

Competing Interests: The authors have declared that no competing interests exist.

* E-mail: lara.coelho@ipec.fiocruz.br

Introduction

Major advances have been achieved in the management and treatment of HIV infected patients. As result the incidence and morbimortality of opportunistic illnesses have dramatically declined in the years that followed combination antiretroviral therapy (cART) introduction [9,17,31,35]. Nonetheless, opportunistic illnesses (OI) still represent a major cause of death and hospitalization in HIV infected patients, in these settings [5,30,34,36].

The incidence of specific OI in HIV infected patients can vary geographically mainly as a result of the differential burden of tropical infectious diseases observed in middle-low income settings [11,47]. One prominent example is tuberculosis with only 22 countries located in Africa, Asia and Latin America (including Brazil) being responsible for more than 80% of all cases worldwide [45].

Brazil is a middle-income country where publically funded universal access to cART, laboratory monitoring with CD4 cell counts and viral load quantification and OI prophylaxis and treatment have been provided since 1996 [29]. Yet, few studies have evaluated trends in the incidence of OI in our setting [11].

In this study, we examine rates and patterns of OIs incidence in an urban clinical cohort in Rio de Janeiro, Brazil, from 1987 to 2012.

Patients and Methods

Ethics Statement

This study was approved by the ethics committee of the Evandro Chagas Clinical Research Institute of the Oswaldo Cruz Foundation (CAAE 0032.0.009.000-10) and was conducted according to the principles expressed in the Declaration of Helsinki. All patient records/information was de-identified prior to analysis.

Study Population

Evandro Chagas Clinical Research Institute (IPEC/Fiocruz) is a reference center for treatment of patients with HIV/AIDS, in Rio de Janeiro, Brazil. As of June 2013, over 5,000 patients have been cared for at IPEC. A longitudinal, observational, clinical database has been maintained on patients receiving care at IPEC since 1986. Cohort procedures have been described and results published [18,19,27]. The database includes socio-demographic, laboratory, clinical, and therapeutic information abstracted from the medical records and is updated periodically by trained staff.

For this study we included all patients 18 years of age or older at cohort entry, who were followed for a period of at least 60 days from 1 January 1987 to 31 October 2012. The start of the observation period was defined based on the first medical appointment at IPEC. Follow-up ended at the date of the first OI for those who presented with an OI during follow-up. For those patients who never experienced an OI during follow-up, the end of follow-up was defined as the date of the last clinic visit, the date of death or study closure, whichever occurred first.

Database Validation

To assess the quality of the OI diagnoses present in the IPEC longitudinal database, we performed a clinical validation of diagnoses by direct comparison of database with chart review. Ten percent of the patients who presented an OI during follow-up (n = 118 patients) were randomly selected for chart review and validation of the first and concomitant OI, that is, those occurring within 30 days of the date of the first OI.

A trained HIV medical specialist used two criteria to validate the diagnoses. The first, which classified diagnoses into certain, probable and possible, took into consideration all forms of complementary exams, including radiological, microbiological and hystopatological, in addition to medical prescriptions. This criterion had already been used by our team in other study [34]. The second criterion was built based on the case definition for HIV-related diseases established by the WHO [43]. According to this criterion, the diagnoses were classified either as definitive or clinical.

The validation showed that 95% of the OI diagnosis were confirmed using either criteria. Out of the confirmed diagnosis, 49% were classified as certain using the first criterion, and 56% were classified as definitive according to second (WHO) criterion.

Although WHO criteria for case definition of HIV-related diseases was applied for the database validation process described above, the selection of the opportunistic illnesses included in the incidence analysis were based on those present in the Center for Disease Control "1993 Revised Classification System for HIV Infection and Expanded Surveillance Case Definition for AIDS Among Adolescents and Adults" (CDC, 1993) [8].

Outcome Measures

The outcome of interest was the occurrence of the first OI after cohort enrollment. Prevalent diagnosis at or up to 30 days of the date of cohort enrollment were excluded from the incidence rate calculation.

The opportunistic illnesses included in the analysis were those in the CDC 1993 definition [8], namely tuberculosis, esophageal candidiasis, toxoplasmosis cerebral, *Pneumocystis jirovecii* pneumonia (PCP), herpes simplex virus, cytomegalovirus disease, extrapulmonar cryptococcosis, Kaposi sarcoma, crypstosporidiosis, isosporosis, non tuberculosis mycobacterium disease, disseminated histoplasmosis, non Hodgkin lymphoma. We excluded from the analysis the following opportunistic illnesses: HIV associated encephalopathy, recurrent bacterial pneumonia, salmonella septicemia and wasting syndrome. The reasons for excluding these diseases were disease-specific, namely the low number of cases in the case of salmonella septicemia, the difficultly in establishing a diagnosis of recurrence in the case of bacterial pneumonia, and the subjective nature of the diagnosis criteria in the case of HIV associated encephalopathy and wasting syndrome.

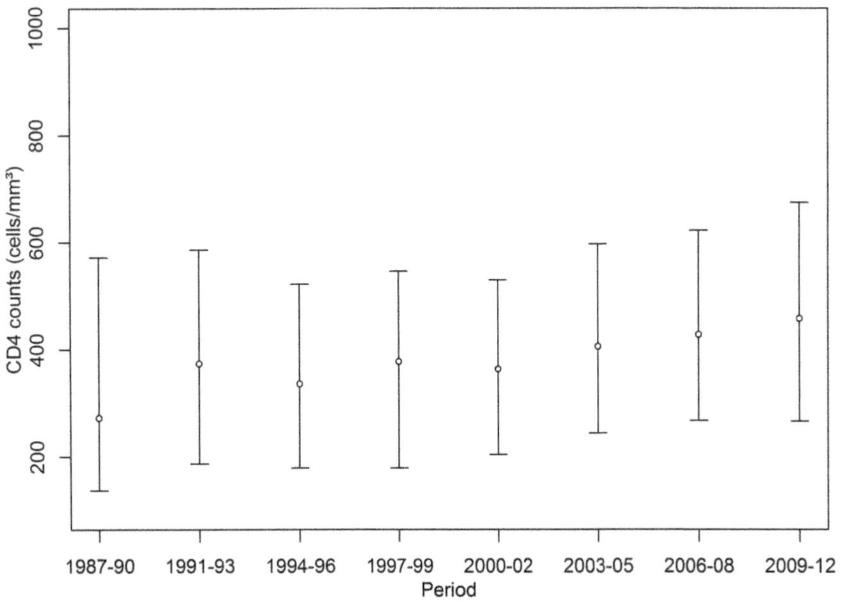

Figure 1. CD4 cell counts of patients under follow-up by calendar period: for each period medians and interquartile ranges are displayed.

Table 1. Characteristics of patients included in the opportunistic illnesses incidence analyses by period of cohort enrollment, IPEC cohort, period 1987–2012.

	1987–1990	1991–1993	1994–1996	1997–1999	2000–2002	2003–2005	2006–2008	2009–2012	p-value
	(n = 186)	(n = 291)	(n = 205)	(n = 243)	(n = 369)	(n = 427)	(n = 933)	(n = 1124)	
Age at enrollment years (median, IQR)	31.9 (28.5,39)	34.7 (28.6,40.6)	33 (28.4,38.8)	33.5 (28.4,38.9)	36.6 (29.6,42.5)	37.1 (30.3,43.2)	35.4 (28.7,43.1)	34.5 (27.9,42.3)	<0.001
Male sex	161 (86.6)	210 (72.2)	113 (55.1)	114 (46.9)	225 (61)	306 (71.7)	615 (65.9)	770 (68.5)	<0.001
Non white race/ethnicity	63 (33.9)	128 (44)	72 (35.1)	106 (43.6)	143 (38.8)	155 (36.4)	467 (50.2)	653 (58.8)	<0.001
Educational level									0.198
0–8 years	78 (47.6)	152 (52.2)	119 (58)	136 (56)	187 (50.8)	208 (48.7)	469 (50.4)	546 (49.1)	
9+ years	86 (52.4)	139 (47.8)	86 (42)	107 (44)	181 (49.2)	219 (51.3)	462 (49.6)	565 (50.9)	
HIV exposure category									<0.001
Heterossexual	31 (16.7)	126 (43.3)	118 (57.6)	140 (57.6)	209 (56.6)	208 (48.7)	525 (56.3)	502 (44.7)	
MSM	126 (67.7)	127 (43.6)	61 (29.8)	66 (27.2)	118 (32)	168 (39.3)	324 (34.7)	452 (40.2)	
IDU	15 (8.1)	20 (6.9)	10 (4.9)	7 (2.9)	6 (1.6)	3 (0.7)	13 (1.4)	9 (0.8)	
Other/Unknown	14 (7.5)	18 (6.2)	16 (7.8)	30 (12.3)	36 (9.8)	48 (11.2)	71 (7.6)	161 (14.3)	
Median baseline CD4 (IQR)	172 (96,225)	251.5 (110.5,674.8)	335.5 (149.2,499.8)	323.5 (148.2,500.5)	220 (96.2,390)	268 (103.2,464.8)	311.5 (112.8,524.5)	310 (107.5,551)	0.009
0–49 cells/mm^3	1 (0.5)	3 (1)	3 (1.5)	14 (5.8)	25 (6.8)	49 (11.5)	94 (10.1)	126 (11.2)	<0.001
50–199 cells/mm^3	6 (3.2)	9 (3.1)	9 (4.4)	34 (14)	69 (18.7)	67 (15.7)	150 (16.1)	191 (17)	
200–349 cells/mm^3	2 (1.1)	8 (2.7)	5 (2.4)	23 (9.5)	45 (12.2)	63 (14.8)	137 (14.7)	155 (13.8)	
350+ cells/mm^3	2 (1.1)	14 (4.8)	17 (8.3)	63 (25.9)	61 (16.5)	115 (26.9)	331 (35.5)	391 (34.8)	
Missing	175 (94.1)	257 (88.3)	171 (83.4)	109 (44.9)	169 (45.8)	133 (31.1)	221 (23.7)	261 (23.2)	
Baseline VL									<0.001
0–399 copies/mm^3	0 (0)	0 (0)	0 (0)	10 (4.1)	11 (3)	33 (7.7)	66 (7.1)	125 (11.1)	
400–4,999 copies/mm^3	0 (0)	1 (0.3)	0 (0)	20 (8.2)	20 (5.4)	27 (6.3)	45 (4.8)	81 (7.2)	
5,000–99,999 copies/mm^3	0 (0)	0 (0)	1 (0.5)	51 (21)	77 (20.9)	101 (23.7)	177 (19)	296 (26.3)	
100,000+ copies/mm^3	0 (0)	0 (0)	0 (0)	39 (16)	86 (23.3)	85 (19.9)	146 (15.6)	196 (17.4)	
Missing	186 (100)	290 (99.7)	204 (99.5)	123 (50.6)	175 (47.4)	181 (42.4)	499 (53.5)	426 (37.9)	
OI at enrollment	41 (22)	47 (16.2)	35 (17.1)	47 (19.3)	100 (27.1)	100 (23.4)	189 (20.3)	325 (28.9)	<0.001
Median time from HIV diagnosis and cohort enrollment, days (IQR)	0 (0,62.5)	33 (0,111)	58 (0,226)	104 (29.5,481.5)	123 (30,848)	260 (45,2370)	110 (24,742)	53 (8.8,574.5)	<0.001

OI: opportunistic illness; MSM: men who had sex with men; IDU: injection drug users; VL: viral load.

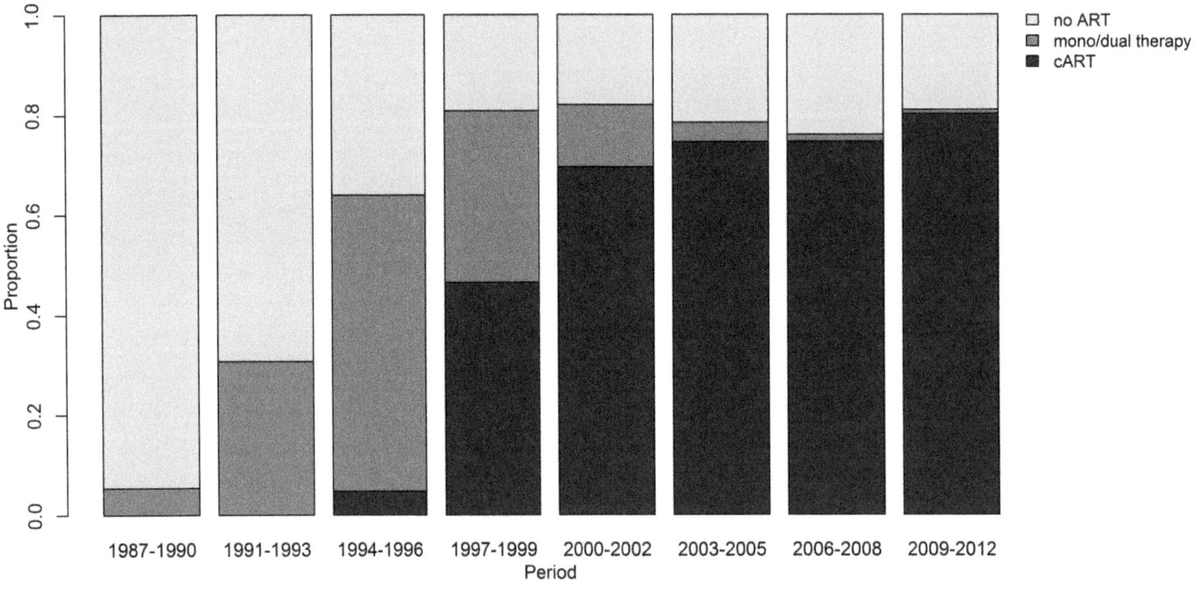

Figure 2. Use of antiretroviral therapy by calendar period.

Statistical Methods

Eight calendar periods were defined a priori as follows: 1987–1990, 1991–1993, 1994–1996, 1997–1999, 2000–2002, 2003–2005, 2006–2008 and 2009–2012. Socio-demographic, behavioral, laboratory, clinical features were compared among all included patients according to date of cohort entry using Kruskal-Wallis test for continuous variables and Chi-square for categorical variables.

We estimated the incidence rates of the first OI in each calendar period. The incidence rate of an OI was defined as the ratio between the number of cases of a specific illness and the number of person-years at risk during that period. Person-years at risk were calculated for each patient as the sum of days at risk by period. Rates were calculated by 1000 person-years with respective 95% confidence intervals (CI) using a Poisson regression model. Trends for overall and specific OI were tested for all OI with frequency above 40 cases during the study period. Incidence rate ratios as a function of calendar period were calculated as the ratio between the incidence rate observed in the most recent period of the study (2009–2012) and the incidence rate observed in first period of the study (1987–1990).

Results

From January 1st 1987 to December 31st 2012 a total of 3378 patients met the study criteria and were included in this analysis, 1119 (33%) presented an OI during follow-up. Age at enrollment increased over the years and male sex predominated in all of the study periods, with an increase in the proportion of women in the 1994–2002 periods. CD4 cell counts at cohort enrollment have increased over the years and in the last period of the study over one third of the patients have CD4 counts at cohort enrollment higher than 350 cells/mm^3 (Table1). Moreover, when analyzing the median of CD4 counts of all patients under follow-up at each study period, we noticed that it had progressively increased over the years, reaching 458 cells/mm^3 in the latter period of the study (Figure 1). The use of antiretroviral therapy also increased over the years, and in the most recent period, almost 80% of the patients were under cART (Figure 2).

During the study period, the incidence rates of overall OIs decreased from 295.4/1000 PY in 1987–1990 to 34.6/1000 PY in 2009–2012, with an incidence rate ratio (IRR) of 0.12 for the period 2009–2012 compared to 1987–1990, $p<0.001$ (Figure 3, Table 2). Incidence rates for specific OIs have also significantly decreased over the years (Table 2). Tuberculosis, esophageal candidiasis, cerebral toxoplasmosis and PCP had the highest incidence rates during the study period.

Tuberculosis was the most incident OI, except for the first study period (1987–1990). An incidence rate over 80.8/1000 PY was observed in 1991–1993, and since then the rates have decreased with an IRR of 0.22 (2012–2009 *vs.* 1987–1990, $p<0.001$) (Figure 3, Table 2). PCP incidence rate was 87.2/1000 PY in 1987–1990, and after that showed the steepest decline over the years, reaching an IRR of 0.03 (2012–2009 *vs.* 1987–1990, $p<0.001$) (Figure 3, Table 2). Cerebral toxoplasmosis was the third most incident OI in 1987–1990 (incidence rate of 43.6/1000 PY), experienced over the years a significant decrease in its incidence rates (IRR = 0.09, 2012–2009 *vs.* 1987–1990, $p<0.001$) and currently persists as the third most incident OI, with an incidence rate of 4.0/1000 PY (Figure 3, Table 2). Esophageal candidiasis was the fourth most incident OI in 1987–1990 with an incidence rate of 33.9/1000 PY, its incidence decreased over the years (IRR = 0.18, 2012–2009 *vs.* 1987–1990, $p<0.001$), and currently it is the second most incident OI (6.1/1000 PY) (Figure 3, Table 2).

Discussion

In this study, we have shown that the incidence rates of OI decreased over the years, with a trend of reduction that began even before cART was made universally available in Brazil. These results are in agreement with those reported from others cohorts and most likely reflect improvements in the general care of HIV infected patients in addition to the use of specific OI preventive measures as well as mono and dual antiretroviral therapy [21,26,31]. The most incident OIs in our casuistic (tuberculosis, esophageal candidiasis, cerebral toxoplasmosis and PCP) are also the most frequent OIs reported in other studies from high-income and low-income settings [2,4,6].

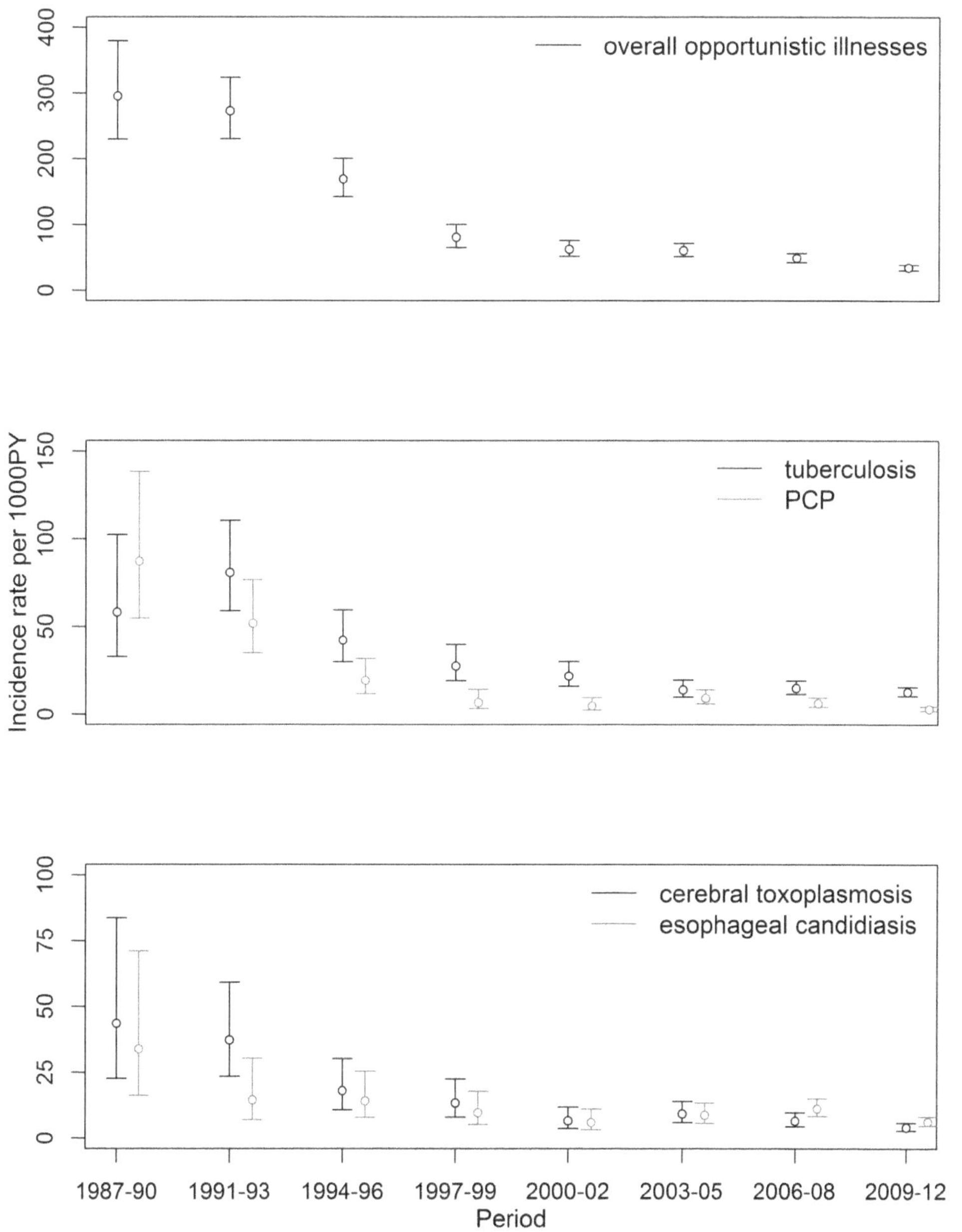

Figure 3. Incidence rates (per 1000 persons-years) and confidence interval for overall opportunistic illnesses, tuberculosis, *Pneumocystis jirovecii* pneumonia, cerebral toxoplasmosis and esophageal candidiasis by calendar period.

Tuberculosis represents the most incident OI in our cohort, with an incidence rate that is currently two-fold higher than the second most incident OI, esophageal candidiasis (12.54/1000 PY vs. 6.08/1000 PY). The 85% reduction observed in tuberculosis incidence rate over the years (1991–1993 *vs.* 2009–2012) is similar to the incidence rate variation observed in multiple cohorts, in both high-income and low-income settings [3,6,15,39], and in our setting it might be a result of overall antiretroviral therapy expansion. In a recently published meta-analysis, the summary estimate of the risk reduction associated with the use of cART across all CD4 counts was 67% (95%CI 61–73) [42]. Randomized clinical trials such as the Cipra HAITI study and the HPTN 052 also showed a 50% reduction after cART initiation among individuals with CD4 cell counts higher than 250 cells/mm^3 and 350 cells/mm^3, respectively [16,41].

HIV and tuberculosis co-infection is a huge challenge for countries with high tuberculosis prevalence, as Brazil, and, in these settings, tuberculosis is still an important cause of severe morbidity [34] and the main cause of death of HIV infected individuals [17,22,45]. Unlike others OIs, tuberculosis can occur in a HIV-infected patient independent of the degree of immunodeficiency [3] and the risk of developing tuberculosis is 20 to 37 times higher in HIV infected persons than in those without HIV infection [44].

In our cohort, tuberculosis prophylaxis has been used for HIV infected patients since 1994 according to national guidelines [28]. In the guidelines, isoniazid prophylaxis is recommended for HIV-infected patients with positive tuberculin skin test (TST) and no history of previous tuberculosis [12]. Previous studies have already shown the protective effect of isoniazid prophylaxis on tuberculosis incidence, independently of cART use [1,14,15], particularly for

Table 2. First opportunistic illness after enrollment in IPEC cohort, absolute numbers and incidence rates per 1000 persons-years for 1987–2012 and by calendar period.

	1987–2012		1987–1990		1991–1993		1994–1996		1997–1999		2000–2002		2003–2005		2006–2008		2009–2012		p-value for trend[a]	IRR[b]
Person-years	**18,137**		**206**		**483**		**780**		**1,047**		**1,694**		**2,317**		**3,877**		**7,735**			
	n	**IR**	**n**	**IR**	**n**	**IR**	**n**	**IR**	**n**	**IR**	**n**	**IR**	**n**	**IR**	**n**	**IR**	**n**	**IR**		
Overall opportunistic illnesses	1119	61,70	61	295,44	132	273,47	132	169,27	85	81,21	107	63,18	142	61,30	192	49,53	268	34,65	<0.01	0.12
Tuberculosis	336	18.53	12	58.12	39	80.80	33	42.32	29	27.71	37	21.85	32	13.81	57	14.70	97	12.54	<0.01	0.22
Esophageal candidiasis	155	8.55	7	33.90	7	14.50	11	14.11	10	9.55	10	5.90	20	8.63	43	11.09	47	6.08	<0.01	0.18
Toxoplasmosis cerebral	143	7.88	9	43.59	18	37.29	14	17.95	14	13.38	11	6.50	21	9.07	25	6.45	31	4.01	<0.01	0.09
Pneumocystis carinii pneumonia	140	7.72	18	87.18	25	51.79	15	19.24	7	6.69	8	4.72	21	9.07	24	6.19	22	2.84	<0.01	0.03
Herpes simplex virus	64	3.53	4	19.37	3	6.22	1	1.28	6	5.73	18	10.63	5	2.16	11	2.84	16	2.07	<0.01	0.11
Cytomegalovirus	58	3.20	1	4.84	10	20.72	13	16.67	2	1.91	7	4.13	7	3.02	6	1.55	12	1.55	<0.01	0.32
Extrapulmonar cryptococcosis	52	2.87	1	4.84	7	14.50	5	6.41	7	6.69	6	3.54	6	2.59	8	2.06	12	1.55	<0.01	0.32
Kaposi Sarcoma	45	2.48	2	9.69	8	16.57	8	10.26	3	2.87	1	0.59	10	4.32	4	1.03	9	1.16	<0.01	0.12
Crypstosporidiosis	31	1.71	2	9.69	4	8.29	17	21.80	0	0.00	1	0.59	3	1.30	2	0.52	2	0.26	-	0.03
Isosporosis	30	1.65	3	14.53	9	18.65	4	5.13	2	1.91	2	1.18	2	0.86	4	1.03	4	0.52	-	0.04
Non tuberculosis mycobacterium	26	1.43	0	0.00	0	0.00	7	8.98	2	1.91	3	1.77	7	3.02	4	1.03	3	0.39	-	0.04[c]
Disseminated histoplasmosis	15	0.83	1	4.84	1	2.07	3	3.85	1	0.96	1	0.59	1	0.43	2	0.52	5	0.65	-	0.13
Non-Hodgkin lymphoma	14	0.77	1	4.84	0	0.00	1	1.28	2	1.91	1	0.59	2	0.86	1	0.26	6	0.78	-	0.16

Diseases with less than 10 cases reported during the study period are not shown (progressive multifocal leukoencephalopathy n = 8, invasive cervical cancer n = 1, coccidioidomycosis n = 1).
[a]Trend was tested for all illnesses with 40 cases of more during the study period.
[b]Incidence rate ratio between 2009–2012 and 19987–1990 periods.
[c]Reference period was 1994–1996 since the IR in previous periods were equal to zero.

those patients with positive TST [32]. Despite the fact that a meta-analysis did not find a reduction in tuberculosis incidence in TST negative patients [1], considering the high risk of false-negative results (up to 66%) in HIV infected patients [7] and operational barriers related to TST implementation and realization, the WHO recommends that in resource-constrained settings TST should not be a requirement for initiating isoniazid prophylaxis [44]. Given that operational barriers and late presentation of HIV-infected patients (that can be associated to false negative TST results) prevail in our cohort, it is possible that isoniazid prophylaxis has been underused, resulting in a high incidence of tuberculosis, even in the most recent periods. Moreover, a recent study conducted in several HIV clinics in Rio de Janeiro showed that efforts to improve coverage of isoniazid prophylaxis to HIV infected patients by training clinicians in tuberculosis prevention resulted in a significant decrease in tuberculosis incidence [14]. It is clear that efforts to properly address the tuberculosis and HIV co-infection burden in our setting are urgently needed.

Cerebral toxoplasmosis was the third most incident OI in our cohort, with and incidence rate that decreased from 43.6/1000 PY in 1987–1990 to 4.0/1000 PY 2009–2012. Both in pre and post cART era, cerebral toxoplasmosis incidence rates observed in our cohort are higher than those observed in other studies both from high and low-middle income countries [23,35,37,38]. Brazilian prevalence of *Toxoplasma gondii* infection is high [13], and specifically in the HIV-infected population this prevalence can reach 80% [46]. A significantly lower Toxoplasma seroprevalence has been estimated in HIV cohorts from high-income settings (11–16%) [20,24]. It is likely that the elevated incidence rates of cerebral toxoplasmosis observed in our cohort is a result of the high burden of toxoplasmosis infection in Brazil.

PCP was the most incident OI in the first period of our study, with incidence rates comparable to those observed in high-income cohorts in pre cART era [25,40]. The decreasing trend in the incidence rate of PCP likely results from the use of chemoprophylaxis and antiretroviral therapy. Currently PCP incidence rate in our cohort is lower than that observed in both in high income and low-middle income settings in the post cART era [10,23,25,33,35].

Esophageal candidiasis incidence rates decreased since the first period of the study, and remained relatively stable after the 2000–2002 period. The rates observed in our study pre and post cART availability are similar to those from high and middle-low income settings [6,25,35], and as well as its incidence rates stabilization observed after 2002 [6].

There are limitations and strengths to our study that should be considered. The clinical database for the cohort is based in chart-abstracted information and thus subject to errors in the process of collecting the data from the medical charts. To address this concern and examine the degree of this limitation, a clinical database validation and chart review was performed and great consistence (95%) between the database and original medical charts was found. Another point worth mentioning is the possible underestimation of OI events due to seek of care elsewhere. However, IPEC provides general multidisciplinary care including inpatient care free of charge with an emergency entrance available and, as such, the likelihood that they resort to IPEC in case of illness is high thus minimizing this potential bias.

In conclusion, the incidence rates of OIs overall and of specific illnesses decreased over the years but they still occur in an unacceptable frequency. Tuberculosis and HIV co-infection represent a challenge for the health care professional and policy makers in places with high tuberculosis burden such as Brazil. Continued efforts to address the tuberculosis-HIV co-infection remain highly relevant and needed. We found that cerebral toxoplasmosis incidence in our setting was higher than that of other settings suggesting that the baseline burden of tropical infectious diseases in a particular place influences the incidence of the disease among the HIV infected population. Knowledge of the current burden of infectious diseases among the HIV and non-HIV infected can help plan control efforts for both populations.

Author Contributions

Conceived and designed the experiments: LC PML BG. Performed the experiments: LC PML. Analyzed the data: LC PML. Contributed reagents/materials/analysis tools: RIM DPC RTA SWC VGV. Wrote the paper: LC PML BG SWC VGV.

References

1. Akolo C, Adetifa I, Shepperd S, Volmink J (2010). Treatment of latent tuberculosis infection in HIV infected persons. Cochrane Database Syst Rev(1): Cd000171.
2. Badri M, Maartens G, Bekker LG, Wood R (2005). The spectrum and prognosis of AIDS-defining illnesses in Cape Town. The Southern African Journal of HIV Medicine 6(2): 11–16.
3. Badri M, Wilson D, Wood R (2002). Effect of highly active antiretroviral therapy on incidence of tuberculosis in South Africa: a cohort study. Lancet 359(9323): 2059–2064.
4. Brodt HR, Kamps BS, Gute P, Knupp B, Staszewski S, et al. (1997). Changing incidence of AIDS-defining illnesses in the era of antiretroviral combination therapy. Aids 11(14): 1731–1738.
5. Buchacz K, Baker RK, Moorman AC, Richardson JT, Wood KC, et al. (2008). Rates of hospitalizations and associated diagnoses in a large multisite cohort of HIV patients in the United States, 1994–2005. Aids 22(11): 1345–1354.
6. Buchacz K, Baker RK, Palella FJ Jr, Chmiel JS, Lichtenstein KA, et al. (2010). AIDS-defining opportunistic illnesses in US patients, 1994–2007: a cohort study. Aids 24(10): 1549–1559.
7. CDC (1991). Purified protein derivative (PPD)-tuberculin anergy and HIV infection: guidelines for anergy testing and management of anergic persons at risk of tuberculosis. MMWR Recomm Rep 40(RR-5): 27–32.
8. CDC (1992). 1993 Revised Classification System for HIV Infection and Expanded Surveillance Case Definition for AIDS Among Adolescents and Adults. MMWR Recomm Rep 41(RR-17).
9. Chaisson RE, Moore RD, Richman DD, Keruly J, Creagh T (1992). Incidence and natural history of Mycobacterium avium-complex infections in patients with advanced human immunodeficiency virus disease treated with zidovudine. The Zidovudine Epidemiology Study Group. Am Rev Respir Dis 146(2): 285–289.
10. Charurat M, Blattner W, Hershow R, Buck A, Zorrilla CD, et al. (2004). Changing trends in clinical AIDS presentations and survival among HIV-1-infected women. J Womens Health (Larchmt) 13(6): 719–730.
11. Coelho L, Veloso VG, Grinsztejn B, Luz PM (2013). Trends in overall opportunistic illnesses, Pneumocystis carinii pneumonia, cerebral toxoplasmosis and Mycobacterium avium complex incidence rates over the 30 years of the HIV epidemic: a systematic review. Brazilian Journal of Infectious Diseases.
12. Conde MB, Melo FA, Marques AM, Cardoso NC, Pinheiro VG, et al. (2009). III Brazilian Thoracic Association Guidelines on tuberculosis. J Bras Pneumol 35(10): 1018–1048.
13. Dubey JP, Lago EG, Gennari SM, Su C, Jones JL (2012). Toxoplasmosis in humans and animals in Brazil: high prevalence, high burden of disease, and epidemiology. Parasitology 139(11): 1375–1424.
14. Durovni B, Saraceni V, Moulton LH, Pacheco AG, Cavalcante SC, et al. (2013). Effect of improved tuberculosis screening and isoniazid preventive therapy on incidence of tuberculosis and death in patients with HIV in clinics in Rio de Janeiro, Brazil: a stepped wedge, cluster-randomised trial. Lancet Infect Dis 13(10): 852–858.
15. Golub JE, Pronyk P, Mohapi L, Thsabangu N, Moshabela M, et al. (2009). Isoniazid preventive therapy, HAART and tuberculosis risk in HIV-infected adults in South Africa: a prospective cohort. Aids 23(5): 631–636.
16. Grinsztejn B, Hosseinipour M, Ribaudo H, Havlir D, Cohen M, et al. (2014). Effects of Early versus Delayed Initiation of Antiretroviral Therapy on HIV Clinical Outcomes: Results from the HPTN 052. Lancet Infect Dis Accepted.
17. Grinsztejn B, Luz PM, Pacheco AG, Santos DV, Velasque L, et al. (2013). Changing mortality profile among HIV-infected patients in Rio de Janeiro, Brazil: shifting from AIDS to non-AIDS related conditions in the HAART era. PLoS One 8(4): e59768.

18. Grinsztejn B, Veloso VG, Friedman RK, Moreira RI, Luz PM, et al. (2009). Early mortality and cause of deaths in patients using HAART in Brazil and the United States. Aids 23(16): 2107–2114.
19. Grinsztejn B, Veloso VG, Pilotto JH, Campos DP, Keruly JC, et al. (2007). Comparison of clinical response to initial highly active antiretroviral therapy in the patients in clinical care in the United States and Brazil. J Acquir Immune Defic Syndr 45(5): 515–520.
20. Israelski DM, Chmiel JS, Poggensee L, Phair JP, Remington JS (1993). Prevalence of Toxoplasma infection in a cohort of homosexual men at risk of AIDS and toxoplasmic encephalitis. J Acquir Immune Defic Syndr 6(4): 414–418.
21. Kaplan JE, Hanson D, Dworkin MS, Frederick T, Bertolli J, et al. (2000). Epidemiology of human immunodeficiency virus-associated opportunistic infections in the United States in the era of highly active antiretroviral therapy. Clin Infect Dis 30 Suppl 1: S5–14.
22. Lawn SD, Harries AD, Anglaret X, Myer L, Wood R (2008). Early mortality among adults accessing antiretroviral treatment programmes in sub-Saharan Africa. Aids 22(15): 1897–1908.
23. Ledergerber B, Egger M, Erard V, Weber R, Hirschel B, et al. (1999). AIDS-related opportunistic illnesses occurring after initiation of potent antiretroviral therapy: the Swiss HIV Cohort Study. Jama 282(23): 2220–2226.
24. Mathews WC, Fullerton SC (1994). Use of a clinical laboratory database to estimate Toxoplasma seroprevalence among human immunodeficiency virus-infected patients. Overcoming bias in secondary analysis of clinical records. Arch Pathol Lab Med 118(8): 807–810.
25. Mocroft A, Sabin CA, Youle M, Madge S, Tyrer M, et al. (1999). Changes in AIDS-defining illnesses in a London Clinic, 1987–1998. J Acquir Immune Defic Syndr 21(5): 401–407.
26. Mocroft A, Youle M, Phillips AN, Halai R, Easterbrook P, et al. (1998). The incidence of AIDS-defining illnesses in 4883 patients with human immunodeficiency virus infection. Royal Free/Chelsea and Westminster Hospitals Collaborative Group. Arch Intern Med 158(5): 491–497.
27. Moreira RI, Luz PM, Struchiner CJ, Morgado M, Veloso VG, et al. (2011). Immune status at presentation for HIV clinical care in Rio de Janeiro and Baltimore. J Acquir Immune Defic Syndr 57 Suppl 3: S171–178.
28. 47.MS (1994). Co-infecção TB/HIV/AIDS: Manual de Normas. P. N. d. DST/AIDS. Brasilia: 1–20.
29. 12.MS (1999). Terapia Anti-retroviral e Saúde Pública. Um balanço da experiência brasileira.
30. Pacheco AG, Tuboi SH, May SB, Moreira LFS, Ramadas L, et al. (2009). Temporal Changes in Causes of Death Among HIV-Infected Patients in the HAART Era in Rio de Janeiro, Brazil. J Acquir Immune Defic Syndr 51(5): 624–630 610.1097/QAI.1090b1013e3181a1094ecf1095.
31. Palella FJ Jr, Delaney KM, Moorman AC, Loveless MO, Fuhrer J, et al. (1998). Declining morbidity and mortality among patients with advanced human immunodeficiency virus infection. HIV Outpatient Study Investigators. N Engl J Med 338(13): 853–860.
32. Pape JW, Jean SS, Ho JL, Hafner A, Johnson WD Jr (1993). Effect of isoniazid prophylaxis on incidence of active tuberculosis and progression of HIV infection. Lancet 342(8866): 268–272.
33. Podlasin RB, Wiercinska-Drapalo A, Olczak A, Beniowski M, Smiatacz T, et al. (2006). Opportunistic infections and other AIDS-defining illnesses in Poland in 2000–2002. Infection 34(4): 196–200.
34. Ribeiro S, Luz PM, Campos D, Moreira R, Japiassu A, et al. (2013). Incidence and determinants of severe morbidity among HIV-infected patients from Rio de Janeiro, Brazil, 2000–2010. Antiviral Therapy.
35. Rojanawiwat A, Tsuchiya N, Pathipvanich P, Pumpradit W, Schmidt W-P, et al. (2011). Impact of the National Access to Antiretroviral Program on the incidence of opportunistic infections in Thailand. International Health 3(2): 101–107.
36. Sackoff JE, Hanna DB, Pfeiffer MR, Torian LV (2006). Causes of death among persons with AIDS in the era of highly active antiretroviral therapy: New York City. Ann Intern Med 145(6): 397–406.
37. Sacktor N, Lyles RH, Skolasky R, Kleeberger C, Selnes OA, et al. (2001). HIV-associated neurologic disease incidence changes:: Multicenter AIDS Cohort Study, 1990–1998. Neurology 56(2): 257–260.
38. San-Andres FJ, Rubio R, Castilla J, Pulido F, Palao G, et al. (2003). Incidence of acquired immunodeficiency syndrome-associated opportunistic diseases and the effect of treatment on a cohort of 1115 patients infected with human immunodeficiency virus, 1989–1997. Clin Infect Dis 36(9): 1177–1185.
39. Santoro-Lopes G, de Pinho AM, Harrison LH, Schechter M (2002). Reduced risk of tuberculosis among Brazilian patients with advanced human immunodeficiency virus infection treated with highly active antiretroviral therapy. Clin Infect Dis 34(4): 543–546.
40. Schwarcz L, Chen MJ, Vittinghoff E, Hsu L, Schwarcz S (2013). Declining incidence of AIDS-defining opportunistic illnesses: results from 16 years of population-based AIDS surveillance. Aids 27(4): 597–605.
41. Severe P, Juste MA, Ambroise A, Eliacin L, Marchand C, et al. (2010). Early versus standard antiretroviral therapy for HIV-infected adults in Haiti. N Engl J Med 363(3): 257–265.
42. Suthar AB, Lawn SD, del Amo J, Getahun H, Dye C, et al. (2012). Antiretroviral therapy for prevention of tuberculosis in adults with HIV: a systematic review and meta-analysis. PLoS Med 9(7): e1001270.
43. 16.WHO (2007). WHO case definitions of HIV for surveillance and revised clinical staging and immunological classification of HIV-related disease in adults and children.
44. 29.WHO (2011). Guidelines for intensified tuberculosis case-finding and isoniazid preventive therapy for people living with HIV in resource-constrained settings.
45. 11.WHO (2012). Global tuberculosis Report.
46. Xavier GA, Cademartori BG, Cunha Filho NA, Farias NA (2013). Evaluation of seroepidemiological toxoplasmosis in HIV/AIDS patients in the south of Brazil. Rev Inst Med Trop Sao Paulo 55(1): 25–30.
47. Yazdanpanah Y, Chene G, Losina E, Goldie SJ, Merchadou LD, et al. (2001). Incidence of primary opportunistic infections in two human immunodeficiency virus-infected French clinical cohorts. Int J Epidemiol 30(4): 864–871.

15

The Increased Effectiveness of HIV Preventive Intervention among Men Who Have Sex with Men and of Follow-Up Care for People Living with HIV after 'Task-Shifting' to Community-Based Organizations: A 'Cash on Service Delivery' Model in China

Hongjing Yan[1¶], Min Zhang[2¶], Jinkou Zhao[1,3]*, Xiping Huan[1,4], Jianping Ding[1,4], Susu Wu[2], Chenchen Wang[2], Yuanyuan Xu[2], Li Liu[2], Fei Xu[2], Haitao Yang[1]*

1 Jiangsu Provincial Center for Disease Control and Prevention, Nanjing, China, **2** Nanjing Municipal Center for Disease Control and Prevention, Nanjing, China, **3** The Global Fund to fight AIDS, Tuberculosis and Malaria, Geneva, Switzerland, **4** Jiangsu Provincial Preventive Medicine Association, Nanjing, China

Abstract

Background: A large number of men who have sex with men (MSM) and people living with HIV/AIDS (PLHA) are underserved despite increased service availability from government facilities while many community based organizations (CBOs) are not involved. We aimed to assess the feasibility and effectiveness of the task shifting from government facilities to CBOs in China.

Methods: HIV preventive intervention for MSM and follow-up care for PLHA were shifted from government facilities to CBOs. Based on 'cash on service delivery' model, 10 USD per MSM tested for HIV with results notified, 82 USD per newly HIV cases diagnosed, and 50 USD per PLHA received a defined package of follow-up care services, were paid to the CBOs. Cash payments were made biannually based on the verified results in the national web-based HIV/AIDS information system.

Findings: After task shifting, CBOs gradually assumed preventive intervention for MSM and follow-up care for PLHA from 2008 to 2012. HIV testing coverage among MSM increased from 4.1% in 2008 to 22.7% in 2012. The baseline median CD4 counts of newly diagnosed HIV positive MSM increased from 309 to 397 cells/μL. HIV tests among MSM by CBOs accounted for less than 1% of the total HIV tests in Nanjing but the share of HIV cases detected by CBOs was 12.4% in 2008 and 43.6% in 2012. Unit cost per HIV case detected by CBOs was 47 times lower than that by government facilities. The coverage of CD4 tests and antiretroviral therapy increased from 71.1% and 78.6% in 2008 to 86.0% and 90.1% in 2012, respectively.

Conclusion: It is feasible to shift essential HIV services from government facilities to CBOs, and to verify independently service results to adopt 'cash on service delivery' model. Services provided by CBOs are cost-effective, as compared with that by government facilities.

Editor: Anil Kumar, University of Missouri-Kansas City, United States of America

Funding: The present study was funded by The Bill & Melinda Gates Foundation; Outstanding Medical Academic Leader Program of Jiangsu Provincial government and Outstanding Medical Academic Leader Program of Jiangsu Provincial Center for Diseases Control and Prevention. The Bill & Melinda Gates Foundation Beijing Representative Office participated in the study design. The other study sponsors had no role in the study design. All study sponsors had no role in data collection, data analysis, data interpretation, or writing of this report.

Competing Interests: The authors have declared that no competing interests exist. Jiangsu Provincial Preventive Medicine Association is affiliated with Jiangsu Provincial Center for Diseases Control and Prevention.

* Email: jinkouzhao@hotmail.com (JZ); yht@jscdc.cn (HY)

¶ HY and MZ are joint first authors on this work.

Introduction

Since the first case of HIV/AIDS was reported in China in 1985, the epidemic has spread to different populations around the country [1,2]. HIV transmission route has also shifted from predominantly injection drug use (IDU) during the late 1980s to early 1990s, to unsafe blood and plasma collection in mid-1990s, and to the sexual contact mode since 2005 [3]. Among new annual infections estimated in 2011, 52.2% were infected through heterosexual contact and 29.4% through homosexual contact [4].

Similar to control programs for other infectious diseases, programs for HIV/AIDS shall follow public health principles, including case finding and surveillance, interrupting transmission, treatment and case management, together with population based monitoring and evaluation [5]. Successful adoption of these public health principles requires a non-stop service chain ranging from preventive intervention to avoid HIV acquisition, to HIV testing to detect the infection, prevention of secondary transmission with positive prevention, follow-up care, preparation and initiation and retention with antiretroviral therapy (ART) [6].

China's central government and local governments have taken various measures to contain the epidemic. These include HIV testing, preventive interventions such as methadone maintenance therapy and behavioral change, prevention of HIV mother-to-child transmission, follow-up care for people living with HIV/AIDS (PLHA) and implementation of free ART [6,7]. These government funded HIV programs are implemented by health and medical professionals within the government structure, primarily through its public health system, namely national - provincial-prefecture- county/district center for disease control and prevention (CDC) system. This arrangement, in the context of the stigma and/illegality being associated with high risk behaviors and with being HIV positive, hindered the acceptability and uptake of relevant HIV program services [8–11]. The difference between the two numbers of 343,000 PLHA cases cumulatively reported through 2011 and 780,000 PLHA estimated in 2011 [4], suggested that large numbers of PLHA have not yet known their HIV positive status and as a result unknowingly transmit the virus to partners. In the meantime HIV counseling and testing services provided by the CDCs and government hospitals are not well used [12,13]. Furthermore, 25.4% of those tested and reported HIV positive cases are not in regular follow-up and 45.8% of PLHA are missed in CD4 testing [14]. AIDS mortality remains high and ranked the first among all infectious diseases in China since 2009 [15]. About 30% of PLHA still initiated ART at very late stage despite increased availability of ART services [16].

In the meantime, other social resources, such as civil society organizations and community-based groups, are yet to be closely involved in the response to the challenging HIV/AIDS epidemic. Internationally, task-shifting from health professionals to lay personnel in community-based organizations (CBOs) has been implemented and proven to be effective in provision of HIV counseling and testing, and HIV care and treatment. Studies have shown a lower unit cost, comparable quality and increased acceptability for these services provided by lay personnel, especially peers [17,18].

Nanjing, the capital city of Jiangsu province, is located in eastern China with a residential population of 6.36 million and a migrant population of 1.75 million [19]. It is also a gay cruising center, where population size of men who have sex with men (MSM) was estimated to be 25,000 in 2008, after the consensus was reached among all relevant stakeholders [20]. This figure was used for all years during the program as there was no any additional estimation effort after 2008. In 2007 the overall HIV/AIDS epidemic of the city was quite low based on HIV/AIDS case surveillance data. As of 2007, the cumulatively reported number of HIV/AIDS cases was about 500, 40.0% due to injection drug use, 22.7% via unprotected heterosexual and 6.5% via unprotected homosexual behaviors. However, a growing HIV epidemic was reported among MSM. HIV prevalence increased from zero in 2003 to 6.6% in 2008, and an HIV incidence of 3.36 per 100 person-years was observed in a cohort study from 2008 to 2010 [21–23]. Only one MSM peer group provided hotline-based health education, and conducted outreach intervention services at gay bars and bathhouse during weekends in 2008. HIV testing targeting high risk population, and pre-ART care and treatment referral were mainly implemented by local CDCs, while CBOs and peer groups were not involved.

In 2008, Nanjing started to pilot shifting selected HIV preventive intervention, follow-up care and support tasks along the service chain for HIV programs from health and medical professionals to CBOs, with support from China-Bill & Melinda Gates Foundation Cooperation Project on HIV Prevention and Care. This article aims to describe this 'task shifting' and present the findings resulted from it.

Methods

Design of the pilot project

After mapping of available CBOs and assessment of their capacity to provide relevant services, two groups of services were selected for 'task shifting' from government health facilities, including local CDCs and hospitals, to CBOs. One group was HIV preventive intervention service centered on HIV testing among high risk populations; the other group was follow-up care and support service for PLHA centered on referral for CD4 tests and ART.

A 'cash on service delivery' model [24] was adopted for the pilot design. Core components most representative of the two service packages were used as the output measure of achievement for CBOs. Following the performance-based funding mechanism, unit price was developed. For HIV preventive intervention service, per most-at-risk population (MARP) mobilized and screened for HIV and syphilis with the testing result informed, 62 Chinese Yuan (CNY) (approximately 10 USD) were paid to the CBOs. The service package provided by CBOs included health education, condom promotion, HIV and syphilis test mobilization, and pre- and post-test counseling. The core indicator was the number of MARP screened for HIV. Per newly confirmed HIV positive case, an additional of 500 CNY (approximately 82 USD) were paid to the CBOs. The service package provided by CBOs included accompanying and referring patients to local CDCs for HIV repeated test and confirmation, providing social and psychological support while waiting for laboratory results. The core indicator was the number of newly HIV positives confirmed with results informed. For follow-up care and support service for PLHA, 300 CNY (approximately 50 USD) were paid to the CBO who provided a package of services for one HIV positive case for a year, including social support, home-based care, CD4 test facilitation, pre-ART counseling and ART referral. The core indicator was the number of PLHA receiving at least one follow up care, one CD4 test and one syphilis testing within a year. Cash was paid to CBOs every six months by Jiangsu Province Preventive Medicine Association (JSPMA), based on verified core indicators retrieved by respective local CDCs and Nanjing Municipal CDC.

Implementation of the pilot project

The pilot project started in July 2008 and ended in December 2012 in Nanjing. HIV preventive intervention services covered MSM, female sex workers (FSW) and IDU in 2008 and 2009. After the mid-term project review in 2010, HIV preventive intervention services focused on MSM only, due to evidence of a growing epidemic among MSM and extremely low case detention rates among FSW and IDU. This article focuses on MSM only for the preventive intervention services. As for the follow-up care and support services for PLHA, only local HIV/AIDS cases (Nanjing residents) were included in the pilot program.

To build capacity for the CBOs selected for service delivery, local CDCs and hospitals as well as well-established CBOs were organized and provided training on HIV knowledge, HIV/sexually transmitted diseases, risk behavior change communication, administering rapid HIV test, maintaining confidentiality and

Table 1. Roles of community-based organizations (CBOs) and government health facilities (GHFs) in the tasks before and after the pilot program in Nanjing, China.

Task	Activities	Role played*			
		Before		After	
		GHFs†	CBOs	GHFs	CBOs
Preventive interventions	Knowledge dissemination	+++	+++	+	+++
	Risk reduction counseling	+++	+	+	+++
	Condom use promotion	+++	+	+	+++
	Referral for testing	+++	–	+	+++
	Rapid HIV testing	+++	–	++	+++
	Notification of test results	+++	–	++	+++
Follow-up care	Social/psychological support	+	+	+	+++
	Home-based care	++	+	++	+++
	CD4 test facilitation	+++	–	++	+++
	Pre-ART counseling	+++	–	++	++
	OI and ART referral	+++	–	++	++
	Drug adherence education	+++	–	++	+++
	Stigma and discrimination reduction	+	+	++	+++

*Role played: Major +++, Medium ++, Minor +, No role–;
†including hospitals and local Center for Disease Control and Prevention.

procedures for referral and follow-up for PLHA according to national guidelines [25]. For CBOs haven't been officially registered and without nurses or physicians, rapid HIV testing and counseling were required to implement by peers under the technical support and supervision by local CDCs to avoid adverse events among those who tested HIV positive or social harm. Following pre-and post-test counseling, the window period and need for repeat testing for recent risk and periodic testing every six months with on-going risk were explained, as well as the information of local HIV laboratory algorithm used and the potential discordant testing results between HIV rapid test and confirmatory test, and the need for further repeated testing in six weeks and follow up by local CDCs. Contents of the prevention with positives, pre-ART counseling and ART referral, ART adherence, stigma and discrimination reduction, and program data collection and reporting were also discussed during the training.

Data collection and verification

Local district CDCs worked with CBOs to collect and enter the programmatic data to the project information reporting system, and compiled and reported the service results to JSPMA every six months. Programmatic data included program management variables such as cost, and performance-based core indicators, such as the number of MARP tested for HIV, the number of newly confirmed HIV positive cases, the number of HIV/AIDS cases received at least one follow up care service within a year and the number of HIV/AIDS patients received at least one CD4 test within a year. These were entered to the web-based national HIV/AIDS information system [26] by local district CDCs. The Nanjing Municipal CDC verified the results of core indicators and shared with JSPMA. JSPMA compared the data from CBOs and Nanjing Municipal CDC, and then paid cash to CBOs based on the verified results.

Table 2. The coverage of HIV testing and HIV detection rate among men who have sex with men, the median CD4 counts among local HIV/AIDS cases, through services by community-based organizations (CBOs), 2008 to 2012,Nanjing, China.

Year	HIV tests performed by CBOs*		Newly detected HIV cases†		Median of CD4 counts‡	
	Number	Coverage %	Number	Rate %	Number of newly diagnosed local cases	Baseline CD4 counts (cells/μL)
2008	1,034	4.1	27	2.6 (27/1,034)	20	309
2009	2,540	10.2	131	5.2 (131/2,540)	98	356
2010	3,297	13.3	192	5.8 (192/3,297)	149	345
2011	4,547	18.2	158	3.5 (158/4,547)	146	357
2012	5,673	22.7	237	4.2 (237/5,673)	220	397

*P value for trend of the coverage, <0.001; the denominator was 25,000 [20];
†P value for the trend of the rate of newly detected HIV positives, <0.001;
‡P value for the trend of median CD4 counts, <0.01.

Table 3. Unit cost per HIV case detected, comparison between government health facilities (GHFs) and community-based organizations (CBOs), 2008 to 2012 (U.S. dollars).

Year	HIV testing		Newly detected HIV cases		Unit cost per HIV case detected					
					CBOs		GHFs			Unit cost ratio, GHFs/CBOs
	CBOs	GHFs	CBOs	GHFs	Pilot program funding	Unit cost†	Government funding	Hospital Charges	Unit cost‡	
2008	1,034	493,015	27	190	12,723	471	381,148	2,261,705	13,910	30
2009	2,540	564,965	131	250	36,554	279	340,492	2,718,544	12,236	44
2010	3,297	556,404	192	210	49,248	257	481,475	2,972,977	16,450	64
2011	4,547	712,192	158	251	59,166	374	543,115	3,576,400	16,412	44
2012	5,673	799,765	237	306	77,086	325	616,557	4,098,931	15,410	47
Total	17,091	3,126,341	745	1,207	234,777	315	2,362,787	15,628,557	14,906	47

†All costs by the CBOs to detect one HIV case.
‡All costs by the government health facilities to detect one HIV case.

Non-programmatic data, including the number of total HIV tests and HIV positive cases confirmed and reported, the number of HIV/AIDS cases receiving CD4 tests and initiating ART and being retained on ART at 12-month follow-up, were obtained from Nanjing Municipal CDC through the web-based national HIV/AIDS information system. CD4 testing was provided free of charge once a year for PLHA who were not on ART and twice a year for those who were on ART according to the national guideline, and the criterion for receiving free ART was based on CD4 counts less then 200 cells/uL prior to and in 2011 and then less then 350 cells/uL in 2012 and afterwards [27]. The registered and alive PLHA was used as denominators to calculate the rates of follow-up care and CD4 counts. The PLHA eligible for ART was used as denominators for ART coverage. The cost data for HIV program jointly funded by Chinese central government, Jiangsu Provincial Government and Nanjing Municipal Government were collected annually from Nanjing Health Bureau. The project was approved by the Ethics Committee of the Chinese Center for Disease Control and Prevention.

Laboratory procedure

HIV rapid test kit (Alere Determine HIV-1/2, Alere Medical Co., Ltd)or enzyme-linked immunosorbent assay (ELISA) kit (Beijing Wantai Biological Pharmacy Enterprise Co., Ltd) were used for HIV screening from finger-prick blood or intravenous blood sample. Blood specimen for screening HIV positive individuals were sent to Nanjing Municipal CDC for confirmation using Western Blot test (HIVBLOT 2.2, Genelabs, Singapore). Following the same testing procedure, CD4 counts were measured using fluorescent activated cell sorter (FACS) analysis with BD FACS Calibur at Jiangsu Provincial CDC in 2008 and 2009, and at the Nanjing Second Hospital, the designated ART hospital in Nanjing since 2010.

Data analysis

Data is presented annually, prior to and after the pilot launch. Data is disaggregated by and compared among service providers over time. Chi-square was used for trend analysis of categorical data while non-parametric analysis was used for the comparison in median CD4 counts across years. Analyses were performed through SPSS 16.0 version. Statistical significance was defined by $P<0.05$.

Results

Roles of government health facilities and CBOs before and after 'task shifting'

The scope of the two tasks shifted from government health facilities to CBOs is presented in Table 1. In HIV preventive intervention service, CBOs assumed the functions of three new tasks related to providing rapid HIV testing and result notification, enhancing the roles in two existing tasks of conducting risk behavior change and communication, while government health facilities shifted four tasks substantially to CBOs. In follow-up care and support service for PLHA, CBOs took responsibility for four new tasks, enhanced the roles in two existing tasks of providing social and family support, while government health facilities shifted partially four tasks to CBOs. The roles of stigma and discrimination reduction were both strengthened in government health facilities and CBOs.

HIV preventive intervention services among MSM

After 'tasks shifting', the number of CBOs providing preventive intervention services among MSM increased from 1 in 2007 to 8

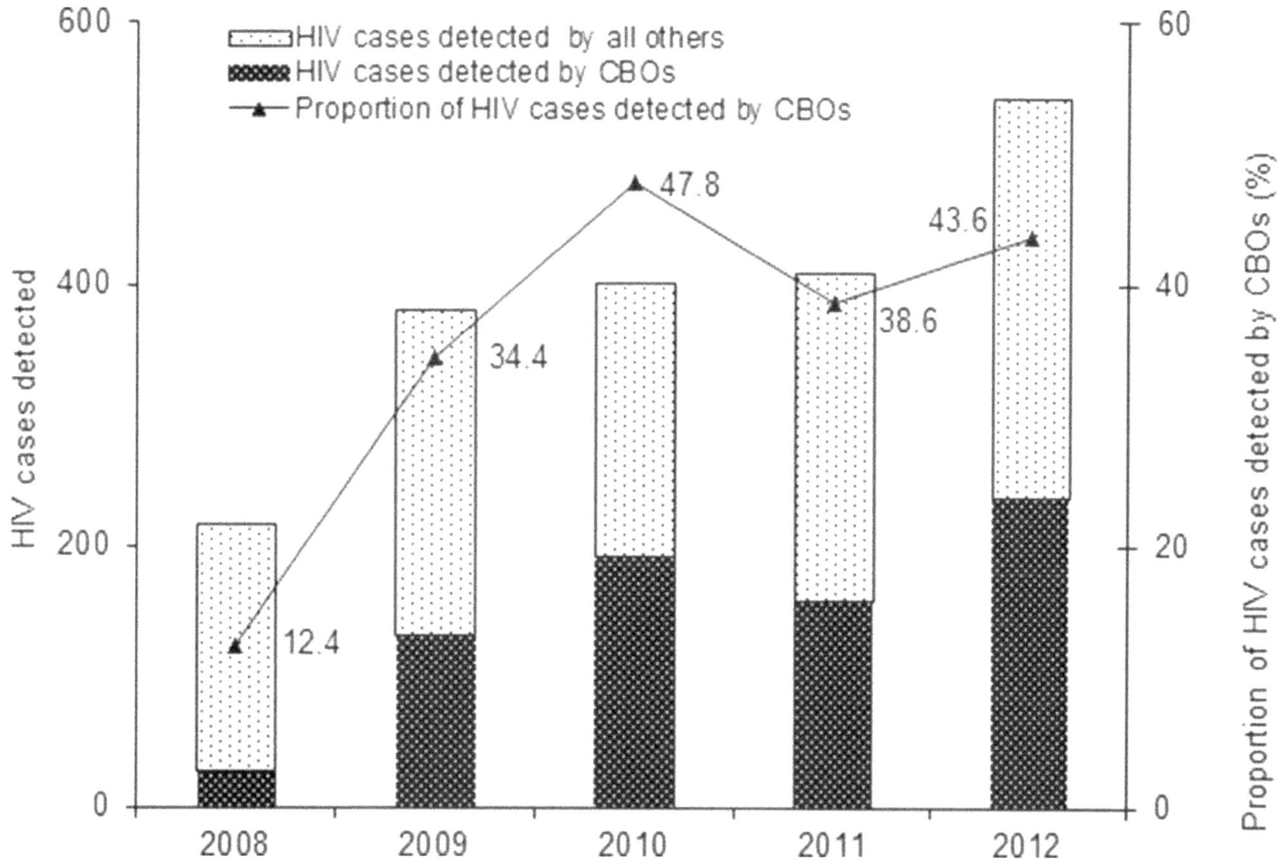

Figure 1. HIV cases detected by community-based organizations (CBOs) and their contribution to the total HIV cases detected, 2008 to 2012, Nanjing, China.

in 2008 and 10 in 2009 and was maintained at 8 since 2010. HIV testing coverage increased from 4.1% in 2008 to 22.7% in 2012 (P-values <0·001), based on the estimated MSM population size of 25,000 in Nanjing in 2008. In accordance with the increasing HIV testing coverage, the confirmed newly diagnosed HIV cases also increased with the detection rate ranged from 2.6% to 5.8% (P-values <0·001). The baseline CD4 counts of these new cases with Nanjing residence showed a rising trend (P-values <0·01), with the median CD4 cell counts from 309 cells/uL in 2008 to 397 cells/uL in 2012 (Table 2).

The share of MSM tested for HIV by CBOs out of the total HIV tests performed by government health facilities was very low, accounting for from 0.2% (1,034 of 493,015) in 2008 to 0.7% (5,673 of 799,765) in 2012. However, the total case detected by CBOs each year was very high. The proportion of the cases detected by CBOs out of the total cases detected in the city increased from 12.4% in 2008 to 43.6% in 2012 (Table 3, Figure 1).

The unit cost per HIV case found through CBOs decreased from 2,874 CNY (approximately 417 USD) in 2008 to 1,984 CNY (approximately 325 USD) in 2012. Compared to that through government health facilities, the unit cost per HIV case found through CBOs was 47 times lower (Table 3).

Follow-up care and support service for PLHA

The number of CBOs providing follow-up care and support service for HIV/AIDS cases living in Nanjing city increased from none in 2007 to 8 in 2012. The percentage of local PLHA receiving follow-up care and support services from CBOs increased from 5.2% in 2008 to 83.5% in 2012 (P-values < 0.01). In the meantime, the rate of the CD4 test and ART coverage in Nanjing increased from 71.1% and 78.6% in 2008 to 86.0% and 90.1% respectively (P-values <0.05).The 12-month ART retention rate maintained above 95% since 2009 despite increased volume of ART cohorts (P-values >0.05) (Table 4).

Discussion

The results along the service chain for HIV prevention and follow-up care program achieved in this pilot, strongly indicate the feasibility of the 'task shifting' from government health facilities to CBOs using a 'cash on service delivery' approach. Mapping of CBO service providers and assessment of capacity of potential CBO service providers, supplemented with timely and targeted capacity building, appeared to well prepare the CBOs to deliver quality services. There were no any social harm events reported as a result of being tested by CBOs. Procedures established for program management through this pilot appeared to achieve the fundamental objective of 'cash on service delivery', ie, performance-based funding. Routine programmatic data generated from CBO services were reported to local CDCs and the program management unit, JSPMA, but actual cash payment made by JSPMA was based on independently verified results through web-based national HIV/AIDS information system, which has been consistently operated since 2005 [26].

Table 4. Local people living with HIV/AIDS (PLHA) covered with follow-up care, tested for CD4, initiated and retained antiretroviral therapy (ART), before and after the task shifting from government health facilities to community-based organizations (CBOs), 2008 to 2012, Nanjing, China.

Year	Enrollment of local PLHA alive	CD4 test†		Number of ART eligibility‡	ART initiation		12 month ART retention rate§ % (n)
		n	%		n	%	
2008	232	165	71.1(165/232)	84	66	78.6(66/84)	95.5(63/66)
2009	400	287	71.0(287/400)	143	108	75.5(108/143)	96.3(104/108)
2010	572	442	77.3(442/572)	261	188	72.0(188/261)	96.3(181/188)
2011	792	596	75.3(596/792)	408	346	84.8(346/408)	97.1(336/346)
2012	1,090	937	86.0(937/1,090)	574	517	90.1(517/574)	97.7(505/517)

†CD4 test defined as PLHA received CD4 tests at least one time within a year.
‡The criterion of ART eligibility is CD4 <200 cells/uL prior to and in 2011, and ≤350 cells/uL in 2012 and afterwards.
§The number of ART initiation was 42 in 2007.
P values for trend analyses: P<0.01 for follow-up care, P<0.05 for CD4 tests, P<0.05 for ART coverage, and P>0.05 for 12-month ART retention rate.

The results also indicate the effectiveness of 'task shifting' from government health facilities to CBOs, as evident by increased coverage, better targeting and early case detection, as well as increased linkage of detected cases to clinical care, which are highly consistent with findings observed from systematically reviewed community-based tasks recommended by WHO [28]. The coverage of HIV testing among MSM performed by CBOs only increased by 5.5 times and reached 22.7% in 2012, which was almost equal to the country progress reported level of coverage of HIV testing among MSM performed by all health facilities and CBOs combined [29]. HIV detection rate by CBOs remained high regardless of the expansion of the HIV testing during the pilot. The proportion of newly diagnosed HIV cases contributed by CBOs increased remarkably from about one tenth in 2008 to nearly half of the total HIV cases reported in 2012, despite a very low share of HIV tests by CBOs out of the total HIV tests performed each year during the pilot. Both these indicated a good targeting at most at risk subgroups among MSM. With services provided by CBOs and health facilities, in accordance with the national new HIV/AIDS prevention and control approach of 'Five expands, six strengthens' [30], coverage of CD4 tests among PLHA increased by about 15%, reached nearly 86% in 2012. The coverage of ART increased from 78.6% in 2008 to 90.1% during the program pilot despite the ART eligibility changed from CD4 <200 cells/μL in 2008 to CD4 ≤350 cells/μL in 2012. Cost-effectiveness was apparent in the pilot, as evident by the 47 times lower unit cost newly diagnosed HIV cases by CBOs compared to that by government health facilities.

In addition, early detection of HIV infection was also found after the greater involvement of CBOs in referral for HIV testing and providing follow-up care services. The median baseline CD4 cell counts increased by about 100 cells/μL in five years and reached nearly 400 cells/μL. This is dramatically different from the current national picture where HIV cases transmitted sexually had a significantly lower median CD4 cell counts than cases infected with other routes of transmission [31]. Early detection of HIV infection reduces not only population level transmission risk, as a result of increased percentage of PLHA knowing their positive status, but provides opportunity for PLHA to receive early treatment to reduce population based viral load in order to achieve more comprehensive HIV prevention [32–33].

We recognize the limitations of our data. First, the population size of MSM we used is data estimated in 2008 and hasn't been updated over time. It may overestimate or underestimate the HIV testing coverage. Second, the data on HIV tests offered by health facilities were not disaggregated by risk groups in the reporting forms, the total number of HIV testing uptake among MSM in the city were not available, thereby CBOs performance on HIV testing and case finding may not be measured accurately. However, the analysis focused on the temporal trend during the pilot. Third, follow-up care and CD4 tests were confined to local resident HIV/AIDS cases in Nanjing, this may not reflect the situation among those temporarily living in Nanjing. These cases may present a different transmission risk portrait from local cases.

Despite limitations, however, this pilot provides evidence that it is feasible to shift tasks from health facilities to CBOs. It is also feasible to adopt 'cash on service delivery' model as services resulting from CBOs can be independently verified. CBOs provided more effective services with a lower cost.

While the Chinese government recognizes the significant role CBOs could play in the response to HIV/AIDS epidemic [7], effective mechanism of preparing CBOs and allocating adequate funds to CBOs to provide essential HIV services to high risk groups and PLHA should be implemented. During the past decade, external funders, such as the Global Fund and Gates Foundation, have been the primary sources of support to CBOs to build up capacity and to provide essential services. This pilot provides operational guidance for Chinese government to shift essential HIV services to CBOs in a time when the external donors started to withdraw the development aid from China [34]. The apparent results, that CBOs can provide effective services at a lower cost, shed light on sustainability of providing essential HIV services globally. International aid on HIV/AIDS appears to be leveling out as a result of internal financial constraints in many high-income donor countries [35] while demands of HIV essential services, such as ART, are increasing.

Acknowledgments

The authors would like to thank the officers from the Jiangsu Provincial Department of Health and the Nanjing Municipal Bureau of Health for their strong political support in implementing this pilot. We also feel grateful for MSM volunteers from community-based organizations and staff from Jiangsu Provincial CDC, Nanjing Municipal CDC and Nanjing Second Hospital who have been involved in the pilot. Special thanks to Jodie Cole and Daniel Prior for their kind proofreading the manuscript.

Author Contributions

Conceived and designed the experiments: HY MZ JZ HY. Performed the experiments: HY MZ JD SW CW XH YX FX LL. Analyzed the data: HY JZ. Wrote the paper: YH JZ. Reviewed and approved the final version of the manuscript: HY MZ JZ XH JD SW CW YX LL FX HY.

References

1. Settle E (2003) AIDS in China: an annotated chronology: 1985–2003. Montreal: China AIDS Survey. Available: http://portal.unesco.org/education/en/file_download.php/82b973698fcdf215528d63d2b6796087AIDSchron_111603.pdf. Accessed 2013 Nov 20.
2. State Council AIDS Working Committee Office, UN Theme Group on HIV/AIDS in China (2004) A joint assessment of HIV/AIDS prevention, treatment and care in China. Beijing: China Ministry of Health. Available: http://www.chinaaids.cn/ddpg/lhpgbg1/zgazbyq/201312/P020131210547942626797.pdf. Accessed 2013 Nov 20.
3. Wu ZY, Sullivan SG, Wang Y, Rotheram-Borus MJ, Detels R (2007) Evolution of China's response to HIV/AIDS. Lancet 369: 679–90.
4. 2011 Estimates for the HIV/AIDS Epidemic in China (2011) Ministry of Health, People's Republic of China. Joint United Nations Programme on HIV/AIDS World Health Organization, Beijing, China. Available: http://www.unaids.org.cn/pics/20130521161757.pdf. Accessed 2013 Nov 20.
5. Thomas RF, Moupali DD, Scott EK, Kelly JH (2005) Applying Public Health Principles to the HIV Epidemic. N Engl J Med 353: 2397–2402.
6. 2012 China AIDS response progress report (2012) Ministry of Health of the People's Republic of China. Available: http://www.unaids.org/en/dataanalysis/knowyourresponse/countryprogressreports/2012countries/ce_CN_Narrative_Report[1].pdf. Accessed 2013 Nov 20.
7. Wu Z, Wang Y, Detels R, Rotheram-Borus MJ (2010) China AIDS policy implementation: reversing the HIV/AIDS epidemic by 2015. Int J Epidemiol 39 Suppl 2: ii1–3.
8. Obermeyer CM, Osborn M (2007) The utilization of testing and counseling for HIV: a review of the social and behavioral evidence. Am J Public Health 97: 1762–74.
9. Du J, Lombardi C, Evans E, Jiang H, Zhao M, et al. (2012) Mixed methods approach to identifying factors related to voluntary HIV testing among injection drug users in Shanghai, China. Int J Infect Dis 16: 498–503.
10. Wang Y, Li B, Pan J, Sengupta S, Emrick CB, et al. (2011) Factors Associated with Utilization of a Free HIV VCT Clinic by Female Sex Workers in Jinan City, Northern China. AIDS Behav 15: 702–710.
11. Wei C, Yan H, Yang C, Raymond HF, Li J, et al. (2014) Accessing HIV testing and treatment among men who have sex with men in China. A qualitative study. AIDS Care 26: 372–8.
12. Ma W, Detels R, Feng Y, Wu Z, Shen L, et al. (2007) Acceptance of and barriers to voluntary HIV counselling and testing among adults in Guizhou province, China. AIDS 21 Suppl 8: 129–35.
13. Xu J, Brown K, Ding G, Wang H, Zhang G, et al. (2011) Factors associated with HIV testing history and HIV-test result follow-up among female sex workers in two cities in Yunnan, China. Sex Transm Dis 38: 89–95.
14. China 2010 UNGASS Country Progress Report (2008–2009) Ministry of Health of the People's Republic of China. Available http://aidsdatahub.org/dmdocuments/china_2010_country_progress_report_en.pdf. Accessed 2013 Nov 24.
15. BBC News (2009) Aids takes deathly toll in China. 2009, February 18th. Available http://news.bbc.co.uk/2/hi/asia-pacific/7896133.stm. Accessed 2013 Nov 20.
16. Wen Y, Zhao D, Dou Z, Ma Y, Zhao Y, et al. (2011) Some patient-related factors associated with late access to ART in China's free ART program. AIDS Care 23: 1226–35.
17. Zachariah R, Ford N, Philips M, Lynch S, Massaquoi M, et al. (2009) Task shifting in HIV/AIDS: opportunities, challenges and proposed actions for sub-Saharan Africa. Trans R Soc Trop Med Hyg 103: 549–58.
18. Broadhead RS, Heckathorn DD, Weakliem DL, Anthony DL, Madray H, et al. (1998) Harnessing Peer Networks as an Instrument for AIDS Prevention: Results from a Peer-Driven Intervention. Public Health Rep 113 Suppl 1: 42–57.
19. Statistical Yearbook of Nanjing Municipality 2011 (2012) Nanjing municipal Bureau Statistics. Available: http://www.njtj.gov.cn/_siteId/4/pageId/71/columnId/8136/articleId/86594/DisplayInfo.aspy. Accessed 2013 Nov 23.
20. Yan H, Tang W, Zhang M, Liu X, Huan X (2010) Combination of multiplier method with qualitative interview to estimate the population size of men who have sex with men in a city of Jiangsu. Ch in J AIDS S TD16, 29–31.
21. Zhang J, Cao N, Jiang J, You Y, Sha Z (2004) Serological Investigation of STIs in 138 Men Who Have Sex with Men. Chin J Dermatol 37: 546–47.
22. Tang W, Huan X, Mahapatra T, Tang S, Li J, et al. (2013) Factors associated with unprotected anal intercourse among men who have sex with men: results from a respondent driven sampling survey in Nanjing, China, 2008. AIDS Behav 17: 1415–22.
23. Yan H, Yang H, Zhao J, Wei C, Li J, et al. (2012) Long-chain peer referral of men who have sex with men: a novel approach to establish and maintain a cohort to measure HIV incidence, Nanjing, China. J Acquir Immune DeficSyndr 59: 177–84.
24. Birdsall N, Savedoff NB (2010) Cash on Delivery: A New Approach to Foreign Aid. Washington, DC:CGD. Available: http://www.cgdev.org/content/publications/detail/1423949/. Accessed 2013 Dec 5.
25. National Centre for AIDS/STD Control and Prevention, Chinese Centre for Diseases Control and Prevention (2012) National technical handbook on HIV rapid antibody test (Version 2011). Beijing: Ministry of Health. Available: http://www.chinaids.org.cn/n16/n1193/n4073/n734019.files/n734018.pdf. Accessed 2013 Dec 5.
26. Mao Y, Wu Z, Poundstone K, Wang C, Qin Q, et al. (2010) Development of a unified web-based national HIV/AIDS information system in China. Int J Epidemiol 39 (Suppl 2): ii79–89.
27. Zhang F, Wang J, Wang F, Lu H, Lu L, et al. (2012) The Chinese national free antiretroviral treatment manual (version 3). People's Medical Publishing House. Available: http://www.chinaaids.cn/zlgh/jswj4/201301/W020131106349229773339.pdf. Accessed 2013 Nov 23.
28. Suthar AB, Ford N, Bachanas PJ, Wong VJ, Rajan JS, et al. (2013) Towards universal voluntary HIV testing and counselling: a systematic review and meta-analysis of community-based approaches. PLoS Med.10: e1001496.
29. Joint United Nations Programme on HIV/AIDS (UNAIDS) (2012) Global report: UNAIDS report on the global AIDS epidemic 2012. Available: http://www.unaids.org/en/media/unaids/contentassets/documents/epidemiology/2012/gr2012/20121120_UNAIDS_Global_Report_2012_with_annexes_en.pdf. Accessed 2013 Dec 2.
30. Ministry of Health, People's Republic of China (2012) 2012 China AIDS response progress report. Beijing: Ministry of Health, 2012. Available: http://www.unaids.org/en/dataanalysis/knowyourresponse/countryprogressreports/2012countries/ce_CN_Narrative_Report[1].pdf. Accessed 2013 Dec 4.
31. Dou Z, Chen RY, Xu J, Ma Y, Jiao JH, et al. (2010) Changing baseline characteristics among patients in the China National Free Antiretroviral Treatment Program, 2002–09. Int J Epidemiol 39 Suppl 2: ii56–64.
32. Marks G, Crepaz N, Senterfitt JW, Janssen RS (2005) Meta-analysis of high-risk sexual behavior in persons aware and unaware they are infected with HIV in the United States: implications for HIV prevention programs. Acquir Immune DeficSyndr 9: 446–53.
33. Jain V, Byonanebye DM, Liegler T, Kwarisiima D, Chamie G, et al. (2014) Changes in Population HIV RNA Levels in Mbarara, Uganda During Scale-Up of HIV Antiretroviral Therapy Access. J Acquir Immune DeficSyndr 65: 327–32.
34. Li H, Kuo NT, Liu H, Korhonen C, Pond E, et al. (2010) From spectators to implementers: civil society organizations involved in AIDS programmes in China. Int J Epidemiol 39 Suppl 2: ii65–71.
35. Vassall A, Remme M, Watts C, Hallett T, Siapka M, et al. (2013) Financing Essential HIV Services: A New Economic Agenda. PLoS Med [Epub ahead of print].

A 10-Year Population Based Study of 'Opt-Out' HIV Testing of Tuberculosis Patients in Alberta, Canada: National Implications

Richard Long[1,2]*, Selvanayagam Niruban[2], Courtney Heffernan[1], Ryan Cooper[1], Dina Fisher[3], Rabia Ahmed[1], Mary Lou Egedahl[1], Rhonda Fur[4]

1 Department of Medicine, University of Alberta, Edmonton, Alberta, Canada, **2** Department of Public Health Sciences, University of Alberta, Edmonton, Alberta, Canada, **3** Department of Medicine, University of Calgary, Calgary, Alberta, Canada, **4** Alberta Health Services, Alberta, Canada

Abstract

Introduction: Compliance with the recommendation that all tuberculosis (TB) patients be tested for human immunodeficiency virus (HIV) has not yet been achieved in Canada or globally.

Methods: The experience of "opt-out" HIV testing of TB patients in the Province of Alberta, Canada is described over a 10-year period, 2003–2012. Testing rates are reported before and after the introduction of the "opt-out" approach. Risk factors for HIV seropositivity are described and demographic, clinical and laboratory characteristics of TB patients who were newly diagnosed versus previously diagnosed with HIV are compared. Genotypic clusters, defined as groups of two or more cases whose isolates of *Mycobacterium tuberculosis* had identical DNA fingerprints over the 10-year period or within 2 years of one another, were analyzed for their ability to predict HIV co-infection.

Results: HIV testing rates were 26% before and 90% after the introduction of "opt-out" testing. During the "opt-out" testing years those <15 or >64 years of age at diagnosis were less likely to have been tested. In those tested the prevalence of HIV was 5.6%. In the age group 15–64 years, risk factors for HIV were: age (35–64 years), Canadian-born Aboriginal or foreign-born sub-Saharan African origin, and combined respiratory and non-respiratory disease. Compared to TB patients previously known to be HIV positive, TB patients newly discovered to be HIV positive had more advanced HIV disease (lower CD4 counts; higher viral loads) at diagnosis. Large cluster size was associated with Aboriginal ancestry. Cluster size predicted HIV co-infection in Aboriginal peoples when clusters included all cases reported over 10 years but not when clusters included cases reported within 2 years of one another.

Conclusion: "Opt-out" HIV testing of TB patients is effective and well received. Universal HIV testing of TB patients (>80% of patients tested) has immediate (patients) and longer-term (TB/HIV program planning) benefits.

Editor: Pascal Launois, World Health Organization, Switzerland

Funding: These authors have no support or funding to report.

Competing Interests: The authors have declared that no competing interests exist.

* E-mail: richard.long@ualberta.ca

Introduction

All tuberculosis (TB) patients ought to be tested for human immunodeficiency virus (HIV), but compliance with this recommendation has not yet been achieved in Canada or globally. In 2010 nationally, and in 2011 internationally, an HIV test result was reported in only 40% of TB patients [1,2]. A lack of compliance was understandable before the availability of highly active anti-retroviral therapy (HAART) and in the context of discrimination, when informed consent and extensive pre- and post-test counseling were advised. More recently, however, these factors have been mitigated and both counseling and testing are considered part of routine medical care. Not knowing the HIV status of prevalent active TB cases has the potential to compromise TB management, outcomes and elimination [2,3]. As such, poor compliance with the recommendation that all TB patients be HIV tested is now indefensible.

In response to two national advisories and the close biological and epidemiological links between HIV and TB, an 'opt-out' approach to HIV testing of TB patients was introduced in Alberta, a Province of Western Canada, in 2002–2003 [4,5]. HIV testing is defined as 'universal' if >80% of incident TB cases were tested annually [6–8]. The 'opt-out' approach implemented in Alberta was patterned after an established program of 'opt-out' HIV testing of prenatal women [9], and is similar to the 'provider-initiated' HIV testing program recommended by the United Nations Programme on HIV/AIDS and World Health Organization (UNAIDS/WHO) in 2004 and 2007 for countries with high co-infection rates [10,11]. This approach is characterized by two stages: 1) patients are briefly informed about the connection between HIV and TB and the clinical and prevention benefits of being tested and 2) the routine testing of TB patients for HIV unless their provider is actively informed of the patient's decision not to be tested.

We describe ten years of experience with universal 'opt-out' HIV testing of TB patients in Alberta. In addition to identifying risk factors for HIV seropositivity, the demographic, clinical and laboratory characteristics of TB patients who were newly diagnosed versus previously diagnosed with HIV are compared. Finally, we describe the extent to which clustering and/or cluster size, markers of recent transmission, predict HIV co-infection in the host using molecular epidemiologic techniques.

Methods

Persons meeting the Canadian case definition for TB [1], and notified in the Province of Alberta (population 3,645,257 in 2011, Statistics Canada) over the 10-year period 2003 to 2012, were identified. In addition to HIV test results the following demographic and clinical information were abstracted from the Provincial TB Registry for each case: age, sex, population group, disease type (new active versus relapse/re-infection), first-line drug resistance, disease site, (respiratory, non-respiratory or both, according to the Canadian TB Standards) and mortality [1]. Population groups in this study include Canadian-born Aboriginal (First Nations [North American Indian], Métis or Inuit according to the Constitution Act of 1982), Canadian-born 'other', foreign-born from sub-Saharan Africa (as per the Canadian International Development Agency at: http://www.acdi-cida.gc.ca/subsaharanafrica) and foreign-born 'other'. The proportion of all TB patients and TB patients aged 15 to 64 years who were HIV tested before and after the introduction of 'opt-out' testing, was related to the timing of two national advisories and the availability of HAART. All HIV testing of TB patients was performed in the Provincial Laboratory for Public Health (ProvLab) using conventional methods. Risk factors for HIV co-infection are described; in a multivariable model an *a priori* set of variables was retained.

For HIV co-infected patients data from individual health records supplements those data abstracted from the TB Registry (see below). HIV co-infected TB patients are divided into those who were known to be HIV-positive in the past and those who were discovered to be HIV positive during the 3 months immediately preceding their date of diagnosis of TB or during the period of active treatment of TB. The window for a "new positive" HIV test permits TB being unmasked or diagnosed during the early investigation and management of HIV [12–14]. TB patients with *known* positive HIV tests were compared to TB patients with *new* positive HIV tests on the basis of age, sex, population group, disease type, CD4 count, viral load (≤ 400 copies/ml – a viral load that is generally associated with controlled HIV infection on antiretroviral therapy [ARV's] and accounts for changing testing methodology; 401–100,000 copies/ml – moderately advanced HIV infection, and >100,000 copies/ml – the recognized cutoff for advanced HIV infection), hepatitis C serology, HIV exposure category and mortality. Results indicate whether TB patients were on ARVs at the time of diagnosis of TB.

Isolates of *M. tuberculosis* from all culture-positive cases of TB diagnosed in the Province of Alberta between 2003 and 2012 are routinely DNA fingerprinted using standardized restriction fragment-length polymorphism (RLFP), supplemented in those isolates with five or fewer copies of the insertion sequence *6110*, by spoligotyping [15,16]. Images were digitalized using the imager video camera system (Appligene, Illkirch, France). Digitalized gel images were analyzed using Gelcompar II computer software (Applied Maths, Kortrijk, Belgium). The analysis was performed on coded specimens in a blinded fashion. All isolates matched as identical by computer were manually confirmed by visually comparing the original autoradiographs. 'Clusters' are defined as two or more case isolates with identical DNA fingerprints over either (i) the entire 10-year "opt-out" testing period or (ii) within two years of one another. For the latter we chronologically ordered the TB cases in each genotypic cluster by the date of diagnosis of each culture-positive case. We assumed that the first case of respiratory TB in a cluster resulted from reactivation of latent TB infection and was the source case patient. Subsequent respiratory and/or non-respiratory cases in the same genotypic cluster likely resulted from recent transmission and rapid progression to disease and were defined as secondary cases if they occurred within 24 months of the sourse case or each other [17,18]. For each definition of a cluster, mean cluster size was compared by age, sex, population group, HIV status and population-group-by-HIV-status-interaction.

Statistical Analysis

Fisher's exact test, where necessary, was used to compare proportions. To compare the demographic and clinical characteristics of HIV-negative and HIV-positive TB patients between 2003 and 2012, odds ratios (OR) with 95% confidence intervals were reported. Purposeful selection method was used to select the variables included in the multivariable logistic regression model [19]. Age, sex, population group, disease type and site, drug resistance, and mortality were tested for potential confounding effect. Wald's test was used to test the significance of each variable in the model. Generalized estimating equation (GEE) with identity link and independent correlation was used to account for clustering with the same strain, to estimate the mean cluster size after adjusting for age, sex, population group and HIV status. A p-value of 0.05 was used as statistically significant. All analyses were conducted using Stata (StataCorp. 2011. Stata Statistical Software: Release 12. College Station, TX: StataCorp LP). This study was approved by the Health Research Ethics Board of the University of Alberta. A waiver of written consent was provided as anonymous, routinely collected surveillance data were used.

Results

Between 1991 and 2002 the proportion of TB patients who were HIV tested averaged 26.1% (see Figure 1). In 1996–1997 the introduction of HAART and in 2002–2003 the introduction of "opt-out" HIV testing, resulted in sharp increases in the proportion of TB patients who were HIV tested. In 2003, and annually thereafter, "universal" HIV testing of TB patients was achieved (average 90.6%; range 74.8% to 100% overall and average 94.9%; range 84.8% to 100% in the age group 15–64 years). Of the 1317 TB patients who were HIV tested between 2003 and 2012, 74 (5.6%) were HIV-positive (see Table 1). Independent of sex or population group, TB patients in the age group 15–64 years were more likely to be HIV tested than TB patients in the age groups 0–14 years or >64 years (94.9% vs. 74.7%, $p<0.001$; and 94.9% vs. 81.3%, $p<0.001$, respectively). CBO were less likely to be HIV tested than other population groups but the difference was not statistically significant after adjustment for age. For patients who did not undergo HIV testing ($n = 136$), the test was not offered in 39 (28.7%), declined in 13 (9.6%), and in the remainder the reason for not testing was unknown. For patients who were not offered the test, 14 (35.9%) were diagnosed with TB at death and 16 (41.0%) were either younger than 15 or older than 64 years of age. For patients who

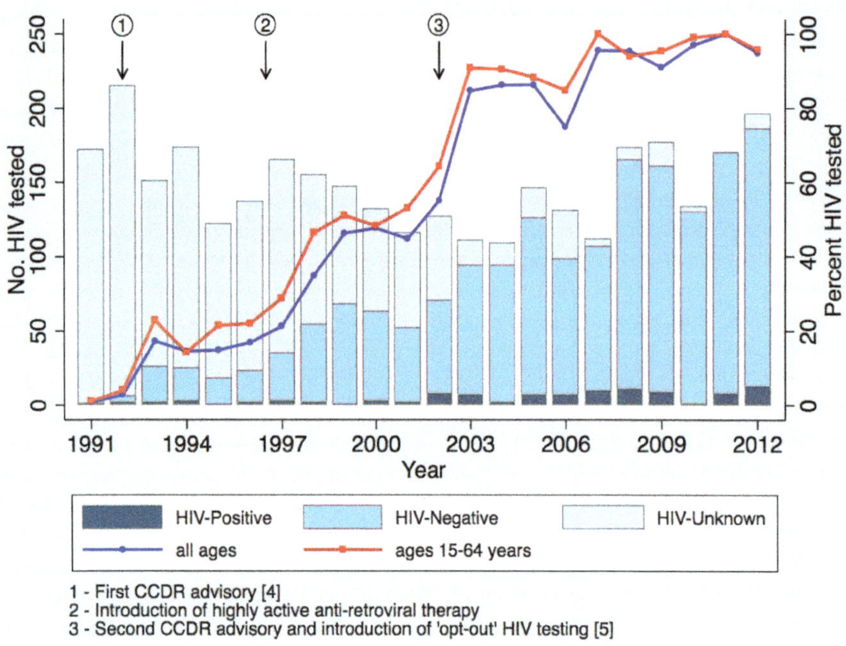

Figure 1. The absolute number of TB patients that were HIV tested (left axis) and the proportion of TB patients who were HIV tested (right axis) by year in Alberta, 1991–2012.

declined HIV testing there was no consistent pattern in their demographic characteristics.

Among HIV tested TB patients in the age group 15–64 years, 72/910 or 7.9% were HIV-positive (see Table 2). This seroprevalence was not significantly different from the one we reported in 1991-2002 (28/342 or 8.2%, $p = 0.87$) when much more selective testing was performed, suggesting, in the absence of major secular trends, that HIV co-infection may have been missed in the earlier era [7]. In the age group 15–64, those aged 35–64 years were more likely than those aged 15–34 years (9.5% vs. 4.7%, $p < 0.001$) to be HIV co-infected in multivariate analysis (see Table 2). Similarly, Canadian-born Aboriginal or foreign-born sub-Saharan

Table 1. HIV status of TB patients in Alberta by demographic group, 2003–2012.

Demographic group		TB Cases	HIV tested*	HIV Positive†
			n (%)	n (%)
Total		1453	1317 (90.6)	74 (5.6)
Age (years)				
	0–14	75	56 (74.7)	01 (1.8)
	15–34	458	443 (96.7)	21 (4.7)
	35–64	577	539 (93.4)	51 (9.5)
	>64	343	279 (81.3)	01 (0.4)
Sex				
	Male	748	685 (91.6)	45 (6.6)
	Female	705	632 (89.6)	29 (4.6)
Population group				
	CBO	154	130 (84.4)	01 (0.8)
	CBA	182	167 (91.8)	16 (9.6)
	FBO	854	771 (90.3)	15 (2.0)
	FBSSA	263	249 (94.7)	42 (16.9)

Abbreviations: CBO = Canadian-born 'Other'; CBA = Canadian-born Aboriginal; FBO = Foreign-born 'Other'; FBSSA = Foreign-born sub-Saharan African.
*Percent of all TB cases.
†Percent of HIV-tested TB cases.

Table 2. Risk Factors for HIV Seropositivity in TB patients aged 15–64 years, Alberta, 2003–2012.

Characteristic		HIV-negative (N = 910)	HIV-positive (%) (N = 72)	Univariate OR (95% CI; p-value)	Multivariate OR (95% CI; p-value)
Age (years)					
	15–34	422	21 (4.7)	1.00	1.00
	35–64	488	51 (9.5)	2.1 (1.24, 3.55; 0.006)	3.3 (1.83, 5.96; <0.001)
Sex*					
	Female	453	29 (6.0)	1.00	1.00
	Male	457	43 (8.6)	1.47 (0.9, 2.4; 0.12)	1.59 (0.94, 2.71; 0.09)
Population Group†					
	CBO	76	1 (1.3)	1.00	1.00
	FBO	535	13 (2.4)		
	CBA	112	16 (12.5)	6.23 (2.96, 13.13; <0.001)	5.42 (2.49, 11.82; <0.001)
	FBSSA	187	42 (18.3)	9.8 (5.24, 18.34; <0.001)	13.9 (7.14, 27.0; <0.001)
Disease Type					
	New Active	853	70 (7.6)	1.00	-
	Relapse/Retreatment	57	2 (3.4)	0.43 (0.1, 1.79; 0.19)	-
Drug Resistance‡					
	No	647	53 (7.6)	1.00	-
	Yes	119	10 (7.8)	1.02 (0.51, 2.07; 0.94)	-
	Unknown	144	9 (5.9)	-	-
Disease Site					
	Respiratory	545	41 (7.0)	1.00	1.00
	Non-respiratory	329	22 (6.3)	0.89 (0.52, 1.52; 0.6)	0.93 (0.52, 1.65; 0.8)
	Both	36	9 (20.0)	3.32 (1.5, 7.37; 0.003)	3.32 (1.29, 8.53; 0.013)
Mortality§					
	No	892	65 (6.8)	1.00	1.00
	Yes	18	7 (30.4)	6.02 (2.39, 15.15; <0.001)	2.80 (0.96, 8.15;0.059)

Abbreviations: CBO = Canadian-born 'Other'; CBA = Canadian-born Aboriginal; FBO = Foreign-born 'Other'; FBSSA = Foreign-born sub-Saharan African.

*By convention, sex was retained in the multivariable model. Its exclusion in the multivariable model did not affect the significance of other variables

†CBO and FBO were combined in the analysis as HIV prevalence rates were similarly low in both groups and the number of CBO cases was small

‡Resistance to one or more first-line drug; cases whose drug resistance pattern was unknown were culture-negative.

§Death before or during the period of active treatment of TB.

Africans were more likely than Canadian-born or foreign-born 'other' (12.5% vs. 2.2% and 18.3 vs. 2.2%, $p<0.001$ and $p<0.001$, respectively) to be HIV co-infected. Finally, patients with respiratory and non-respiratory TB combined were more likely than patients with respiratory TB alone (20.0% vs. 7.0%, $p=0.01$), and patients reported as a TB death were more likely than patients not reported as a TB death (30.4% vs. 6.8%, $p=0.043$) to be HIV co-infected. In contrast, HIV positive and negative TB patients did not differ by sex, disease type and presence of drug resistance.

Of the 74 TB patients determined to be HIV co-infected in 2003-2012, 38 (51.4%) were known to have been HIV-positive prior to the diagnosis of TB and 36 (48.6%) were discovered to be HIV-positive at the time of diagnosis of TB (see Table 3). Those with known HIV positivity and those with new HIV positivity did not differ with respect to age, sex, population group, exposure category or mortality in univariate analysis. With respect to other characteristics, however, there were notable differences between groups. Compared to known HIV-positive cases, new HIV-positive cases were more likely to have respiratory TB in combination with non-respiratory TB, a low CD4 count ($<200\times10^6$/L) and a high viral load (>100,000 HIV RNA copies/ml); odds ratios and 95% confidence intervals 2.71(1.04, 6.99), 7.65(1.92, 30.5), and 12.7(1.32, 121.5), respectively. In patients with an ARV utilization history, 14 of 34 (41.2%) with known HIV positivity and none of 31 (0.0%) with new HIV positivity, were on ARV's at the time of diagnosis of TB (see Figure S1). TB patients with new HIV positivity were less likely than TB patients with known HIV positivity to be HCV positive, 8.6% vs 28.6% (0.23; 0.06, 0.94). In data that is not shown, HCV positivity was strongly correlated with IDU, 11 of 13 (84.6%) with IDU versus 0 of 36 (0.0%) without IDU, were HCV positive ($p<0.0001$). And IDU was strongly correlated with population group; of the 53 HIV positive TB patients whose exposure category was known, 11/14 (78.6%) Aboriginal peoples versus 2/39 (5.1%) persons of other population groups, reported IDU ($p<0.001$).

Of the 1453 patients diagnosed with TB between 2003 and 2012, 228 (15.7%) were culture-negative, 18 (1.2%) were culture-positive for MTB complex species other than *M. tuberculosis* and 1207 (83.1%) were culture-positive for *M. tuberculosis* (see Figure

Table 3. Demographic and clinical characteristics of HIV co-infected TB patients according to the date of diagnosis of HIV relative to the date of diagnosis of TB*.

Characteristics		Total	Known HIV(+ve)*	New HIV(+ve)*	Odds ratio (95% CI; p-value)
		n	n (%)	n (%)	
No. assessed (%)		74	38	36	-
Age (years)					
	<35	22	14 (36.8)	08 (22.2)	0.49 (0.17, 1.36, 0.17)
	≥35	52	24 (63.2)	28 (77.8)	1.00
Sex					
	Female	29	18 (47.4)	11 (30.6)	1.00
	Male	45	20 (52.6)	25 (69.4)	2.04 (0.79, 5.31, 0.14)
Population group					
	CBO	01	01 (2.6)	0 (0.0)	Included with FBO
	CBA	16	10 (26.3)	06 (16.7)	0.36 (0.09, 1.51, 0.16)
	FBO	15	05 (13.2)	10 (27.8)	1.00
	FBSSA	42	22 (57.9)	20 (55.6)	0.54 (0.17, 1.77, 0.31)
Disease site					
	Respiratory	42	26 (68.4)	16 (44.4)	1.00
	Non-Respiratory	23	09 (23.7)	14 (38.9)	2.71 (1.04, 6.99, 0.04)
	Both	09	03 (7.9)	06 (16.7)	Included with Non-Resp
CD4 count †					
	<200	43	17 (44.7)	26 (72.2)	7.65 (1.92, 30.5, 0.004)
	≥200	18	15 (39.5)	03 (8.3)	1.00
	Unknown	13	06 (15.8)	07 (19.4)	-
HIV RNA (copies/ml) ‡					
	≤400	7	06 (15.8)	01 (2.8)	1.00
	401–100,000	21	14 (36.8)	7 (19.4)	3.0 (0.30, 30.0, 0.35)
	>100,000	28	09 (23.7)	19 (52.8)	12.7 (1.32, 121.5, 0.03)
	Unknown	18	09 (23.7)	09 (25.0)	-
Hepatitis C					
	Pos	13	10 (28.6)	03 (8.6)	0.23 (0.06, 0.94, 0.04)
	Neg	57	25 (71.4)	32 (91.4)	1.00
	Unknown	04	03 (7.9)	01 (2.8)	-
Exposure category §					
	HSS	36	17 (44.7)	19 (52.8)	1.00
	IDU	13	10 (26.3)	03 (8.3)	0.27 (0.06, 1.14, 0.07)
	Other	04	03 (7.9)	01 (2.8)	0.30 (0.03, 3.14, 0.31)
	Unknown	21	08 (21.1)	13 (36.1)	
Mortality					
	No death	66	33 (86.8)	33 (91.7)	1.00
	Died	08	05 (13.2)	03 (8.3)	0.6 (0.13, 2.72, 0.51)

abbreviations: CBO Canadian-born 'other'; CBA Canadian-born Aboriginal; FBO foreign-born 'other'; FBSSA foreign-born sub-Saharan African; IDU injection drug use; HSS heterosexual sex.

*The date of diagnosis of TB is defined as the start date of treatment; see text for definition of "known" vs. "new" HIV-positive

†Refers to the number of CD4 receptor-bearing lymphocytes $\times 10^6$/L; only measurements made up to three months before or one month after the start date of treatment of TB were accepted. If multiple measurements were made in this time period the measurement closest to the date of diagnosis of TB was used.

‡Quantitative HIV viral loads were assessed in the Provincial Laboratory for Public Health; only measurements made up to three months before or one month after the start date of treatment of TB were accepted. If multiple measurements were made in this time period the measurement closest to the date of diagnosis of TB was used.

§2 HSS also listed 'transfusion'; 10 IDU also listed 'heterosexual'; 'other' exposure categories included 2 men who have sex with men, and 2 vertical exposure.

S2). HIV co-infection varied by culture status; 5/228 (2.2%) if culture-negative, 3/18 (16.7%) if culture-positive for MTB complex species other than *M. tuberculosis* and 65/1207 (5.4%) if culture-positive for *M. tuberculosis*. Of the *M. tuberculosis* isolates, 1202 (99.7%) were DNA fingerprinted (65 [5.4%] from HIV-positive patients, 1042 [86.7%] from HIV-negative patients and

95 [7.9%] from HIV-unknown patients). Of the 1107 HIV tested cases with DNA fingerprinted isolates 759 cases exhibited unique fingerprint patterns (non-clustered cases) and 348 (31.4%) clustered cases were dispersed among 104 clusters, when the analysis of clustering was unconstrained by time; i.e. any genotypic match over 10 years was accepted. Eighteen clusters (96 cases) involved one or more HIV-positive case (median cluster size 3.5 [2–16] cases); 86 clusters (252 cases) involved HIV-negative cases only (median cluster size 2.0 [2–18] cases), $p<0.03$ (see Figure 2). Only one cluster involved both CBA and FBSSA cases. Using the same unconstrained cluster analysis mean cluster size did not differ by age, sex or HIV status (see Table 4). Mean cluster size was, however, much larger in Aboriginal peoples compared to other population groups, and within Aboriginal peoples, larger in those who were HIV-positive compared to those who were HIV-negative. When the cluster analysis was constrained by time (i.e. clustered cases had to have occurred within 24 months of one another [see Methods], thus better reflecting recent transmission, cluster size was again much larger in Aboriginal peoples, but within Aboriginal peoples an HIV interactive effect was no longer seen.

Discussion

In the time period and jurisdiction of this study, the routine 'opt-out' HIV testing of TB patients was very well received, with only 9.4% of incident TB cases not being tested. Similar to experience in the United States, TB patients at the extremes of age (<15 and >64 years) were less likely to be tested [20]. In those who were HIV tested the prevalence of HIV was 5.6%, almost identical to the rate estimate made for Canada by the WHO in 2007 (5.7%) [21]. In the age group 15–64 years, which included 97.3% of the co-infected patients, HIV was more common in those aged 35–64 years, Canadian-born Aboriginal or foreign-born sub-Saharan African (HIV prevalence's 12.5% and 18.3%, respectively), those with combined respiratory and non-respiratory TB, and those who died. Compared to patients with known HIV positivity, patients with new HIV positivity at the time of diagnosis of TB, had more advanced HIV disease (lower CD4 counts; higher viral loads). Median cluster size was greater when clusters contained one or more HIV-positive case than when clusters contained HIV-negative cases only. Mean cluster size was greater in HIV-positive versus HIV-negative Aboriginal peoples.

In the WHO's package of collaborative TB/HIV activities aimed at reducing the burden of TB/HIV, TB patients are recommended to be HIV tested [22,23]. Quite appropriately, UN/AIDS/WHO pronouncements on provider-initiated ('opt-out') HIV counseling and testing of TB patients have focused on countries with high co-infection rates where the potential return on HIV testing of TB patients is greatest in terms of preventing morbidity, mortality and sustained transmission [10,11,24]. Despite some difficulties in implementation such as the structural and personal factors described by Pope et al. in South Africa [25,26], a remarkable 69% of TB patients in the African Region had a documented HIV test result in 2011 [2]. In high income countries such as Canada co-infection rates are lower, limiting the potential impact of screening, but the resources necessary to maximize the clinical and prevention benefits of screening are more readily available. Since 1989 in the US and 1992 in Canada, national advisories have recommended universal HIV testing of TB patients [4,5,27]. In Alberta, the availability of ART in 1996–1997 and the introduction of 'opt-out' HIV testing in 2002–03, the latter facilitated by centralized clinical and laboratory TB services [28], resulted in universal HIV testing of TB patients. Though the prevalence of HIV co-infection was low at the extremes of age and in those who were Canadian-born non-Aboriginal or foreign-born from countries other than those in sub-Saharan Africa, rates in all of these groups were still >0.1%, the rate above which testing is considered cost-effective [29,30]. Nationally, it is unknown whether the low proportion of TB patients with a reported HIV test result is due to a failure to record the test result, to offer the test, or to the test being declined, once offered [1]. Differences in the organization of TB programs in Canada's provinces and territories and perhaps some under-appreciation of TB as a clinical opportunity for HIV testing [31], may otherwise explain the low proportion of TB patients that are HIV tested in Canada.

Universal HIV testing of TB patients allowed us to further refine our understanding of the risk factors for co-infection of TB patients in Alberta and by extrapolation, other major immigrant-receiving provinces of Canada. As in earlier analyses, age and population group emerged as significant risk factors [7,8]. Higher HIV co-infection rates in middle-aged versus young adult TB patients is understood to reflect not only age at HIV acquisition

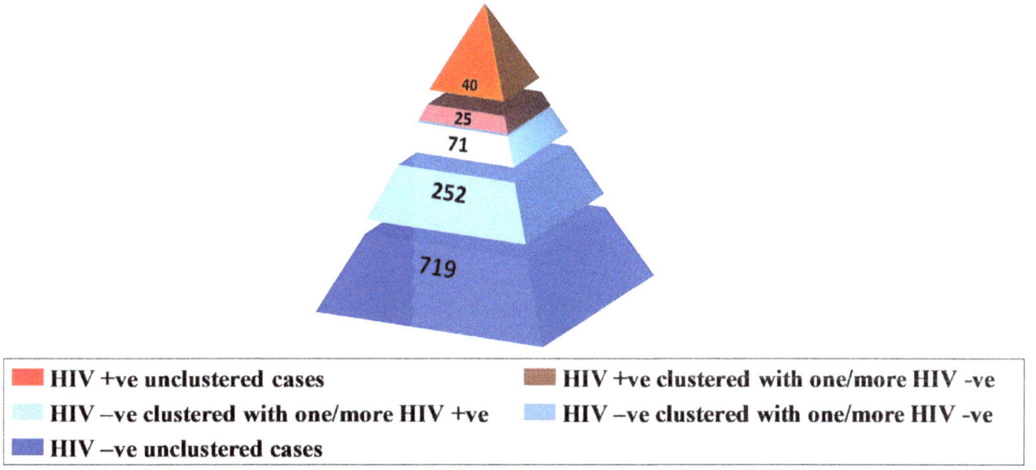

Figure 2. TB patients in Alberta who were culture-positive for *Mycobacterium tuberculosis*, whose isolates were DNA fingerprinted, and who were HIV tested (n = 1107) by clustering.

Table 4. Mean cluster size by demographic group, HIV status and population group-HIV status interaction in Alberta, 2003–2012.

Characteristics		Clustering with no time frame		Clustering with 2-yr time frame	
		Cluster size	Overall	Cluster size	Overall
		Mean (SE)	Significance*	Mean (SE)	Significance*
Age			0.23		0.45
	<15 years	3.50 (0.56)		2.7 (0.5)	
	15–34 years	2.58 (0.16)		2.08 (0.15)	
	35–64 years	2.63 (0.15)		2.1 (0.13)	
	>64 years	2.33 (0.21)		1.89 (0.18)	
Sex			0.15		0.13
	Male	2.69 (0.13)		2.18 (0.12)	
	Female	2.43 (0.14)		1.93 (0.12)	
Population group			<0.0001		<0.0001
	CBA	6.88 (0.25)		5.38 (0.23)	
	CBO & FBO	1.82 (0.12)		1.49 (0.11)	
	FBSSA	1.98 (0.23)		1.61 (0.2)	
HIV Status			0.54		0.51
	HIV-negative	2.57 (0.10)		2.07 (0.09)	
	HIV-positive	2.38 (0.58)		1.82 (0.52)	
Population group by	HIV-status interaction		0.017		0.11
	CBA HIV-negative	6.76 (0.26)		5.3 (0.24)	
	CBA HIV-positive	8.81 (0.78)		6.58 (0.7)	
	CBO & FBO HIV-negative	1.85 (0.12)		1.52 (0.1)	
	CBO & FBO HIV-positive	1.34 (0.83)		1.02 (0.75)	
	FBSSA HIV-negative	2.02 (0.24)		1.64 (0.21)	
	FBSSA HIV-positive	1.34 (0.53)		1.15 (0.47)	

Abbreviations: CBA Canadian-born Aboriginal; CBO Canadian-born 'other'; FBO foreign-born 'other'; FBSSA foreign-born sub-Saharan African.
*Significance of difference between categories obtain from Wald chi-squared test in multivariate analysis.

but more immunologically advanced disease and therefore higher risk of TB associated with years of living with HIV (see below). The latest recommendations of the CDC and the US Preventive Services Task Force, which are in turn based upon evidence that earlier initiation of ART (when CD4 counts are between 200 and 500×10^6/L), is associated with reduced risk for AIDS-related events or deaths [30,32], suggests that broader, more inclusive testing is the direction Canada should be taking. In this regard, the US has for some time now recommended HIV testing of TB contacts [33]; more recently this has been shown to be feasible, using either conventional or point-of-care testing methods [34,35].

The high HIV prevalence in Aboriginal TB patients is especially troubling; Aboriginal peoples in Canada are known to be at higher risk for latent TB infection and the penetration of HIV into this subpopulation has the potential to aggravate what is already an unsatisfactory state of TB control [1]. Though HIV testing is part of the immigration medical examination in Canada, it is unlikely to result in the exclusion of the applicant [36]. The high HIV co-infection rate in immigrants to Alberta from sub-Saharan Africa with TB is not altogether unexpected [24]. The prevalence does, however, add weight to the argument that all immigrants and refugees with HIV infection ought to be referred for medical surveillance for both HIV and TB as a condition of entry to Canada. That TB patients with combined respiratory and non-respiratory TB or TB patients that died, were more likely to be HIV co-infected was not surprising [1,7,20].

Though the number of HIV co-infected TB patients was relatively small, representing a potential study limitation, a new diagnosis of HIV was just as common as a known diagnosis of HIV. Within the limitations of the data (small numbers; missing data) those with a new diagnosis of HIV and therefore without ART, were as expected, more likely to be immunosuppressed and to have both respiratory and non-respiratory disease combined. This notwithstanding, many of those known to have been HIV positive in the past were immunosuppressed and not on ARVs at the time of diagnosis of TB. The reasons for this and the possibility that TB may have been prevented in these patients and those with a new diagnosis of HIV, had they been HIV tested earlier as a TB contact, will be explored in a separate communication. Screening persons with HIV for TB at regular intervals, allowing for earlier diagnosis and treatment of TB, might lower mortality [37]. Diagnosing HIV in contacts followed by treatment with ART and TB preventive therapy might prevent TB [38]. As expected, HCV was closely associated with IDU, placing this subpopulation of the HIV co-infected at greater risk of anti-TB drug induced liver injury [39]. That IDU was commonly reported in HIV-positive Aboriginal TB patients suggests that efforts to prevent IDU-related HIV infection might also prevent TB in this population group.

In earlier studies HIV was shown to increase the risk of belonging to a cluster of TB cases [40,41], but not to affect the size of clusters [42]. More recently, in a study from San Francisco, median cluster size was shown to be larger when clusters involved one or more HIV-positive case than when clusters involved HIV-negative cases only; within the homeless population HIV was judged to be a key factor sustaining TB transmission [17,43]. In Alberta, where being of Aboriginal ancestry is well known to be associated with clustering [44], cluster size was much larger in Aboriginal peoples, but within Aboriginal peoples there was no HIV interactive effect. In earlier studies in Alberta no association between Beijing strains and either transmission or HIV was found[18,45]. In contrast to HIV endemic countries, where most TB in HIV-positive persons is thought to result from recent transmission [46], the large proportion of 'un-clustered' HIV-positive patients (almost all foreign-born) in our study suggests that reactivation TB is the predominate pathogenic mechanism for HIV-related TB in high income immigrant-receiving countries. Dual control measures would appear to be indicated based on population groups, emphasizing prevention of transmission in Aboriginal peoples and treatment of latent infection in the foreign-born.

Supporting Information

Figure S1 Anti-retroviral (ARV) utilization history of HIV co-infected TB patients according to date of diagnosis of HIV.

Figure S2 Culture Status and HIV status of TB Patients in Alberta, 2003–2012.

Acknowledgments

The authors are very grateful to the staff of the TB Program Evaluation and Research Unit, University of Alberta, the Public Health TB clinics (Calgary, Edmonton, and Provincial), the HIV/AIDS clinics (North and South), and the Provincial Laboratory for Public Health in Alberta, for their assistance in preparing this manuscript.

Author Contributions

Conceived and designed the experiments: RL SN CH DF RC. Performed the experiments: RL SN CH RC. Analyzed the data: RL SN CH RC DF RA MLE RF. Contributed reagents/materials/analysis tools: RL SN CH MLE RF. Wrote the paper: RL SN CH RC DF RA MLE RF.

References

1. The Canadian Tuberculosis Standards, 7th Edition. Menzies D, Ed. (2013) Can Respir J 20(Suppl A): 1A–174A.
2. World Health Organization. Global Tuberculosis Report 2012. Available: http://apps.who.int/iris/bitstream/10665/75938/1/9789241564502_eng.pdf. Accessed: 2014 May 14
3. UNAIDS Report on the Global AIDS Epidemic 2012. Global Report. Available: http://www.unaids.org/en/media/unaids/contentassets/documents/epidemiology/2012/gr2012/20121120_unaids_global_report_2012_with_annexes_en.pdfhttp://www.unaids.org/en/media/unaids/contentassets/documents/epidemiology/2012/gr2012/20121120_UNAIDS_Global_Report_2012_en.pdf.
4. Canadian Thoracic Society, Tuberculosis Directors of Canada, Department of National Health and Welfare in consultation with the provincial and territorial epidemiologists, AIDS coordinators and HIV caregivers (1992) Guidelines for the identification, investigation and treatment of individuals with concomitant tuberculosis and HIV infection. CCDR 18: 155–160.
5. The Canadian Tuberculosis Committee of the Centre for Infectious Disease Prevention and Control, Population and Public Health Branch, Health Canada (2002) Recommendations for screening and prevention of tuberculosis in patients with HIV and for screening for HIV in patients with tuberculosis and in their contacts. CCDR 28(ACS-7): 1–6.
6. Horsburgh C, Feldman S, Ridzon R (2000) Practice Guidelines for the treatment of tuberculosis. CID 31: 633–639.
7. Sturtevant D, Preiksaitis J, Singh A, Houston S, Gill J, et al. (2009) The feasibility of using an 'opt-out' approach to achieve universal HIV testing of tuberculosis patients in Alberta. Can J Public Health 100: 116–120.
8. Long R, Boffa J (2010) High HIV-TB co-infection rates in marginalized population: evidence from Alberta in support of screening TB patients for HIV. Can J Public Health 101: 202–204.
9. Jayaraman G, Preiksaitis J, Larke B (2003) Mandatory reporting of HIV infection and opt-out prenatal screening for HIV infection: Effect on testing rates. CMAJ 168:679–682.
10. UNAIDS/WHO (2004) Policy statement on HIV testing. Available: http://data.unaids.org/una-docs/hivtestingpolicy_en.pdf. Accessed: 2014 May 14
11. WHO/UNAIDS (2007) Guidance on provider-initiated HIV testing and counseling in health facilities. Available: http://whqlibdoc.who.int/publications/2012/9789241503006_eng.pdf. Accessed: 2014 May 14
12. Girardi E, Sabin CA, Monforte A d'A, Hogg B, Phillips AN, et al. (2005) Incidence of tuberculosis among HIV-infected patients receiving highly active antiretroviral therapy in Europe and North American. CID 41: 1772–1782.
13. Brinkhof MW, Egger M, Boulle A, May M, Hosseinpour M, et al. (2007) Tuberculosis after initiation of antiretroviral therapy in low-income and high-income countries. CID 45: 1518–1521.
14. Manabe YC, Breen R, Perti T, Girardi E, Sterling TR (2009) Unmasked tuberculosis and tuberculosis immune reconstitution inflammatory disease: a disease spectrum after initiation of antiretroviral therapy. J Infect Dis 199: 437–444.
15. Van Embden JDA, Cave MD, Crawford JT, Dale JW, Eisenach KD, et al. (1993) Strain identification of *Mycobacterium tuberculosis* by DNA fingerprinting: recommendations for a standardized methodology. J Clin Microbiol 31: 406–409.
16. Dale JW, Brittain D, Cataldi AA, Cousins D, Crawford JT, et al. (2001) Spacer oligonucleotide typing of bacteria of the *Mycobacterium tuberculosis* complex: recommendations for standardized nomenclature. Int J Tuberc Lung Dis 5: 216–219.
17. DeRiemer K, Kawamura LM, Hopewell PC, Daley CL (2007) Quantitative impact of human immunodeficiency virus infection on tuberculosis dynamics. Am J Respir Crit Care Med 176: 936–944.
18. Langlois-Klassen D, Senthilselvan A, Chui L, Kunimoto D, Saunders D, et al. (2013) Transmission of *Mycobacterium tuberculosis* Beijing strains, Alberta, Canada, 1991–2007. Emerg Infect Dis 19: 701–711.
19. Hosmer DW Jr, Lemeshow S (2004) Applied Logistic Regression. 2nd Ed. John Wiley and Sons, Toronto, 2004.
20. Centre for Disease Control (CDC) (2010) Mortality among patients with tuberculosis and association with HIV status-United States, 1993–2008. MMWR 59: 1509–1513.
21. World Health Organization (2009) Global tuberculosis control, 2009: epidemiology, strategy, financing. Geneva: World Health Organization. WHO/HTM/TB/2009.411
22. Policy on collaborative TB/HIV activities (2010) Geneva. World Health Organization, 2004 (WHO/HTM/TB/2004.330;WHO/HTM/HIV/2004.1)
23. World Health Organization (2012) WHO policy on collaborative TB/HIV activities: guidelines for national programmes and other stakeholders. Geneva, 2012 (WHO/HTM/TB/2012.1).
24. Chaisson RE, Martinson NA (2008) Tuberculosis in Africa-Combating an HIV-driven crisis. N Engl J Med 358: 1089–1092.
25. Pope DS, Atkins S, DeLuca AN, Hausler H, Hoosain E, et al. (2010) South African TB nurses' experiences of provider-initiated HIV counseling and testing in the Eastern Cape Province: a qualitative study. AIDS Care 22: 238–245
26. Pope DS, DeLuca AN, Kali P, Hausler H, Sheard C, et al. (2008) A cluster randomized trial of provider initiated (Opt-out) HIV counseling and testing of tuberculosis patients in South Africa. J Acquir Immune Defic Syndr 48: 190–195.
27. Centre for Disease Control (CDC) (1989) Tuberculosis and immunodeficiency virus infection: Recommendations of the Advisory Committee for the Elimination of Tuberculosis (ACET). MMWR 38(14): 236–238, 243–250.
28. Jensen M, Lau A, Langlois-Klassen D, Boffa J, Manfreda J, et al. (2012) Eliminating tuberculosis: a population-based study of TB epidemiology and innovative service delivery in Canada. Int J Tuberc Lung Dis 16: 43–49
29. Sanders GE, Bayoumi AM, Holodniy M, Owens DK (2008) Cost-effectiveness of HIV screening in patients older than 55 years of age. Ann Intern Med 148: 889–903.
30. Moyer VA, on behalf of the U.S. Preventive Services Task Force (2013) Screening for HIV: U.S. Preventive Services Task Force Recommendation Statement. Ann Intern Med PMID: 23698471.
31. Long R. Langlois-Klassen D (2013) A clinical opportunity for routine HIV testing. CMAJ 185: 587.
32. Branson BM, Handsfield HH, Lampe MA, Janssen RS, Taylor AW, et al. (2006) Revised recommendations for HIV testing of adults, adolescents, and pregnant women in health-care settings. MMWR Recomm Rep 55: 1–17.
33. Centers for Disease Control (1994) Revised Guidelines for HIV Counseling, Testing and Referral. MMWR 50 (RR-19): 1–58.

34. Gardner A, Naureckas C, Beckwith C, Losikoff P, Martin C, et al. (2012) Experiences in implementation of routine human immunodeficiency virus testing in a US tuberculosis clinic. Int J Tuberc Lung Dis 16: 1241–1246.
35. Person AK, Goswami ND, Bissett DJ, Turner DS, Baker AV, et al. (2010) Pairing QuantiFERON TB Gold In-Tube with opt-out HIV testing in a tuberculosis contact investigation in the SouthEastern United States. AIDS Patient Care and STDs 24: 539–546.
36. Zencovich M, Kennedy K, MacPherson DW, Gushulak BD (2006) Immigration medical screening and HIV infection in Canada. Int J STD and AIDS 17: 813–16.
37. Reid A, Scano F, Getahun H (2006) Towards universal access to HIV prevention, treatment, care and support: the role of tuberculosis/HIV collaboration. Lancet Infect Dis 6: 483–495.
38. Akolo C, Adetifa I, Shepperd S, Volmink J (2010) Treatment of latent tuberculosis infection in HIV infected persons. Cochrane Database Syst Rev Jan 20: CD000171.
39. Staples CT, Rimland D, Dudas D (1999) Hepatitis C in the HIV (Human Immunodeficiency Virus) Atlanta V.A. (Veterans Affairs Medical Center) Cohort Study (HAVACS): The Effect of Coinfection on Survival. CID 29: 150–154.
40. Alland D, Kalkut GE, Moss AR, McAdam RA, Hahn JA, et al. (1994) Transmission of tuberculosis in New York city: an analysis by DNA fingerprinting and conventional epidemiological methods. N Engl J Med 330: 1710–1716.
41. Jasmer RM, Hahn JA, Small PM, Daley CL, Behr MA, et al. (1999) A molecular epidemiological analysis of tuberculosis trends in San Francisco, 1991-1997. Ann Intern Med 130: 971–978.
42. Giordano T, Soini H, Teeter L, Adams G, Musser J, et al. (2004) Relating the size of molecularly defined clusters of tuberculosis to the duration of symptoms. CID 38: 10–6.
43. Mohtashemi M, Kawamura LM (2010) Empirical evidence for synchrony in the evolution of TB cases and HIV + contacts among the San Francisco homeless. PloS One 5: e 8851.
44. Kunimoto D, Sutherland K, Manfreda J, Wooldrage K, Fanning A, et al. (2004) Transmission characteristics of tuberculosis in the foreign–born and Canadian-born population of Alberta, Canada. Int J Tuberc Lung Dis 8: 1213–1220.
45. Langlois-Klassen D, Kunimoto D, Saunders LD, Chui L, Boffa J, et al. (2013) A Population based cohort study of *Mycobacterium tuberculosis* Beijing strains: An emerging public health threat in an immigrant-receiving country? PLoS One 7: e38431. doi:10.1371/journal. pone. ee38431.
46. Houben RMGJ, Crampin AC, Ndhlovu R, Sonnenberg P, Godfrey-Faussett P, et al. (2011) Human immunodeficiency virus associated tuberculosis more often due to recent infection than reactivation of latent infection. Int J Tuberc Lung Dis 15: 24–31.

17

High Uptake of Systematic HIV Counseling and Testing and TB Symptom Screening at a Primary Care Clinic in South Africa

Annelies Van Rie[1]*, Kate Clouse[1], Colleen Hanrahan[1], Katerina Selibas[2], Ian Sanne[2], Sharon Williams[3], Peter Kim[3], Jean Bassett[4]

1 Department of Epidemiology, University of North Carolina at Chapel Hill, Chapel Hill, North Carolina, United States of America, **2** Clinical HIV Research Unit, University of the Witwatersrand, Johannesburg, South Africa, **3** National Institute of Allergy and Infectious Diseases, National Institutes of Health, Bethesda, Maryland, United States of America, **4** Witkoppen Health and Welfare Center, Johannesburg, South Africa

Abstract

Background: Timely diagnosis and treatment of tuberculosis (TB) and HIV is important to reduce morbidity and mortality, and break the cycle of ongoing transmission.

Methods: We performed an implementation research study to develop a model for systematic TB symptom screening and HIV counseling and testing (HCT) for all adult clients at a primary care clinic and prospectively evaluate the 6-month coverage and yield, and 18-month sustainability at a primary care clinic in Johannesburg, South Africa.

Results: During the first 6 months, 26,515 visits occurred among 12,078 adults. The proportion of adults aware of their HIV status was 43.7% at the start of the first visit, increased to 84.6% at the end of the first visit, and to 90% at end of any visit during the first 6 months. During these 6 months, 1042 clients were newly diagnosed with HIV. HIV prevalence was 22.9% among those newly tested, and 58.9% among all adult clinic clients. High coverage of systematic HCT was sustained across all 18 months. Coverage of systematic HIV-stratified TB symptom screening during first 6-months was also high (89.6%) but only 35.0% of those symptomatic were screened by sputum. During these 6-months, 90 clients had a positive Xpert MTB/RIF assay, corresponding to a TB prevalence of 0.4% among all 23,534 clients TB symptom-screened and 2.8% among the 3,284 clients with a positive TB symptom screen. The initial high coverage of TB symptom screening was not sustained, with coverage of TB symptom screening dropping after the first six months to 70% and assessment by sputum dropping to 15%.

Conclusion: Routine, systematic HCT and HIV-stratified TB symptom screening is feasible at primary care level. Systematic HCT doubled the proportion of clients with known HIV status. While HCT was sustainable, coverage of systematic TB screening dropped significantly after the first 6 months of implementation.

Editor: Nitika Pant Pai, McGill University Health Centre, McGill University, Canada

Funding: This work was supported by PEPFAR and the National Institutes of Health grant UM1 AI069463, and by the United States Agency for International Development grants to Right to Care: 674-A-00-08-00007 and 674-A-12-00020, and to Witkoppen Health and Welfare Center: 674-A-12-00033. The funders had no role in data collection, analysis, or decision to publish.

Competing Interests: The authors have declared that no competing interest exists.

* Email: Vanrie@email.unc.edu

Introduction

The global burden of tuberculosis (TB) and human immunodeficiency virus (HIV) remains enormous. In 2012, there were an estimated 35.3 million people living with HIV (PLWH), 2.3 million new HIV infections, 1.3 million AIDS deaths, 8.6 million new cases of TB, and 1.3 million TB deaths, including 320,000 among PLWH [1,2]. In sub-Saharan Africa, there is a high prevalence of undiagnosed TB in the community [3–5], many people are unaware of their HIV status [6], and people often enter care at advanced stages of disease [7], suggesting that the current public health approach to diagnosis of TB and HIV is insufficient.

HIV counseling and testing (HCT) is predominantly delivered through voluntary counseling and testing or provider-initiated counseling and testing (PICT). Even though the World Health Organization (WHO) recommends PICT for all people visiting a health facility [8], PICT in health care facilities in high burden countries is mainly targeted at individuals presenting for antenatal, TB or STI care [9]. Alternative approaches such as testing contacts of index cases, mobile testing, door-to-door testing, and school-based testing can increase HIV case finding [10]. A similar situation holds for TB, with suboptimal case finding using the conventional approach of passive case finding among people presenting to health facilities with symptoms suggestive of TB [1,11]. In pursuit of a more active approach to TB case detection, the WHO recommends intensified case finding among PLWH and close contacts of individuals with infectious TB [12,13]. Mobile TB screening, door-to-door screening, school-based programs, and community sputum collection point programs have been evaluated but are not routinely implemented [4,14,15].

Despite high rates of missed TB and HIV case finding at health facilities [16–19], few studies have evaluated the impact of systematic TB symptom screening and HCT for all clients, independent of the presence of risk factors. We aimed to develop a primary care model for systematic TB and HIV screening for all adults presenting to a primary care clinic. We evaluated the model's impact on knowledge of HIV status of clinic clients, HIV and TB case finding, and assessed feasibility and sustainability at a primary care clinic in Johannesburg, South Africa.

Methods

Ethics statement

The study was approved by the Institutional Review Board of the University of North Carolina at Chapel Hill, USA, and the Human Research Ethics Committee of the University of the Witwatersrand, Johannesburg, South Africa. Clinic clients provided written consent for use of routine clinic data for research purposes.

Study setting

The prospective implementation research study took place at the Witkoppen Health and Welfare Centre (WHWC), a primary care clinic serving Diepsloot, a densely populated informal settlement community. Diepsloot, located in northern Johannesburg, is the 5th most deprived of the 420 geopolitical subdivisions of Gauteng Province, South Africa [20].

Prior to the intervention, clinic clients were referred for HIV counseling and testing either through self-request (voluntary HCT) or by their provider (PICT) who targeted clients of antenatal care, tuberculosis and sexually transmitted disease services. Symptom screening for the presence of prolonged cough and weight loss was initiated by the care provider at time of clinical evaluation, either systematically among PLWH or as part of targeted clinical assessment in others. Collection of sputum was performed if requested by the nurse or doctor.

Development of a primary care model for integrated routine screening for TB and HIV

Model development first involved meetings with the clinic leadership to discuss preliminary findings [18], map current patient flow, and identify possibilities for re-allocation of space and distribution of new tasks. Meetings were then held to receive input from clinic staff routinely involved in TB and HIV care and treatment. To establish the final model, an iterative process was implemented over a 12-month period using participatory quality improvement methods. Once the final model was developed, the TB symptom screening and HCT activities became routine clinic activities and were no longer supported or monitored by research staff.

Data collection

All data were collected as part of routine patient care. Data used in the analysis were retrieved from paper-based medical files and clinic registers, as well as electronic clinic records and laboratory data. Clinic files of all adults (age ≥18 years) visiting the clinic between 30 Jan 2012 and 27 July 2012 were reviewed and data were collected on age, gender, pregnancy status, nationality, employment, HIV status (known positive, negative test result in prior 3 month period, unknown), outcome of HCT (positive, negative, not done), CD4 count if newly diagnosed with HIV, outcome of HIV-stratified TB symptom screening (positive, negative, not done), collection of sputum (if positive symptom screen), and Xpert MTB/RIF result.

To determine long-term sustainability, an additional file review was performed for 162 clients randomly selected among those visiting the clinic between January 28 to February 1, 2013 and 142 clients visiting the clinic during July 29 to August 2, 2013.

Statistical analysis

Characteristics of clinic clients are described using proportions for categorical variables, and medians and interquartile ranges (IRQ) for continuous variables. Detailed analysis of uptake and results of HCT by prior HCT status was performed for all clinic clients at the time of their first visit to the clinic during the six-month period. To determine changes in weekly HIV and TB screening outcomes of all visits (including repeat visits by some clinic clients), linear regression modeling techniques were used, incorporating an autoregressive error model to correct for the time-series structure and autocorrelation. The model output consists of a slope estimate (β) corresponding to an increase or decrease per week during the 6-month period. For example, a β of 0.001 corresponds to an increase of 0.1% per week. Log-binomial regression modeling was used to identify factors associated with testing outcomes, with results presented as crude risk ratios (RR) and 95% confidence intervals (95%CI).

Results

Model development for integrated systematic screening for TB and HIV at primary care

During the iterative, 12-month participatory process, changes were made to leverage existing space and staff, simplify patient flow and reduce waiting times. Conditions agreed upon between investigators and clinic staff were to: (1) integrate activities into current clinic activities instead of creating separate screening officers [21] (2) make HIV counseling part of routine care and perform HIV testing in those with unknown HIV status unless the client refuses, (3) have HCT precede TB screening to allow HIV-stratified TB symptoms screening, and (4) perform HCT and TB symptom screening during the time people wait to see a nurse or clinician so that results are available at time of clinical evaluation. Two TB symptom checklist stamps were developed to guide health care workers in performing a rapid HIV-stratified TB screen. For PLWH, symptoms suggestive of TB were cough, fever, night sweats and loss of weight for any duration [12]. For HIV-negative individuals, prolonged (≥2 weeks) cough or fever, night sweats and substantial weight loss were considered suggestive of active TB.

The final model involved staff across the spectrum of clinic personnel. The administrative staff registering clinic clients at presentation reviewed the client's file to determine the individual's need for HCT. People who visited WHWC for the first time and returning clients without documented HIV-infected status or a documented HIV negative test performed more than three months prior were judged in need of HCT and referred for group HIV pretest counseling. Lay counselors performed HIV pretest counseling in small groups throughout the morning prior to a client's clinical evaluation. At the end of the group session, people were invited for one-on-one rapid HIV testing and post-test counseling in a private setting. Upon completion of post-test counseling, the counselor placed the appropriate TB symptom screen stamp in the patient's clinic file. It was then the task of the clinic staff performing the routine assessment of vitals (weight, temperature, blood pressure and pregnancy test) to complete the information in the TB symptom screen stamp and to follow the simple algorithm to determine which individuals had a positive TB symptom screen. The same staff decided whether collection of a sputum sample was indicated. Between July 1, 2011 and July 31,

2012, Xpert MTB/RIF assay was performed at point-of-care, with the goal to have the result ready by the time the patient was seen by the nurse or doctor. After August 1, 2012, sputum samples were transported to a centralized laboratory for analysis. If the first-line clinic staff did not request a sputum sample, the nurse of doctor could still request this upon completion of the history-taking and clinical exam.

Clinic population

A total of 26,515 visits by 12,078 adults occurred at the clinic during the 6-month period (30 Jan 2012 to 27 July 2012) after the model was finalized as described above. The majority (69.5%) of clinic clients were women, 16.8% of whom were pregnant (Table 1). Ages of clients spanned the entire adult range, with a median age of 35 years (IQR 28-43), and 13.7% being 50 years or older. Almost one in three (32.3%) were not of South African nationality, and half (51.7%) were unemployed.

Uptake of HIV counseling and testing

At time of arrival for the first clinic visit during the 6-month period, 41.2% (95%CI: 40.3–42.0%) of the 12,078 adults were known HIV positive, 2.5% (95%CI: 2.2–2.8%) had a documented HIV negative test within the past 3 months, and 54.7% (95%CI: 53.8–55.6%) had an unknown HIV status (Table 2). Of those with unknown HIV status, the vast majority (88.2%) had never been tested for HIV at WHWC. Of those with unknown status, 74.8% (95%CI: 73.6–75.9%) were tested during their first clinic visit. The proportion tested was higher for those never previously tested at WHWC (77.9%, 95% CI 76.8–79.0%) compared to those tested more than 3 months ago (51.7%, 95% CI 48.2–55.2%). All except one person with a prior negative HIV test had a repeat negative HIV test. Among the 4537 tested for the first time at the clinic, 1041 new cases of HIV were detected (22.9%, 95% CI 21.7–24.2%). The number needed to test to identify one new case of HIV was 4.7 among all 4940 clients tested and 6.3 among all 6603 clients who received pretest counseling. By the end of the first clinic visit during the 6-month period, 84.6% (95% CI 83.9–85.2%) of all adult clients were aware of their HIV status, of which 58.9% were HIV positive. Failure to receive a documented HIV status during the first clinic visit was not associated with gender (RR 0.97, 95%CI: 0.93–1.02) but was higher among younger clients (age<40 years, RR 1.25, 95% CI 1.19–1.30) and those with foreign nationality (RR 1.10, 95% CI 1.05–1.15).

To assess sustainability, we assessed changes over time in the proportion of clients knowledgeable of their HIV status by the end of *any* clinic visit (i.e. first and repeat visits) (Figure 1). During the 6-month period, 90.0% (95%CI: 89.7–90.4%) of clients were aware of their HIV status by the end of any visit. This proportion did not change during the 6-month period ($\beta = 0.000$) and remained similar 6 and 12 months later (92.6%, $p = 0.27$ and 86.0%, $p = 0.12$), suggesting long-term sustainability of routine HCT.

While the HIV prevalence among newly-tested clients at *any* visit decreased from an estimated 19.5% (95%CI: 10.5–28.3) to 16.4% (95%CI: 7.5–25.3) during the 6-month period (Figure 1), HIV prevalence among clients newly tested when visiting the clinic for the *first* time was 22.9% and increased from an estimated 19.5% (95%CI: 10.5–28.3) to 23.1% (95% CI: 11.4%–34.8%).

The median CD4 value at the time of a new HIV diagnosis was 260 cells/µl (IQR 136–412). Newly-diagnosed men had more advanced disease compared to women (221 CD4 cells/µl, IQR: 94–352 among men vs. 295 cells/µl, IQR: 169–427 among women, $p < 0.001$).

Table 1. Characteristics of clients seeking care at a primary care clinic in Johannesburg, South Africa.

	Overall	Male	Female
Number of clinic visits	26515	7831	18684
Number of individual clinic clients, n (%)	12078	3687 (30.5)	8391 (69.5)
Number of visits per client, median (range)	2 (1–11)	2 (1–11)	2 (1–10)
Age at first visit			
Median (IQR)	35 (28–43)	36 (30–44)	34 (27–43)
18–29 years	3799 (31.5)	920 (24.2)	2879 (34.3)
30–39 years	4221 (35.0)	1375 (37.3)	2846 (33.9)
40–49 years	2407 (19.9)	876 (23.8)	1531 (18.3)
≥50 years	1651 (13.7)	516 (14.0)	1135 (13.5)
Pregnancy status at first visit, n (%)*			
Pregnant	—	—	1360 (16.8)
Not pregnant	—	—	6729 (83.2)
Nationality, n (%)#			
Born in South Africa	8172 (67.8)	2395 (65.1)	5777 (68.9)
Born outside of South Africa	3890 (32.3)	1285 (34.9)	2605 (31.1)
Employment status at first visit, n (%)**			
Employed	5827 (48.3)	1966 (53.4)	3861 (46.0)
Not employed	6246 (51.7)	1717 (46.6)	4529 (54.0)

IQR: interquartile range;
* pregnancy status missing in 302 (3.6%) of women;
#nationality missing in 16 (0.1%) individuals;
** employment status missing in 5 (0.0) individuals.

Table 2. Uptake and results of HIV counseling and testing among 12,078 individuals visiting a primary care clinic in Johannesburg, South Africa.

	Overall		Male		Female	
	N*	%*	N*	%*	N*	%*
HIV status at start of first visit						
Known positive	4972	41.2	1481	40.2	3491	41.6
Known negative (test ≤3 m)	304	2.5	51	1.4	253	3.0
Unknown	6603	54.7	2103	57.0	4500	53.6
Prior tested (>3 m)	779	11.8	134	6.4	645	14.3
Not tested previously	5824	88.2	1969	93.6	3855	85.7
Clinic file not found	199	1.7	52	1.4	147	1.8
Outcome of HCT (among those with unknown HIV status)						
Not tested	1663	25.2	592	28.2	1071	23.8
Tested	4940	74.8	1511	71.9	3429	76.2
All tested						
HIV positive	1042	21.1	354	23.4	688	20.1
HIV negative	3898	78.9	1157	76.6	2741	79.9
Prior test (>3 m) negative						
Tested	403	51.7	58	43.3	345	53.5
HIV positive	1	0.2	0	0.0	1	0.3
HIV negative	402	99.8	58	100.0	344	99.7
Not tested previously						
Tested	4537	77.9	1453	73.8	3084	80.0
HIV positive	1041	22.9	354	24.4	687	22.3
HIV negative	3496	77.1	1099	75.6	2397	77.7
Initial CD4 count if newly diagnosed with HIV						
Median (IQR) cells/μl	268	136–412	221	94–352	295	169–427
<50 cells/μl	87	8.3	46	13.0	41	6.0
50–199 cells/μl	262	25.1	109	30.8	153	22.2
200–350 cells/μl	283	27.2	92	26.0	191	27.8
>350 cells/μl	330	31.7	86	24.3	244	35.4
Missing	80	7.7	21	5.9	59	8.6
HIV status at end of clinic visit						
Known	10216	84.6	3043	82.5	7173	85.5
Known positive	6014	58.9	1835	60.3	4179	58.3
Known negative	4202	41.1	1208	39.7	2994	41.7
Unknown	1862	15.4	644	17.5	1218	14.5

* N and % unless indicated otherwise the estimated proportion.

Uptake of HIV-stratified TB symptom screening

Information on completion of a TB symptom screen was available for 26,279 clinic visits during the 6-month period (Table 3). A TB symptom screen was performed at 89.6% (95% CI 89.2–89.9%) of the visits (Figure 2). Of the 23,534 symptom screens performed, 14.0% (95% CI 13.5–14.4%) were positive. Among the 3284 visits with a positive TB symptom screen, a sputum specimen was collected in 1150 (35.0%, 95%CI: 33.4–36.7%), of which 90 (8.0%, 95% CI 6.5–9.7%) were positive for *Mycobacterium tuberculosis* on Xpert MTB/RIF. Overall, 90 cases of TB were detected, corresponding to a 7.8% case detection among the 1150 cases screened by sputum, 2.7% case detection rate among the 3284 clients with a positive symptom screen and 0.4% case detection among all 23534 clients screened for TB symptoms.

There was no difference in TB symptom screening by gender (RR 1.00. 95%CI: 0.99–1.01), but men were more likely to be investigated by sputum (RR 1.45, 95%CI: 1.31–1.62) and were twice as likely to test positive for *M. tuberculosis* (RR 2.24, 95%CI: 1.53–3.26). HIV-positive clients were more likely to be screened for TB symptoms (94.4%) compared to HIV-negative clients (84.3%); those with unknown HIV status were least likely to be screened (70.6%). Case detection rate was similar among the three groups (7.5%, 8.7% and 7.9% for HIV-positive, HIV-negative and HIV-unknown, respectively). The number of clients needed to symptom screen to identify one case of TB was 262 overall, 131 for male clients, 448 for female clients, 317 for HIV infected clients,

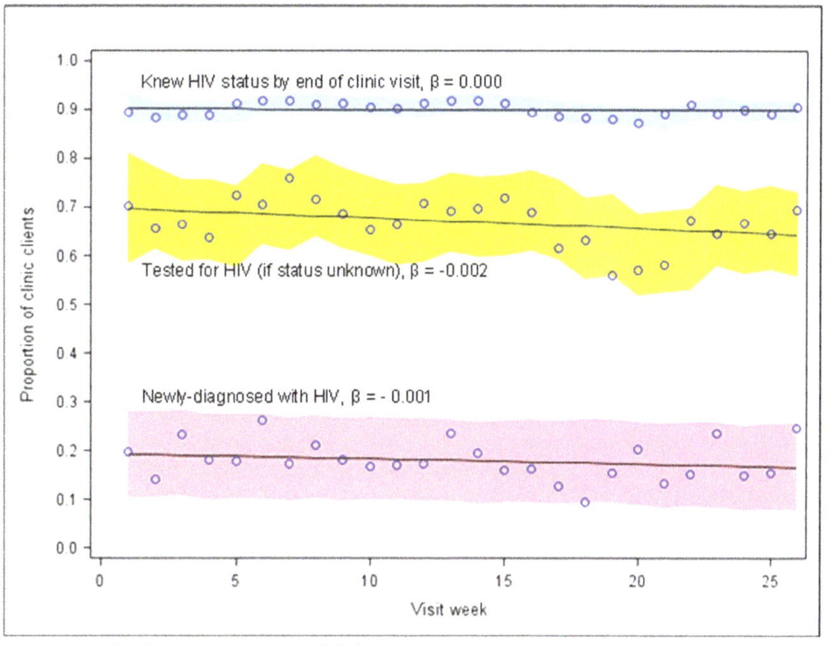

Figure 1. Systematic HIV counseling and testing at primary care clinic in Johannesburg, South Africa: coverage, case detection and sustainability over a 26-week period.

239 for HIV uninfected clients and 116 for clients with unknown HIV status.

During the 6-month period, an increase over time was observed for the uptake of TB symptom screening (from an estimated 84.7 (95%CI: 79.1–90.3%) to 93.5% (95%CI: 88.2–98.7%), $\beta = 0.004$) and the proportion of TB suspects investigated by sputum (from an estimated 19.9% (95%CI: 9.5–38.9%) to 49.8% (95%CI: 34.1–65.4%), $\beta = 0.012$) (Figure 3). Associated with the increase in the proportion of clients assessed by sputum, the proportion Xpert MTB/RIF positive among those assessed by sputum decreased ($\beta = -0.003$) from an estimated 12.6% (95%CI: 4.3–24.7%) to 5.3% (95%CI: 0.0–17.5%).

TB screening coverage was not sustained long-term, with significantly lower proportion of clients screened for TB symptoms 6 and 12 months later (68.5% and 71.0%, respectively, $p<0.001$), and significantly lower proportion of TB suspects assessed by sputum 6 and 12 months later (15.3% and 13.6%, respectively, $p = 0.090$).

Discussion

In this study, the first to our knowledge to implement and evaluate a primary care model for integrated systematic HIV counseling and testing and TB symptom screening, we achieved high rates of TB symptom screening and HCT when implemented for all adult clients at a primary care clinic in South Africa, with 89.6% being screened for TB symptoms and 84.6% of people being aware of their HIV status by the end of their first clinic visit. Six months of systematic screening for HIV and TB resulted in the detection of 1042 cases of HIV, corresponding to a 22% HIV prevalence among those with unknown status, and 90 new cases of TB, corresponding to a 2.7% TB prevalence rate among those with a positive symptom screen.

Missed opportunities for HIV testing at health facilities are common, and only testing those perceived to be at high risk of HIV can miss large numbers of PLWH [19]. Implementation of routine HCT doubled the proportion of individuals knowledgeable about their HIV status, from 43.7% at the start of the clients' first clinic visit to 84.6% by the end of the clinic visit. HCT uptake was higher than that reported for other facility-based HCT approaches, and similar to the 80–85% uptake achieved in community-based HCT programs [10].

HIV prevalence among those with unknown HIV status who accepted testing was 19.5%, slightly higher but not statistically different from the 16.1% estimated population HIV prevalence in Gauteng Province in 2011 [22]. This is in contrast with results of a meta-analysis, which found that the HIV positivity rate at facility-based HCT was, on average, double that of community-based HCT [10]. Despite high uptake, HCT did not result in high proportions of diagnoses at early stages of disease, with only 31.7% diagnosed at CD4 count >350 cells/µl, substantially lower than the 40.2% estimate in a meta-analysis of individuals diagnosed with CD4 count >350 through community-based HCT [10]. Taken together, these data suggest that systematic HIV testing at facility levels can reach similar case finding rates as community-based HCT but captures individuals at more advanced level of disease progression.

Reports of missed opportunities for TB case finding at primary care clinics suggest that TB case finding should not be limited to passive case finding or PLWH [17]. We achieved high (89.6%) coverage of HIV-stratified TB symptom screening of all clinic clients, suggesting operational feasibility under programmatic conditions. The proportion of individuals with positive symptom screen assessed by sputum (35%) was lower than expected, in part due to the frequent occurrence of unproductive cough. This is similar to findings at primary care clinics in Botswana, where only 35.3% of those with a positive symptom screen were referred for sputum smear microscopy or X-ray [23]. The TB case finding yield was relatively low, with 90 cases detected, representing 2.8% of the 3,284 clients with a positive TB symptom screen and 0.4%

Table 3. Uptake and results of TB symptom screening and sputum testing during 26,279 clinic visits at a primary care facility in Johannesburg, South Africa.

	All visits		Male		Female		HIV-positive		HIV-negative		HIV-unknown	
	N	%	N	%	N	%	N	%	N	%	N	%
Screened for TB symptoms at visit*												
No	2745	10.5	803	10.3	1942	10.5	952	5.6	1023	15.7	770	29.4
Yes	23534	89.6	6962	89.7	16572	89.5	16181	94.4	5502	84.3	1851	70.6
Presence of TB symptoms among those screened												
No	20250	86.1	5778	83.0	14572	87.3	14145	87.4	4690	85.2	1415	76.5
Yes	3284	14.0	1184	17.0	2100	12.7	2036	12.6	812	14.8	436	23.5
Investigation by sputum among those with positive symptom screen												
No	2134	65.0	726	61.3	1408	67.0	1355	66.5	547	67.4	232	53.2
Yes	1150	35.0	458	38.7	692	33.0	681	33.5	265	32.6	204	46.8
Xpert result among those investigated by sputum**												
Negative	1030	89.8	393	86.0	637	92.3	609	89.7	238	89.8	183	90.2
Positive	90	7.9	53	11.6	37	5.4	51	7.5	23	8.7	16	7.9
Error or invalid	27	2.4	11	2.4	16	2.3	19	2.8	4	1.5	4	2.0

* Clinic file could not be located for 229 patients;

** Excludes 3 missing Xpert results.

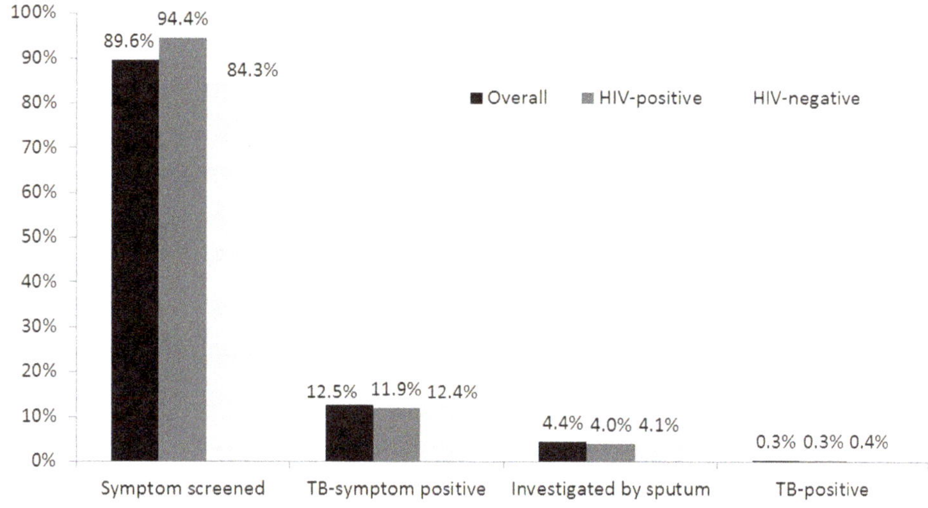

Figure 2. The TB screening cascade observed at 26,279 clinic visits at a primary care clinic in Johannesburg, South Africa. Black bars represent screenings in all clinic clients, dark grey bars represent screenings in HIV-positive clinic clients, and light grey bars represent screenings in HIV-negative clinic clients.

of the 23,534 clients screened. Operational feasibility but low yield of systematic TB symptom screening was also observed in other studies. In Botswana, 926 (8%) of 11,799 clinic clients had a positive symptom screen, 327 (35.3%) were referred for examinations (sputum smear microscopy or X-ray), and 19 (13.4% of those tested, 0.2% of those screened) were diagnosed with TB [23]. In outpatient departments of 32 hospitals in Swaziland [11], 14,998 (6%) of 251,867 clients screened positive and were tested using Xpert, 1499 (10% of those tested, 0.6% of those screened) were diagnosed with TB. In Afghanistan, 22,228 (2.5%) of 889,120 clinic attendees systematically screened for TB at 47 health facilities were tested with smear microscopy of whom 1986 were diagnosed with TB (8.9% of those tested, 0.2% of those screened) [11].

In contrast to our findings of sustainability of systematic HCT, the high coverage of systematic TB screening was not sustained long term. The proportion of individuals symptom screened dropped from 89.6% to about 70% and the proportion with positive symptom screen assessed by sputum dropped from 35% to about 15%. Several factors may have contributed to this observation. First, whereas systematic HIV testing is part of a South Africa national testing campaign, systematic TB symptom

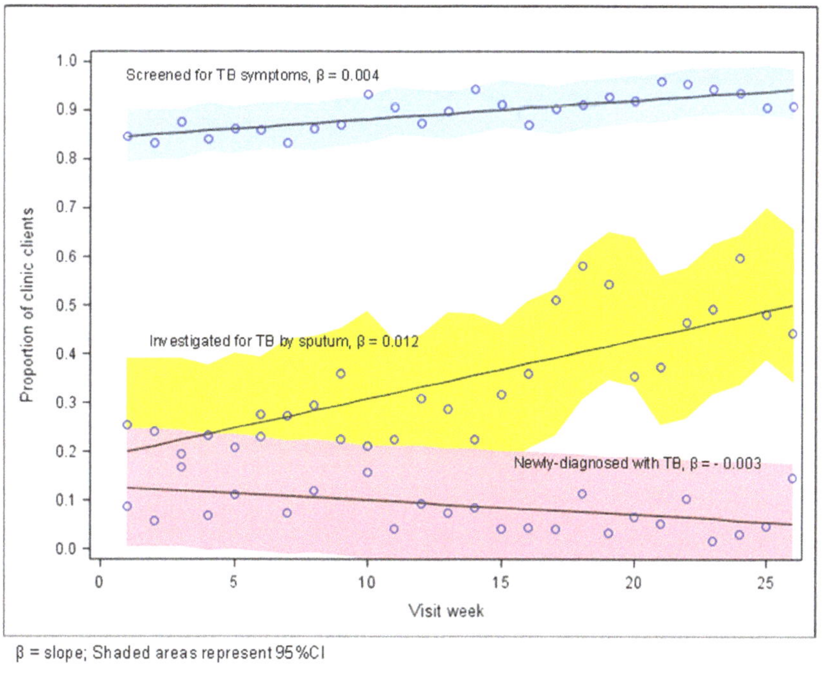

Figure 3. Systematic TB symptom screening and assessment at primary care clinic in Johannesburg, South Africa: coverage, case detection, and sustainability over a 26-week period.

screening in all clinic clients is not recommended by the South African Department of Health. Second, the number needed to screen to detect one case is much higher for TB than HIV (262 versus 6), possibly resulting in a perception of higher effectiveness and thus stronger motivation for the health care workers to test for HIV compared to TB. Third, while Xpert MTB/RIF was performed at point-of-care during the study period, samples were sent to a centralized laboratory after the first 6 months. Lack of immediate feedback on sputum results may further have decreased the motivation of the clinic staff to collect sputum for evaluation.

The large sample size, pragmatic approach and the evaluation under real-world conditions using non-research clinic staff to perform all activities are important strengths of our study. The interpretation of the findings however needs to take some limitations into account. The study was a single-site observational study without a control group. The impact of the intervention on HIV and TB diagnoses could therefore not be estimated as the proportion of new HIV and TB diagnoses that would have been made under standard of care was not known. We also do not know if missed diagnoses occurred among those who were not tested for HIV, those with a negative TB symptom screen, and clients with a positive symptom screen who were not assessed by sputum. Inclusion of a historical control using routine clinic statistics could provide some insights but would have inherent limitations due to differences in time periods assessed and use of different data collection standards. Finally, the available data did not allow us to estimate cost effectiveness of the program, or to assess the impact of the intervention on individual morbidity and mortality or transmission of TB and HIV at population level.

Conclusion

To date, efforts to curb the TB/HIV epidemic have focused on TB screening for PLWH and HCT for people diagnosed with active TB. While outreach screening activities have been shown to be effective, these programs require infrastructure development, complicate linkage to care, and sustainability under programmatic conditions of such programs can be hard to obtain. Improving TB and HIV case finding at health facilities may be a more affordable and sustainable first step to increase case finding in high burden settings. Key features likely contributing to our program's success were full integration of TB symptom screening and HCT into routine clinic activities, distribution of tasks across a range of clinic personnel, and timing of HCT and TB symptom screening during the time clinic clients waited to see a nurse or physician. Future research is needed to explore the epidemiological and contextual factors that improve the effectiveness of different tools and approaches to systematic TB screening at primary care.

Acknowledgments

We are deeply grateful to all patients and staff at Witkoppen Health and Welfare Center. We would also like to thank members of the research team: Veronica Modise, Bridgette Moatlhodi, and Violet Molepo. We thank Pierre Barker and Michèle Youngleson of the Institute for Healthcare Improvement for guidance and support regarding the use of quality improvement methods.

Author Contributions

Conceived and designed the experiments: AVR PK SW IS JB. Performed the experiments: JB KC CH KS. Analyzed the data: KC AVR CH. Wrote the paper: AVR KC CH JB PK. Collected data: KS CH.

References

1. WHO (2013) Global Tuberculosis Report Geneva, Switzerland.
2. UNAIDS (2012) Report on the Global AIDS Epidemic. UNAIDS.
3. Ayles H, Schaap A, Nota A, Sismanidis C, Tembwe R, et al. (2009) Prevalence of tuberculosis, HIV and respiratory symptoms in two Zambian communities: implications for tuberculosis control in the era of HIV. PLoS One 4: e5602.
4. Corbett EL, Bandason T, Duong T, Dauya E, Makamure B, et al. (2010) Comparison of two active case-finding strategies for community-based diagnosis of symptomatic smear-positive tuberculosis and control of infectious tuberculosis in Harare, Zimbabwe (DETECTB): a cluster-randomised trial. Lancet 376: 1244–1253.
5. Wood R, Middelkoop K, Myer L, Grant AD, Whitelaw A, et al. (2007) Undiagnosed tuberculosis in a community with high HIV prevalence: implications for tuberculosis control. Am J Respir Crit Care Med 175: 87–93.
6. WHO, UNAIDS, UNICEF (2011) Global HIV/AIDS repsonse. Epidemic update and health sector progress towards universal access. Progress report 2011.
7. Braitstein P, Brinkhof MW, Dabis F, Schechter M, Boulle A, et al. (2006) Mortality of HIV-1-infected patients in the first year of antiretroviral therapy: comparison between low-income and high-income countries. Lancet 367: 817–824.
8. WHO (2007) Guidance on provider-initiated HIV testing and counseling in health facilities Geneva.
9. Roura M, Watson-Jones D, Kahawita TM, Ferguson L, Ross DA (2013) Provider-initiated testing and counselling programmes in sub-Saharan Africa: a systematic review of their operational implementation. AIDS 27: 617–626.
10. Suthar AB, Ford N, Bachanas PJ, Wong VJ, Rajan JS, et al. (2013) Towards Universal Voluntary HIV Testing and Counselling: A Systematic Review and Meta-Analysis of Community-Based Approaches. PLoS Med 10: e1001496.
11. Uplekar M, Creswell J, Ottmani SE, Weil D, Sahu S, et al. (2013) Programmatic approaches to screening for active tuberculosis. Int J Tuberc Lung Dis 17: 1248–1256.
12. WHO (2010) Guidelines for intensified tuberculosis case finding and isoniazid preventive therapy for people living with HIV in resource-contrained settings. Geneva, Switzerland: World Health Organization.
13. WHO (2012) Recommendations for investigating contacts of persons with infectious tuberculosis in low- and middle-income countries. World Health Organization. WHO/INT/TB/2012.9 WHO/INT/TB/2012.9.
14. Kranzer K, Lawn SD, Meyer-Rath G, Vassall A, Raditlhalo E, et al. (2012) Feasibility, yield, and cost of active tuberculosis case finding linked to a mobile HIV service in Cape Town, South Africa: a cross-sectional study. PLoS Med 9: e1001281.
15. Ayles H, Muyoyeta M, Du Toit E, Schaap A, Floyd S, et al. (2013) Effect of household and community interventions on the burden of tuberculosis in southern Africa: the ZAMSTAR community-randomised trial. Lancet.
16. Bassett IV, Wang B, Chetty S, Giddy J, Losina E, et al. (2010) Intensive tuberculosis screening for HIV-infected patients starting antiretroviral therapy in Durban, South Africa. Clin Infect Dis 51: 823–829.
17. Claassens MM, Jacobs E, Cyster E, Jennings K, James A, et al. (2013) Tuberculosis cases missed in primary health care facilities: should we redefine case finding? Int J Tuberc Lung Dis 17: 608–614.
18. Voss De Lima YP-S, Sanne I, Van Rie A (2010) Routine screening for TB and HIV by health care workers ar primary care clinics. Lille, France. The International Unions Against Tuberculosis and Lung Diseases. pp. S111.
19. Fetene NW, Feleke AD (2010) Missed opportunities for earlier HIV testing and diagnosis at the health facilities of Dessie town, North East Ethiopia. BMC Public Health 10: 362.
20. De Wet T, Patel L, Korth M, Forrester C (2008) Johannesburg Poverty and Livelihoods Study. Johannesburg: Centre for Social Development in Africa, University of Johannesburg.
21. Khan AJ, Khowaja S, Khan FS, Qazi F, Lotia I, et al. (2012) Engaging the private sector to increase tuberculosis case detection: an impact evaluation study. Lancet Infect Dis 12: 608–616.
22. Health SANDo (2012) The National Antenatal Sentinel HIV and Syphilis Prevalence Survey, South Africa, 2011. Pretoria.
23. Bloss E, Makombe R, Kip E, Smit M, Chirenda J, et al. (2012) Lessons learned during tuberculosis screening in public medical clinics in Francistown, Botswana. Int J Tuberc Lung Dis 16: 1030–1032.

Developing Content for a mHealth Intervention to Promote Postpartum Retention in Prevention of Mother-To-Child HIV Transmission Programs and Early Infant Diagnosis of HIV

Thomas A. Odeny[1,2*], Maya Newman[3], Elizabeth A. Bukusi[1,4,5], R. Scott McClelland[2,4,6,7], Craig R. Cohen[8], Carol S. Camlin[8,9]

1 Center for Microbiology Research, Kenya Medical Research Institute, Nairobi, Kenya, **2** Department of Epidemiology, University of Washington, Seattle, Washington, United States of America, **3** School of Medicine, University of Washington, Seattle, Washington, United States of America, **4** Department of Global Health, University of Washington, Seattle, Washington, United States of America, **5** Department of Obstetrics and Gynecology, University of Washington, Seattle, Washington, United States of America, **6** Department of Medicine, University of Washington, Seattle, Washington, United States of America, **7** Institute of Tropical and Infectious Diseases, University of Nairobi, Nairobi, Kenya, **8** Department of Obstetrics, Gynecology and Reproductive Sciences, University of California San Francisco, San Francisco, California, United States of America, **9** Center for AIDS Prevention Studies, University of California San Francisco, San Francisco, California, United States of America

Abstract

Background: Maternal attendance at postnatal clinic visits and timely diagnosis of infant HIV infection are important steps for prevention of mother-to-child transmission (PMTCT) of HIV. We aimed to use theory-informed methods to develop text messages targeted at facilitating these steps.

Methods: We conducted five focus group discussions with health workers and women attending antenatal, postnatal, and PMTCT clinics to explore aspects of women's engagement in postnatal HIV care and infant testing. Discussion topics were informed by constructs of the Health Belief Model (HBM) and prior empirical research. Qualitative data were coded and analyzed according to the construct of the HBM to which they related. Themes were extracted and used to draft intervention messages. We carried out two stages of further messaging development: messages were presented in a follow-up focus group in order to develop optimal phrasing in local languages. We then further refined the messages, pretested them in individual cognitive interviews with selected health workers, and finalized the messages for the intervention.

Results: Findings indicated that brief, personalized, caring, polite, encouraging, and educational text messages would facilitate women bringing their children to clinic after delivery, suggesting that text messages may serve as an important "cue to action." Participants emphasized that messages should not mention HIV due to fear of HIV testing and disclosure. Participants also noted that text messages could capitalize on women's motivation to attend clinic for childhood immunizations.

Conclusions: Applying a multi-stage content development approach to crafting text messages – informed by behavioral theory – resulted in message content that was consistent across different focus groups. This approach could help answer "why" and "how" text messaging may be a useful tool to support maternal and child health. We are evaluating the effect of these messages on improving postpartum PMTCT retention and infant HIV testing in a randomized trial.

Editor: Claire Thorne, UCL Institute of Child Health, University College London, United Kingdom

Funding: This work was supported by the National Institutes of Health Office of the Director, Fogarty International Center, Office of AIDS Research, National Cancer Center, National Eye Institute, National Heart, Blood, and Lung Institute, National Institute of Dental and Craniofacial Research, National Institute on Drug Abuse, National Institute of Mental Health, National Institute of Allergy and Infectious Diseases, and National Institutes of Health Office of Women's Health and Research through the Fogarty International Clinical Research Scholars and Fellows Program at Vanderbilt University (R24 TW007988) and the American Relief and Recovery Act. TAO was a Fogarty International Clinical Research Fellow. CSC was supported by a Research Scientist Development Award from the National Institute of Mental Health (K01MH093205). The funders had no role in study design, data collection and analysis, decision to publish, or preparation of the manuscript.

Competing Interests: Craig R. Cohen declares the following: Financial competing interests include but are not limited to: Paid employment or consultancy: Dr. Cohen served as a paid consultant for CerMed Inc. to help them develop a barrier contraceptive/HIV prevention device. This consultancy ended in 2012. Research grants (from any source, restricted or unrestricted): Dr. Cohen has active grants from the US NIH, CDC, and Bill & Melinda Gates Foundation. Travel grants and honoraria for speaking or participation at meetings: Dr. Cohen received a travel grant to consult with Gynuity on a study they conducted to investigate infections following medical abortion in the US. Non-financial Professional interests: Acting as an expert witness: Dr. Cohen has served as an expert witness on a case in New York City involving a malpractice suit of a woman who died after delivery due to infectious complications. Membership in a government or other advisory board: Dr. Cohen was a non-paid consultant on a WHO panel to assess the risk of hormonal contraception and HIV acquisition in women. All other authors have declared that no competing interests exist.

* Email: odeny@uw.edu

Introduction

Early diagnosis of HIV among infants born to HIV-positive mothers is a critical component of prevention of mother-to-child transmission of HIV (PMTCT) [1]. The World Health Organization (WHO) recommends that infants of HIV-infected women undergo HIV testing at six weeks. WHO estimates that in low- and middle-income countries in 2010, only 28% of HIV-exposed infants were tested for HIV within two months after birth [2]. Similarly, a high proportion of HIV-positive pregnant women are not retained in PMTCT programs after delivery [1,3–5]. One potential solution for improving maternal retention in PMTCT programs and increasing the rates of early infant HIV diagnosis is the use of mobile phone technology for health (mHealth). We have previously used text messaging to improve clinic return rates for other HIV prevention interventions [6]. The United Nations Children's Fund encourages PMTCT programs to utilize mobile phones in health interventions because of the high levels of access among enrolled mothers [7]. Mobile phones have successfully been used to support other aspects of HIV care and treatment. For example, two recent randomized controlled trials found that mobile phone text message interventions significantly improve adherence to antiretroviral therapy [8–10]. Despite strong evidence of efficacy, to our knowledge the theoretical foundations for these interventions have not been reported in the literature. This makes it difficult to interpret *why* the interventions were efficacious [11], and *how* they can best be transferred to other regions. Further, the authors of both landmark trials concede that mHealth interventions that affect behavior change in one context might not work in another [12]. SMS interventions, like other health behavioral interventions, need a theoretical framework to explain how each aspect of the intervention relates to each construct of the theory; in other words, a causal framework illustrating why a particular intervention is hypothesized to be successful [13,14]. If the theory can explain the *why*, then it might be possible to apply and adapt the framework to other health behaviors in other populations [11,15,16]. Despite a rich foundation in theory that has been developed to understand HIV-related sexual risk behavior change interventions [17], the application of behavioral theory to SMS intervention studies for HIV is nascent. Further, the qualitative process of developing SMS interventions in the HIV field is rarely documented. We address this gap by describing our process of developing a theory-informed SMS intervention. Our aim was to develop a set of individually tailored, culturally appropriate text messages targeted at improving uptake of infant HIV testing rates and maternal retention in PMTCT programs.

Methods

Setting

This study was conducted in the Nyanza region of Kenya, an area with high adult HIV prevalence in general (14%), and among pregnant women in particular (18%) [18,19]. Study participants were recruited from among patients and providers at health facilities supported by Family AIDS Care and Education Services, a President's Emergency Plan for AIDS Relief /Centers for Disease Control funded program which is implemented as a collaboration between the Kenya Medical Research Institute and and the University of California San Francisco [20]. These health facilities all offer PMTCT services, including testing for infant HIV infection.

Sampling design and participants

Purposive sampling was used to recruit participants for five focus group discussions (FGD). These groups were selected to represent the population of women who would be potential recipients of the text messages, and health workers who would interact with them routinely. General announcements were made asking women to take part in discussions to help design culturally appropriate, educational text messages for improving early infant diagnosis of HIV. Health workers at maternal and child health (MCH) clinics were approached in person by a member of the study team and invited to participate. Between eight and ten participants each were recruited for four different focus groups: health workers from maternal and child health clinics; women attending antenatal clinics; women attending postnatal clinics; women enrolled in PMTCT programs. Eight other women representing each of these four groups were recruited for a fifth follow up FGD to further develop, refine and pretest messages. We also purposively recruited four clinic staff members to participate in cognitive interviews for a final pretesting of messages. They were selected to represent both clinical and community health service providers with experience working in the study region.

Data collection

After completing their clinic visit or clinic duties for health workers, participants were brought to a private room where trained moderators led the discussions in English, Kiswahili, and Dholuo, the primary languages spoken in this region. In addition to a moderator, each focus group had a note-taker documenting the discussion in detail. All participants gave oral consent to participate in the study and were then assigned identification numbers that were used in place of their real names. Participant demographic information was then collected on a separate form, distinguishing each woman by her assigned identification number. Participants received a transport reimbursement of KSh250 (approximately US$3) and refreshments during the discussion.

The content of the study's structured focus group discussion guide was informed by the Health Belief Model [13,21,22], as well as findings of prior empirical research on factors that may influence attendance at postpartum clinic appointments and infant testing. We referred to the Family Health International handbook on focus group research [23]. The moderator introduced the project and described how the participants' general experiences and opinions would be helpful to design the SMS intervention, then introduced a series of topics approximately organized according to the constructs of the HBM, but permitting additional topics to emerge in the discussion. The first topic, *perceived susceptibility*, explored participants' perceptions of the risk of their (or others') children being HIV positive, and the risks associated with failure to attend maternal and child health clinics for early infant testing. Questions for the second topic, *perceived severity*, elicited participants' perceptions of the consequences of failure to attend clinic after delivery, and the consequences of HIV testing for infants. The third topic, *perceived benefits*, explored participants' beliefs about the reasons why women should return to clinic and bring their children for HIV testing following delivery, and their perceptions of the potential positive benefits of doing so. We further probed about the kinds of things that may need to be done in order for women to understand those benefits. For the fourth area, *perceived barriers*, we sought to determine the material costs, assumed by the mother, of returning to clinic after delivery and bringing her child for HIV testing. We also asked women to describe what might prevent them from returning to the clinic for themselves or their infant. We then probed about the kinds of assistance that women would need in order to help them overcome these challenges, whether related to incentives or messages of reassurance. The final discussion topic addressed both *cues to action* and *self-efficacy* [24,25]. To develop the best potential "cues to action", we asked participants specific questions concerning the kinds of text messages that would potentially help women and their families understand more about the importance of postnatal clinic visits and HIV testing for their children, including their content, timing, and frequency. To explore aspects of "self-efficacy", we asked participants what sorts of messages may best encourage women and elicit their self-confidence in their ability to attend postnatal clinic visits and bring their newborns in for HIV testing. Finally, before closing the discussion and thanking participants, the guide allowed participants to offer other ideas, besides sending messages, to help women return for post-natal clinic visits and bring their infants for HIV testing [13,22,26]. The focus group discussion questions are displayed in Table 1.

Data analysis, message development, and pretesting

Audio recordings from the FGDs were transcribed and then translated into English. The data were first coded and analyzed according to the construct of the HBM to which they were related. From these broad themes, sub-themes emerged through the context of the discussion that were used to design a sequence of focused text messages. The first draft of proposed messages were developed from the major themes and subthemes by a team of content experts. The team comprised a behavioral scientist and two physician-epidemiologists with expertise in the fields of HIV prevention and treatment, and experience in text messaging interventions for HIV prevention. The draft interventional SMS messages were then pretested in a follow-up focus group with systematically selected participants from each of the four groups (health workers from maternal and child health clinics, women attending antenatal, postnatal, and PMTCT clinics) in order to develop the optimal wording and phrasing of the messages in the

Table 1. Focus group discussion questions grouped by Health Belief Model constructs.

Perceived susceptibility
What do people think about women visiting clinics after giving birth?
What do people think about bringing children for HIV testing soon after birth?
In your community, who makes decisions about these things in a family? The husband? The wife? Or another family member?
Perceived severity
Why do some women fail to return to clinic after giving birth?
Why do you think some women fail to bring their children back to clinic for HIV testing after birth?
What are some of the consequences of failing to return to clinic after giving birth?
What are some of the consequences of failing to bring infants for HIV testing after birth?
What things can be done to help women return to the clinic after giving birth?
What things can be done to help women bring their infants for HIV testing?
Perceived benefits
What are some of the reasons why women should return to clinic after giving birth?
What are the potential positive results of returning to clinic after giving birth?
What are some of the reasons why women would want to bring infants for HIV testing after birth?
What are the potential positive results of bringing infants for HIV testing after birth?
What kinds of things may need to be done in order for women to understand the benefits of returning to clinic and bringing their infants for HIV testing?
Perceived barriers
What are some of the material costs related to returning to clinic after delivery and bringing infants for HIV testing? By material costs, I mean cost of transport, time taken away from work or other duties, and such like things, distance that you have to travel, and similar things.
What things would women worry about that would prevent them from returning to clinic, or prevent them from bringing their infants for HIV testing?
What kind of assistance would women need in order to help them overcome these challenges? Incentives? Reassurance?
Cues to action & Self-efficacy
If we were to send pregnant women SMS text messages, what are the kinds of messages that would help them and their families understand more about post-natal clinic visits and HIV testing for their infants? When should these messages be sent? What time in the post-partum period? What time of day? How frequently?
What kinds of messages would help them understand the importance of post-natal clinic visits and HIV testing for their infants?
What kinds of messages would help them understand the consequences of failure to attend clinic and/or bringing their infants for HIV testing? When should these messages be sent? What time in the post-partum period? What time of day? How frequently?
What kinds of messages do you think women may want to receive to help them better understand the potential benefits of returning to clinic and bringing their infants for HIV testing? When should these messages be sent? What time in the post-partum period? What time of day? How frequently?
Are there specific messages that you think women should receive to help them overcome material and psychological challenges that prevent them from either returning to clinic after delivery or bringing their infants for HIV testing? When should these messages be sent? What time in the post-partum period? What time of day? How frequently?
Apart from just sending messages, what are the other things that can be done to help women return for post-natal clinic visits and bring their infants for HIV testing?

three languages. We used a cognitive interviewing approach [27] for two stages of pretesting of the messages. First, participants were shown written examples on an easel notepad of different SMS messages (in English, Kiswahili, and Dholuo) to be used in the third trimester of pregnancy and the postpartum period. Participants were asked to comment on their understanding of and feelings toward the messages, as well as how to improve the text. During the discussion, the moderator edited the messages on the easel notepad in order for all the participants to see the changes and agree on the most appropriate text for each of the messages in all three languages. Participants were invited to write on the easel pad if they wished to edit the messages themselves. Following the development of the messages in the focus groups, we carried out a second pretesting of the messages in individual cognitive interviews with selected volunteer clinicians and non-clinical program staff members. These individuals included an expert in community liaison, a nurse experienced in providing clinical and community HIV prevention services, a local social scientist, and a community mobilizer/community health worker. Each individual further refined the messages, ensured that the word count was within the limits for a typical SMS, and ascertained that the translations between the three languages retained the same meaning. Their suggestions were then reviewed by the initial team of content experts, resulting in a final set of messages. The review of messages by health workers was limited to ensuring that the word count for SMS was acceptable, and that intended meanings were not lost in translation to the local languages.

Ethical review

This study was approved by the Ethical Review Committees of the Kenya Medical Research Institute, the Human Subjects Division at the University of Washington, and the University of California San Francisco Committee on Human Research. All participants provided oral informed consent. The ethical committees approved of this consent procedure. A waiver of the requirement to obtain written documentation of consent was allowed by the ethical review committees because the research presented no more than minimal risk of harm to subjects and involved no procedures for which written consent is normally required outside of the research context. In order to provide subjects with the required consent-related information about the research, we provided both an oral explanation of the research and a written information sheet. Specifically, the focus group moderator read out consent-related information to participants from an information sheet. Participants were informed that participation would be voluntary, discussions would be confidential, and that they could withdraw from the focus group at any time with no negative repercussions. The moderator then gave each participant a copy of the information sheet, which contained all consent-related information about the study including descriptions of the purpose of the focus groups, topics to be discussed, and expected risks and benefits. Participants were then individually asked for permission to take part in the discussion as part of the oral informed consent process.

Results

Participant characteristics

We conducted five focus group discussions, with a total of 41 participants. The median age was 28 years (inter-quartile range [IQR] 24–31), 34 (83%) were married, 39 (95%) were Christian, 27 (66%) were employed, and 24 (59%) had at least secondary-level education. The median number of living children reported was one (IQR 0–2). Participant characteristics for each focus group are summarized in Table 2.

Perceived susceptibility to, and severity of HIV and other childhood illnesses

In this high HIV prevalence area of Kenya, women often perceive themselves and their infants to be highly susceptible to HIV and other illnesses:

> *"When a mother fails to attend the clinics, she may be HIV positive yet she will just go and give birth then goes ahead to breastfeed this child. This is likely to cause HIV transmission to the child..." – 22 year old married participant (postnatal clinic)*
>
> *"If we leave out the issue of HIV, there are lots of things that can harm the baby... if he is not immunized with polio vaccine or the others which we know, the child may grow up in poor health and at the end he may even become paralyzed ..." – 35 year old married participant (PMTCT clinic)*

Fears of returning to clinic, and perceived consequences of failure to return

Participants noted that infant illness was the main consequence of failure to return to clinic after delivery. Women were aware of the severity of HIV infection for their infants. However, fears of HIV and of disclosure keep many women from returning to clinic for postpartum visits and infant HIV testing. Many women associate the clinic with learning one's HIV status,

Table 2. Participant characteristics.

	Health worker (n = 9)	Antenatal clinic attendees (n = 8)	Postnatal clinic attendees (n = 8)	*PMTCT clinic attendees (n = 8)	Mixed focus group (n = 8)	Overall (n = 41)
Characteristic	**n (%)**	**n (%)**	**n (%)**	**n (%)**	**n (%)**	**n (%)**
Age – median (inter-quartile range)	30 (29–40)	25 (21–28)	30 (28–36)	23 (21–25)	30 (28–36)	28 (24–31)
Married	4 (44)	7 (88)	8 (100)	7 (88)	8 (100)	34 (83)
Religion – Christian versus Other	9 (100)	8 (100)	7 (88)	8 (100)	7 (88)	39 (95)
Education – secondary or higher	9 (100)	4 (50)	3 (38)	5 (63)	3 (38)	24 (59)
Living children – median (inter-quartile range)	2 (0–2)	0 (0–2)	2 (1–4)	1 (1–2)	2 (1–4)	1 (1–2)

*PMTCT, Prevention of mother-to-child transmission of HIV.

and even death. Those who have yet to disclose their status to their partners fear they will have to reveal that they are positive if they go to the clinic for delivery or postpartum visits.

> *"On many occasions I see people prefer mostly the traditional birth attendant...these ones do not ask you about your status... If I go back to hospital I will discover the baby's status and know mine again. Therefore, I would rather stay there to avoid much stress." – 27 year old participant (antenatal clinic)*

Several HIV-positive women reported fearing that if they return to the clinic to have their child tested, they will learn that their infant is also HIV-positive. These women discussed how knowing that HIV infection tends to exact a more severe toll on children may make women feel anxious or psychologically disturbed. Participants were aware that HIV positive children who fail to return to clinic for HIV diagnosis are more likely to fall sick and require hospitalization than those who return to clinic and undergo early infant HIV diagnosis. This also leads to higher financial costs:

> *"...the consequence of not going to the clinic is that you may require to use more money, you may even require to sell a cow if you had one, if the baby is in the ward for treatment. This implies that you ought to have gone to hospital to avoid using a lot of money..." – 28 year old participant (antenatal clinic)*

Most participants identified, in particular, lack of information, transport costs, religious beliefs, fear of HIV testing, and fear of disclosure of HIV status, as important barriers to postnatal clinic attendance. In addition, young mothers may be unaware of the importance of antenatal, delivery, and postpartum care, or may be dissuaded by other mothers who never took their children to a clinic.

Participants reported that some women might opt to visit traditional healers due to the cost and time necessary to travel to a clinic and to take time off of work. Participants felt that women worry about the long queues at the clinic and having to wait for hours to be seen by a clinician, often missing work or leaving other children at home. Many women live in remote areas and travel long distances to arrive at the clinic. Moreover, participants complained that the line to wait to be seen at the clinic can be six to eight hours.

> *"These nurses ... are not ready to serve you. When it is time for lunch they slip away ... leaving you there waiting. Such kind of things can discourage one and make her become reluctant in going to the clinic because when you come you cannot get the appropriate services." – 35 year old participant (PMTCT clinic)*

While lack of information, cost, travel time, and wait time impede many women from attending, participants noted that failure to go to the clinic may result in complications that require hospitalization which ultimately accrues a significantly higher cost for the family.

Perceived benefits

Benefits of returning to clinic after birth. The majority of participants recognized infant and maternal wellness as the central positive outcomes of returning to clinic after giving birth. They identified immunization and HIV testing for infants, nutritional counseling and maternal health assessment as benefits of clinic return. Participants also noted that the clinic teaches HIV-positive women about family planning methods and how to exclusively breastfeed to minimize HIV transmission.

> *"If you bring the baby to the clinic, you do so to check on his status. First of all you get information that when you deliver, you bring the baby to the clinic and you are taught how to take care of him, what to do if you have to breastfeed him even when you have to be away from home...." – 30 year old participant (PMTCT clinic)*
>
> *"Another fact that I think is making these mothers to come is family planning. I realize that a good number of them are starting to practice family planning methods...." – 29 year old female nurse (health worker)*

Participants noted that in addition to detecting early childhood illness, if a child is identified as HIV-positive, then the clinic team can discuss and apply necessary medical interventions. If the child is found to be HIV-negative, then it is important to continue educating the mother and monitoring the child to prevent mother-to-child transmission.

Finally some women highlighted that a child is "innocent" and at the whims of his caregivers to provide the optimum care, and therefore should have the opportunity to be tested for HIV to enable early and preventative treatment.

> *"It is never a good thing, especially for the innocent child—because for you, you may have known your status then decline to take the baby there to be tested so that when found positive, he may be put on care early enough, together with the appropriate treatment. That way, you make a mistake for the baby, because if he is infected, you will neglect his health just like that. And if he is not infected, maybe he has been born free of HIV but [the] breastfeeding and mixed feeding you do to him will compromise his health. This is not good— it may have a bad outcome." – 36 year old participant (PMTCT clinic)*

Perceived barriers: health systems and structural

Participants cited a range of practical, social, and psychological barriers many women face in attending clinic during the postpartum period. Participants identified poor communication between patients and healthcare workers as a barrier to getting a referral to a clinic closer to one's home. Participants explained that when nurses and clinical officers take the time to talk with and explain to women the specific reasons for coming back to the clinic, they often do. Yet, participants explained that the care in the clinic is often given without sympathy, and the medical personnel can be unfriendly and discouraging:

> *"... we need friendly grounds. When I get to the clinic and realize I'm being treated unfairly, I may not come. You know we are also like babies, we also need people who care.... So the kind of clinic we may want to have are those that have friendly nurses to treat us well.... Let them understand each one of us because we are different." – 27 year old participant (antenatal clinic)*

"I think one issue that can make these mothers remember to come back to clinic, we have to be friendly to them.... 'Cause if you talk to her rudely or you are cruel to her, she might not feel like coming back, so we have to be friendly." – 43 year old female nurse (health worker)

In addition to recommending that clinic staff should be more warm and compassionate to patients, participants offered numerous suggestions for how to help women overcome many of these material barriers that challenge women's ability to get to clinic. Participants suggested increasing the number of staff at the clinic to reduce wait times, building more health facilities to improve accessibility, and sending text message reminders.

Providing cues to action and enhancing self-efficacy

The majority of participants identified education of pregnant women as one of the things that could be done to help women return to clinic after birth. Participants suggested that health workers should provide information and motivate women early in the pregnancy about the importance and reasons to return for infant testing, as well as the potential consequences of failing to return.

"If they know the reason why they are coming then they will be coming. [If] the right information is given, a return date is given, that by this date you are supposed to come back, then they will be able to come." – 24 year old female nurse (health worker)
"I think the mothers who do not want to bring their babies to the clinic should be given appropriate education on the benefits of taking the baby to the clinic, and what might happen if they do not take them." – 32 year old participant (postnatal)

Moreover, participants felt that health workers should emphasize the importance of involving and educating the partners in the decision to return to the clinic for infant testing to help remind and support the mothers to ensure the safety of the child.

"Involving the partners ...I used to see in another clinic, whereby when the mother comes for the first antenatal clinic visit they type some letters. Like every woman takes a letter to the husband, so that the next visit the husband accompanies the partner to the clinic." – 40 year old female nurse (health worker)
"I feel it may be possible for a man to take responsibility of telling the woman to go to the clinic when the woman discloses her status to him so that he also joins in." – 36 year old participant (PMTCT clinic)

Potential channels of information

Participants offered many suggestions regarding methods that can be used to provide important information for women, including phone reminders (text messages and phone calls) from the clinic.

"If they have disclosed maybe you can text a message like maybe a reminder. Maybe she was supposed to come to the clinic today and by evening she's not come, so you are going through the files and you've realized she's not come. So you can send a message like, "Hi, you were supposed to report to the clinic today. Why didn't you make it?" – 31 year old female clinical officer (health worker)
"What could remind a mother who has delivered or an expectant mother to come back to the hospital is just to take the phone numbers of the patients. I mean we should avail them at the PMTCT office so that if you miss your appointment, it makes it easy for them to call and remind you" – 36 year old participant (PMTCT clinic)

Some participants suggested that nurses communicate and work with traditional birth attendants to help urge women to go to the clinic after they have delivered. Several women suggested other forms of community involvement, such as through "mentor mothers" who can identify with the pregnant woman and inspire them through their own experience of taking their children to be tested, as well as through community gatherings of mothers (e.g., led by a chief or at a church) expressing the importance of going to the clinic after delivery.

"The use of mentor mothers can go a long way because they are living examples. It is easier for someone to identify with someone who has the same problem as them. The mentor mothers are positive who have success stories of how they took care of their children and how the children turned out negative." – 29 year old female nurse (health workers)
"The nurses can get in touch with the traditional birth attendants to invite the mothers who are not willing to go the clinic." – 23 year old participant (postnatal clinic)

Participants' recommendations for messaging content

Table S1 contains a selection of quotes offered by focus group participants to support the inclusion of major themes into intervention text messages. In addition to exploring these topics, FGDs incorporated participants' specific suggestions for the content of text messages and schedule for their delivery in the intervention. Participants preferred messages that congratulated women on their delivery and those that had a personal touch. They suggested that text messages that were caring, polite, and encouraging would persuade women to return to clinic after giving birth. As one 27-year old woman mentioned, "First of all I may really want someone to congratulate me because this journey is really long, to reach the destination is no joke...I'll feel happy 'cause we all need to be congratulated for the success." Other comments included:

"Everybody would wish to be loved...Meaning, the first word you use must sound loving... You may use words like 'please', 'kindly' and others like these. It could be one word that can generalize the others and after putting it that way, she will say for sure this person has talked to me politely and humbly." – 35 year old participant (PMTCT clinic)
"...Being polite is very important... when you speak with people they associate hospitals—sadly, government hospitals – with people that are rude.... They need that touch; we need to be polite to the person who is coming. That will make the person come back." – 30 year old male doctor (health worker)

Several participants emphasized the importance of brief educational messages. One 20-year old woman said, "... it should be an educative message and should be precise, I mean very short," and a 35-year old participant noted that, "You know SMS is a brief statement and you cannot make it too long. You just have to look for few words which can comfort someone or sound polite."

According to most participants, potential messages should begin with a greeting, include the woman's name, congratulate her, ask if she has attended clinic, and give a brief educational message or appointment reminder, as illustrated in the following quotes:

"You should be positive, you know; somehow, a positive message trying to convince them why it is important for them to come. Also important for someone to take a message very seriously: that personal touch. If you could put someone's name, like say she's called Mary. Use the name 'Dear Mary'..." – 30 year old male doctor (health worker)

"You know if one calls you by name you know at least they recognize you and it is not like they sent the SMS for granted. So that would mean they know me and want me to go. In the first place, that would motivate me to go." – 27 year old participant (antenatal clinic)

There was consensus that messages should be sent in the daytime, preferably during regular work hours.

"Definitely during the day." – 40 year old nurse (health worker)

"...Office hours, eight or seven to six. I think that's going to be the best time, reason being that you know when you get a message and you don't know the number, people usually call back." – 30 year old male doctor (health worker)

"Any time from eight to eight because at night people sleep early and so they do not even bother to read." – 27 year old participant (antenatal clinic)

Participants suggested that women may need to receive messages a few days before the appointment date to enable them to prepare. One 22-year old woman said, "Not immediately but when her appointment date is close by, maybe three days to, or one week to." Other illustrative quotes were:

"It should be sent a day before, like it should be sent today if you were to go tomorrow to enable you to prepare early." – 24 year old participant (postnatal clinic)

"I would prefer to be reminded maybe three days in advance so that one may prepare herself even financially." – 27 year old participant (antenatal clinic)

Participants emphasized that text messages should not mention HIV or HIV testing as a reason for clinic return.

"But you should not send one like this, 'Please come; bring the baby for HIV test. ' No!" – 22 year old participant (antenatal clinic)

"I believe that an SMS...can land anywhere...A message has no secret so if I tell you that you are HIV positive kindly come for testing, you know that one will demoralize me and I may faint, because that is my status which I wouldn't have wanted to share with another person." – 27 year old participant (antenatal clinic)

In addition to SMS messages, women also suggested using other media, such as educational posters at marketplaces and messages over radio and television, which would be sure to reach women without phones and those in rural areas. Moreover, some participants proposed working with community leaders, such as the chief or an elder to help remind people.

The research team utilized these findings to craft a set of text messages and a schedule for their delivery. The first draft of interventional SMS text messages was presented in follow-up FGDs with selected participants from each of the groupings in order to develop optimal phrasing in local languages. On the basis of findings of this first stage of pretesting, we then further refined the messages, and pretested them in individual cognitive interviews [27] with selected volunteer clinicians and non-clinical program staff members. After a final stage of analysis and refinement, the messages were finalized for the intervention. Table 3 contains the final set of text messages. A total of 14 text messages were developed to be sent during the third trimester of pregnancy (weeks 28, 30, 32, 34, 36, 38, 39, and 40), and weekly for the first six weeks after delivery. Messages were personalized by having an option to insert the recipient's name (or their infant's name) and were translated into Kiswahili and Dholuo.

Discussion

In this study, we used a multi-stage content development approach to crafting SMS text messages, informed by behavioral theory and prior empirical research. We found that applying this careful and theoretically informed approach resulted in message content that was consistent across different focus groups. We identified certain key themes that we felt would be useful in the design of text messaging content, as they may facilitate women's self-confidence and perceived self-efficacy to attend clinic, reduce or minimize potential fears, and provide "cues to action". These included maximizing "a personal touch" in messaging, encouragement and validation of the patient, and content that suggested that health care workers were caring and loving toward their patients. Participants held a strong consensus that personalized and caring messages would provide a stimulus to trigger women to take the necessary action of attending clinic. For women who fear knowing the HIV status of their children, such messages could potentially reduce their fears and increase their confidence.

It emerged that reminders about immunizations might help build on women's already clear sense of susceptibility to disease and knowledge of the benefits of treatment. This mix of perceived susceptibility and benefit of immunization can be leveraged to get women back to the clinic, with SMS text messages functioning as "cues to action". In other cases, findings pointed to stigma as a major barrier to follow-up. Participants unanimously recommended to never use the word "HIV" or other terminology that would suggest HIV testing or infection. The high level of perceived HIV stigma expressed by the participants in our study is consistent with prior research among pregnant women in the Nyanza region [19]; a recent study among women attending antenatal clinics found that 32% anticipated break-up of their relationship, and 45% anticipated losing their friends, if they were to test HIV positive. Women who anticipated negative responses from male partners were especially likely to refuse HIV testing. Our study further suggests that the decision to have infants tested for HIV is intertwined with other issues related to testing and disclosure faced by women, who must often navigate between their fears of HIV/AIDS stigma, the threat of violence from male partners, and their desire to protect their infants from HIV infection. At the same time, many participants felt that involvement of male partners

Table 3. Intervention text messages.

Gestation Week	Message
28	Hi [name]! Congratulations for visiting clinic this week! Please call or flash 0788100133 if you have questions about your pregnancy. We're here to help you!
30	Hi [name]. We wish you a good and healthy pregnancy. We are here to support you during this journey. If you have questions please call or flash 0788100133
32	Hi [name]! We would like to wish you a good day. Please remember that if you have questions about your pregnancy, you can call or flash 0788100133
34	Good day [name]! Have you visited the mother and child care clinic lately? If not, please feel welcome to visit. Call or flash 0788100133 for questions
36	Greetings [name]! We are here for you if you have any questions about your pregnancy. Please call or flash or send a please call me to 0788100133
38	Hello [name]! Have you planned where you will deliver your baby? Please call or flash 0788100133 if you have questions or want to discuss your options
39	Hi [name], We wish you a healthy pregnancy and safe delivery! If you would like to plan your delivery, call or flash or send please call me to 0788100133
40	Hi [name], We wish you a healthy pregnancy and safe delivery! If you would like to plan your delivery, call or flash or send please call me to 0788100133
Weeks after delivery	
1	Dear [name], congratulations on the birth of baby [babyname]! We treasure you both! If you have questions about baby's health please call or flash 0788100133
2	Dear [name], your baby [boy/girl] will need immunization at 6 weeks of age to prevent childhood diseases and grow healthy and strong. Please call or flash 0788100133 to find out more about baby's clinic schedule. Thank you
3	Hi [name]! How are you & baby [babyname]? We know you're working hard to care for [babyname]. If you have any fever, pain or bleeding, please come to clinic
4	Dear [name], your baby [boy/girl] is now one month old. Congratulations! Please remember to have enough rest and sleep to keep yourself healthy
5	Hi [name]! How are you and baby [babyname]? Your baby needs to be immunized to prevent childhood diseases. Kindly bring baby to clinic next week. See you then!
6	Hi [name]! This week, please bring baby [babyname] to clinic for important immunizations to prevent childhood diseases and make sure [babyname] grows up healthy and strong. You will also be counselled on how to keep your baby [boy/girl] healthy

greatly enhances the support that pregnant and postpartum women need with regard to clinic attendance, and that male partners may even take the responsibility of reminding women about clinic visits. Involving male partners could also potentially help to reduce stigma as it could permit a safer space in which marital partners can learn each other's status, and support each other with disclosure and coping with the community around them [19]. In sum, text messaging interventions need to be designed in a way that supports the involvement of men as partners, while being sensitive to the reality that women are at risk of domestic violence.

In the end, our SMS text messaging intervention was designed carefully to minimize women's fears of HIV testing and risks of disclosure – no text messages referred to HIV testing directly. We encouraged women to visit the clinic as scheduled, and provided them a service for texting or calling to ask questions or receive additional information from a clinician. Further, we ensured that text messages were brief and began with a greeting. Messages sent in the post-partum period congratulated mothers and encouraged them to get their children immunized. We also provide a description of the process used to craft these messages (summarized in Figure 1) that would permit replication in other settings.

This study had several limitations. First, given the limited financial resources available, we recruited participants passively and only included women who were present at the clinics. This might have resulted in more informed, motivated women being included. Women who fail to attend clinic might have different perceptions about the use of text messages to improve clinic return and uptake of early infant diagnosis. Similarly, FGD responses may be biased in favor of participants willing to participate in group activities and therefore more likely to have disclosed their status. Second, we did not involve men in any of the patient discussion groups, or have a separate discussion with men. It emerged that male involvement may be a strong determinant of women's ability to make decisions surrounding their health and that of their children. However, our focus group with health workers included male providers who were able to give both professional and personal opinions. Third, participants were all recruited from urban clinics. Women from rural areas also stand to benefit from interventions to improve clinic return, and their input would be useful in crafting messaging content. Finally, although participants generally agreed on the preferred time of day for receiving messages, no consensus emerged regarding the frequency of messages. Other studies have shown that less frequent messages have a stronger association with good clinical outcomes [9]. This informed our final decision to use two-weekly intervals during pregnancy, and weekly intervals after delivery. Our findings might be important for dissemination and implementation practice as relates to mHealth interventions to support HIV programs, providing a model for a multi-stage, theoretically-informed approach to SMS messaging content development. Using theory-based methods could help to answer the "why"

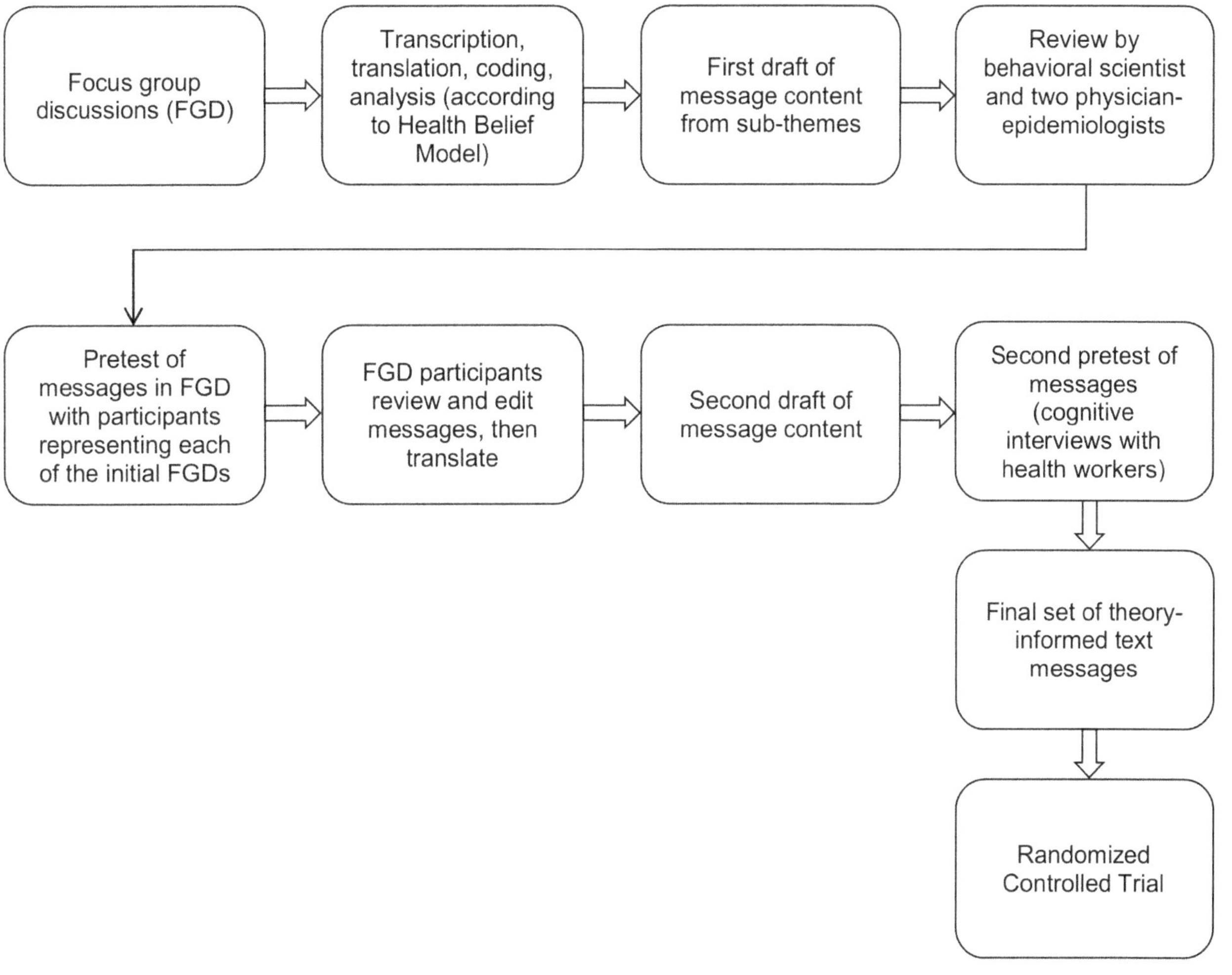

Figure 1. Process of crafting and refining text message content. HBM, Health Belief Model; FGD, Focus Group Discussion.

when such interventions are successful. Insight from theory-based research could therefore help to understand the effectiveness of mHealth interventions and inform expansion and replication in different regions and settings.

Conclusions

Text messages may prove useful as a tool to promote and support clinic attendance for pregnant and postpartum women, and to improve the rates of early infant diagnosis. Involving potential message recipients in the design of the intervention by having them craft and refine the actual content of messages, and underpinning the process on sound behavioral theory, resulted in more relevant content for engaging the target audience. Importantly, since our process of crafting these messages was founded on a theoretical framework, it is possible to explain *how* and *why* they can potentially result in behavior change. This also makes it possible for our intervention, and our methods of intervention development, to be adapted for use in other regions and in different contexts. We are evaluating the effect of these messages on improving retention in postpartum HIV care for mother-infant pairs in a randomized trial [28].

Supporting Information

Table S1 Representative recommendations offered by focus group participants.

Acknowledgments

We thank the Director, Kenya Medical Research Institute, for permission to publish this work. We would like to thank the following study staff members: Perez Ochwal, Patrick Mbullo, and Joel Odondi. We thank Eliud Akama, Lisa Abuogi, Patrick Oyaro, and the staff of the Family AIDS Care and Education Services for their collaboration.

Author Contributions

Conceived and designed the experiments: TAO EAB RSM CRC CSC. Performed the experiments: TAO MN RSM CSC. Analyzed the data: TAO MN RSM CSC. Contributed reagents/materials/analysis tools: TAO EAB CRC. Contributed to the writing of the manuscript: TAO MN EAB RSM CRC CSC. Conceptualized, designed, interpreted results: TAO EAB RSM CRC CSC. Collected and analyzed data: TAO MN RSM CSC. Drafted manuscript or revised it critically for important intellectual content: TAO MN EAB RSM CRC CSC. Read and approved the final manuscript: TAO MN EAB RSM CRC CSC.

References

1. Perez F, Orne-Gliemann J, Mukotekwa T, Miller A, Glenshaw M, et al. (2004) Prevention Of Mother To Child Transmission Of Hiv: Evaluation Of A Pilot Programme In A District Hospital In Rural Zimbabwe. Bmj (Clinical Research Ed) 329: 1147.
2. Unaids (2011) Epidemic Update And Health Sector Progress Towards Universal Access. Global Hiv/Aids Response.
3. Nassali M, Nakanjako D, Kyabayinze D, Beyeza J, Okoth A, et al. (2009) Access To Hiv/Aids Care For Mothers And Children In Sub-Saharan Africa: Adherence To The Postnatal Pmtct Program. Aids Care 21: 1124–1131.
4. Manzi M, Zachariah R, Teck R, Buhendwa L, Kazima J, et al. (2005) High Acceptability Of Voluntary Counselling And Hiv-Testing But Unacceptable Loss To Follow Up In A Prevention Of Mother-To-Child Hiv Transmission Programme In Rural Malawi: Scaling-Up Requires A Different Way Of Acting. Trop Med Int Health 10: 1242–1250.
5. Rawizza H, Meloni S, Oyebode T, Sagay S, Adewole I, et al. (2012) Evaluation Of Loss To Follow-Up Within The Pmtct Care Cascade In A Large Art Program: Nigeria. 19th Conference On Retroviruses And Opportunistic Infections Paper #1017. Seattle, Washington, Usa.
6. Odeny Ta, Bailey Rc, Bukusi Ea, Simoni Jm, Tapia Ka, et al. (2012) Text Messaging To Improve Attendance At Post-Operative Clinic Visits After Adult Male Circumcision For Hiv Prevention: A Randomized Controlled Trial. Plos One 7: E43832.
7. Elhadj As (2010) Opening Remarks By Unicef Regional Director Elhadj As Sy At The Global Fund Pmtct Meeting. Http//Www.Unicef.Org/Esaro/5440_6380.Html.
8. Lester Rt, Ritvo P, Mills Ej, Kariri A, Karanja S, et al. (2010) Effects Of A Mobile Phone Short Message Service On Antiretroviral Treatment Adherence In Kenya (Weltel Kenya1): A Randomised Trial. Lancet 376: 1838–1845.
9. Pop-Eleches C, Thirumurthy H, Habyarimana Jp, Zivin Jg, Goldstein Mp, et al. (2011) Mobile Phone Technologies Improve Adherence To Antiretroviral Treatment In A Resource-Limited Setting: A Randomized Controlled Trial Of Text Message Reminders. Aids (London, England) 25: 825.
10. Horvath T, Azman H, Kennedy Ge, Rutherford Gw (2012) Mobile Phone Text Messaging For Promoting Adherence To Antiretroviral Therapy In Patients With Hiv Infection. Cochrane Database Of Systematic Reviews (Online) 3: Cd009756.
11. Chi Bh, Stringer Js (2010) Mobile Phones To Improve Hiv Treatment Adherence. Lancet 376: 1807.
12. Thirumurthy H, Lester Rt (2012) M-Health For Health Behaviour Change In Resource-Limited Settings: Applications To Hiv Care And Beyond. Bulletin Of The World Health Organization 90: 390.
13. Glanz K, Rimer Bk (1997) Theory At A Glance: A Guide For Health Promotion Practice: U.S. Dept. Of Health And Human Services Public Health Service National Institutes Of Health National Cancer Institute.
14. The Pme (2013) A Reality Checkpoint For Mobile Health: Three Challenges To Overcome. Plos Med 10: E1001395.
15. Coomes Cm, Lewis Ma, Uhrig Jd, Furberg Rd, Harris Jl, et al. (2012) Beyond Reminders: A Conceptual Framework For Using Short Message Service To Promote Prevention And Improve Healthcare Quality And Clinical Outcomes For People Living With Hiv. Aids Care 24: 348–357.
16. Riley Wt, Rivera De, Atienza Aa, Nilsen W, Allison Sm, et al. (2011) Health Behavior Models In The Age Of Mobile Interventions: Are Our Theories Up To The Task? Transl Behav Med 1: 53–71.
17. Catania Ja, Kegeles Sm, Coates Tj (1990) Towards An Understanding Of Risk Behavior: An Aids Risk Reduction Model (Arrm). Health Educ Q 17: 53–72.
18. (2010) Kenya Demographic And Health Survey 2008-09. Calverton, Maryland: Kenya National Bureau Of Statistics (Knbs) And Icf Macro.
19. Turan Jm, Bukusi Ea, Onono M, Holzemer Wl, Miller S, et al. (2011) Hiv/Aids Stigma And Refusal Of Hiv Testing Among Pregnant Women In Rural Kenya: Results From The Mamas Study. Aids Behav 15: 1111–1120.
20. Lewis Kulzer J, Penner Ja, Marima R, Oyaro P, Oyanga Ao, et al. (2012) Family Model Of Hiv Care And Treatment: A Retrospective Study In Kenya. J Int Aids Soc 15: 8.
21. Rosenstock I, Strecher V, Becker M (1994) The Health Belief Model And Hiv Risk Behavior Change; Diclemente Rj, Peterson Jl, Editors: Springer.
22. Janz Nk, Becker Mh (1984) The Health Belief Model: A Decade Later. Health Education Quarterly 11: 1.
23. Mack N, Woodsong C, Macqueen Km, Guest G, Namely E (2005) Qualitative Research Methods: A Data Collector's Field Guide. Research Triangle Park, North Carolina: Family Health International.
24. Bandura A, Mcclelland Dc (1977) Social Learning Theory.
25. Bandura A (1989) Perceived Self-Efficacy In The Exercise Of Control Over Aids Infection. In: Mays Vm, Albee Gw, Schneider Sf, Editors.Primary Prevention Of Aids: Psychological Approaches.London: Sage Publications, Inc. Pp. 128–141.
26. Rosenstock Im, Strecher Vj, Becker Mh (1988) Social Learning Theory And The Health Belief Model. Health Education Quarterly 15: 175.
27. Tourangeau R (1984) Cognitive Sciences And Survey Methods. In: Jabine T, Straf M, Tanur J, Tourangeau R, Editors.Cognitive Aspects Of Survey Methodology: Building A Bridge Between Disciplines: Report Of The Advanced Research Seminar On Cognitive Aspects Of Survey Methodology: National Academies. Pp.73–100.
28. Odeny T, Bukusi E, Cohen C, Camlin C, Yuhas K, et al. (2014) Texting Improves Testing: A Randomized Trial Of 2-Way Sms To Increase Postpartum Pmtct Retention And Infant Hiv Testing. Aids: In Press.

19

Antiretroviral Therapy Uptake, Attrition, Adherence and Outcomes among HIV-Infected Female Sex Workers

Elisa Mountain[1]*, Sharmistha Mishra[1,2,3], Peter Vickerman[4], Michael Pickles[1], Charles Gilks[5], Marie-Claude Boily[1]

1 Department of Infectious Disease Epidemiology, Imperial College London, London, United Kingdom, **2** Division of Infectious Diseases, St. Michael's Hospital, University of Toronto, Toronto, Canada, **3** Li Ka Shing Knowledge Institute, University of Toronto, Toronto, Canada, **4** School of Social and Community Medicine, University of Bristol, Bristol, United Kingdom, **5** School of Population Health, University of Queensland, Brisbane, Australia

Abstract

Purpose: We aimed to characterize the antiretroviral therapy (ART) cascade among female sex workers (FSWs) globally.

Methods: We systematically searched PubMed, Embase and MEDLINE in March 2014 to identify studies reporting on ART uptake, attrition, adherence, and outcomes (viral suppression or CD4 count improvements) among HIV-infected FSWs globally. When possible, available estimates were pooled using random effects meta-analyses (with heterogeneity assessed using Cochran's Q test and I^2 statistic).

Results: 39 studies, reporting on 21 different FSW study populations in Asia, Africa, North America, South America, and Central America and the Caribbean, were included. Current ART use among HIV-infected FSWs was 38% (95% CI: 29%–48%, $I^2 = 96\%$, 15 studies), and estimates were similar between high-, and low- and middle-income countries. Ever ART use among HIV-infected FSWs was greater in high-income countries (80%; 95% CI: 48%–94%, $I^2 = 70\%$, 2 studies) compared to low- and middle-income countries (36%; 95% CI: 7%–81%, $I^2 = 99\%$, 3 studies). Loss to follow-up after ART initiation was 6% (95% CI: 3%–11%, $I^2 = 0\%$, 3 studies) and death after ART initiation was 6% (95% CI: 3%–11%, $I^2 = 0\%$, 3 studies). The fraction adherent to ≥95% of prescribed pills was 76% (95% CI: 68%–83%, $I^2 = 36\%$, 4 studies), and 57% (95% CI: 46%–68%, $I^2 = 82\%$, 4 studies) of FSWs on ART were virally suppressed. Median gains in CD4 count after 6 to 36 months on ART, ranged between 103 and 241 cells/mm^3 (4 studies).

Conclusions: Despite global increases in ART coverage, there is a concerning lack of published data on HIV treatment for FSWs. Available data suggest that FSWs can achieve levels of ART uptake, retention, adherence, and treatment response comparable to that seen among women in the general population, but these data are from only a few research settings. More routine programme data on HIV treatment among FSWs across settings should be collected and disseminated.

Editor: Nicolas Sluis-Cremer, University of Pittsburgh, United States of America

Funding: This work was funded by the Canadian Foundation for AIDS Research (CANFAR) (grant # 023-015), and UNAIDS. The funders had no role in study design, data collection and analysis, decision to publish, or preparation of the manuscript.

Competing Interests: The authors have declared that no competing interests exist.

* Email: elisa.mountain08@imperial.ac.uk

Introduction

By reducing HIV viral load and helping to restore immune function, antiretroviral therapy (ART) has led to substantial reductions in HIV-attributable mortality and morbidity and has greatly improved the quality of life for people living with HIV. Evidence also indicates that individuals on effective ART are less likely to transmit HIV [1–5]. This evidence has sparked great interest in ART-based HIV prevention approaches, including 'Treatment as Prevention' (TasP), which aims to expand ART coverage among HIV-infected individuals in order to help reduce HIV transmission at a population level [6].

Successful treatment can sustain viral suppression and lead to immunological improvement among those that are HIV-infected, but requires that individuals engage and remain in the HIV care cascade. This cascade involves a series of actions, starting with HIV screening/testing, and followed by linkage to HIV care after HIV diagnosis, retention in pre-ART care prior to ART initiation, initiation of ART once eligible for treatment, retention on treatment once ART is started, and then maintenance of good ART adherence in order to achieve viral suppression and immunological improvement [7–9]. However, evidence indicates that many individuals are lost at each stage of the cascade, and many individuals are diagnosed late, only initiating ART at the onset of symptoms [8–11].

Female sex workers (FSWs) are a population at high risk of acquiring and transmitting HIV infection, and in many HIV epidemics bear a disproportionately larger burden of HIV [12–14]. Worldwide, the HIV prevalence among FSWs is 12%, ranging between 1.7% in the Middle East and North Africa to 36.9% in Sub-Saharan Africa, and FSWs have a pooled odds ratio of HIV infection compared to women in the general population of 14 [13]. Thus, FSWs remain a key population for HIV prevention strategies. Ensuring high levels of ART uptake, adherence and retention among FSWs, would provide not only individual benefits to HIV-infected FSWs, but could also help reduce HIV transmission at the population level [15,16].

With the high burden of HIV among FSWs and the potential merits of expanding ART in populations at high risk of transmitting HIV [15,17], it is crucial to understand the extent to which FSWs currently access ART, and continue ART with good adherence. We conducted a systematic review to summarise the existing information on the following events in the HIV care cascade among FSWs globally: ART uptake, ART attrition, adherence, and treatment response (viral suppression and CD4 count improvements).

Methods

Our systematic review and meta-analysis was conducted and reported in accordance with PRISMA and MOOSE guidelines (see Checklist S1) [18,19].

Search Strategy

Our search strategy was conducted in three stages. First, we searched PubMed, Embase and MEDLINE for studies published up until 10th March 2014. The search terms (keywords and medical subject heading terms) reflected three key domains: HIV/AIDS, FSWs and ART (see Table 1 for combinations of search terms used). There were no language restrictions. Following removal of duplicate references, abstracts were screened for exclusion. If studies were not excluded after abstract screening, the full text of the article was retrieved and evaluated for eligibility. Second, we hand-searched the reference lists of all eligible studies and relevant review articles identified in the database search for additional publications. Finally, for completion, whenever an eligible study analysed data from a specific FSW cohort, a supplementary database search was conducted, using the name and location of the FSW cohort and corresponding author names as search terms, to find any additional publications. Authors were contacted for additional information and supplementary data when needed. One reviewer conducted the search, reviewed abstracts, and evaluated full text articles for eligibility. Any queries on article eligibility were discussed and resolved with other team members.

Inclusion and Exclusion Criteria

We included observational or intervention studies with a sample size of at least 10 FSWs that reported estimates or sufficient data to derive the following ART cascade outcomes: ART uptake (specifically the fraction of all HIV-infected individuals or the fraction of all ART-eligible individuals, who either initiated ART within a specified follow-up period, currently use ART, or ever used ART (no time-frame for ART initiation specified)), ART attrition (specifically the fraction using ART who were either lost-to-follow-up, died or discontinued ART, or the fraction of treatment-experienced individuals no longer on ART), ART adherence (specifically the fraction achieving a predefined threshold of adherence e.g. ≥90%, ≥95%, 100%), viral suppression (specifically the fraction with undetectable plasma viral load following ART initiation), and CD4 counts at and/or after ART initiation (specifically the median CD4 count, median CD4 count gain, or fraction with CD4 counts <200, 200–499 or >500 cells/mm^3). We included studies which reported on the same study population if the studies provided estimates of different ART cascade outcomes for that study population or provided estimates for that study population on the same ART cascade outcome over different time periods.

We included studies that enrolled active or former FSWs, women who engage in sex work or transactional sex, or women who exchange sex for money, drugs or gifts. "Active" FSWs were defined as women who either reported sex work as their employment at enrolment, or within the previous 6 months. "Former" FSWs were those that either reported sex work as a former occupation at enrolment, reported transactional sex more than 6 months ago, or were no longer sexually active. We excluded review articles, mathematical modelling studies, qualitative studies and conference/oral/poster abstracts.

Data Extraction

One reviewer extracted data from included articles, and any queries during data extraction were discussed and resolved with other team members. Variables extracted included study characteristics (e.g. study design, study period and sample size of FSWs), participant characteristics (e.g. HIV status and illicit drug use), outcome estimates (or the data to calculate them), and the time period over which estimates were measured. Exact binomial confidence intervals (CI) for proportions were derived when not provided. Each study could provide information on multiple ART cascade outcomes and/or on the same ART cascade outcome over different time periods. Multiple studies could provide different ART cascade estimates for the same study population.

We also extracted information on ART initiation criteria and ART administration in order to provide a background to the local context for included studies. To assess risk of bias in included

Table 1. Search Terms Used For Search Strategy.

Domain	Search Terms
HIV	"HIV" OR "human immunodeficiency virus" OR "AIDS" OR "acquired immune deficiency syndrome"
	AND
FSWs	"FSW" OR "FSWs" OR "CSW" OR "CSWs" OR "commercial sex" OR "female sex worker*" OR "commercial sex work*" OR "sex-work*" OR "sexwork*" OR "sex work*" OR "prostitute*" OR "prostitution" OR "transactional sex" OR "paid sex" OR "money for sex" OR "sex for money" OR "paid for sex" OR "sex in exchange for money" OR (("core group" OR "high risk" OR "high-risk" OR highrisk") AND ("female*" OR "women" or "woman"))
	AND
ART	"ART" OR "antiretroviral*" OR "anti-retroviral*" OR "HAART" OR "highly active antiretroviral therapy" OR "cART" OR "combined antiretroviral therapy"

studies, we also extracted the following study characteristics: study setting and recruitment, type of sampling, and outcome measurement methods. No studies were excluded from the systematic review or meta-analysis on the basis of this assessment, but the potential impact of these characteristics on study results was considered when interpreting overall findings.

Data Analysis

We firstly describe key characteristics of all included studies and the total number that provide estimates for the different ART cascade outcomes. We then summarise the results from different studies for each outcome. Given that several studies could provide information on the same study population, we give both the number of studies (N_s) and the number of independent study populations (N_p) when summarising the study characteristics and ART cascade outcome estimates.

All available study estimates are presented on forest plots in the main text and are also reported in Tables S1–S5. On all forest plots, study estimates are grouped by country income (high-income (HI) versus low- and middle-income (LMI)), and ordered by study-period, follow-up period, or time on ART.

For each outcome with at least 2 study estimates available from different study populations, we calculated an overall pooled estimate, and when possible performed sub-group meta-analyses by country income (i.e. HI versus LMI). These results are reported in the main text and are also presented on forest plots. As time period of data collection could influence HIV treatment outcomes, in particular ART uptake outcomes, we did additional sub-group analyses for ART uptake outcomes in order to address this issue. If the time period of data collection for any estimates of ART uptake spanned the pre-HAART and HAART era, sub-group meta-analyses were performed if possible by year of data collection (i.e. data collected in the pre-HAART to HAART era versus data collected in the HAART era) for that ART uptake outcome. These results are reported in the main text. We did not pool study estimates for outcomes relating to median CD4 count. For all other outcomes, we pooled study estimates using a DerSimonian and Laird random effects model on the logit scale, and then back-transformed the overall pooled estimate to the original scale. We assessed heterogeneity across study-estimates using the Cochran Q homogeneity test, which assesses whether differences in study estimates are due to chance alone (typically a p-value <0.1 or <0.05 indicates heterogeneity between study estimates), and the I^2 statistic, which measures the percentage of variation across study estimates that is due to heterogeneity rather than chance (the higher the I^2 value the greater the heterogeneity between study estimates) [20,21]. Meta-analyses were conducted using the 'meta' package in R (Version 3.0.0).

When pooling estimates, we only included study estimates with sample sizes of at least 10 FSWs. Study estimates with an unknown numerator and denominator were not included in any pooled estimates, and for ART uptake outcomes any study estimates with an unknown study period were not included in pooled estimates. If a study provided estimates of an outcome over different time-periods, we only used one estimate (the most recent estimate from each study) for pooling. If more than one study reported estimates of a given outcome for the same study population, we only used one estimate per study population (the study estimate with the largest sample size) for pooling. Study estimates that were included in overall or subgroup pooled estimates are indicated in forest plots and tables with a star symbol (*).

Results

Search Results and Study Characteristics

The search strategy and process of article selection is described in Figure 1. Of 3081 unique publications identified in our original search, 28 met the inclusion criteria (Figure 1). Additional studies were then identified from the supplementary database search ($N_s = 9$) and reference lists ($N_s = 2$) (Figure 1). In total, 39 studies ($N_s = 39$) identified in the search were eligible to be included in our review (Figure 1), providing data on 21 independent FSW study populations ($N_p = 21$) and at least 4,700 HIV-infected FSWs [22–60]. Table 2 summarises the key characteristics of the 39 included studies and their reported outcomes. Figure 2 shows the geographical location of the study settings. Study characteristics that were extracted to help assess risk of bias are shown in Table S6.

The majority of the 39 included studies were prospective cohort ($N_s = 24$, $N_p = 11$) or cross-sectional ($N_s = N_p = 12$) studies. There were also a small number of intervention ($N_s = N_p = 2$) and retrospective case-control ($N_s = N_p = 1$) studies. Twenty-four studies were conducted in five African countries: Benin ($N_s = N_p = 1$), Burkina Faso ($N_s = 5$, $N_p = 1$), Kenya ($N_s = 16$, $N_p = 3$), Rwanda ($N_s = N_p = 1$), and Zimbabwe ($N_s = N_p = 1$). Six studies were conducted in two North American countries: Canada ($N_s = 4$, $N_p = 3$) and United States ($N_s = N_p = 2$). Six studies were conducted in four Asian countries: India ($N_s = N_p = 3$), Russia ($N_s = N_p = 1$), Thailand ($N_s = N_p = 1$), and Vietnam ($N_s = N_p = 1$). Two studies were conducted in two Central America and Caribbean countries: Dominican Republic ($N_s = N_p = 1$), and El Salvador ($N_s = N_p = 1$), and one study was conducted in South America: Brazil ($N_s = N_p = 1$). Twenty-four studies (62%) had fewer than 150 HIV-infected FSW participants, and four studies enrolled HIV-infected FSWs who were also injecting drug users (IDUs) (Table 2).

Of the 39 eligible studies included, 26 reported ART uptake outcomes, 10 reported ART attrition outcomes, 9 reported on adherence to ART, 6 reported on viral suppression, and 17 reported on CD4 counts at and/or after ART initiation (Table 2 and Tables S1–S5). Criteria for ART initiation were reported by only 16 studies, the majority of which reported a CD4 count threshold for ART initiation of 200 cells/mm^3 ($N_s = 11$) [28–30,32,37–39,44,46,51,54]. Other CD4 count thresholds used for ART initiation were CD4 count <250 cells/mm^3 ($N_s = 2$), CD4 count <350 cells/mm^3 ($N_s = 1$), and any CD4 count ($N_s = 1$) [23,42,48,60], and in one other study the ART initiation criteria changed from CD4 count <200 cells/mm^3 to CD4 count <350 cells/mm^3 during the study period ($N_s = 1$) [56]. Other details on ART administration were provided in some studies. For example, studies in Rwanda and India report that ART has been provided free of charge to those with HIV through government ART programmes and ART centres, since 2003 and 2004, respectively [40,42,46]. Studies in Canada also report that ART is provided free of charge through provincial drug treatment programmes, and in the United States, free ART is provided to all those living with HIV [23,45,48]. In 2005, an ART programme was initiated in the Nairobi FSW cohort in Kenya, as part of the U.S. Presidents Emergency Plan for AIDS Relief (PEPFAR), and FSWs received ART through the research clinic [34]. From 2004, FSWs enrolled in the Mombasa FSW cohort in Kenya received ART through either the study research clinic or other clinics in the area, and FSWs enrolled in the Yérélon FSW cohort in Burkina Faso received ART through either the study research clinic or the Bobo-Dioulasso University Teaching Hospital [29,32,33,37–39,49,51,54,56,57]. In another study in Mombasa, FSWs received

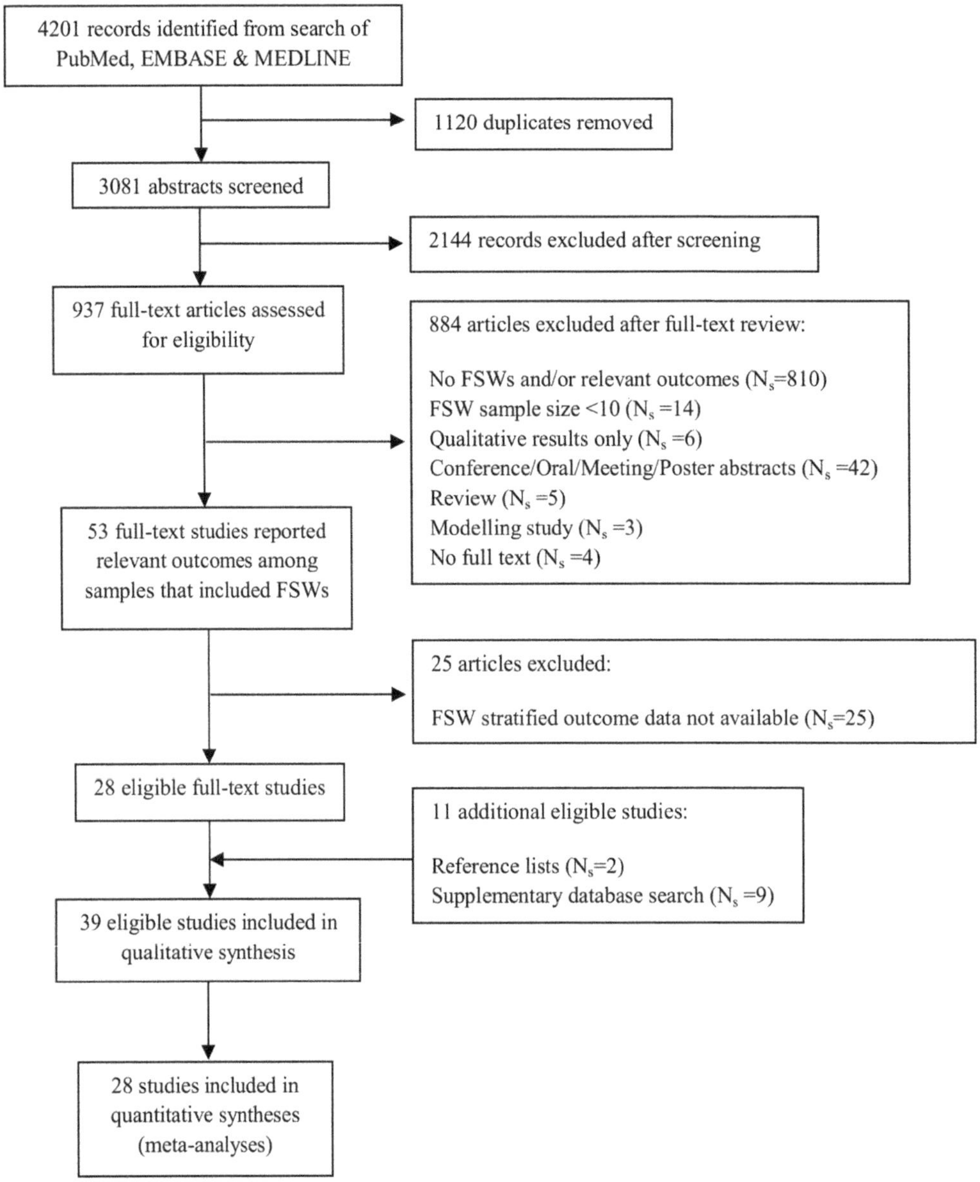

Figure 1. Flow diagram of search strategy and study selection process. FSW = female sex worker, ART = antiretroviral therapy, N_s = number of studies.

ART at the study research clinic, whilst in Benin FSWs accessed ART at a medical center dedicated to FSWs [44,60].

ART Uptake

Estimates of ART uptake (either ART initiation within specified follow-up periods, current ART use, or ever use of ART (no time-frame for ART initiation specified)), among ART-eligible or all HIV-infected FSWs, were available from 26 studies reporting on 20 independent study populations in Asia, Africa, North America, South America, and Central America and the Caribbean [22,24,32–34,36–38,40–43,45–50,52–55,57–60] (Figures 3, 4, 5, Table S1). CD4 count criteria for ART initiation were reported by only 8 of these studies (CD4 count ≤200 cells/mm^3 ($N_s = 5$), CD4 count ≤250 cells/mm^3 ($N_s = 1$), CD4 count <350 cells/mm^3 ($N_s = 1$) and any CD4 count ($N_s = 1$)) (Table S1).

Estimates of ART initiation among all HIV-infected FSWs were provided by 6 studies reporting on 4 independent study populations in Asia and Africa ($N_s = 6$, $N_p = 4$) (Figure 3A, Table S1A). Across these 6 studies, 0.4% to 48% of HIV-infected FSWs initiated ART, during follow-up periods which varied between 4 months to 16 years ($N_s = 6$, $N_p = 4$) (Figure 3A, Table S1A). The overall pooled estimate for ART initiation among HIV-infected FSWs, when pooling only one estimate per study population, was 19% (95%CI: 10%–35%, $I^2 = 96\%$, $N_s = N_p = 4$) (Figure 3A). Pooled estimates were lower for studies which collected data on HIV-infected FSWs between the pre-HAART and HAART era (6%; 95%CI: 0%–51%, $I^2 = 96\%$, $N_s = N_p = 2$) than for studies which collected data on HIV-infected FSWs in the HAART era alone (37%; 95%CI: 20%–58%, $I^2 = 91\%$, $N_s = N_p = 2$).

One study in Rwanda provided estimates of ART initiation among ART-eligible FSWs (Figure 3B, Table S1B). In this study,

Table 2. Study Characteristics and Outcomes Reported.

Study Population	Country/ Population Code	Study [Reference]	Study Design	Study Period	FSW Sample Size	FSW Characteristics	ART Cascade Outcomes				
							Uptake	Attrition	Adherence	VS	CD4
Abriendo Puertas Intervention Project	Dominican Republic 1	Donastorg *et al*, 2014 [53][a]	CS	2012–2013	268	Active, HIV +ve, Drug use (24%)	✓	✓	✓	✓	
ACCESS cohort	Canada 1	Reddon *et al*, 2011 [45][c]	PC	2005–2011	88	Active, HIV +ve, IDU	✓				
Canadian Co-infection Cohort	Canada 2	Cox *et al*, 2014 [58][a]	PC	2003–2013	43	Active, HIV +ve, IDU or crack	✓				
Chiang Rai Health Club FSW Cohort	Thailand 1	Kilmarx *et al*, 2000 [22]	PC	1991–1998	194	Active, HIV +ve	✓				
El Salvador FSW and MSM Study	El Salvador 1	Dennis *et al*, 2013 [52]	CS	2008	848	Active, HIV +ve (5%)	✓				
FSW and GP Comparative Study	Benin 1	Diabaté *et al*, 2011 [44]	PC	2008–2010	53	Active, HIV +ve, On ART					✓
FSW Focus Group Study	India 1	Chakrapani *et al*, 2009 [46][a]	CS	2007	19	Active, HIV +ve	✓				
HERMITAGE RCT Cohort	Russia 1	Tyurina *et al*, 2013 [59][a]	PC	2007–2011	42	Active, HIV +ve, Risky drinkers	✓				
Maka Project Partnership/WISH Drop-In Centre Society	Canada 3	Deering *et al*, 2009 [23][a]	PDI	2007–2008	20	Active + Former, HIV +ve, IDU (40%)			✓		
		Shannon *et al*, 2005 [24]	CS	2003	159	Active + Former, HIV +ve (21%), IDU (57%)	✓	✓			
Karnataka Multi-District FSW Study	India 2	Jadhav *et al*, 2013 [55]	CS	2011	603	Active, HIV +ve	✓				
Mombasa FSW cohort	Kenya 1	Balkus *et al*, 2013 [49]	PC	1993–2010	282	Active, HIV +ve, *T.vaginalis* infection	✓				
		Day et al, 2013 [51]	PC	2004–2010	159	Active, HIV +ve, On ART		✓			✓
		Graham *et al*, 2013 [54]	PC	1993–2009	306	Active, HIV +ve	✓				
		Graham *et al*, 2012 [29][b]	PC	2005–2009	102	Active + Former, HIV +ve, On ART		✓			✓
		Graham *et al*, 2011 [26]	PC	2004–2008	36	Active, HIV +ve, On ART, Genital ulcers					✓
		Masese *et al*, 2011[25]	PC	2004–2008	41	Active, HIV +ve, On ART, T.*vaginalis* infection		✓	✓		✓
		McClelland *et al*, 2011 [33][c]	CS	1993–2006	571	Active, HIV +ve	✓				

Table 2. Cont.

Study Population	Country/ Population Code	Study [Reference]	Study Design	Study Period	FSW Sample Size	FSW Characteristics	ART Cascade Outcomes				
							Uptake	Attrition	Adherence	VS	CD4
		Gitau *et al*, 2010 [31]	PC	2004–2008	30	Active, HIV +ve, On ART, Cervicitis infection					✓
		Graham *et al*, 2010 [28][b]	PC	2005–2008	102	Active + Former, HIV +ve, On ART		✓		✓	✓
		McClelland *et al*, 2010 [32][a]	PC	1993–2008	966	Active, HIV +ve	✓				✓
		Graham *et al*, 2009 [27]	PC	2004–2008	134	Active, HIV +ve, On ART					✓
		Graham *et al*, 2007 [30][a]	PC	2004	21	Active, HIV +ve, On ART			✓		✓
Multicentre Vietnam Study	Vietnam 1	Dean *et al*, 2011 [43][a]	CS	2008–2009	147	Active, HIV +ve	✓			✓	
Multicity Study of YPLH	USA 1	Comulada *et al*, 2003 [48][a]	CS	1999–2000	21	Active + Former, HIV +ve	✓	✓	✓		
Multisite Zimbabwe FSW Study	Zimbabwe 1	Cowan *et al*, 2013 [50]	CS	2009	836	Active, HIV +ve (57%)	✓				
Nairobi FSW cohort	Kenya 2	Mawji *et al*, 2012 [35][a]	RCC	2001–2006	62	Active, HIV +ve, On ART					✓
		McKinnon *et al*, 2010 [34][a]	PC	1986–2009	607	Active, HIV +ve	✓				✓
		Lester *et al*, 2009 [36]	CS	Not reported	57	Active, HIV +ve	✓				
North Mombasa Clinic Cohort	Kenya 3	Graham *et al*, 2013 [60][a]	PC	2005–2011	108	Active, HIV +ve	✓	✓	✓		
Payana FSW Cohort	India 3	Becker *et al*, 2012 [40][a]	PC	2008–2009	45	Active, HIV +ve, Died during follow-up	✓				
Port of Imbutiba Sex Worker Study	Brazil 1	Schuelter-Trevisol *et al*, 2007 [47]	CS	2003–2004	90	Active, HIV +ve (4%), Illicit Drug Users (52%)	✓				
Project HOPE	USA 2	Kalokhe *et al*, 2012 [41][c]	CS	2006–2010	46	Active, HIV +ve, Crack cocaine use	✓				
Project Ubuzima FSW HIV incidence study	Rwanda 1	Braunstein *et al*, 2011 [42]	PC	2006–2008	141	Active + Former, HIV +ve	✓		✓		✓
Yerelon FSW Cohort	Burkina Faso 1	Low et al, 2014 [56]	PC	2004–2011	199	Active, HIV +ve, On ART				✓	✓
		Low et al, 2014 [57]	PC	2007–2011	258	Active, HIV +ve	✓				

Table 2. Cont.

Study Population	Country/ Population Code	Study [Reference]	Study Design	Study Period	FSW Sample Size	FSW Characteristics	ART Cascade Outcomes				
							Uptake	Attrition	Adherence	VS	CD4
		Huet *et al*, 2011 [39]	PC	2003–2007	47	Active, HIV +ve, On ART		✓	✓	✓	✓
		Konate *et al*, 2011 [38]	PDI	2003–2005	658	Active, HIV +ve	✓	✓	✓	✓	✓
		Low *et al*, 2011 [37]	PC	2003–2006	767	Active, HIV +ve	✓				✓

FSW – female sex worker, ART – antiretroviral therapy, HIV – human immunodeficiency virus, VS – viral suppression, MSM – men who have sex with men, GP – general population, IDU – injecting drug user, PC – prospective cohort, CS – cross-sectional, RCT – randomised controlled trial, RCC – retrospective case-control, PDI – peer driven intervention, YPLH – young people living with HIV, HERMITAGE – HIV's Evolution in Russia – Mitigating Infection Transmission and Alcoholism in a Growing Epidemic, WISH – Women's Information and Safe House, HOPE – Hospital visit is an Opportunity for Prevention and Engagement, ACCESS – AIDS Care Cohort to evaluate Exposure to Survival Services.

[a]Additional data or clarifications were provided by corresponding author/s.

[b]Corresponding author confirmed that participants were FSWs from the Mombasa FSW cohort.

[c]Outcome data is based on entire cohort rather than subset of participants in referenced study; in some cases this data was provided by study authors.

87% of ART-eligible (CD4 <350 cells/mm^3) FSWs enrolled in HIV care reported initiating ART within 12 to 36 months of their HIV diagnosis [42] (Figure 3B, Table S1B).

Estimates of current ART use among all HIV-infected FSWs were provided by 18 studies reporting on 16 independent study populations in Asia, Africa, North America, South America, and Central America and the Caribbean ($N_s = 18$, $N_p = 16$) (Figure 4, Table S1A). Across these 18 studies, the fraction of HIV-infected FSWs currently using ART ranged between 0% and 72% ($N_s = 18$, $N_p = 16$) (Figure 4, Table S1A). The overall pooled estimate for current ART use among HIV-infected FSWs, when pooling only one estimate per study population and pooling only those estimates with a known time period of data collection measured among at least 10 FSWs, was 38% (95% CI: 29%–48%, $I^2 = 96\%$, $N_s = N_p = 15$) (Figure 4). Pooled estimates were similar for LMI countries (39%; 95% CI: 27%–53%, $I^2 = 97\%$, $N_s = N_p = 9$) and HI countries (35%; 95% CI: 20%–55%, $I^2 = 87\%$, $N_s = N_p = 6$) (Figure 4). Removing the one LMI country estimate where data on HIV-infected FSWs was collected between the pre-HAART and HAART era had a marginal impact on the pooled estimate for LMI countries (42%; 95% CI: 29%–57%, $I^2 = 97\%$, $N_s = N_p = 8$).

Estimates of ever ART use (i.e. no time-frame for ART initiation specified) among HIV-infected FSWs were provided by five studies reporting on 5 independent study populations in Asia, Africa, North America, and Central America and the Caribbean. Across these 5 studies, the fraction of HIV-infected FSWs who had ever used ART ranged between 14% and 91% ($N_s = N_p = 5$) (Figure 5, Table S1A). The overall pooled estimate of ever ART use among HIV-infected FSWs was 54% (95% CI: 21%–84%, $I^2 = 98\%$, $N_s = N_p = 5$). Pooled estimates were lower for LMI countries (36%; 95% CI: 7%–81%, $I^2 = 99\%$, $N_s = N_p = 3$) than HI countries (80%; 95% CI: 48%–94%, $I^2 = 70\%$, $N_s = N_p = 2$) (Figure 5).

Treatment Attrition

Estimates of treatment attrition (either treatment discontinuation, loss-to-follow-up on ART, death on ART, or ART-experienced but no longer on ART), were available from 10 studies reporting on 6 independent study populations in Africa, North America, and Central America and the Caribbean [24,25,28,29,38,39,48,51,53,60] (Figure 6, Table S2).

Treatment discontinuation was reported by 2 studies reporting on the same study population in Kenya ($N_s = 2$, $N_p = 1$) (Figure 6A, Table S2). In this Kenyan cohort, estimates of treatment discontinuation among FSWs starting ART, increased from 4% at 6 months to 10% at 12 months [28,29] (Figure 6A, Table S2).

Estimates of loss-to-follow-up among FSWs on ART were provided by 6 studies reporting on 3 independent study populations in Kenya and Burkina Faso ($N_s = 6$, $N_p = 3$) (Figure 6B, Table S2). Across the three different study populations, estimates of loss-to-follow-up after ART initiation were similar, ranging between 3% and 10% after varying times on ART ($N_s = 6$, $N_p = 3$) (Figure 6B, Table S2). In one of the Kenyan cohorts, loss-to-follow-up increased from 3% after 3 months to 6% after 12 months on ART [28,29], whilst in the Burkina Faso cohort 4% were lost-to-follow-up after 32 months on ART [38,39]. The overall pooled estimate of loss-to-follow-up on ART, when pooling the most recent study estimate per study population, was 6% (95% CI: 3%–11%, $I^2 = 0\%$, $N_s = N_p = 3$) (Figure 6B).

Estimates of death among FSWs on ART were provided by 6 studies reporting on 3 independent study populations in Kenya and Burkina Faso ($N_s = 6$, $N_p = 3$) (Figure 6C, Table S2). Across

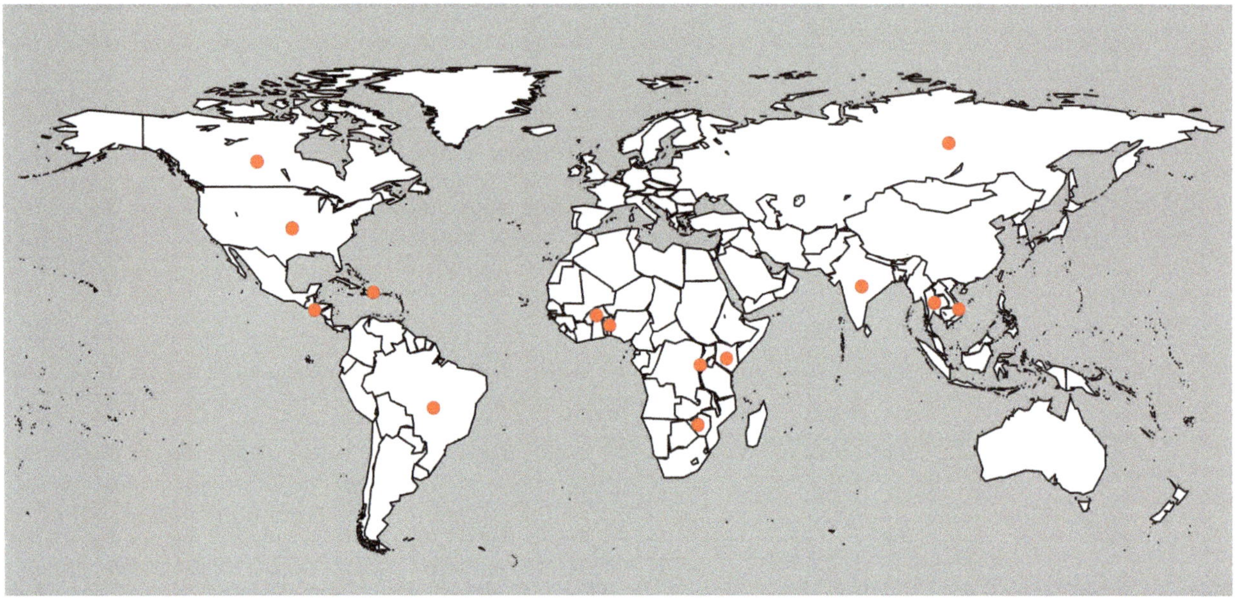

Figure 2. Map of Study Locations. Red dots highlight the countries where included studies were conducted.

the three different study populations, the fraction of FSWs who died after varying times on ART ranged between 0% and 8.5% ($N_s = 6$, $N_P = 3$) (Figure 6C, Table S2). In two of the study populations in Kenya and Burkina Faso the fraction of FSWs who died whilst on ART increased over time [28,29,38,39,51] (Figure 6C, Table S2). The overall pooled estimate of death on ART, when pooling the most recent study estimate per study population, was 6% (95% CI: 3%–11%, $I^2 = 0\%$, $N_s = N_P = 3$) (Figure 6C). In one of the Kenyan cohorts, total attrition from ART, due to treatment discontinuation, loss-to-follow-up and

Population	Follow-up	n/N	Estimate (%) and 95% CI
A. Among all HIV +ve			
Low and Middle Income			
Thailand 1 [22]	1991-1998	3/194	1.6 (0.3-4.5)*
Kenya 1 [33]	1993-2006 [a]	108/571	18.9 (15.8-22.4)
Kenya 1 [32]	1993-2008 [a]	197/966	20.4 (17.9-23.1)*
Kenya 1 [54]	4-24 months [a b]	1/232	0.4 (0.0-2.4)
	>24 months [a b]	10/159	6.3 (3.1-11.3)
Burkina Faso 1 [38]	2003-2005	47/169	27.8 (21.2-35.2)*
Rwanda 1 [42]	12-36 months [c]	57/120	47.5 (38.3-56.8)*
Overall (I^2 = 95.6%, p<0.001, N_p =4*)			**19.4 (9.6-35.4)**
B. Among all ART-eligible			
Low and Middle Income			
Rwanda 1 [42]	12-36 months [c]	34/39 [d]	87.2 (72.6-95.7)

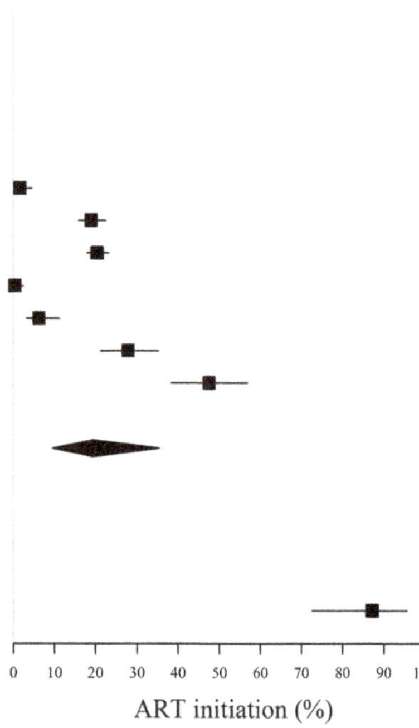

Figure 3. Forest plot of ART initiation among (A) all HIV-infected FSWs and (B) all ART-eligible FSWs. Study estimates are grouped by country income and ordered by follow-up period. The star symbol (*) highlights the individual study estimates (one per study population) included in the pooled overall estimate. I^2 and p-values are the measures of heterogeneity used. [a] ART was provided to FSWs in the Kenyan cohort from 2004, [b] Follow-up refers to months since HIV-diagnosis, study recruitment occurred between 1993 and 2009, [c] Follow-up refers to months since HIV-diagnosis, study recruitment occurred between 2006 and 2008. [d] N refers to HIV-infected ART-eligible FSWs who had enrolled in HIV care following HIV diagnosis. ART = antiretroviral therapy, FSW = female sex workers, CI = confidence interval, n = number of FSWs with each outcome, N = sample size of FSWs available for each outcome, N_P = number of independent study populations.

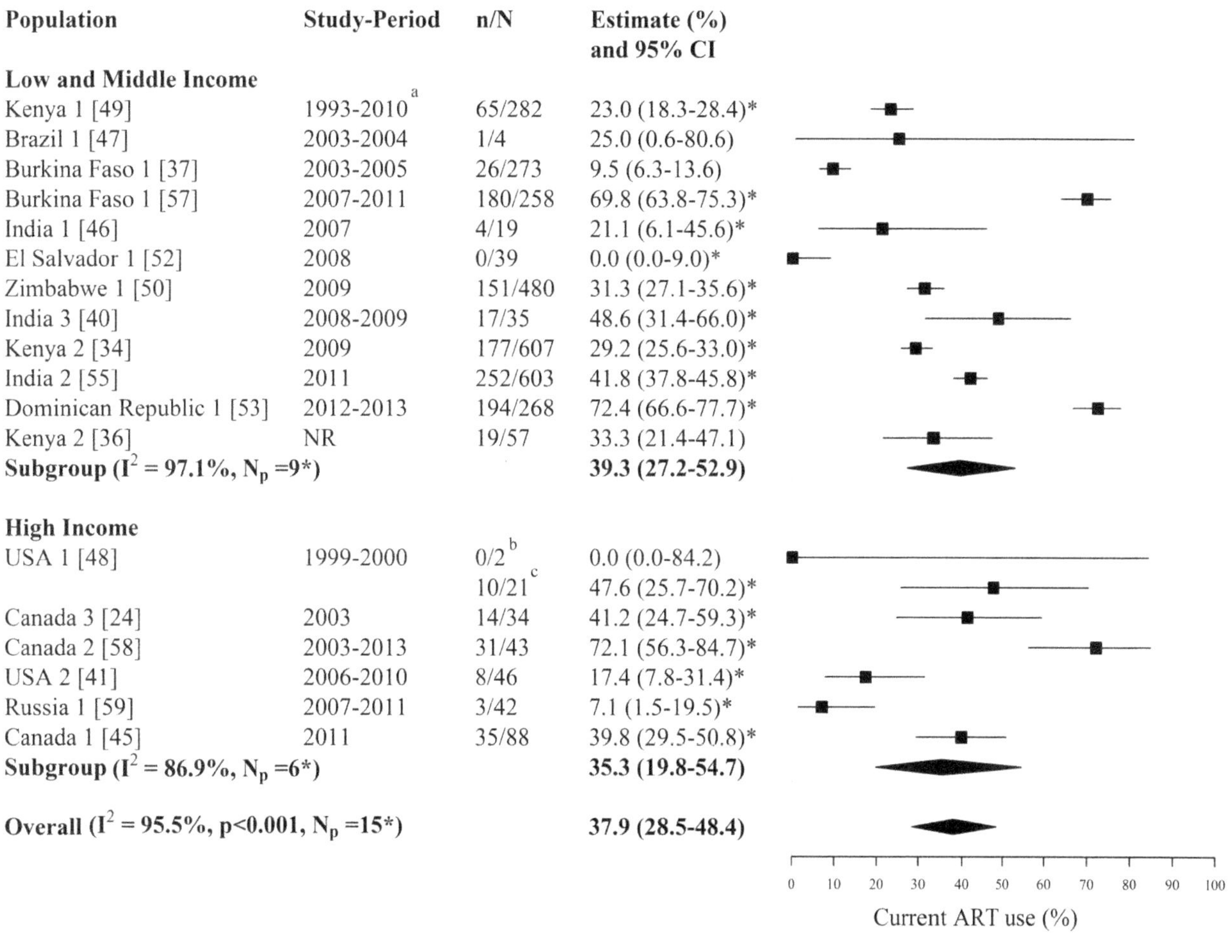

Figure 4. Forest plot of current ART use among HIV-infected FSWs. Study estimates are grouped by country income and ordered by study-period. The star symbol (*) highlights the study estimates (one per study population) included in the pooled overall or subgroup estimates. Only study estimates with a known time period of data collection which were measured among at least 10 FSWs were used for pooling. I^2 and p-values are the measures of heterogeneity used. [a] ART was provided to FSWs in the Kenyan cohort from 2004, [b] Sample is 'active' FSWs, [c] Sample is 'active' and 'former' FSWs. ART = antiretroviral therapy, FSW = female sex workers, CI = confidence interval, NR = not reported, n = number of FSWs with each outcome, N = sample size of FSWs available for each outcome, N_p = number of independent study populations.

mortality, was 10% and 21%, after 6 and 12 months on ART, respectively [28,29].

Estimates of the number of treatment-experienced FSWs that reported no longer receiving ART, were provided by 3 studies reporting on 3 independent study populations in Canada, USA and Dominican Republic ($N_s = 3$, $N_p = 3$) (Figure 6D, Table S2). Across these three studies, the fraction of treatment-experienced FSWs that reported no longer receiving ART ranged between 8% and 47%, with an overall pooled estimate of 26% (95% CI: 6%–65%, $I^2 = 93.3\%$, $N_s = N_p = 3$) (Figure 6D). The pooled estimate for HI countries (43%; 95% CI: 29%–58%, $I^2 = 0\%$, $N_s = N_p = 2$), was higher than the single LMI country estimate (8%, 95% CI: 4%–12%, $N_s = N_p = 1$) (Figure 6D, Table S2).

Adherence

Estimates of adherence (i.e. the fraction achieving a predefined threshold of adherence) were available from 9 studies, reporting on 7 independent study population in Africa, North America, and Central America and the Caribbean [23,25,30,38,39,42,48,53,60] (Figure 7, Table S3). Among these 9 studies, three reported the availability of adherence counselling [23,38,39], one study reported the use of directly observed therapy [30], and one study reported that monthly support groups were used to promote adherence [60] (Table S3). The fraction of FSWs adherent to treatment was consistently high, ranging from 67% to 100% ($N_s = 9$, $N_p = 7$), across the varying time periods, adherence thresholds (≥90%, ≥95% and 100%), recall periods (past 3 days, past 4 days, past week, past 30 days, past month, and since ART initiation), and methods of assessment (self-report, pill count and visual analog scale) (Figure 7, Table S3). Estimates of the fraction of FSWs 100% adherent to ART were highest shortly after starting directly observed therapy (91% after 28 days on ART [30]) and at the end of a peer-driven intervention (90.4% [23]) (Figure 7, Table S3). Estimates of the fraction of FSWs ≥95% adherent to ART increased from 83% after 6 months on ART to 100% after 36 months on ART in a cohort in Burkina Faso [38,39] (Figure 7, Table S3). For LMI countries, the pooled estimate of adherence, when pooling only one estimate per study population and pooling only those estimates with a known numerator and denominator, was 76% (95% CI: 68%–83%, $I^2 = 36\%$, $N_s = N_p = 4$) (Figure 7).

Viral Suppression

Estimates of viral suppression (i.e. the fraction on ART with undetectable plasma viral load), were available from 6 studies

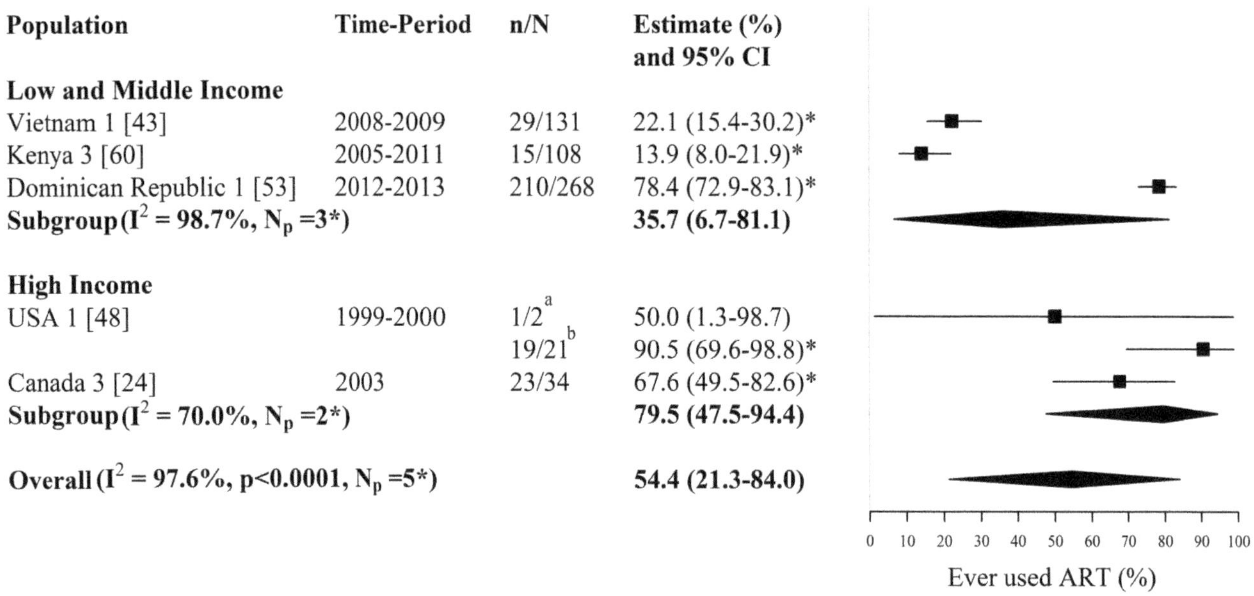

Figure 5. Forest plot of ever ART use among HIV-infected FSWs. Study estimates are grouped by country income and ordered by time-period. The star symbol (*) highlights the study estimates (one per study population) included in the pooled overall or subgroup estimates. I^2 and p-values are the measures of heterogeneity used. [a] Sample is 'active' FSWs, [b] Sample is 'active' and 'former' FSWs. ART = antiretroviral therapy, FSW = female sex workers, CI = confidence interval, n = number of FSWs with each outcome, N = sample size of FSWs available for each outcome, N_p = number of independent study populations.

reporting on 4 independent study populations in Asia, Africa, and Central America and the Caribbean [28,38,39,43,53,56] (Figure 8, Table S4). The fraction of FSWs on ART virally suppressed, ranged between 40%–82% (N_s = 6, N_p = 4), across varying time periods and definitions of viral suppression (≤50 copies/mm^3, ≤100 copies/mm^3, ≤180 copies/mm^3, ≤300 copies/mm^3) (Figure 8, Table S4). The lowest study estimate of viral suppression (40%) was reported in the Kenyan study population after 3 months on ART [28], which increased to 73% after 6 months on ART [28] (Figure 8, Table S4). In the Burkina Faso study population, the high fraction of FSWs virally suppressed (79%–88%) after 6 to 36 months on ART, corresponded to similarly high levels of treatment adherence seen over the same time periods for these FSWs (Figure 7 & 8, Tables S3 & S4) [38,39]. The overall pooled estimate of viral suppression, when pooling one estimate per study population, was 57% (95% CI: 46%–68%, I^2 = 82%, N_s = N_p = 4) (Figure 8).

CD4 Counts at and/or after ART Initiation

Information on CD4 counts at and/or after ART initiation (either median CD4 count, median CD4 count gain, or fraction with CD4 counts >500, 200–499 or <200 cells/mm^3), were available from 17 studies reporting on 5 independent study populations in Africa [25–32,34,35,37–39,42,44,51,56] (Figures 9 &10, Table S5). Across the studies, the CD4 count criteria for ART initiation was either ≤200 cells/mm^3 or not reported, with one study reporting a change in ART initiation criteria from CD4 count <200 cells/mm^3 to CD4 count <350 cells/mm^3 (Table S5).

Median CD4 counts at and/or after ART initiation were provided by 14 studies reporting on 5 independent study populations in Benin, Kenya, Burkina Faso, and Rwanda (N_s = 14, N_p = 5) (Figure 9A & 9B, Table S5A). Across 4 of these study populations, the median CD4 count ranged between 121 and 205 cells/mm^3 at ART initiation (N_s = 12, N_p = 4), and 204 to 343 cells/mm^3 after 1 to 36 months on ART (N_s = 9, N_p = 4) (Figure 9A & 9B, Table S5A).

Median gains in CD4 count following ART initiation, were provided by 5 studies reporting on 4 independent study populations in Benin, Kenya, Burkina Faso, and Rwanda (N_s = 5, N_p = 4) (Figure 9C, Table S5A). Across 3 of these study populations, median gains in CD4 counts after 6 to 36 months on ART, ranged between 103 and 241 cells/mm^3 (N_s = 4, N_p = 3) (Figure 9C, Table S5A).

Estimates of the fraction of FSWs with CD4 counts <200, 200–499 or >500 cells/mm^3 at and/or after ART initiation were provided by 2 studies reporting on 2 independent study populations in Kenya and Burkina Faso (N_s = 2, N_p = 2) (Figure 10, Table S5B). In the Kenyan study, the fraction of FSWs with CD4 counts ≤200 cells/mm^3, decreased from 90% at ART initiation to 11% after 24 months on ART [32] (Figure 10A, Table S5B). When pooling the most recent study estimates from the 2 study populations, the overall pooled fractions of FSWs on ART with CD4 counts <200 cells/mm^3, 200–499 cells/mm^3, and >500 cells/mm^3, were 22% (95% CI: 5%–66%, I^2 = 88%, N_s = N_p = 2), 63% (95% CI: 28%–89%, I^2 = 89%, N_s = N_p = 2), and 13% (95% CI: 7%–22%, I^2 = 0%, N_s = N_p = 2), respectively [32,37] (Figure 10).

Discussion

Despite the recent momentum to scale-up ART coverage worldwide, there is a concerning lack of published data on HIV treatment among FSWs [61]. We found only thirty-nine studies, from fourteen different countries in Africa, Asia, North America, South America, and Central America and the Caribbean that reported information on the ART cascade among FSWs (Figure 2). Of these studies, the majority reported estimates of either current ART use or median CD4 counts at and/or after

Population	Time on ART	n/N	Estimate (%) and 95% CI
A. Treatment Discontinuation			
Low and Middle Income			
Kenya 1 [28]	6 months	4/102	3.9 (1.1-9.7)
Kenya 1 [29]	12 months	10/102	9.8 (4.8-17.3)
B. LFU on ART			
Low and Middle Income			
Kenya 1 [28,29]	3 months	3/102	2.9 (0.6-8.4)
	6 months	4/102	3.9 (0.1-9.7)
	12 months	6/102	5.9 (2.2-12.4)*
Kenya 1 [25]	10 months (m)	2/41	4.9 (0.6-16.5)
Burkina Faso 1 [38,39]	32 months (m)	2/47	4.3 (0.5-14.5)*
Kenya 3 [60]	NR	1/10	10.0 (0.3-44.5)*
Overall (I^2 = 0%, p=0.77, N_p =3*)			**5.8 (3.0-10.8)**
C. Deaths on ART			
Low and Middle Income			
Kenya 1 [28,29]	3 months	2/102	2.0 (0.2-6.9)
	6 months	2/102	2.0 (0.2-6.9)
	12 months	5/102	4.9 (1.6-11.1)*
Kenya 1 [51]	41 months (m)	7/159	4.4 (1.8-8.9)
Burkina Faso 1 [38,39]	12 months	3/47	6.4 (1.3-17.5)
	36 months	4/47	8.5 (2.4-20.4)*
Kenya 3 [60]	NR	0/10	0.0 (0.0-30.9)*
Overall (I^2 = 0%, p=0.67, N_p =3*)			**6.2 (3.3-11.2)**
D. No Longer on ART			
Low and Middle Income			
Dominican Republic 1 [53]	NR	16/210	7.6 (4.4-12.1)*
High Income			
Canada 3 [24]	NR	9/23	39.1 (19.7-61.5)*
USA 1 [48]	NR	9/19	47.4 (24.5-71.1)*
Subgroup (I^2 = 0%, p=0.59, N_p =2*)			**42.9 (28.9-58.1)**
Overall (I^2 = 93.3%, p<0.0001, N_p =3*)			**26.0 (6.4-64.6)**

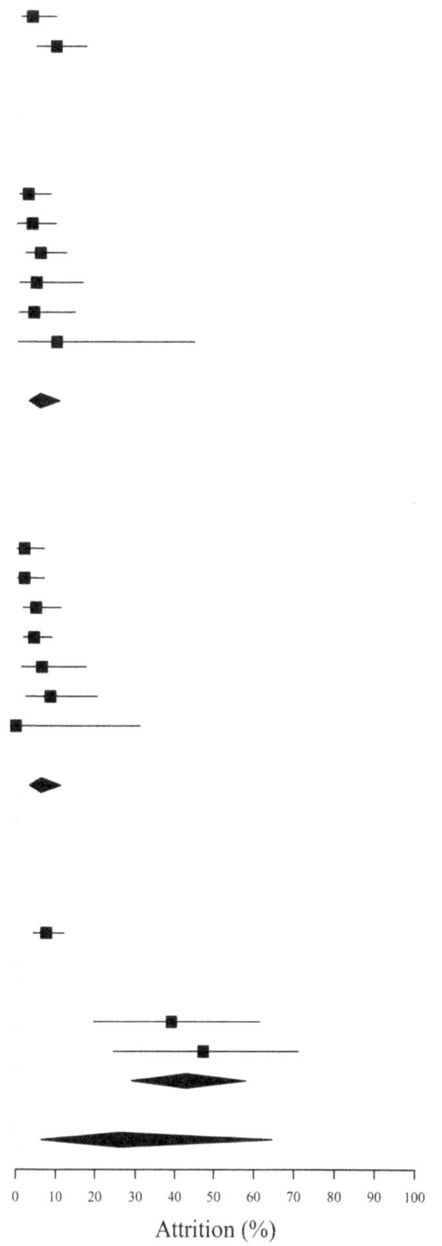

Figure 6. Forest plot of treatment attrition among HIV-infected FSWs, including (A) treatment discontinuation (B) loss to follow-up on ART (C) death on ART and (D) ART-experienced but no longer on ART. Study estimates are grouped by country income and ordered by time on ART. The star symbol (*) highlights the study estimates (one per study population) included in the pooled overall or subgroup estimates. For studies providing estimates over multiple time-periods, only one estimate was used for pooling (the most recent estimate from that study). I^2 and p-values are the measures of heterogeneity used. ART = antiretroviral therapy, FSW = female sex workers, CI = confidence interval, NR = not reported, n = number of FSWs with each outcome, N = sample size of FSWs available for each outcome, N_p = number of independent study populations, m = median, LFU = lost to follow-up.

ART initiation, with very few providing estimates of treatment attrition, adherence and viral suppression among FSWs.

ART uptake among HIV-infected FSWs was particularly variable across the different studies and settings. Pooled estimates of ART initiation in HIV-infected FSWs were higher among studies which collected data on HIV-infected FSWs exclusively in the HAART era versus studies which collected data spanning the pre-HAART and HAART eras, and pooled estimates of ever

Population	Time on ART	Threshold, Method Assessed, Recall Period	n/N	Estimate (%) and 95% CI
Low and Middle Income				
Kenya 1 [30]	28 days	100%, PC, month	19/21	90.5 (69.6-98.8)
Kenya 1 [25]	10 months (m)	95%, PC, month	21/31	67.7 (48.6-83.3)*
Burkina Faso 1 [38,39]	6 months	95%, PC, 30-day	NR	83.3 (67.2-93.6)
	12 months	95%, PC, 30-day	NR	92.1 (78.6-98.3)
	36 months	95%, PC, 30-day	NR	100.0 (54.1-100.0)
Rwanda 1 [42]	NR	100%, SR, 3-day	49/57	86.0 (74.2-93.7)*
		100%, SR, all ART use	38/57	66.7 (52.9-78.6)
Dominican Republic 1 [53]	NR	100%, SR, 4-day	155/210	73.8 (67.3-79.6)*
Kenya 3 [60]	NR	95%, VAS, 30-day	8/10	80.0 (44.4-97.5)*
Subgroup (I^2 = 35.5%, p=0.2, N_p =4*)				**76.2 (67.8-83.0)**
High Income				
Canada 3 [23]	NR (PDI Start)	100%, SR, week	NR	87.2
	NR (PDI End)	100%, SR, week	NR	90.4
USA 1 [48]	NR	90%, SR, 3-day	6/9	66.7 (29.9-92.5)

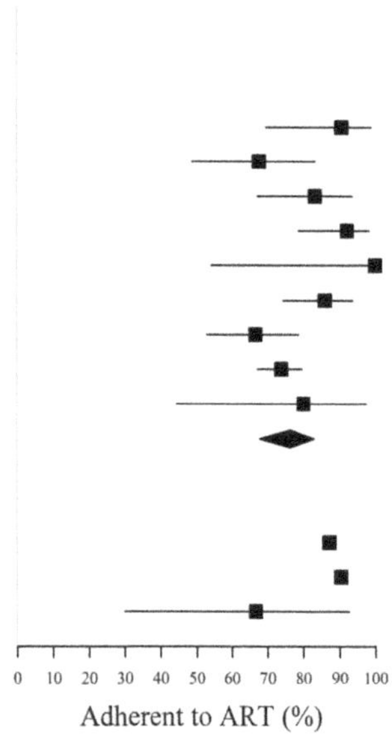

Figure 7. Forest plot of ART adherence among HIV-infected FSWs. Study estimates are grouped by country income and ordered by time on ART. The star symbol (*) highlights the study estimates (one per study population) included in the pooled overall or subgroup estimates. Only study estimates with a known sample size of at least 10 FSWs were used for pooling. For studies providing estimates over multiple time-periods, only one estimate was used for pooling (the most recent estimate from that study). I^2 and p-values are the measures of heterogeneity used. ART = antiretroviral, FSW = female sex workers, CI = confidence interval, NR = not reported, n = number of FSWs with each outcome, N = sample size of FSWs available for each outcome, N_p = number of independent study populations, m = median, PDI = peer driven intervention, PC = pill count, SR = self-report, VAS = visual analog scale.

ART use among HIV-infected FSWs were higher in high-income countries compared to low- and middle-income countries. Conversely, pooled estimates of current ART use among HIV-infected FSWs were similar between high-income countries and low- and middle-income countries. However, there was substantial between-study heterogeneity for all pooled estimates of ART uptake. Varied study periods, different follow-up times and different ART eligibility criteria across studies could all contribute to the variability in study estimates. Nevertheless, pooled estimates of current ART use among HIV-infected FSWs are similar to estimates of current ART use among HIV-infected women in Burkina Faso (27%) and among HIV-infected female IDUs in Canada (30%) [62,63]. Likewise, in the one study in Rwanda that reported ART initiation among ART-eligible FSWs, the propor-

Population	Time on ART	Definition of Viral Suppression	n/N	Estimate (%) and 95% CI
Low and Middle Income				
Kenya 1 [28]	3 months	<100 copies/ml	39/97	40.2 (30.4-50.7)
	6 months	<100 copies/ml	69/95	72.6 (62.5-81.3)*
Burkina Faso 1 [38,39]	6 months	<300 copies/ml	27/34	79.4 (62.1-91.3)
	12 months	<300 copies/ml	27/35	77.1 (59.8-89.6)
	18 months	<300 copies/ml	24/30	80.0 (61.4-92.3)
	24 months	<300 copies/ml	7/8	87.5 (47.4-99.7)
	30 months	<300 copies/ml	9/12	75.0 (42.8-94.5)
	32 months (m)	<300 copies/ml	36/47	76.7 (61.4-88.2)
	36 months	<300 copies/ml	18/22	81.8 (59.7-94.8)
Burkina Faso 1 [56]	3.4 years (m)	<300 copies/ml	84/174	48.3 (40.7-56.0)*
Vietnam 1 [43]	NR	<180 copies/ml	13/29	44.8 (26.5-64.3)*
Dominican Republic 1 [53]	NR	<50 copies/ml	115/193	59.6 (52.3-66.6)*
Overall (I^2 = 82%, p=0.0008, N_p =4*)				**57.4 (45.7-68.2)**

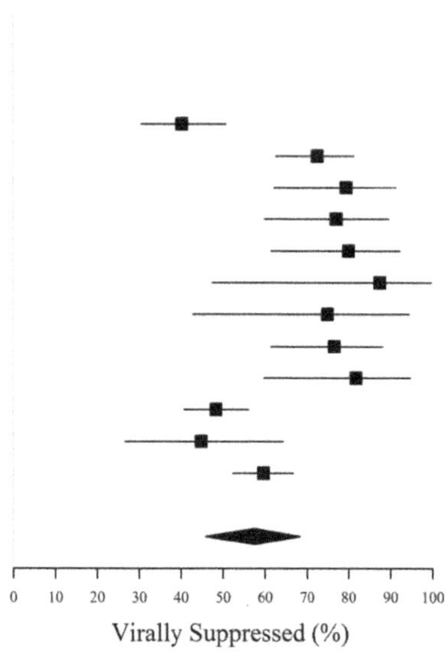

Figure 8. Forest plot of viral suppression among HIV-infected FSWs on ART. Study estimates are grouped by country income and ordered by time on ART. The star symbol (*) highlights the study estimates (one per study population) included in the pooled overall estimate. For studies providing estimates over multiple time-periods, only one estimate was used for pooling (the most recent estimate from that study). I^2 and p-values are the measures of heterogeneity used. ART = antiretroviral, FSW = female sex workers, CI = confidence interval, NR = not reported, n = number of FSWs with each outcome, N = sample size of FSWs available for each outcome, N_p = number of independent study populations, m = median.

Population	Time on ART	ART Eligibility Criteria	N	Estimate (cells/mm³) and IQR
A. Median at ART initiation				
Low and Middle Income				
Benin 1 [44]	ART initiation	CD4 count<200	53	134 (67-175)
Kenya 1 [29]	ART initiation	CD4 count<200	102	124
Kenya 1 [26]	ART initiation	NR	36	125 (76-168)
Kenya 1 [27]	ART initiation	NR	134	127 (79-165)
Kenya 1 [25]	ART initiation	NR	31	126 (68-159)
Kenya 1 [30]	ART initiation	CD4 count<200	21	121 (58-161)
Kenya 1 [51]	ART initiation	CD4 count<200	159	132 (80-180)
Kenya 2 [35]	ART initiation	NR	62	205
Kenya 2 [34]	ART initiation	NR	79	180
Burkina Faso 1 [38,39]	ART initiation	CD4 count<200	47	147 (79-183)
Burkina Faso 1 [56]	ART initiation	CD4 count<200 then <350	163	177 (122-228)
B. Median after ART initiation				
Low and Middle Income				
Kenya 1 [30]	28 days	CD4 count<200	19	204 (131-277)
Kenya 1 [29]	3 months	CD4 count<200	97	238
	6 months	CD4 count<200	95	236
	12 months	CD4 count<200	88	240
Kenya 1 [26]	5 months (m)	NR	36	241 (158-312)
Burkina Faso 1 [38,39]	6 months	CD4 count<200	43	234 (180-327)
	12 months	CD4 count<200	41	306 (249-381)
	36 months	CD4 count<200	22	343 (230-553)
Kenya 1 [25]	10 months (m)	NR	31	241 (161-292)
Benin 1 [44]	12 months	CD4 count<200	53	212
Kenya 1 [31]	15 months (m)	NR	30	308 (238-395)
Kenya 2 [34]	697 days (m)	NR	79	339
Rwanda 1 [42]	NR	CD4 count<350	57	441 (309-619)
			34	354 (213-456)[a]
C. Median gain				
Low and Middle Income				
Kenya 1 [28]	6 months	CD4 count<200	95	109 (66-176)
Benin 1 [44]	12 months	CD4 count<200	53	103 (25-178)
Burkina Faso 1 [38,39]	6 months	CD4 count<200	43	132 (41-196)
	12 months	CD4 count<200	41	177 (105-255)
	18 months	CD4 count<200	33	172 (121-309)
	24 months	CD4 count<200	29	221 (98-295)
	30 months	CD4 count<200	26	241 (87-319)
	36 months	CD4 count<200	22	230 (90-400)
Rwanda 1 [42]	NR	CD4 count<350	57	139 (34-261)

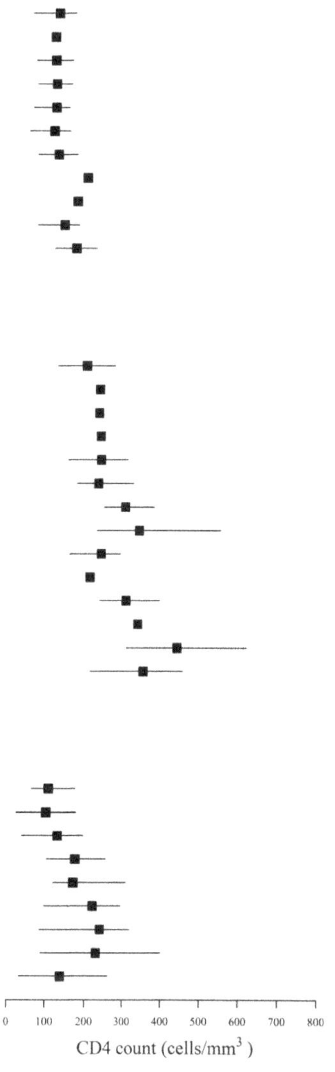

Figure 9. Forest plot of (A) median CD4 count and (B) median gains in CD4 count among HIV-infected FSWs on ART and starting ART. Study estimates are grouped by country income and ordered by time on ART. [a] N refers to a subset of FSWs who were eligible for ART upon HIV diagnosis and enrolled in HIV care following HIV diagnosis. ART = antiretroviral, FSW = female sex workers, CI = confidence interval, NR = not reported, N = sample size of FSWs available for each outcome, N_p = number of independent study populations, m = median, IQR = interquartile range.

tion of ART-eligible FSWs in HIV care initiating ART was similar to the proportion of ART-eligible individuals in the Rwandan general population initiating ART (71%) [42].

Data from two African FSW research cohorts suggest that treatment discontinuation, loss to follow-up on ART, and mortality on ART among FSWs may be low, at least over the first few years of ART use [25,28,29,38,39]. However, these studies were conducted in research contexts where there is likely to be intensive follow-up of participants, and thus better retention on treatment. Even so, total treatment attrition after one year on ART in one of the African FSW cohorts was similar to that found in the sub-Saharan African general population after 12 months on ART (23%) [64]. In addition estimates of loss to follow-up and death on ART among FSWs are similar to if not better than estimates of loss to follow-up and death among women on ART enrolled in cohort studies in South Africa and Tanzania, where 17.5% and 25.6% were loss to follow-up, respectively, and 4.1% and 12.8% died on ART, respectively [65,66]. Only three studies in Dominican Republic, Canada and the USA reported on the fraction of ART-experienced FSWs that were no longer on ART, and there was substantial between-study heterogeneity. Although the proportion of FSWs in the Dominican Republic that reported ever but not current ART use was similar to that reported by women from the general population in the USA (9%) [67], the two cross-sectional studies in North America found much higher proportions of FSWs self-reporting that they were previously but no longer on ART [24,48]. However, the sample size of FSWs in these two North American studies was very small.

Population	Time on ART	n/N	Estimate (%) and 95% CI
A. CD4 count<200			
Low and Middle Income			
Kenya 1 [32]	ART initiation [a]	115/118	89.8 (83.3-94.5)
	6 months	37/111	33.3 (24.7-42.9)
	12 months	26/92	28.3 (19.4-38.6)
	18 months	13/65	20.0 (11.1-31.8)
	24 months	6/56	10.7 (4.5-21.9)*
Burkina Faso 1 [37]	NR	10/25	40.0 (21.1-61.3)*
Overall (I^2 = 88.0%, p=0.004, N_p =2*)			**22.2 (5.0-66.4)**
B. CD4 count 200-499			
Low and Middle Income			
Kenya 1 [32]	ART initiation [a]	13/128	10.2 (5.5-16.7)
	6 months	72/111	64.9 (55.2-73.7)
	12 months	64/92	69.6 (59.1-78.7)
	18 months	43/65	66.2 (53.4-77.4)
	24 months	44/56	78.6 (65.6-88.4)*
Burkina Faso 1 [37]	NR	11/25	44.0 (24.4-65.1)*
Overall (I^2 = 88.7%, p=0.003, N_p =2*)			**63.4 (27.7-88.7)**
C. CD4 count >500			
Low and Middle Income			
Kenya 1 [32]	ART initiation [a]	0/128	0.0 (0.0-2.8)
	6 months	2/111	1.8 (0.2-6.4)
	12 months	2/92	2.2 (0.3-7.6)
	18 months	9/65	13.9 (6.5-24.6)
	24 months	6/56	10.7 (4.0-21.8)*
Burkina Faso 1 [37]	NR	4/25	16.0 (4.5-36.1)*
Overall (I^2 = 0%, p=0.507, N_p =2*)			**12.5 (6.9-21.8)**

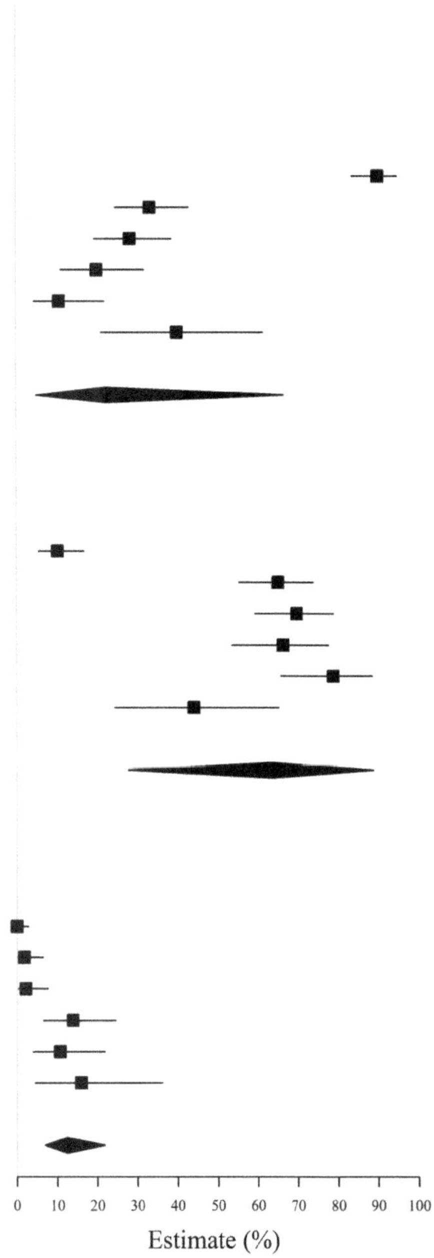

Figure 10. Forest plot of the fraction of HIV-infected FSWs on ART and starting ART with (A) CD4 counts <200 cells/mm^3 (B) CD4 counts 200–499 cells/mm^3 and (C) CD4 counts >500 cells/mm^3. Study estimates are grouped by country income and ordered by time on ART. The star symbol (*) highlights the study estimates (one per study population) included in the pooled overall estimates. For studies providing estimates over multiple time-periods, only one estimate was used for pooling (the most recent estimate from that study). I^2 and p-values are the measures of heterogeneity used. [a] ART initiation criteria is CD4 count <200 cells/mm^3. ART = antiretroviral, FSW = female sex workers, CI = confidence interval, NR = not reported, n = number of FSWs with each outcome, N = sample size of FSWs available for each outcome, N_p = number of independent study populations.

Adherence among FSWs, in the few studies where it was measured, was found to be consistently high despite different methods of assessment, recall periods and adherence thresholds. The pooled estimate of adherence among FSWs is similar to that reported for the general population in sub-Saharan Africa, where 77% were estimated to be ≥80% adherent [68], and is also similar to if not better than that reported for women in the general population, where 62% were estimated to be ≥90% adherent [69]. Adherence counselling in 4 studies [23,38,39,44], monthly support groups in one study [60], and directly administered therapy in another study [30], could have contributed to the high adherence seen in these FSW study populations.

Limited data also indicate that overall just over half of FSWs initiating ART are achieving viral suppression, which is much lower than the pooled estimate of ART adherence seen among FSWs. However, there was considerable between-study heterogeneity in the pooled estimate of viral suppression, and the varied limits of viral load detection used to define viral suppression, which ranged from <50 copies/ml to <300 copies/ml, may have influenced the results. The cohort of FSWs in Burkina Faso which used the highest limit of viral load detection to define viral suppression (<300 copies/ml), had the highest estimates of viral suppression, and these were comparable to estimates of viral suppression (defined as viral load <400 copies/ml) seen among women from the general population in South Africa, where 87%–93% of women were virally suppressed after 12 to 36 months on ART [70]. The FSWs in Burkina Faso, who had the highest levels of viral suppression, also had high levels of adherence [38,39]. Thus, the lower estimates of viral suppression could also reflect lower adherence rates among FSWs in those study settings.

For a number of FSWs, improvements in CD4 count were also achieved within 6 to 24 months of ART initiation, and these were comparable to the median gains in CD4 count achieved among women in the general population from South Africa and the UK after 6 to 12 months on ART [70,71].

To date, this is the first study to systematically review and quantify the ART cascade among FSWs globally, which builds on a limited review already undertaken by the authors [15]. Available data indicate that FSWs can achieve promising levels of ART uptake, adherence, retention, and treatment response, at least in the short-term and in these research settings, which in some cases may even be comparable to that seen in the general population over similar time-periods. However, there are a number of limitations to this systematic review. In particular, the review and meta-analysis were limited by the scarcity and heterogeneity of eligible studies. The included studies, the majority of which had small sample sizes of HIV-infected FSWs, reported data on only twenty-one different FSW study populations from only fourteen countries in Asia, Africa, North America, South America, and Central America and the Caribbean, which limits the generalizability of these findings to FSWs elsewhere (Figure 2). Most of the included studies were also research cohorts, thus these results are of limited generalizability to FSWs in other routine programme (non-research) settings. FSWs enrolling in research cohorts may be more motivated to adhere to and remain on treatment, and there are likely to be a number of other HIV prevention and support services available to FSWs in these cohorts, which coupled with intense follow-up and intensive adherence counselling, could help to improve ART uptake, retention, adherence and treatment outcomes among FSWs in these studies [72,73]. Our pooled analyses are also limited by the heterogeneity between studies, but still provide useful overall estimates of engagement in HIV treatment among FSWs. Study periods were particularly variable across studies, and this is likely to influence HIV treatment outcomes, in particular ART uptake. The time periods of data collection spanned 24 years across the different study settings, and in some studies collection of data on HIV-infected FSWs started in the pre-HAART era. To address this issue, whenever possible we conducted sub-group analyses for ART uptake outcomes by time-period of data collection (i.e. data collected in the pre-HAART to HAART era versus HAART era alone). We found that this had an effect on pooled estimates of ART initiation, and although substantial between-study heterogeneity remained, this could indicate that it might not be appropriate to aggregate all data on ART uptake regardless of study period. In the majority of cohort studies, follow-up time on ART was also relatively short, so long term attrition and treatment outcomes in FSWs remain unknown. Lack of reporting on local ART eligibility criteria also made it more difficult to interpret estimates of ART uptake. In addition, adherence to medication was most frequently measured by either self-reports or pill counts, both of which are prone to biases, such as social desirability and recall bias (Table S6). Different types of recruitment settings and sampling methods may have also introduced selection bias into the included studies. However, it was difficult to fully assess risk of selection bias as very few studies reported sampling methodology (Table S6). Some studies reported using random samples, whilst a few others reported the use of non-probability sampling methods, such as snowball sampling and convenience sampling. Snowball sampling and convenience sampling are commonly used when studying hard-to-reach populations, but are likely to have introduced bias into the selection of participants [74]. A couple of studies also reported the use of respondent-driven sampling, which is a type of snowball sampling that aims to reduce bias by taking into account the non-random patterns of participant recruitment [74]. The different recruitment settings and strategies also highlight the diversity of FSW samples across studies (Table S6). Pooled estimates may mask the potential differences in HIV treatment and care across the varied contexts and settings of sex work. It is also possible that women who do not self-identify as FSWs may have been missed at study recruitment, so in some cases outcome data is likely to be restricted to self-identifying FSWs. Thus, results may not be generalizable to indirect FSWs, who may not have been captured in these samples. Publication bias may have also affected our summary estimates, but due to the small numbers of studies that reported each outcome we could not explore this in a meaningful way. In addition, as we did not search for available data in the grey literature (our review focussed on peer-reviewed published literature), we have likely excluded some ART data that may have been available, for example, from reports of integrated biological and behavioural assessment (IBBA) surveys among FSWs.

Despite the limitations, the results from this review are encouraging, and show that even though FSWs are considered a hard population to reach for HIV prevention and care, research cohorts in particular have achieved success at enrolling and retaining FSWs on ART with good adherence and treatment response. Importantly, this review also has important public health implications since it highlights large gaps in the spatial distribution of ART cascade estimates among FSWs (Figure 2) and the paucity of data on the ART cascade among FSWs in routine (non-research) programme settings. These data gaps are concerning, and impede our understanding of 'real-life' HIV treatment and care among FSWs and potential feasibility and effectiveness of targeting FSWs for expanded ART prevention strategies. It is crucial that routine programme data on HIV care and treatment among FSWs is collected and disseminated, in order to better characterise ART cascade outcomes among FSWs (see Box S1 for a summary of our recommendations for future data collection). In particular, information on the percentage of all HIV-infected FSWs receiving ART, and how this evolves over time is needed. Estimates of ART use are likely to be affected by ART initiation criteria, HIV testing policies and testing uptake, as well as rates of linkage to and retention in HIV care prior to ART initiation. So in order to interpret data on ART uptake among FSWs, information on the evolution of ART eligibility criteria over time, the CD4 count at which FSWs are diagnosed and started treatment, as well as the percentage of HIV-infected FSWs who receive HIV testing and are linked to HIV care is required. Furthermore, gathering additional short and long-term data on treatment retention, adherence and viral suppression among FSWs, using standardised indicators is crucial. In 2010, the WHO recommended a number of different early warning indicators to use for monitoring of HIV drug resistance in national ART programmes, which included the following ART care indicators: % of patients receiving ART lost to follow-up at 12 month, % of patients retained on first-line ART at

12 months, % of patients with 100% on-time drug pickups during the first 12 months of ART or during a specified time period, % patient adherence to antiretroviral therapy by pill count or other standardized measure, and % of patients with viral load <1000 copies/mm^3 at 12 months [75]. Gathering and reporting data on these types of ART care indicators for sex workers in routine surveys of sex workers, existing sex worker programmes, and new research studies of HIV care and treatment among FSWs, could help to better characterise the ART cascade among FSWs in different settings and contexts.

When scaling up ART programmes for FSWs, it will also be important to elucidate and overcome the barriers that FSWs face to initiating ART, remaining on treatment and adhering to ART. Many individual-level and structural-level barriers, such as stigma, discrimination, violence, and drug-use, often prevent FSWs from accessing HIV services and practicing HIV prevention and harm reduction, and these barriers may also influence the ability of FSWs to traverse through the HIV care cascade [76–79]. In two of the studies included in this systematic review, FSWs reported that inability to attend regular medical appointments, potential loss of wages from visiting ART centres, prior negative experiences with the health care system, the stigmatizing attitude of medical staff, and fear of adverse consequences as a result of others knowing their HIV status and occupation, were some of the factors that prevented them from initiating ART [24,46]. In three of the studies included in this systematic review, FSWs also reported that running out of pills, not being at home to take pills, feelings of sickness when taking pills, and potential loss of clients if seen taking ART during work hours, were factors that prevented them from adhering to treatment [42,44,46]. Another qualitative study among FSWs in Zimbabwe also found that discrimination from medical staff, shame, and anxiety about being known to be a sex worker, reduced the ability of FSWs to attend HIV treatment services [80]. Travelling times to health clinics and additional financial costs were also reported as barriers to treatment [80]. It is essential that new or ongoing HIV intervention and ART programmes among FSWs try to address the structural and social barriers to HIV treatment that FSWs' face. For example, *Abriendo Puertas*, is an ongoing integrated HIV care and prevention intervention for FSWs in Dominican Republic, that aims to promote HIV care and preventative behaviours among FSWs [53]. This intervention has four key components, including individual counselling and education, peer HIV service navigation and support, clinical care health provider sensitisation training, and community solidarity and mobilisation, which together aim to provide a multi-level response to the social and structural factors that prevent FSWs engaging and remaining in care and adhering to treatment [53]. In Zimbabwe, the Sisters with a Voice (SWV) programme, which provides free STI/HIV services and assisted referrals to ART centers for FSWs, has also initiated numerous measures to try and reduce the stigma, discrimination and barriers that FSWs face at public health clinics, including training and sensitisation for nurses at public ART centers and community mobilisation among FSWs [80].

In conclusion, existing studies in a limited number of research settings indicate that it is it is feasible to enrol and retain FSWs on ART with good adherence, at least in the short-term and in these research contexts. However, there is an evident gap in global data on ART cascade outcomes among FSWs. More data, particularly long-term data, from a larger number of FSW study populations and non-research settings, needs to be collected and disseminated. When scaling-up ART programmes for FSWs, the barriers to HIV care and treatment that they face also need to be addressed.

Supporting Information

Table S1 ART uptake outcomes.

Table S2 Treatment attrition outcomes.

Table S3 Adherence to ART.

Table S4 Viral Suppression.

Table S5 CD4 Counts at and/or after ART Initiation.

Table S6 Risk of Bias Assessment.

Box S1 Recommendations for Future Data Collection.

Checklist S1 PRISMA Checklist.

Acknowledgments

We would like to sincerely thank the following authors who responded to our inquiries about relevant papers, provided additional data, or provided clarifications on study information: Susan Graham (University of Washington), Scott McClelland (University of Washington), Barbra Richardson (University of Washington), Lyle McKinnon (University of Manitoba), Marissa Becker (University of Manitoba), Leigh Anne Shafer (University of Manitoba), Thomas Kerr (British Columbia Centre for Excellence in HIV/AIDS), Kathleen Deering (British Columbia Centre for Excellence in HIV/AIDS), Ameeta Kalokhe (Emory University School of Medicine), Gabriel Cardenas (University of Miami Miller School of Medicine), Lan Anh Nguyen Thi (National Institute of Hygiene and Epidemiology), Robert Dubrow (Yale School of Public Health), Scott Comulada (UCLA Center for Community Health), Mary Jane Rotheram (Semel Institute and the Department of Psychiatry, UCLA), Deanna Kerrigan (John Hopkins Bloomberg School of Public Health), Joseph McGowan (North Shore University Hospital), Denise Jamieson (Centers for Disease Control and Prevention), Joseph Cox (Public Health Department, Montreal Health and Social Services Agency), Emilie Maurais (Public Health Department, Montreal Health and Social Services Agency), Jeffrey Samet (Boston University School of Medicine/Boston Medical Center), Carly Bridden (Boston University School of Medicine/ Boston Medical Center), Emily Kate Sisson (Boston University), Brandon Marshall (Brown University), Evan Wood (British Columbia Centre for Excellence in HIV/AIDS), Ann Dennis (Univeristy of North Carolina), Jaimie Meyer (Yale University School of Medicine), Souleymane Diabaté (University of Québec), Iris Semini (World Bank), Donald Mercante (LSU Health Sciences Center New Orleans), Patti Gravitt (John Hopkins Bloomberg School of Public Health), Laurent Michel (Centre Pierre Nicole), Ellie Schoenbaum (Albert Einstein College of Medicine), Suzanne Ohmit (University of Michigan) and Sadeep Shrestha (University of Alabama at Birmingham. We would also like to thank Juan Vesga (Imperial College London), Romain Silhol (Imperial College London) and Jennifer Tsang (University of Toronto) for their help with translating non-English language publications. SM is supported by a Canadian Institutes of Health Research Fellowship and a Royal College of Physicians and Surgeons of Canada Detweiler Fellowship.

Author Contributions

Conceived and designed the experiments: EM MCB PV SM MP. Analyzed the data: EM SM MCB. Conducted the literature search, data extraction and meta-analysis: EM. Drafted the article: EM. Provided input into article draft: SM MCB. Critically reviewed and edited the article: SM MCB MP PV CG.

References

1. Quinn TC, Wawer MJ, Sewankambo N, Serwadda D, Li C, et al. (2000) Viral load and heterosexual transmission of human immunodeficiency virus type 1. Rakai Project Study Group. New England Journal of Medicine 342: 921–929.
2. Castilla J, Del Romero J, Hernando V, Marincovich B, Garcia S, et al. (2005) Effectiveness of highly active antiretroviral therapy in reducing heterosexual transmission of HIV. Journal of Acquired Immune Deficiency Syndromes: JAIDS 40: 96–101.
3. Donnell D, Baeten JM, Kiarie J, Thomas KK, Stevens W, et al. (2010) Heterosexual HIV-1 transmission after initiation of antiretroviral therapy: a prospective cohort analysis. Lancet 375: 2092–2098.
4. Cohen MS, Chen YQ, McCauley M, Gamble T, Hosseinipour MC, et al. (2011) Prevention of HIV-1 infection with early antiretroviral therapy. N Engl J Med 365: 493–505.
5. Baggaley RF, White RG, Hollingsworth TD, Boily MC (2013) Heterosexual HIV-1 infectiousness and antiretroviral use: systematic review of prospective studies of discordant couples. Epidemiology 24: 110–121.
6. Wilson DP (2012) HIV treatment as prevention: natural experiments highlight limits of antiretroviral treatment as HIV prevention. PLoS Medicine/Public Library of Science 9: e1001231.
7. Hull MW, Wu Z, Montaner JSG (2012) Optimizing the engagement of care cascade: a critical step to maximize the impact of HIV treatment as prevention. Current Opinion in HIV & AIDS 7: 579–586.
8. Kranzer K, Govindasamy D, Ford N, Johnston V, Lawn SD (2012) Quantifying and addressing losses along the continuum of care for people living with HIV infection in sub-Saharan Africa: a systematic review. Journal of the International AIDS Society 15: 17383.
9. Hallett TB, Eaton JW (2013) A Side Door Into Care Cascade for HIV-Infected Patients? Journal of Acquired Immune Deficiency Syndromes: JAIDS 63 Suppl 2: S228–232.
10. Rosen S, Fox MP (2011) Retention in HIV care between testing and treatment in sub-Saharan Africa: a systematic review. PLoS Medicine/Public Library of Science 8: e1001056.
11. Mugglin C, Estill J, Wandeler G, Bender N, Egger M, et al. (2012) Loss to programme between HIV diagnosis and initiation of antiretroviral therapy in sub-Saharan Africa: systematic review and meta-analysis. Trop Med Int Health.
12. Boily MC, Lowndes C, Alary M (2002) The impact of HIV epidemic phases on the effectiveness of core group interventions: insights from mathematical models. Sexually Transmitted Infections 78 Suppl 1: i78–90.
13. Baral S, Beyrer C, Muessig K, Poteat T, Wirtz AL, et al. (2012) Burden of HIV among female sex workers in low-income and middle-income countries: a systematic review and meta-analysis. Lancet Infect Dis 12: 538–549.
14. Vickerman P, Foss AM, Pickles M, Deering K, Verma S, et al. (2010) To what extent is the HIV epidemic in southern India driven by commercial sex? A modelling analysis. AIDS 24: 2563–2572.
15. Delva W, Eaton JW, Meng F, Fraser C, White RG, et al. (2012) HIV treatment as prevention: optimising the impact of expanded HIV treatment programmes. PLoS Medicine/Public Library of Science 9: e1001258.
16. Alary M, Lowndes CM, Van de Perre P, Behanzin L, Batona G, et al. (2013) Scale-up of combination prevention and antiretroviral therapy for female sex workers in West Africa: time for action. AIDS 27: 1369–1374.
17. Kato M, Granich R, Duc Bui D, Tran HV, Nadol P, et al. (2013) The potential impact of expanding antiretroviral therapy and combination prevention in Vietnam: Towards elimination of HIV transmission. J Acquir Immune Defic Syndr.
18. Moher D, Liberati A, Tetzlaff J, Altman DG (2010) Preferred reporting items for systematic reviews and meta-analyses: the PRISMA statement. Int J Surg 8: 336–341.
19. Stroup DF, Berlin JA, Morton SC, Olkin I, Williamson GD, et al. (2000) Meta-analysis of observational studies in epidemiology - A proposal for reporting. Jama-Journal of the American Medical Association 283: 2008–2012.
20. Pereira TPN, Salantic G, Ioannidisc J (2010) Critical interpretation of Cochran's Q test depends on power and prior assumptions about heterogeneity. Research Synthesis Methods 1: 149–161.
21. Engels EA, Schmid CH, Terrin N, Olkin I, Lau J (2000) Heterogeneity and statistical significance in meta-analysis: an empirical study of 125 meta-analyses. Statistics in Medicine 19: 1707–1728.
22. Kilmarx PH, Limpakarnjanarat K, Kaewkungwal J, Srismith R, Saisorn S, et al. (2000) Disease progression and survival with human immunodeficiency virus type 1 subtype E infection among female sex workers in Thailand. Journal of Infectious Diseases 181: 1598–1606.
23. Deering KN, Shannon K, Sinclair H, Parsad D, Gilbert E, et al. (2009) Piloting a peer-driven intervention model to increase access and adherence to antiretroviral therapy and HIV care among street-entrenched HIV-positive women in Vancouver. AIDS Patient Care & Stds 23: 603–609.
24. Shannon K, Bright V, Duddy J, Tyndall MW (2005) Access and utilization of HIV treatment and services among women sex workers in Vancouver's Downtown Eastside. Journal of Urban Health 82: 488–497.
25. Masese LN, Graham SM, Gitau R, Peshu N, Jaoko W, et al. (2011) A prospective study of vaginal trichomoniasis and HIV-1 shedding in women on antiretroviral therapy. BMC Infectious Diseases 11: 307.
26. Graham SM, Masese L, Gitau R, Richardson BA, Mandaliya K, et al. (2011) Genital ulceration does not increase HIV-1 shedding in cervical or vaginal secretions of women taking antiretroviral therapy. Sex Transm Infect 87: 114–117.
27. Graham SM, Masese L, Gitau R, Mwakangalu D, Jaoko W, et al. (2009) Increased risk of genital ulcer disease in women during the first month after initiating antiretroviral therapy. Journal of Acquired Immune Deficiency Syndromes: JAIDS 52: 600–603.
28. Graham SM, Masese L, Gitau R, Jalalian-Lechak Z, Richardson BA, et al. (2010) Antiretroviral adherence and development of drug resistance are the strongest predictors of genital HIV-1 shedding among women initiating treatment. Journal of Infectious Diseases 202: 1538–1542.
29. Graham SM, Jalalian-Lechak Z, Shafi J, Chohan V, Deya RW, et al. (2012) Antiretroviral treatment interruptions predict female genital shedding of genotypically resistant HIV-1 RNA. Journal of Acquired Immune Deficiency Syndromes: JAIDS 60: 511–518.
30. Graham SM, Holte SE, Peshu NM, Richardson BA, Panteleeff DD, et al. (2007) Initiation of antiretroviral therapy leads to a rapid decline in cervical and vaginal HIV-1 shedding. AIDS 21: 501–507.
31. Gitau RW, Graham SM, Masese LN, Overbaugh J, Chohan V, et al. (2010) Effect of acquisition and treatment of cervical infections on HIV-1 shedding in women on antiretroviral therapy. AIDS 24: 2733–2737.
32. McClelland RS, Graham SM, Richardson BA, Peshu N, Masese LN, et al. (2010) Treatment with antiretroviral therapy is not associated with increased sexual risk behavior in Kenyan female sex workers. AIDS 24: 891–897.
33. McClelland L, Wanje G, Kashonga F, Kibe L, McClelland RS, et al. (2011) Understanding the context of HIV risk behavior among HIV-positive and HIV-negative female sex workers and male bar clients following antiretroviral therapy rollout in Mombasa, Kenya. AIDS Educ Prev 23: 299–312.
34. McKinnon LR, Kimani M, Wachihi C, Nagelkerke NJ, Muriuki FK, et al. (2010) Effect of baseline HIV disease parameters on CD4+ T cell recovery after antiretroviral therapy initiation in Kenyan women. PLoS ONE [Electronic Resource] 5: e11434.
35. Mawji E, McKinnon L, Wachihi C, Chege D, Thottingal P, et al. (2012) Does antiretroviral therapy initiation increase sexual risk taking in Kenyan female sex workers? A retrospective case-control study. BMJ Open 2: e000565.
36. Lester RT, Yao XD, Ball TB, McKinnon LR, Omange WR, et al. (2009) HIV-1 RNA dysregulates the natural TLR response to subclinical endotoxemia in Kenyan female sex-workers. PLoS ONE [Electronic Resource] 4: e5644.
37. Low AJ, Clayton T, Konate I, Nagot N, Ouedraogo A, et al. (2011) Genital warts and infection with human immunodeficiency virus in high-risk women in Burkina Faso: a longitudinal study. BMC Infectious Diseases 11: 20.
38. Konate I, Traore L, Ouedraogo A, Sanon A, Diallo R, et al. (2011) Linking HIV prevention and care for community interventions among high-risk women in Burkina Faso–the ARNS 1222 "Yerelon" cohort. Journal of Acquired Immune Deficiency Syndromes: JAIDS 57 Suppl 1: S50–54.
39. Huet C, Ouedraogo A, Konate I, Traore I, Rouet F, et al. (2011) Long-term virological, immunological and mortality outcomes in a cohort of HIV-infected female sex workers treated with highly active antiretroviral therapy in Africa. BMC Public Health 11: 700.
40. Becker ML, Mishra S, Satyanarayana, Gurav K, Doshi M, et al. (2012) Rates and determinants of HIV-attributable mortality among rural female sex workers in Northern Karnataka, India. Int J STD AIDS 23: 36–40.
41. Kalokhe AS, Paranjape A, Bell CE, Cardenas GA, Kuper T, et al. (2012) Intimate partner violence among HIV-infected crack cocaine users. AIDS Patient Care & Stds 26: 234–240.
42. Braunstein SL, Umulisa MM, Veldhuijzen NJ, Kestelyn E, Ingabire CM, et al. (2011) HIV diagnosis, linkage to HIV care, and HIV risk behaviors among newly diagnosed HIV-positive female sex workers in Kigali, Rwanda. Journal of Acquired Immune Deficiency Syndromes: JAIDS 57: e70–76.
43. Dean J, Ta Thi TH, Dunford L, Carr MJ, Nguyen LT, et al. (2011) Prevalence of HIV type 1 antiretroviral drug resistance mutations in Vietnam: a multicenter study. AIDS Research & Human Retroviruses 27: 797–801.
44. Diabaté S, Zannou DM, Geraldo N, Chamberland A, Akakpo J, et al. (2011) Antiretroviral Therapy among HIV-1 Infected Female Sex Workers in Benin: A Comparative Study with Patients from the General Population. World Journal of AIDS 1: 94–99.
45. Reddon H, Wood E, Tyndall M, Lai C, Hogg R, et al. (2011) Use of North America's first medically supervised safer injecting facility among HIV-positive injection drug users. AIDS Educ Prev 23: 412–422.
46. Chakrapani V, Newman PA, Shunmugam M, Kurian AK, Dubrow R (2009) Barriers to free antiretroviral treatment access for female sex workers in Chennai, India. AIDS Patient Care & Stds 23: 973–980.
47. Schuelter-Trevisol F, da Silva MV, Oliveira CM, Rodrigues R (2007) HIV genotyping among female sex workers in the State of Santa Catarina. Revista Da Sociedade Brasileira de Medicina Tropical 40: 259–263.
48. Comulada WS, Swendeman DT, Rotheram-Borus MJ, Mattes KM, Weiss RE (2003) Use of HAART among young people living with HIV. Am J Health Behav 27: 389–400.
49. Balkus JE, Richardson BA, Mochache V, Chohan V, Chan JD, et al. (2013) A prospective cohort study comparing the effect of single-dose 2 G metronidazole

on trichomonas vaginalis infection in HIV-seropositive versus HIV-seronegative women. Sexually Transmitted Diseases 40: 499–505.

50. Cowan FM, Mtetwa S, Davey C, Fearon E, Dirawo J, et al. (2013) Engagement with HIV Prevention Treatment and Care among Female Sex Workers in Zimbabwe: A Respondent Driven Sampling Survey. PLoS ONE 8.
51. Day S, Odem-Davis K, Mandaliya K, Jerome K, Jaoko W, et al. (2012) Hepatitis b virus co-infection in human immunodeficiency virus positive female sex workers in mombasa, Kenya: A prospective cohort study. Journal of Investigative Medicine 60 (1): 195–196.
52. Dennis AM, Murillo W, De Maria Hernandez F, Guardado ME, Nieto AI, et al. (2013) Social network-based recruitment successfully reveals HIV-1 transmission networks among high-risk individuals in El Salvador. Journal of Acquired Immune Deficiency Syndromes 63: 135–141.
53. Donastorg Y, Barrington C, Perez M, Kerrigan D (2014) Abriendo Puertas: Baseline Findings from an Integrated Intervention to Promote Prevention, Treatment and Care among FSW Living with HIV in the Dominican Republic. PLoS One 9: e88157.
54. Graham SM, Rajwans N, Jaoko W, Estambale BB, McClelland RS, et al. (2013) Endothelial activation biomarkers increase after HIV-1 acquisition: plasma vascular cell adhesion molecule-1 predicts disease progression. AIDS 27: 1803–1813.
55. Jadhav A, Bhattacharjee P, Raghavendra T, Blanchard J, Moses S, et al. (2013) Risky Behaviors among HIV-Positive Female Sex Workers in Northern Karnataka, India. AIDS Res Treat 2013: 878151.
56. Low AJ, Konate I, Nagot N, Weiss HA, Kania D, et al. (2014) Cervicovaginal HIV-1 shedding in women taking antiretroviral therapy in burkina faso: A longitudinal study. Journal of Acquired Immune Deficiency Syndromes 65: 237–245.
57. Low AJ, Konate I, Nagot N, Weiss HA, Mabey D, et al. (2014) Neisseria gonorrhoeae and Chlamydia trachomatis infection in HIV-1-infected women taking antiretroviral therapy: a prospective cohort study from Burkina Faso. Sex Transm Infect 90: 100–103.
58. Cox J, Maurais E, Hu L, Moodie EEM, Law S, et al. (2014) Correlates of drug use cessation among participants in the Canadian HIV-HCV Co-infection Cohort. Drug and Alcohol Dependence 137: 121–128.
59. Tyurina A, Krupitsky E, Cheng DM, Coleman SM, Walley AY, et al. (2013) Is cannabis use associated with HIV drug and sex risk behaviors among Russian HIV-infected risky drinkers? Drug and Alcohol Dependence 132: 74–80.
60. Graham SM, Mugo P, Gichuru E, Thiong'o A, Macharia M, et al. (2013) Adherence to antiretroviral therapy and clinical outcomes among young adults reporting high-risk sexual behavior, including men who have sex with men, in coastal Kenya. AIDS and behavior 17: 1255–1265.
61. Mehta M, Semitala F, Lynen L, Colebunders R (2012) Antiretroviral treatment in low-resource settings: what has changed in the last 10 years and what needs to change in the coming years? Expert Rev Anti Infect Ther 10: 1287–1296.
62. Bila B, Egrot M (2009) Gender asymmetry in healthcare-facility attendance of people living with HIV/AIDS in Burkina Faso. Social Science & Medicine 69: 854–861.
63. Tapp C, Milloy MJ, Kerr T, Zhang R, Guillemi S, et al. (2011) Female gender predicts lower access and adherence to antiretroviral therapy in a setting of free healthcare. Bmc Infectious Diseases 11.
64. Fox MP, Rosen S (2010) Patient retention in antiretroviral therapy programs up to three years on treatment in sub-Saharan Africa, 2007–2009: systematic review. Tropical Medicine & International Health 15 Suppl 1: 1–15.
65. Maskew M, Brennan AT, Westreich D, McNamara L, MacPhail AP, et al. (2013) Gender Differences in Mortality and CD4 Count Response Among Virally Suppressed HIV-Positive Patients. Journal of Womens Health 22: 113–120.
66. Mosha F, Muchunguzi V, Matee M, Sangeda RZ, Vercauteren J, et al. (2013) Gender differences in HIV disease progression and treatment outcomes among HIV patients one year after starting antiretroviral treatment (ART) in Dar es Salaam, Tanzania. Bmc Public Health 13.
67. Hughes AJ, Mattson CL, Scheer S, Beer L, Skarbinski J (2014) Discontinuation of antiretroviral therapy among adults receiving HIV care in the United States. Journal of acquired immune deficiency syndromes (1999) 66: 80–89.
68. Mills EJ, Nachega JB, Buchan I, Orbinski J, Attaran A, et al. (2006) Adherence to antiretroviral therapy in sub-Saharan Africa and North America: a meta-analysis. JAMA 296: 679–690.
69. Ortego C, Huedo-Medina TB, Santos P, Rodriguez E, Sevilla L, et al. (2012) Sex differences in adherence to highly active antiretroviral therapy: A meta-analysis. Aids Care-Psychological and Socio-Medical Aspects of Aids/Hiv 24: 1519–1534.
70. Cornell M, Schomaker M, Garone DB, Giddy J, Hoffmann CJ, et al. (2012) Gender Differences in Survival among Adult Patients Starting Antiretroviral Therapy in South Africa: A Multicentre Cohort Study. Plos Medicine 9.
71. Barber TJ, Geretti AM, Anderson J, Schwenk A, Phillips AN, et al. (2011) Outcomes in the first year after initiation of first-line HAART among heterosexual men and women in the UK CHIC Study. Antiviral Therapy 16: 805–814.
72. Jean K, Anglaret X, Moh R, Lert F, Dray-Spira R (2012) Barriers to HIV testing in Cote d'Ivoire: the role of individual characteristics and testing modalities. PLoS One 7: e41353.
73. McMahon JH, Elliott JH, Hong SY, Bertagnolio S, Jordan MR (2013) Effects of physical tracing on estimates of loss to follow-up, mortality and retention in low and middle income country antiretroviral therapy programs: a systematic review. PLoS ONE [Electronic Resource] 8: e56047.
74. Heckathorn DD (2002) Respondent-driven sampling II: Deriving valid population estimates from chain-referral samples of hidden populations. Social Problems 49: 11–34.
75. WHO (2011) Global HIV/AIDS response: epidemic update and health sector progress towards universal access: progress report 2011. WHO, Geneva, Switzerland.
76. Ghimire L, Smith WCS, van Teijlingen ER (2011) Utilisation of sexual health services by female sex workers in Nepal. Bmc Health Services Research 11.
77. Lazarus L, Deering KN, Nabess R, Gibson K, Tyndall MW, et al. (2012) Occupational stigma as a primary barrier to health care for street-based sex workers in Canada. Culture Health & Sexuality 14: 139–150.
78. Phrasisombath K, Thomsen S, Sychareun V, Faxelid E (2012) Care seeking behaviour and barriers to accessing services for sexually transmitted infections among female sex workers in Laos: a cross-sectional study. Bmc Health Services Research 12.
79. Shannon K, Kerr T, Allinott S, Chettiar J, Shoveller J, et al. (2008) Social and structural violence and power relations in mitigating HIV risk of drug-using women in survival sex work. Social Science & Medicine 66: 911–921.
80. Mtetwa S, Busza J, Chidiya S, Mungofa S, Cowan F (2013) "You are wasting our drugs": health service barriers to HIV treatment for sex workers in Zimbabwe. Bmc Public Health 13.

20

γδ T Cells Are Involved in Acute HIV Infection and Associated with AIDS Progression

Zhen Li[1]❡, Wei Li[2]❡, Ning Li[3], Yanmei Jiao[2], Dexi Chen[2], Lianxian Cui[1], Yu Hu[1], Hao Wu[2]*, Wei He[1]*

1 Department of Immunology, School of Basic Medicine, Peking Union Medical College; National Key Laboratory of Medical Molecular Biology, Institute of Basic Medical Sciences, Chinese Academy of Medical Sciences, Beijing, China, **2** Center for Infectious Diseases, Beijing You'an Hospital, Capital Medical University, Beijing, China, **3** Beijing You'an Hospital, Capital Medical University, Beijing, China

Abstract

Background: Early diagnosis is vital to HIV control. γδ T cells play critical roles in viral infections, but their activation in acute HIV infected patients and follow up to 18 months has not been described.

Methods: Changes in γδ T cells, including subsets, function and activation, in treated and untreated acutely HIV-infected patients ($n = 79$) were compared by cytotoxicity assay and flow cytometry with healthy controls ($n = 21$) at month 0, 6, 12 and 18.

Results: In acutely HIV-infected patients, Vδ1 cell proportion was elevated ($P = 0.027$) with Vδ2 population reduced ($P = 0.002$). Effector and central memory γδ T cell factions were decreased ($P = 0.006$ and $P = 0.001$, respectively), while proportion of terminal γδ T cells increased ($P = 0.002$). γδ T cell cytotoxicity was compromised over time. Fraction of IL-17-producing cells increased ($P = 0.008$), and IFN-γ-producing cells were unaffected ($P = 0.115$). Elevation of a microbial translocation marker, sCD14, was associated with γδ T cell activation ($P = 0.001$), which increased in a time-dependent manner, correlating with CD4/CD8 T cell activation set-points and CD4 counts. Antiretroviral therapy did not affect these changes.

Conclusions: γδ T cell subpopulation and functions change significantly in acute HIV infection and over time. Early γδ T cell activation was associated with CD4/CD8 T cell activation set-points, which predict AIDS progression. Therefore, γδ T cell activation represents a potential surrogate marker of AIDS progression.

Editor: R. Keith Reeves, Beth Israel Deaconess Medical Center, Harvard Medical School, United States of America

Funding: This work was supported by Twelve-five Project for Control and Prevention of Major Infectious Diseases [2012ZX10001-006], National Natural Science Foundation of China [81371332], and Beijing Key Laboratory [BZ0089]. The funders had no role in study design, data collection and analysis, decision to publish, or preparation of the manuscript.

Competing Interests: The authors have declared that no competing interests exist.

* Email: wuhao90000@gmail.com (HW); suprahe@126.com (WH)

❡ These authors contributed equally to this work.

Introduction

Human γδ T cells are distinct from αβ T cells, and generally lack CD4 or CD8 antigen expression [1]. These cells represent approximately 3–4% of peripheral T cells in the blood, and are composed predominantly of two subsets, depending on expression of the Vδ1 or Vδ2 gene [2–5].Vδ1 T cells respond to antigens from bacterial pathogens [6]. Vδ2 T cells are believed to be activated by several chemical compounds, some of which are produced by activated host cells in response to pathogenic infections [7]. Vδ2 T cells can be further divided into four subtypes: naïve (Tnaïve), central memory (TCM), effector memory (TEM) and terminally differentiated (TEMRA), based on differential surface expression of CD45RA and CD27 [8,9]. Specific Tnaïve and TCM cells are located in the lymph nodes and possess distinct functions [10–12]. TEM and TEMRA are located preferentially at inflammatory sites and perform effector functions [10].

Functionally, γδ T cells produce interleukin 17 (IL-17), interferon gamma (IFN-γ), and other secreted protein factors after activation [13,14]. IL-17 is thought to be important for maintaining intestinal mucosal integrity and controlling microbial translocation [15]. IFN-γ levels are elevated in many proinflammatory events, and microbial translocation [16]. Furthermore, γδ T cells are involved in the recruitment of neutrophils in bacterial infections [17]. Reports indicate that, the cytotoxic activity of γδ T lymphocytes against human neuroblastoma cells, Burkitt's lymphoma cells and various cancer cell lines (human colon carcinoma, erytholeukemia, human neuroepithelioma and renal adenocarcinoma) is augmented upon activation [18,19].

It has been reported that, in all stages of HIV infections, gut functions are compromised, leading to enteropathy, which is commonly observed in HIV-infected patients. The permeability of the mucosal barrier is significantly elevated [20,21], which may result in translocation of microbial products into the systemic circulation, leading to immune stimulation. A number of studies have described the use of soluble CD14 (sCD14) as a marker of microbial translocation, and even as a predictive marker of disease progression in HIV infection [22–24].

The γδ T cell responses to HIV infection are complicated and not well-elucidated [25,26]. Previous reports have indicated increased levels of Vδ1 cells and decreased levels and function of Vδ2 cells in chronically HIV-infected patients [26,27]. Furthermore, changes in the Vδ2 T cell population correlated positively with CD4 T cell counts and negatively with viral loads [26].

The therapeutic efficacy of antiretroviral therapy (ART) on Vδ2 T cell recovery in HIV patients is controversial and inconclusive. A report in 2004 indicated partial recovery of the Vδ2 T cell population following long-term HIV-suppressive therapy [28]. However, a subsequent study demonstrated that ART failed to restore the Vδ2 repertoire in HIV-infected men [29].

In this study, we aimed to characterize the changes in γδ T cells, including subsets, function and activation status, in acutely HIV-infected patients who were followed from acute infection up to 18 months, and to define their possible correlation with other serum parameters, microbial translocation and AIDS progression.

Methods

Study subjects

The protocol for this study was approved by the Beijing You'an Hospital Ethics Committee and the Guidelines for Human Experimentation (PR. China) were followed throughout. Upon admission, all patients provided written informed consent for their information and clinical samples (blood and plasma) to be stored and used for research.

Seventy-nine homosexual men with acute HIV infection were enrolled in a prospective study (co-inclusion in the Beijing PRIMO cohort) conducted in Beijing You'an Hospital, Beijing, PR. China. Acute HIV infection was defined by a negative enzyme-linked immunosorbent assay (ELISA), and at least one of the following criteria: less than three bands on HIV Western blot (HIV BLOT2.2, 11039, Diagnostic Biotechnology Pte, Singapore), a positive p24 test or detectable plasma HIV-RNA. The estimated date of infection was calculated as follows: 2 weeks before onset of symptoms or 4 weeks before the first positive Western blot. All 79 enrolled HIV-infected patients were diagnosed early during the acute stage of HIV infection (median of estimated time post-infection: 41 days) and transmitted by homosexual activity. At baseline (day 0 of enrollment), all patients were treatment-naïve. During the follow-up times, some of the patients (11/79) started combination antiretroviral treatment (ART), based on CD4 cell counts (e.g. <350/μL according to WHO recommendations) with or without clinical symptoms, and the consensus of both physicians and patients. Patients who were treated during the study received a combination of AZT, 3TC, and EFV or LPV/r. The courses of their treatment were not influenced by the authors for the purpose of this study. Most of them (68/79) were still untreated [CD4 counts: >350/μL (n = 48), <350/μL (n = 20)]. Twenty-one male homosexual healthy subjects were included as controls (HC). The ages of all groups were matched.

Blood samples were collected from patients at baseline (day 0 of enrollment), month 6, month 12 and month 18. Plasma samples were also collected from all healthy volunteers. All tests were performed at baseline. In addition, CD38/HLA-DR antigen expression and the cytotoxicity activity of γδ T cells were determined at baseline, month 6, month 12 and month 18.

Cell culture

Peripheral blood mononuclear cells (PBMCs) were isolated by Ficoll-Hypaque (TBD, Tianjin, China) centrifugation. The expansion of γδ T cells was performed as previously described [30]. Briefly, 24-well plates were coated with 500 μL purified anti-γδTCR antibody (IMMU510, 1 mg/mL; Immunotech, Beckman Coulter, Fullerton, CA, USA) at 37°C for 2 h. PBMCs were then added to the antibody-coated wells and cultured in RPMI 1640 medium supplemented with 10% FCS and 200 IU/mL recombinant human IL-2 (Beijing Read United Cross Pharmaceutical, Beijing, China). The culture medium was replaced every other day. The trypan blue exclusion method was employed to assess cell viability.

Antibodies and flow cytometry

Antibodies (Abs) used in this study were as follows: mouse phycoerythin (PE)-conjugated anti-human CD38 (HIT2) Ab, mouse allophycocyanin (APC)-conjugated anti-human HLA-DR (L243) Ab, mouse phycoerythin-cyanin7(PE-cy7)-conjugated anti-human CD3 (HIT3a) Ab, mouse peridinin-chlorophyll-protein complex cyanine 5.5 (PerCP-cy5.5) conjugated anti-human CD27 (O323) Ab, mouse APC-conjugated anti-human CD45RA (HI100) Ab were purchased from Biolegend (San Diego, CA, USA). Mouse Fluorescein isothiocyanate (FITC)-conjugated anti-human pan TCRγδ Ab, mouse PE-conjugated anti-human pan TCRγδ (IMMU510) Ab and mouse FITC-conjugated anti-human pan $V\delta_2$TCR (IMMU389) Ab were purchased from Immunotech (Beckman Coulter, Fullerton, CA, USA). Mouse FITC-conjugated anti-human pan $V\delta_1$TCR (TS8.2) Ab was purchased from Pierce (USA). Mouse PE-conjugated anti-human IL-17A (SCPL1362) Ab and mouse PE-conjugated anti-human IFN-γ (B27) Ab were purchased from BD Pharmingen (San Diego, CA, USA). The isotype control antibodies were purchased from the corresponding company, respectively.

Cells were stained with appropriate target Abs and isotype Abs using conventional surface- and/or intracellular staining methods. When both surface and intracellular staining was required, cells were first fixed and permeabilized using BD Cytofix/Cytoperm Fixation and Permeabilization Solution (BD Pharmingen), followed by staining for intracellular proteins. Cells were then washed extensively with PBS to remove excess Ab, stained for extracellular targets, and fixed with 2% formaldehyde. Fluorescence was evaluated with a FACSCalibur flow cytometer, and data were analyzed using FlowJo software (Tree Star, Ashland, OR, USA).

Cytotoxicity

The CytoTox 96 Non-Radioactive Cytotoxicity Assay (Promega, Madison, WI, USA), based on the colorimetric detection of released lactate dehydrogenase (LDH), was used according to the manufacturer's instructions. Tumor cells used as target cells were seeded into a 96-round well plate (5×10^4 cells/well). Expanded γδ T cells (effector cells) were added directly to individual wells at different effector/target (E/T) ratios. The plate was incubated at 37°C for 4 h before supernatants were collected and LDH activity was determined. Controls for spontaneous LDH release from effector and target cells, the target maximum release, as well as the culture medium background were assayed simultaneously. The cytotoxicity was calculated as follows: %Cytotoxicity = (Experimental-Effector spontaneous-Target spontaneous)/(Target maximum-Target spontaneous) ×100%.

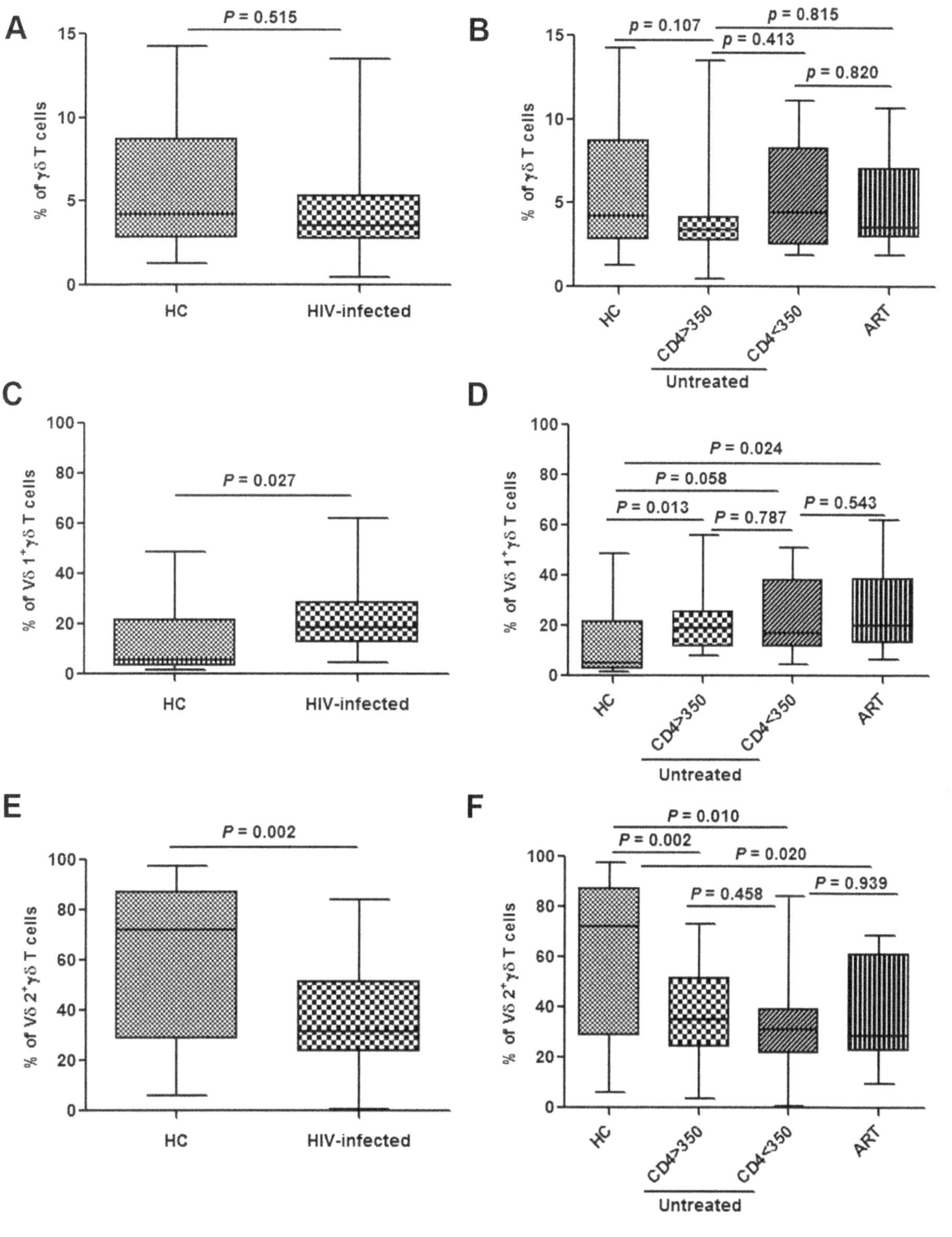

Figure 1. Changes in different subpopulations of γδ T cells in acutely HIV-infected patients. Frequencies of total γδ T cells, Vδ1 γδ T and Vδ2 γδ T cells were analyzed in healthy controls (HC) and acutely HIV-infected subjects at baseline (**A, C, E**). The patients were then subdivided based on the administration of antiretroviral therapy (ART) and CD4 levels (< or >than 350/μL). The frequencies were re-analyzed and compared with HC (**B, D, F**).

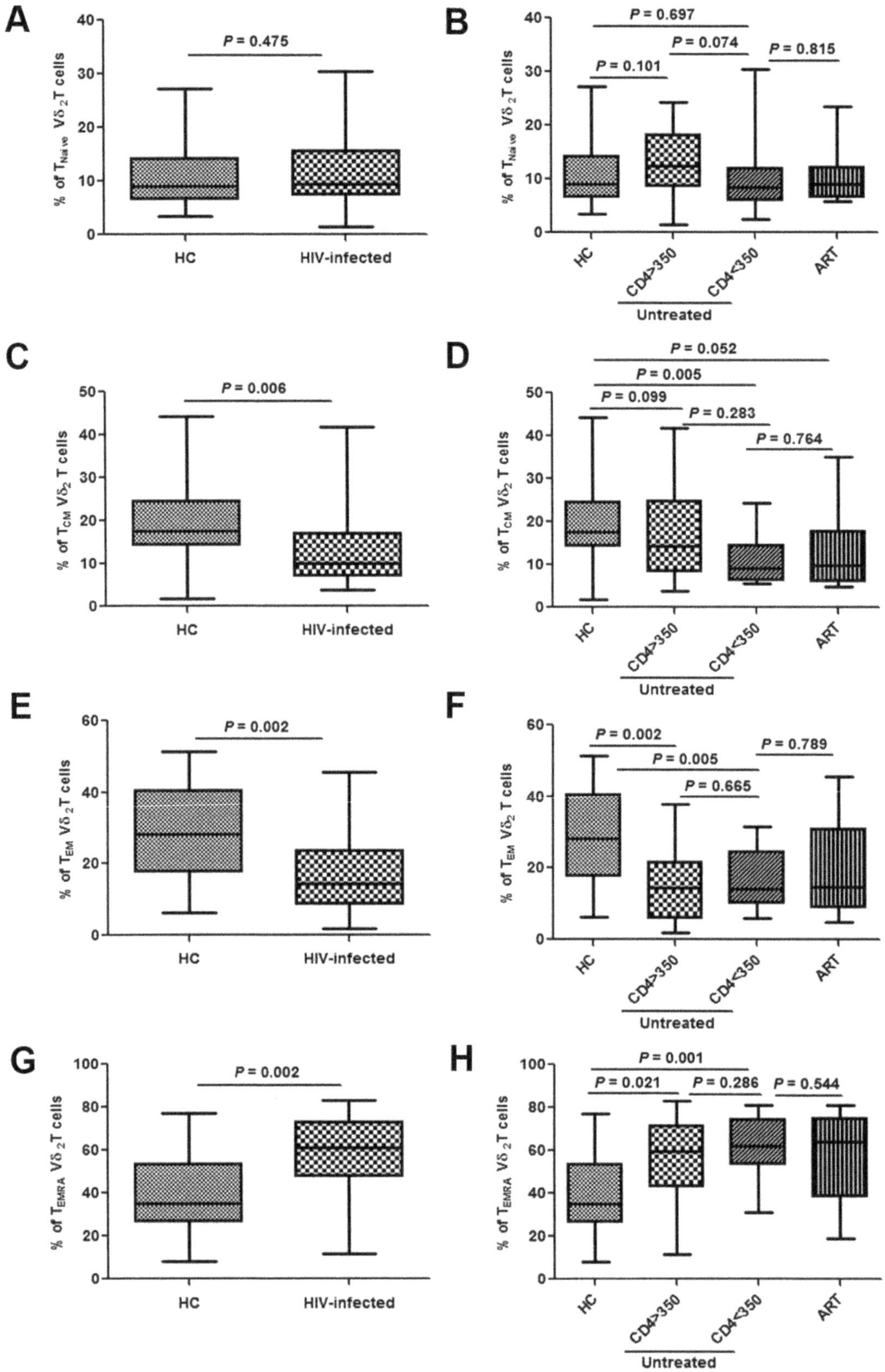

Figure 2. Changes in subpopulations of Vδ2γδ T cells in acutely HIV-infected patients. Frequencies of Tnaïve, TCM, TEM and TEMRA cells were analyzed in healthy controls (HC) and acutely HIV-infected subjects at baseline (**A, C, E, G**). The patients were then subdivided based on the administration of antiretroviral therapy (ART) and CD4 levels (< or >than 350/μL). The frequencies were re-analyzed and compared with HC (**B, D, F, H**).

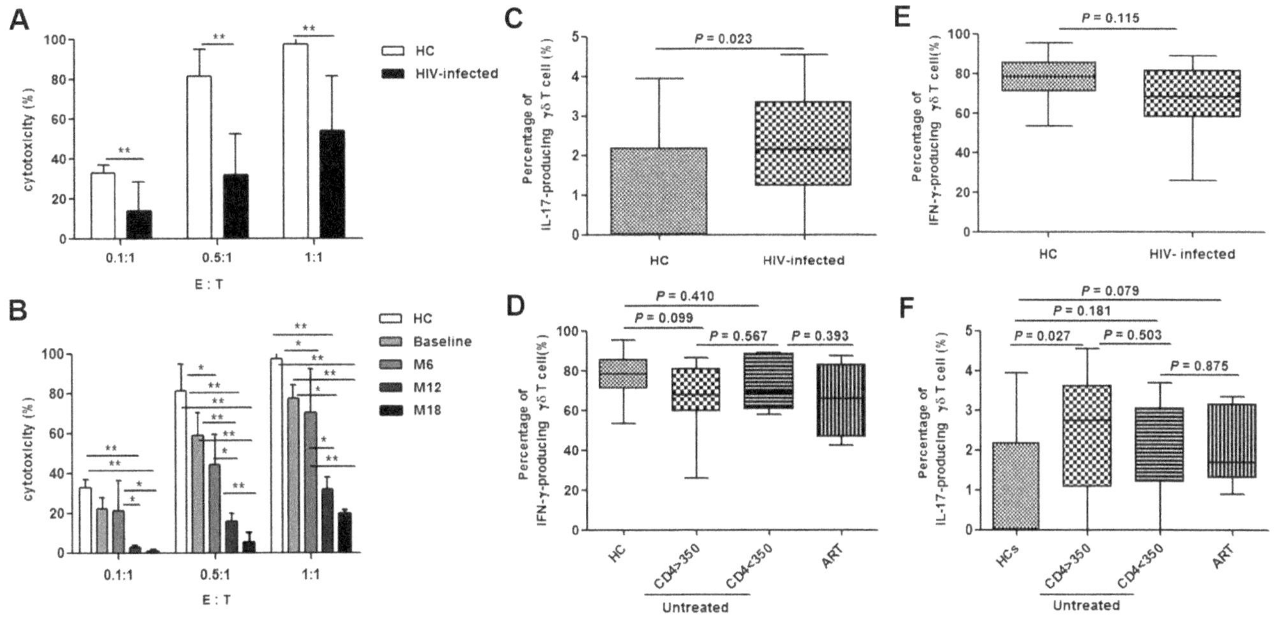

Figure 3. Altered functions of γδ T cells in acute HIV infection. Cytotoxicity (%) was assessed at different effector (E, γδ T cells) to target (T, Daudi cells) ratios (0.1:1, 0.5µ1 and 1:1) at baseline (**A**). Subsequently, longitudinal follow-up analysis of cytotoxicity was conducted at different time-points [baseline, month 6 (M6), month 12 (M12) and month 18 (M18)] (**B**). Frequencies of IFN-γ- and IL-17-producing γδ T cells were analyzed in healthy controls (HC) and acutely HIV-infected subjects at baseline (**C, E**). The patients were then subdivided based on the administration of antiretroviral therapy (ART) and CD4 levels (< or >than 350/µL). The frequencies were re-analyzed and compared with HC (**D, F**). *: $P<0.05$, **: $P<0.01$.

Quantification of plasma lipopolysaccharide (LPS), LPS-binding protein (LBP) and soluble CD14 (sCD14)

Commercially available ELISA kits were used in this study following manufacturers' instructions for measuring plasma concentrations of LBP (Cell Sciences, MA, USA) and sCD14 (soluble CD14) (R&D Systems, MN, USA). Plasma LPS levels were quantified using a *Limulus amebocyte* lysate (LAL) assay (Hycult Biotech, UDEN, Netherlands).

Statistical analysis

Non-parametric tests were used to avoid the impact of potential outlier values in a small study. Comparisons between groups were performed using the Mann-Whitney test. The Wilcox on matched pairs test was used to estimate the changes in the different variables throughout the follow-up. The Spearman's non-parametric correlation was used to estimate the association of two continuous variables of interest. *P*-values below 0.05 were considered statistically significant. Data of patients on ART were compared only with data of untreated patients with CD4 counts lower than 350/µL.

Results

Changes in γδ T cell subpopulations in acutely HIV-infected patients

Compared with healthy subjects, there was no marked difference in the fraction of γδ T cells in acutely HIV-infected patients (**Fig. 1A**). Nor were there any differences between patients with different CD4 counts, or those who did or did not receive ART (**Fig. 1B**). To characterize the changes in γδ T cells subpopulations in acutely HIV-infected patients, we first analyzed changes in the Vδ1 and Vδ2 subtypes. The proportion of Vδ1 cells among γδ T cells was elevated ($P=0.027$), while the Vδ2 population was significantly reduced ($P=0.002$) (**Fig. 1C and 1E**). However, there were no significant differences in both the proportions of Vδ1 and Vδ2 cells between patients with different CD4 counts (both $P>0.05$). Furthermore, Initiation of ART failed to bring about Vδ2 subtype recover, and had no effect on the Vδ1 population (**Fig. 1D and 1F**).

Changes in the levels of Vδ2 γδ T subgroups in acutely HIV-infected patients were investigated by analysis of the expression of surface CD27 and CD45RA antigens [8,9]. There was no difference in the proportion of naïve Vδ2γδT cells (CD27+/CD45RA+) observed ($P=0.475$), on which CD4 levels and ART showed no impact (**Fig. 2A and 2B**). The fractions of the TEM (effector memory Vδ2 γδ T cells, CD27−/CD45RA−) and TCM (central memory Vδ2 γδ T cells, CD27+/CD45RA−) populations were significantly decreased in acutely HIV-infected patients ($P=0.002$ and $P=0.006$, respectively), while the proportion of TEMRA (terminal Vδ2 γδ T cells, CD27−/CD45RA+) was increased ($P=0.002$) (**Fig. 2C, 2E, and 2G**). CD4 levels and the initiation of ART showed no correlation with these changes (**Fig. 2D, 2F, and 2H**).

Compromised γδ T cell functions in acutely HIV-infected patients

The cytotoxic activity of γδ T cells in the acute stage of HIV infection was analyzed at baseline, month 6, 12 and 18. Compared with data from healthy controls, γδ T cell cytotoxicity was gradually compromised in acutely HIV-infected patients over time (**Fig. 3A and 3B**). Furthermore, the fraction of IL-17-producing γδ T cells was elevated ($P=0.023$), while the fraction of IFN-γ-producing γδ T cells was unchanged ($P=0.115$) (**Fig. 3C and 3E**). These changes were not affected by CD4 counts or the initiation of ART (**Fig. 3D and 3F**).

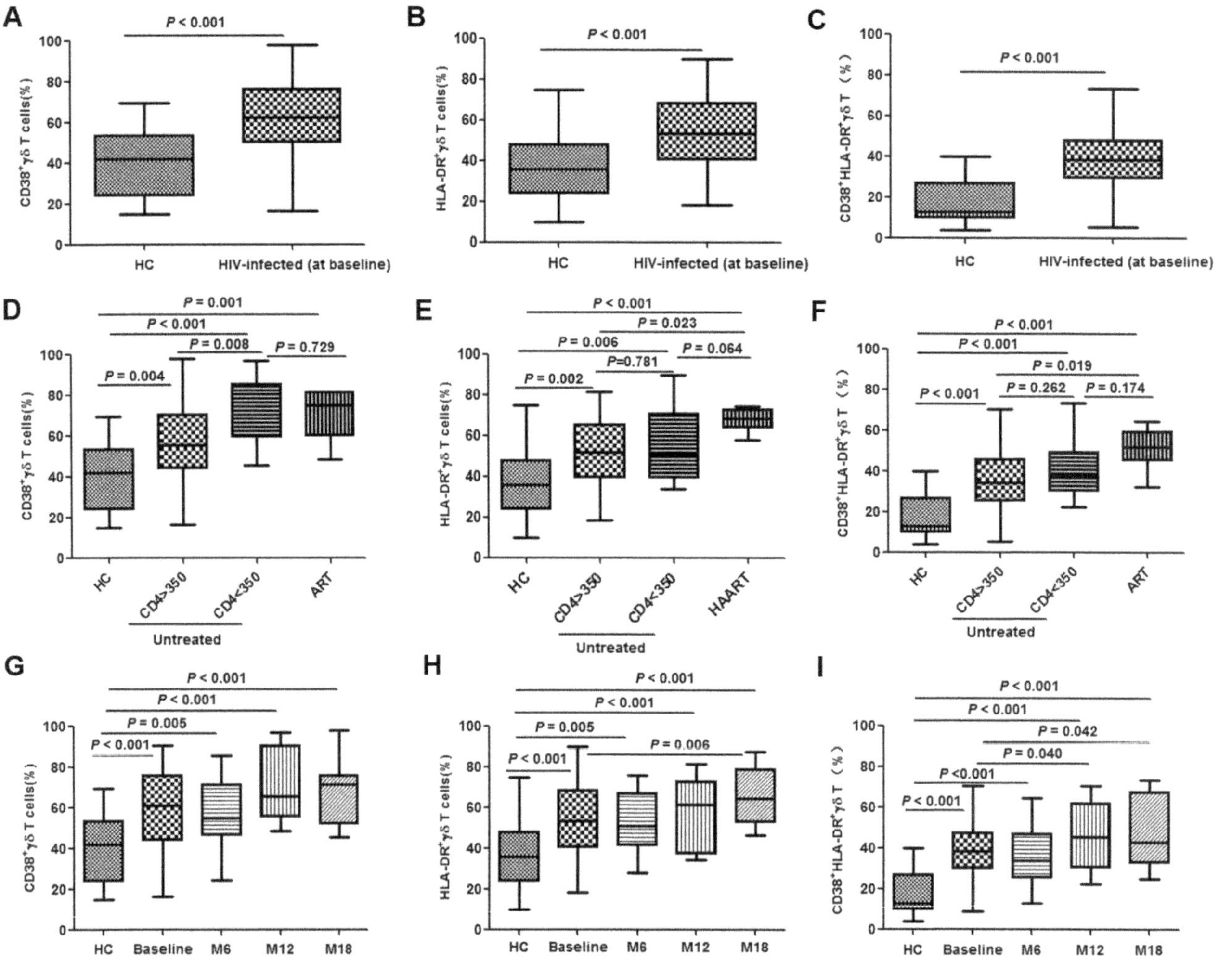

Figure 4. Activation of γδ T cells in acute HIV infection. Activation of γδ T cells was determined by analysis of CD38 and HLA-DR expression. Frequencies of CD38+, HLA-DR+ and CD38+/HLA-DR+ γδ T cells were tested in healthy controls (HC) and acutely HIV-infected subjects at baseline (**A–C**). The patients were then subdivided based on the administration of antiretroviral therapy (ART) and CD4 levels (< or >than 350/μL). The frequencies were re-analyzed and compared with HC (**D–F**). Longitudinal follow-up of γδ T cell activation in patients with acute HIV infection was conducted at baseline, month 6 (M6), month 12 (M12) and month 18 (M18). Frequencies of CD38+, HLA-DR+ and CD38+/HLA-DR+ γδ T cells were tested in healthy controls (HC) and acutely HIV-infected subjects at baseline (**G–I**).

Activation of γδ T cells

CD38 and HLA-DR are used as surrogate markers of γδ T cell activation [31,32]. Compared with healthy controls, the proportions of CD38+ or HLA-DR+ γδ T cells (single-positive and double-positive) were significantly elevated in acutely HIV-infected patients (all P<0.001) (**Fig. 4A–C**). For patients with a CD4 count of less than 350/μL, the fraction of CD38+ γδ T cells was higher than for those with a CD4 count of greater than 350/μL(P = 0.008) (**Fig. 4D**); however, this CD4-dependent change was not evident in HLA-DR+ or double-positive cells (P = 0.781 and 0.262, respectively) (**Fig. 4E and 4F**). No significant differences were observed among patients on ART compared with untreated patients with a CD4 count of less than 350/μL (**Fig. 4D–F**).

To further characterize the activation of γδ T cells, CD38 and HLA-DR expression was determined at different time-points (baseline and months 6, 12, and 18). Steady increases in the fractions of all three groups of γδ T cells (CD38+, HLA-DR+ and CD38+/HLA-DR+) were observed over time, except for CD38+ cells, which showed a marginal reduction at month 6 (**Fig. 4G–I**).No correlation was detected between γδ T cell activation and baseline viral load (data not shown).

Correlations between early γδ T cell activation and CD4/CD8 T cell activation set-point

Activation of CD4/CD8 cells was determined on the basis of CD38 and HLA-DR surface marker expression at month 6 after baseline, when the T cell activation set-point of most patients should have been established [33]. Correlation analysis was performed by comparing CD4/CD8 activation at month 6 and γδ T cell activation at baseline. CD4 and CD8 T cell activation set-points were both positively correlated to γδ T cell activation (**Fig. 5A–B and 5E–F**). If HLA-DR alone was used, the CD8 T cell set-point was correlated (P = 0.006), but not the CD4 T cell activation set-point (P = 0.490) (**Fig. 5C and 5D**). These data demonstrated that early activation of γδ T cells was positively correlated withCD4 and CD8 T cell activation set-points.

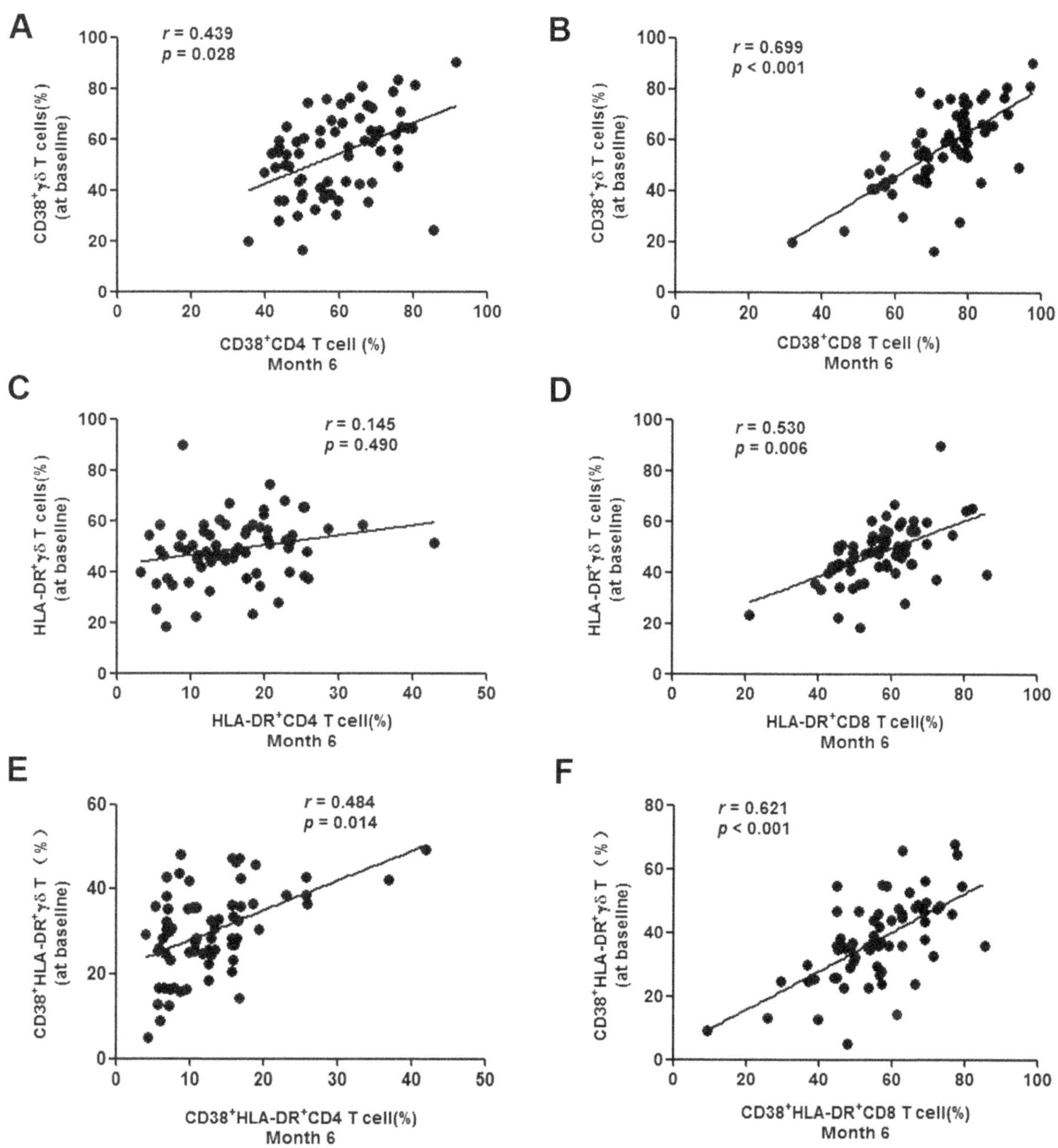

Figure 5. Correlation between early γδ T cell activation and CD4/CD8 T cell activation set-point. Correlation analysis of the proportion of CD38+/CD4+ T cells (**A**) or CD38+/CD8+ T cells (**B**) at month 6 after baseline and CD38+ γδ T cells frequency at baseline was performed by Spearman's rank correlation, where coefficients 'r' and corresponding *P*-values are indicated on each panel. Similar correlation analysis of the proportion of HLA-DR+ (**C, D**) and CD38+/HLA-DR+ cells (**E, F**) and CD4+ or CD8+ T cells at month 6 and γδ T cells at baseline was performed.

Microbial translocation versus γδ T cells

Microbial translocation in acute HIV infection was determined by analysis of the serum levels of LPS (lipopolysaccharides), LBP (LPS-binding protein) and sCD14 (soluble CD14). Only sCD14 levels were found to be elevated in acutely HIV-infected patients compared with those of healthy subjects ($P = 0.001$) (**Fig. 6A–C**). The levels of LPS and LBP did not differ between ART-treated and untreated patients, or between patients with different CD4 count levels (**Fig. 6D–E**). However, the sCD14 level in ART-treated patients was significant elevated compared with untreated patients with CD4>350 cells/μl ($P = 0.003$). Correlation analysis also showed no association between sCD14 levels and the total γδ T cell population ($P = 0.062$) (data not shown); however, further investigation demonstrated positive correlations between sCD14 levels and different γδ T subgroups. Statistical analysis indicated that sCD14 levels were positively correlated withCD38+/HLA-DR+ ($P = 0.002$) and HLA-DR+ ($P = 0.011$), but not with CD38+ ($P = 0.105$) (**Fig. 6G**). Fractions of Tnaïve, TCM and TEM were not correlated with sCD14 levels (all $P>0.05$) (**Fig. 6J**). Proportions of Vδ1, Vδ2 and IL-17 levels were not associated with sCD14 levels (all $P>0.05$) (**Fig. 6H, I, K**).The fraction of IFN-γ-producing γδ T cells was negatively correlated with sCD14 levels ($P = 0.046$) (**Fig. 6L**). Furthermore, sCD14 was associated with LPS levels ($P = 0.034$) (data not shown).

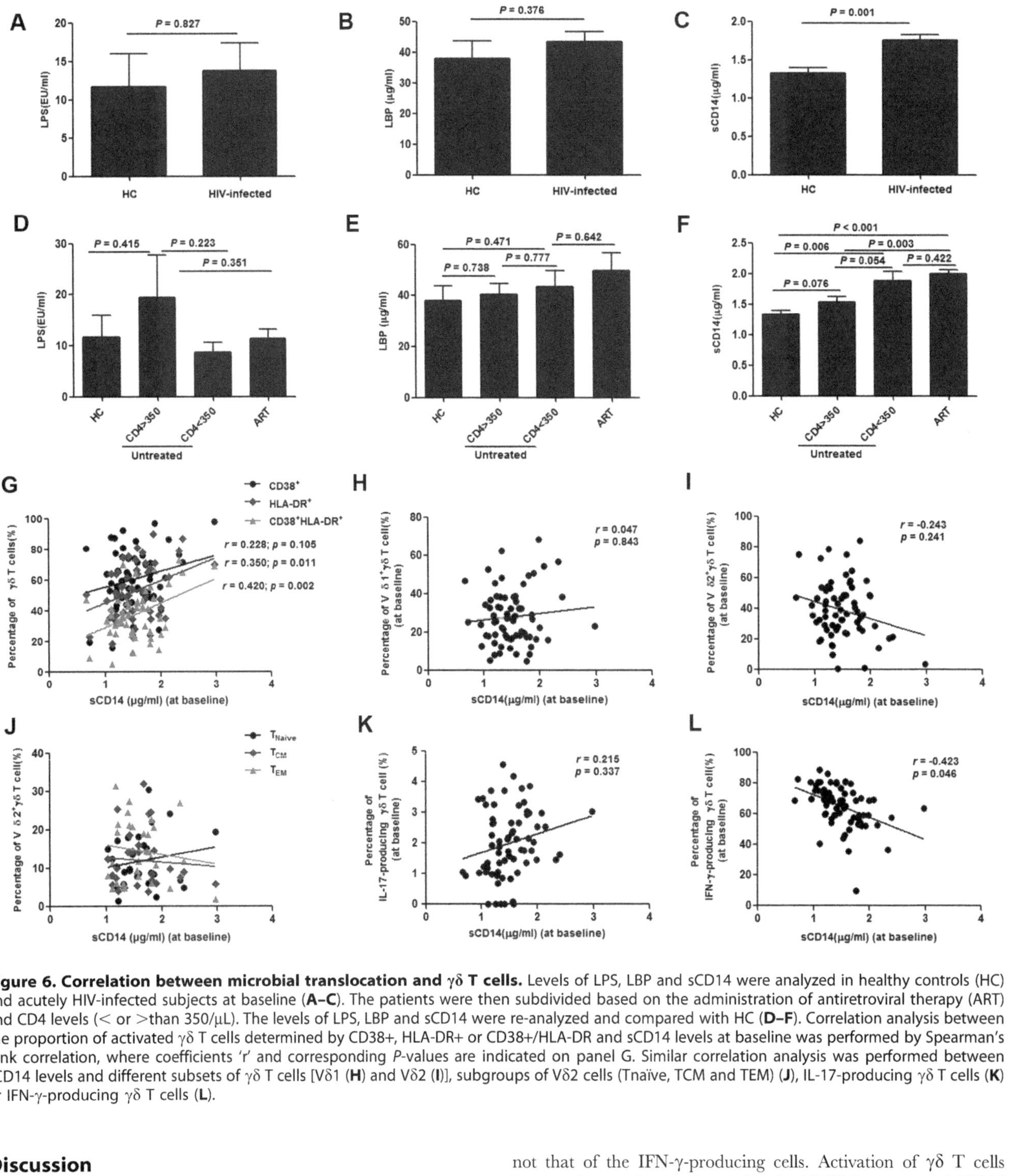

Figure 6. Correlation between microbial translocation and γδ T cells. Levels of LPS, LBP and sCD14 were analyzed in healthy controls (HC) and acutely HIV-infected subjects at baseline (**A–C**). The patients were then subdivided based on the administration of antiretroviral therapy (ART) and CD4 levels (< or >than 350/µL). The levels of LPS, LBP and sCD14 were re-analyzed and compared with HC (**D–F**). Correlation analysis between the proportion of activated γδ T cells determined by CD38+, HLA-DR+ or CD38+/HLA-DR and sCD14 levels at baseline was performed by Spearman's rank correlation, where coefficients 'r' and corresponding *P*-values are indicated on panel G. Similar correlation analysis was performed between sCD14 levels and different subsets of γδ T cells [Vδ1 (**H**) and Vδ2 (**I**)], subgroups of Vδ2 cells (Tnaïve, TCM and TEM) (**J**), IL-17-producing γδ T cells (**K**) or IFN-γ-producing γδ T cells (**L**).

Discussion

There is an increasing body of evidence indicating that γδ T cells play critical roles in HIV infections [25]. In this study conducted in a male homosexual population, we show that the proportion of Vδ1 cells among γδ T cells was elevated in acutely HIV-infected patients, while the Vδ2 population was significantly reduced. Among theVδ2γδT cells, the fractions of TCM and TEM cells were significantly decreased, while the proportion of TEMRA was increased. In term of γδ T cell functions, cytotoxicity was compromised significantly in acutely HIV-infected patients over time. The fraction of IL-17-producing cells was elevated, but not that of the IFN-γ-producing cells. Activation of γδ T cells increased over time and correlated withCD4 counts and CD4/CD8 T cell activation set-points. In acute HIV infection, levels of the microbial translocation marker, sCD14, were significantly elevated, regardless ofCD4 counts. However, sCD14 levels exhibited a positive association withCD38/HLA-DR and HLA-DR expression and a negative association with the fraction of IFN-γ-producing γδ T cells. Initiation of ART had no impact on any of these changes.

It has been shown that the Vδ2 population is depleted in chronically HIV-infected patients [25]. Our data indicated that this is an early event, occurring before the remarkable reduction in the total γδ T cell count, since baseline data showed no significant change in the fraction of γδ T cells among the total T cell population (**Fig. 1A, 1C and 1E**). Our results also demonstrated that there were no significant changes in the proportion of Tnaïve cells in the Vδ2 cell population. The fractions of TEM and TCM cells were decreased, while the TEMRA fraction was elevated, which indicated increased aging of Vδ2 cells in acute HIV infection (**Fig. 2**).

Activated γδ T cells are the subtype of this population of cells that function in response to HIV infections, and therefore, were the primary target cell population of this study. Our data showed a gradual increase in γδ T cell activation, along with compromised γδ T cell cytotoxicity over time, in addition to an elevation in the fraction of IL-17-producing γδ T cells in acute HIV infection (**Fig. 3, 4, 5**).These observations indicated that early initiation of ART failed to bring about recovery of the γδ T cell populations and their functions, which is consistent with a previous report [29], although additional studies are required to confirm this. More importantly, we found a positive correlation between baseline γδ T cell activation and CD4/CD8 T cell activation set-points (**Fig. 5**), which were used to predict subsequent CD4 T cell loss, disease progression and outcome [32,34]. It can therefore be speculated that activation of γδ cells represents a surrogate marker for disease progression and outcome.

Our results indicated potential associations between γδ T cell activation and levels of sCD14, a monocyte activation marker, which is also commonly used as an indicator of microbial translocation (**Fig. 6**). The level of sCD14 is used to predict mortality and disease progression in chronic HIV patients [24,33], in addition to other disorders, such as different cancers and hemodialysis [35,36]. Microbial translocation results in the release of bacterial products, such as LPS and LBP, which in turn activate monocytes in various clinical situations [37,38]. LPS and LBP levels have been shown to be increased in chronic HIV infection, but not in the acute stage. Furthermore, it has been reported that microbial translocation is not observed in primary HIV infection, although sCD14 levels are elevated [33,39]. Therefore, even though sCD14 levels were found to be elevated in acute HIV infection in our study, an association of γδ T cell activation with microbial translocation remains to be established.

No differences were observed between patients on early ART and untreated patients in any aspect investigated in this study. Although there are reports indicating that ART does not bring about recovery of the γδ T cell depletion, this conclusion is controversial. Our study was conducted in only 11 patients on ART, and two treatment plans including two different protease inhibitors; therefore, a larger study with a more stringent design is required to confirm this conclusion.

In conclusion, in acute HIV infections, a significant shift in the proportions and functions of the various γδ T cell subgroups was observed. Elevation of the microbial translocation marker, sCD14, was associated with γδ T cell activation. More importantly, early γδ T cell activation was associated with CD4 and CD8 T cell activation set-points, which predict AIDS progression. Therefore, γδ T cell activation represents a potential surrogate marker of AIDS progression. This conclusion requires confirmation in larger prospective cohort studies.

Author Contributions

Conceived and designed the experiments: WL WH HW. Performed the experiments: ZL YJ LC YH. Analyzed the data: WL NL ZL YJ HW LC. Contributed reagents/materials/analysis tools: NL DC. Contributed to the writing of the manuscript: WL WH.

References

1. Constant P, Davodeau F, Peyrat MA, Poquet Y, Puzo G, et al. (1994) Stimulation of human gamma delta T cells by nonpeptidic mycobacterial ligands. Science 264: 267–270.
2. Dik WA, Pike-Overzet K, Weerkamp F, de Ridder D, de Haas EF, et al. (2005) New insights on human T cell development by quantitative T cell receptor gene rearrangement studies and gene expression profiling. J Exp Med 201: 1715–1723.
3. Hayday AC (2000) [gamma][delta] cells: a right time and a right place for a conserved third way of protection. Annu Rev Immunol 18: 975–1026.
4. Xi X, Guo Y, Chen H, Xu C, Zhang H, et al. (2009) Antigen specificity of gammadelta T cells depends primarily on the flanking sequences of CDR3delta. J Biol Chem 284: 27449–27455.
5. Bukowski JF, Morita CT, Brenner MB (1999) Human gamma delta T cells recognize alkylamines derived from microbes, edible plants, and tea: implications for innate immunity. Immunity 11: 57–65.
6. Vincent MS, Roessner K, Sellati T, Huston CD, Sigal LH, et al. (1998) Lyme arthritis synovial gamma delta T cells respond to Borrelia burgdorferi lipoproteins and lipidated hexapeptides. J Immunol 161: 5762–5771.
7. Sanders JM, Ghosh S, Chan JM, Meints G, Wang H, et al. (2004) Quantitative structure-activity relationships for gammadelta T cell activation by bisphosphonates. J Med Chem 47: 375–384.
8. Battistini L, Caccamo N, Borsellino G, Meraviglia S, Angelini DF, et al. (2005) Homing and memory patterns of human gammadelta T cells in physiopathological situations. Microbes Infect 7: 510–517.
9. Qin G, Liu Y, Zheng J, Xiang Z, Ng IH, et al. (2012) Phenotypic and functional characterization of human gammadelta T-cell subsets in response to influenza A viruses. J Infect Dis 205: 1646–1653.
10. Dieli F, Poccia F, Lipp M, Sireci G, Caccamo N, et al. (2003) Differentiation of effector/memory Vdelta2 T cells and migratory routes in lymph nodes or inflammatory sites. J Exp Med 198: 391–397.
11. Eberl M, Engel R, Beck E, Jomaa H (2002) Differentiation of human gamma-delta T cells towards distinct memory phenotypes. Cell Immunol 218: 1–6.
12. Ribot JC, deBarros A, Pang DJ, Neves JF, Peperzak V, et al. (2009) CD27 is a thymic determinant of the balance between interferon-gamma- and interleukin 17-producing gammadelta T cell subsets. Nat Immunol 10: 427–436.
13. Fenoglio D, Poggi A, Catellani S, Battaglia F, Ferrera A, et al. (2009) Vdelta1 T lymphocytes producing IFN-gamma and IL-17 are expanded in HIV-1-infected patients and respond to Candida albicans. Blood 113: 6611–6618.
14. Battistini L, Borsellino G, Sawicki G, Poccia F, Salvetti M, et al. (1997) Phenotypic and cytokine analysis of human peripheral blood gamma delta T cells expressing NK cell receptors. J Immunol 159: 3723–3730.
15. Brenchley JM, Douek DC (2012) Microbial translocation across the GI tract. Annu Rev Immunol 30: 149–173.
16. Santos-Oliveira JR, Regis EG, Giacoia-Gripp CB, Valverde JG, Alexandrino-de-Oliveira P, et al. (2013) Microbial translocation induces an intense proinflammatory response in patients with visceral leishmaniasis and HIV type 1 coinfection. J Infect Dis 208: 57–66.
17. Shibata K, Yamada H, Hara H, Kishihara K, Yoshikai Y (2007) Resident Vdelta1+ gammadelta T cells control early infiltration of neutrophils after Escherichia coli infection via IL-17 production. J Immunol 178: 4466–4472.
18. Schilbach K, Geiselhart A, Handgretinger R (2001) Induction of proliferation and augmented cytotoxicity of gammadelta T lymphocytes by bisphosphonate clodronate. Blood 97: 2917–2918.
19. Thedrez A, Harly C, Morice A, Salot S, Bonneville M, et al. (2009) IL-21-mediated potentiation of antitumor cytolytic and proinflammatory responses of human V gamma 9V delta 2 T cells for adoptive immunotherapy. J Immunol 182: 3423–3431.
20. Kotler DP, Gaetz HP, Lange M, Klein EB, Holt PR (1984) Enteropathy associated with the acquired immunodeficiency syndrome. Ann Intern Med 101: 421–428.
21. Epple HJ, Schneider T, Troeger H, Kunkel D, Allers K, et al. (2009) Impairment of the intestinal barrier is evident in untreated but absent in suppressively treated HIV-infected patients. Gut 58: 220–227.
22. Romero-Sanchez M, Gonzalez-Serna A, Pacheco YM, Ferrando-Martinez S, Machmach K, et al. (2012) Different biological significance of sCD14 and LPS in HIV-infection: importance of the immunovirology stage and association with HIV-disease progression markers. J Infect 65: 431–438.
23. Wittkop L, Bitard J, Lazaro E, Neau D, Bonnet F, et al. (2013) Effect of cytomegalovirus-induced immune response, self antigen-induced immune response, and microbial translocation on chronic immune activation in successfully treated HIV type 1-infected patients: the ANRS CO3 Aquitaine Cohort. J Infect Dis 207: 622–627.
24. Sandler NG, Wand H, Roque A, Law M, Nason MC, et al. (2011) Plasma levels of soluble CD14 independently predict mortality in HIV infection. J Infect Dis 203: 780–790.

25. Li H, Chaudhry S, Poonia B, Shao Y, Pauza CD (2013) Depletion and dysfunction of Vgamma2Vdelta2 T cells in HIV disease: mechanisms, impacts and therapeutic implications. Cell Mol Immunol 10: 42–49.
26. Li H, Peng H, Ma P, Ruan Y, Su B, et al. (2008) Association between Vgamma2Vdelta2 T cells and disease progression after infection with closely related strains of HIV in China. Clin Infect Dis 46: 1466–1472.
27. Zheng NN, McElrath MJ, Sow PS, Mesher A, Hawes SE, et al. (2011) Association between peripheral gammadelta T-cell profile and disease progression in individuals infected with HIV-1 or HIV-2 in West Africa. J Acquir Immune Defic Syndr 57: 92–100.
28. Bordon J, Evans PS, Propp N, Davis CE Jr, Redfield RR, et al. (2004) Association between longer duration of HIV-suppressive therapy and partial recovery of the V gamma 2 T cell receptor repertoire. J Infect Dis 189: 1482–1486.
29. Hebbeler AM, Propp N, Cairo C, Li H, Cummings JS, et al. (2008) Failure to restore the Vgamma2-Jgamma1.2 repertoire in HIV-infected men receiving highly active antiretroviral therapy (HAART). Clin Immunol 128: 349–357.
30. Zhou J, Kang N, Cui L, Ba D, He W (2012) Anti-gammadelta TCR antibody-expanded gammadelta T cells: a better choice for the adoptive immunotherapy of lymphoid malignancies. Cell Mol Immunol 9: 34–44.
31. Sodora DL, Silvestri G (2008) Immune activation and AIDS pathogenesis. AIDS 22: 439–446.
32. Deeks SG, Kitchen CM, Liu L, Guo H, Gascon R, et al. (2004) Immune activation set point during early HIV infection predicts subsequent CD4+ T-cell changes independent of viral load. Blood 104: 942–947.
33. Chevalier MF, Petitjean G, Dunyach-Remy C, Didier C, Girard PM, et al. (2013) The Th17/Treg ratio, IL-1RA and sCD14 levels in primary HIV infection predict the T-cell activation set point in the absence of systemic microbial translocation. PLoS Pathog 9: e1003453.
34. Karim R, Mack WJ, Stiller T, Operskalski E, Frederick T, et al. (2013) Association of HIV clinical disease progression with profiles of early immune activation: results from a cluster analysis approach. AIDS 27: 1473–1481.
35. Alunno A, Bartoloni E, Bistoni O, Nocentini G, Ronchetti S, et al. (2012) Balance between regulatory T and Th17 cells in systemic lupus erythematosus: the old and the new. Clin Dev Immunol 2012: 823085.
36. Braga WM, Atanackovic D, Colleoni GW (2012) The role of regulatory T cells and TH17 cells in multiple myeloma. Clin Dev Immunol 2012: 293479.
37. Adib-Conquy M, Cavaillon JM (2007) Stress molecules in sepsis and systemic inflammatory response syndrome. FEBS Lett 581: 3723–3733.
38. Munoz C, Carlet J, Fitting C, Misset B, Bleriot JP, et al. (1991) Dysregulation of in vitro cytokine production by monocytes during sepsis. J Clin Invest 88: 1747–1754.
39. Brenchley JM, Price DA, Schacker TW, Asher TE, Silvestri G, et al. (2006) Microbial translocation is a cause of systemic immune activation in chronic HIV infection. Nat Med 12: 1365–1371.

21

Differential MicroRNA Expression Profile between Stimulated PBMCs from HIV-1 Infected Elite Controllers and Viremic Progressors

Lander Egaña-Gorroño[1], Tuixent Escribà[1], Nicolas Boulanger[1,4], Alberto Crespo Guardo[2], Agathe León[3], Manel Enric Bargalló[2], Felipe Garcia[3], José María Gatell[3], Montserrat Plana[2]❡, Mireia Arnedo[1]*❡, HIV Controllers Consortium of the AIDS Spanish Network¶

1 Group of Genomics and Pharmacogenomics, AIDS Research Group, Catalan project for the development of an HIV vaccine (HIVACAT), Institut d'Investigacions Biomèdiques August Pi i Sunyer (IDIBAPS), Hospital Clínic de Barcelona, Barcelona, Spain, **2** Immunopathology and Cellular Immunology, AIDS Research Group, Catalan project for the development of an HIV vaccine (HIVACAT), Institut d'Investigacions Biomèdiques August Pi i Sunyer (IDIBAPS), Hospital Clínic de Barcelona, Barcelona, Spain, **3** Department of Infectious Diseases, Hospital Clínic de Barcelona, University of Barcelona, Barcelona, Spain, **4** Centro Nacional de Análisis Genómico, Scientific Park of Barcelona, Barcelona, Spain

Abstract

Background: The emerging relationship between microRNAs (miRNA) and viral-control is a topic of interest in the field of HIV. Host-genome might play an important role in the control of viremia. The aim of this study was to assess the specific miRNA profile that could contribute to the control of HIV replication in Elite Controllers

Results: After adequate normalization, expression profile of 286 human miRNAs (hsa-miR) was evaluated in phytohaemagglutinin-stimulated PBMCs from 29 individuals classified in 4 groups: 8 elite controllers (EC; viral load < 50 cp/ml without treatment), 8 viremic progressors (VP; VL>5000 cp/ml without treatment), 8 patients under antiretroviral treatment (ART; VL<200 cp/ml) and 5 uninfected individuals (HIV-) through TaqMan Array Human microRNA Cards v3.0. A differential expression pattern consisting of 23 miRNAs became significantly different when comparing EC and VP. Profiling analysis segregated the population in two different blocks: while EC and HIV- clustered together in the same block (EC/HIV-_block 1), VP and ART individuals clustered together in a second block (VP/ART_block 2). Two inversely expressed miRNA patterns were determined within those two blocks: a set of 4 miRNAs (hsa-miR-221, -27a, -27b and -29b) was up-expressed in EC/HIV-_block and down-expressed in VP/ART_block while 19 miRNAs were down-expressed in block 1 and up-expressed in block 2. Differential miRNAs were successfully validated through individual RT-qPCR assays.

Conclusions: Profile in EC resembled HIV- and differentially clusters with VP and ART. Therefore, differential clustering does not rely on undetectable viremia.

Editor: Sebastien Pfeffer, French National Center for Scientific Research - Institut de biologie moléculaire et cellulaire, France

Funding: This work was partially supported by HIVACAT (HIV Vaccine Research and Development Programme in Catalonia), Fundación para la Investigación y la Prevención del Sida en España (FIPSE 09), Fondo Europeo para el Desarrollo Regional (FEDER), Fondo de Investigación Sanitaria FIS, FIS PI070291, PI12/00969, Red de Investigación en Sida (RIS), Instituto de Salud Carlos III (ISCIII-RETIC RD06/0006/0000). M. Arnedo and M. Plana are researchers from the Institut d'Investigacions Biomediques August Pi i Sunyer (IDIBAPS) and are supported by the Spanish Health of the ISCIII (Instituto de SaludCarlos III) and the Health Department of the Catalan Government (Generalitat de Catalunya). L. Egaña-Gorroño is a recipient of a pre-doctoral grant from the ISCIII (FI10/00174). The funders had no role in study design, data collection and analysis, decision to publish, or preparation of the manuscript.

Competing Interests: The authors have declared that no competing interests exist.

* Email: marnedo@clinic.ub.es

❡ These authors contributed equally to this work.

¶ Membership of the HIV Controllers Consortium of the AIDS Spanish Network is provided in the Acknowledgments.

Introduction

The control of human immunodeficiency virus (HIV) replication is an intrinsic feature present in a subset of infected individuals known as Elite Controllers (EC). Contrary to viremic progressors (VP), who register high levels of viral load and exhibit a dramatic loss of CD4+ T-cells, more than 60% of EC have the ability to maintain high T-cell-counts and undetectable viral load (HIV RNA <50 copies/ml) in the absence of antiretroviral therapy (ART) [1–3]. The mechanisms associated with this extreme control of the viremia remains elusive [4]. However, the presence of a low viral reservoir or the existence of a potent CD8+ T-cell response, mainly against the structural protein *gag*, could partially explain this control [5].

There has been an effort to identify molecular, immunological and virological mechanisms leading to the susceptibility of HIV-1 infection, control of viral replication, and disease progression [6–8]. Genetically, EC have been shown to describe a composite of *CCR5* delta-32 gene deletion and/or certain class-I HLA alleles, such as HLA-B*57, that discriminate them from progressors [9–11]. However to date, there has been no clear explanation to why some subjects can control viremia in the absence of antiretroviral treatment and others cannot, even when carrying the same protective alleles. In addition, genome-wide associations studies and transcriptome analyses have been performed aiming to determine specific DNA variants and gene expression patterns present in HIV controllers [12–17]. Furthermore, the discovery of a growing class of small RNAs, termed microRNAs (miRNAs), has opened a new field of research and revealed the possibility to identify plausible miRNA profiles in the context of diseases, including HIV/AIDS and vaccines.

miRNAs are approximately 19–25 nucleotide long single-strand noncoding RNAs capable of regulating gene expression at the post-transcriptional level [18–20]. They pair to the messages of protein-coding genes, usually through imperfect base-pairing with the 3'-untranslated region causing translational repression and/or mRNA destabilization, which is sometimes through direct mRNA cleavage [21–23]. To date, thousands of miRNAs have been identified in a wide diversity of organisms including humans, leading to an actively expanding research field [24]. After over a decade of investigation of miRNAs, it is now clear that these non-coding RNA molecules serve a fundamental role in the regulation of gene expression; even though specific regulation and function of miRNAs is still largely unknown.

The expression profile and role of host miRNAs in the scenario of HIV-infection and AIDS progression has become a topic of interest. Several miRNAs have been described to interact either with the immune system related genes [25,26] or the viral genes [27–29]. Despite recent studies have reported cellular miRNA profiles in several cohorts of HIV-infected patients [30–33], further studies are required in order to better understand the role of miRNAs in the field of HIV/AIDS. The assessment of how a specific miRNA profile could influence the different progression of HIV disease may be useful for understanding the basis of viral and immunological control for future functional therapeutic approaches. Thus, the aim of our study was to determine if there was a specific differential miRNA profile of Elite Controllers.

Materials and Methods

Study population

Samples were obtained from HIV-1-infected patients followed-up at the HIV Unit of the Hospital Clinic of Barcelona (Barcelona, Spain) between 1999 and 2009. Samples of non-infected donors, as a control group, were also obtained. The study was approved by the Institutional Ethics Committee and all participants gave written informed consent for miRNA profiling. Twenty-nine individuals, classified in 4 groups, were included in the study: HIV-negative individuals (HIV-; n = 5), Elite Controllers (EC; n = 8; viral load <50 cp/ml and CD4+ cell count >450 cells/mm^3 for more than six years of follow-up in the absence of ART), Viremic Progressors (VP; n = 8; viral load >5000 cp/ml and CD4+ cell count >400 cells/mm^3 for more than one year of follow-up in the absence of ART) and HIV-infected patients under antiretroviral treatment (ART; n = 8; viral load <50 cop/ml and CD4+ cell count >450 cells/mm^3 for more than one year of follow-up). Medians were used to show central tendencies and interquartile ranges (IQR = upper quartile Q3-lower quartile Q1) were calculated as measures of variability and statistical dispersion in each group.

Table 1. Baseline characteristics of the study participants.

	Screening Cohort				Validation Cohort			
Participant characteristics	**HIV- (n = 5)**	**VP (n = 8)**	**EC (n = 8)**	**ART (n = 8)**	**HIV- (n = 8)**	**VP (n = 14)**	**EC (n = 13)**	**ART (n = 14)**
Age, years*	34 (9)	42.5 (8)	48 (28)	46 (2)	32 (7)	38 (7.75)	49 (20.5)	47 (18.75)
Men/women, n men (%)	2 (40)	7 (87.5)	7 (87.5)	6 (75)	3 (37.5)	13 (92.9)	8 (61.5)	12 (85.7)
Presumed mode of HIV transmission, n (%)								
MSM	N/A	6 (75)	5 (71.5)	3 (37.5)	N/A	12 (85.7)	5 (38.5)	9 (64.3)
heterosexual	N/A	2 (2)	0 (0)	4 (50)	N/A	1 (7.15)	3 (23.1)	2 (14.3)
Other/Unknwon	N/A	-	2 (28.5)	1 (12.5)	N/A	1 (7.15)	5 (38.5)	3 (21.5)
Time since HIV diagnosis, years*	N/A	9 (3.75)	13 (8)	16 (3)	N/A	4.5 (5.25)	10 (8)	9 (9.5)
HIV viral load (log)*	N/A	4.6 (5.12)	1.6 (0.27)	1.56 (0.09)	N/A	4.27 (0.35)	1.57 (0.01)	1.57 (0.01)
CD4+ T-cell count (cells/µl)*	N/A	606 (281)	687 (297)	962.5 (887)	N/A	626.5 (158)	715 (597)	772.5 (354)
Nadir CD4+ T-cell count (cells/µl)*	N/A	466 (88)	600 (332)	348.5 (288)	N/A	445.5 (238)	523.5 (296)	342.5 (193)
Time of exposure to ART, years*	N/A	N/A	N/A	15.5 (1)	N/A	N/A	N/A	6 (10.25)

VP, viremic progressors; EC, elite controller; ART, antiretroviral therapy; MSM, men who had sex with men; *; median [interquartile range = upper quartile (Q3) - lower quartile (Q1)]; N/A, not applicable.

RNA isolation and quality control

Peripheral blood mononuclear cells (PBMCs) were either isolated from fresh blood by Ficoll-Hypaque gradient centrifugation or used after thawing. PBMCs (20×10^6 cells) were cultured in RPMI medium containing 10% FBS and 2% gentamycin. Cells were stimulated with 1 ug/ml of phytohaemagglutinin (PHA; Sigma-Aldrich, St. Louis, Mo, USA) for 72 hours, washed in PBS (1×) and pelleted for RNA extraction. Total RNA (enriched for small RNA) was isolated according to manufacturer's instructions using the mirVana miRNA isolation Kit (Ambion, Huntingdon, UK). RNA concentration was calculated using NanoDrop technology ND-1000 (Thermo Scientific, Waltham, MA, USA). RNA integrity was then evaluated using RNA 6000 Nano LabChips on an Agilent 2100 Bioanalyzer (Agilent Technologies, Santa Clara, CA, USA). All chips were prepared according to the manufacturer's instructions at the Genomic platform of the CCiTUB (Centres Científics i Tecnològics University of Barcelona) located at the Barcelona Science Park (PCB). Total RNA degradation was evaluated by reviewing the electropherograms and the RNA integrity number (RIN) of each sample. Only samples with preserved 18S and 28S peaks and RIN values greater than 7 were selected for miRNA profile analysis.

miRNA profiling using TaqMan low-density arrays (TLDA)

RNA (1 to 350 ng in 3 µl) was reverse transcribed using the miRNA reverse transcription kit in combination with the stem-loop Megaplex primer pool (Applied Biosystems, Foster City, CA, USA), allowing simultaneous reverse transcription of 381 small RNAs. miRNA expression profiles were acquired using TaqMan Array Human microRNA Card A v2.0 (Applied Biosystems, Foster City, CA, USA), containing 384 human miRNAs (hsa-miR). Reactions were performed using the Applied Biosystems 7900HT Fast Real-time PCR system. Reaction volumes contained: 50 µl of cDNA sample (30 to 1000 ng) in RNase-free water and 50 µl of (2×) TaqMan Universal PCR Master Mix. Thermocycler conditions were as follows: 94.5°C hot-start for 10 min, followed by 40 cycles of 97°C for 30 s and 59.7°C for 1 min.

Accessibility of array data

Raw data and sets of filtered and global mean normalized data from TaqMan low-density arrays (TLDA) were deposited with the Gene Expression Omnibus (GEO, [34]) and are accessible at Series number GSE57323.

TLDA data analysis

TLDAs were run in the in the 7900HT Fast Real-time PCR system using the SDS software v.2.3 (Applied Biosystems, Foster City, CA, USA) and raw Ct (cycle threshold: the number of cycles required for the fluorescent signal to cross the threshold) values of the expression of each individual miRNA were obtained using automatic thresholding of all the processed data together with the StatMiner Software (Integromics, Granada, Spain). Those miRNAs with Ct values >35 and not amplified wells were omitted from the analysis. Moreover, miRNAs that were not expressed in more than 25% of the samples, belonging to each group of study, were also excluded from the analysis. For each individual sample, global mean normalization strategy [35,36] was performed calculating the ΔCt values for each miRNA ($\Delta Ct = Ct_{target\ miRNA} - mean\ Ct_{all\ assessed\ miRNAs}$). A non-parametric Mann-Whitney U test was run in MEV software V4.5 [37] for statistical comparisons between group-pairs. Benjamini-Hochberg correction test was applied as an estimated false discovery rate (FDR) of 5%, controlling for the expected proportion of incorrectly rejected null hypotheses [38]. Samples were clustered, comparing EC and VP, by their miRNA expression profiles using the hierarchical clustering algorithm of the software. The Euclidean distance-metric hierarchical cluster represented up-expressed miRNAs in red tones and down-expressed miRNAs in green tones. Fold change ($\log_2$) expression of differentially expressed individual miRNAs in EC and VP relative to HIV- and ART were calculated as $2^{-\Delta\Delta Ct}$ ($\Delta\Delta Ct = \Delta Ct_{EC\ or\ VP} - \Delta Ct_{HIV-\ or\ ART}$). A fold change value closer to "0" would indicate a similar expression level compared to reference group, whereas a positive/negative value would represent an up/down-expressed level. Two-way analysis of variance (ANOVA) tests were performed for global comparisons and Bonferroni post-tests for replicate-means comparisons using GraphPad Prism 5.0.

Validation of results

Those differentially expressed miRNAs with a significance p-value ≤0.001 were re-assessed through individual RT-qPCR assay (Applied Biosystems, Foster City, CA, USA). Furthermore, in order to strengthen the observed expression profiles, a validation cohort consisting of 8 HIV-, 13 EC, 14 VP and 14 ART new patients was added to the study. Individual RT-qPCR assays of the differentially expressed miRNAs of interest were performed in this validation cohort.

RNA (10 ng) was reverse transcribed in 15 µl according to manufacturer's recommendations using TaqMan miRNA reverse transcription kit (Applied Biosystems, Foster City, CA, USA). miRNA expression assays were carried out using TaqMan primers and probes (Applied Biosystems, Foster City, CA, USA) for endogenous control small RNAs RNU44 (ID 001094) and RNU48 (ID 001006) and target miRNAs. Relative quantifications (RQ) were performed using the Applied Biosystems 7900HT Fast Real-time PCR system. Reaction volumes contained: 7.67 µl of water, 1 µl of TaqMan primer/probe mix for target or endogenous control small RNA, 10 µl of (2×) Universal master mix (Applied Biosystems, Foster City, CA, USA) and 1.33 µl of cDNA at a final concentration of 10 ng. Thermocycler conditions were as follows: 95°C hot-start for 10 min, followed by 40 cycles of 95°C for 15 s and 60°C for 1 min. Raw Ct values were exported from the SDS software v.2.3 to the RQ Manager v1.2 softwear (Applied Biosystems, Foster City, CA, USA) for ΔCt ($\Delta Ct = Ct_{target\ miRNA} - mean\ Ct_{endogenous\ small\ RNAs}$) value determination as the normalization method. Fold change ($\log_2$) expression levels of the individual miRNAs in EC, VP, ART, relative to HIV-, were calculated as $2^{-\Delta\Delta Ct}$ ($\Delta\Delta Ct = \Delta Ct_{EC,\ VP,\ ART} - \Delta Ct_{HIV-}$). One-way analysis of variance (ANOVA) tests were performed for global comparisons and Turkey post-hoc tests for pair comparisons using GraphPad Prism 5.0 (GraphPad Software, La Jolla, CA, USA).

Results

Characteristics of the study participants

Characteristics of the study participants of the screening and the validation cohorts are shown in Table 1. None of them was co-infected by hepatitis C virus (HCV). After seven years of follow-up all the participants from the EC group maintained viral load < 50 cp/ml and CD4+ cell count >450 cells/mm^3. A heterogeneous distribution of HLA-B57*01 was observed and none of them showed the *CCR5* delta-32 gene deletion (data not shown). No statistically significant differences were observed in any comparison except in the time since HIV diagnosis ($p = 0.002$) and time of exposure to antiretroviral therapy ($p = 0.002$) between the ART groups of the screening and the validation cohorts.

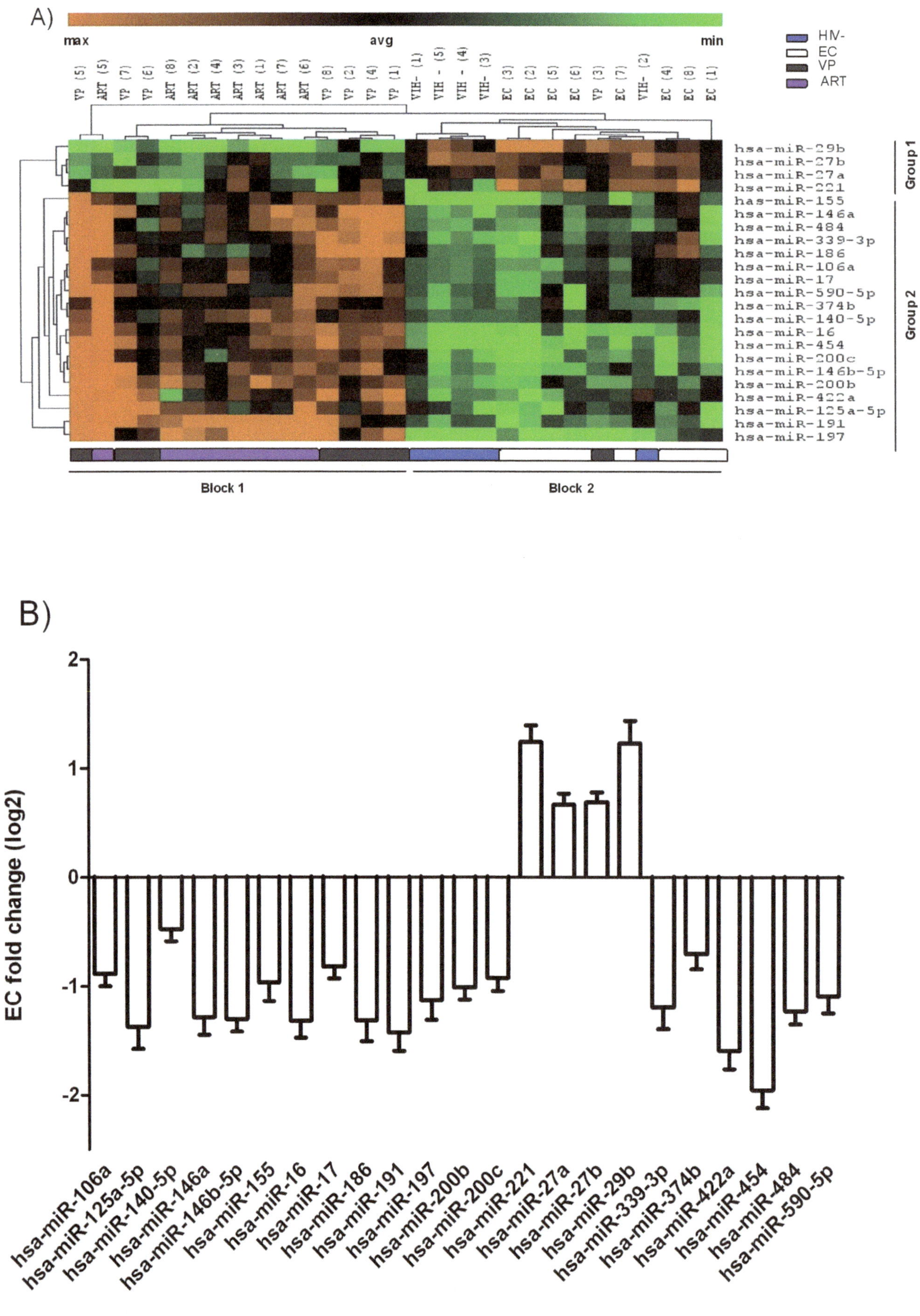
A)
max
avg
min
HIV-
EC
VP
ART
VP (5)
ART (5)
VP (7)
VP (6)
ART (8)
ART (2)
ART (4)
ART (3)
ART (1)
ART (7)
ART (6)
VP (8)
VP (2)
VP (4)
VP (1)
VIH- (1)
VIH - (5)
VIH - (4)
VIH- (3)
EC (3)
EC (2)
EC (5)
EC (6)
VP (3)
EC (7)
VIH- (2)
EC (4)
EC (8)
EC (1)
hsa-miR-29b
hsa-miR-27b
hsa-miR-27a
hsa-miR-221
has-miR-155
hsa-miR-146a
hsa-miR-484
hsa-miR-339-3p
hsa-miR-186
hsa-miR-106a
hsa-miR-17
hsa-miR-590-5p
hsa-miR-374b
hsa-miR-140-5p
hsa-miR-16
hsa-miR-454
hsa-miR-200c
hsa-miR-146b-5p
hsa-miR-200b
hsa-miR-422a
hsa-miR-125a-5p
hsa-miR-191
hsa-miR-197
Group 1
Group 2
Block 1
Block 2
B)
EC fold change (log2)
2
1
0
-1
-2
hsa-miR-106a
hsa-miR-125a-5p
hsa-miR-140-5p
hsa-miR-146a
hsa-miR-146b-5p
hsa-miR-155
hsa-miR-16
hsa-miR-17
hsa-miR-186
hsa-miR-191
hsa-miR-197
hsa-miR-200b
hsa-miR-200c
hsa-miR-221
hsa-miR-27a
hsa-miR-27b
hsa-miR-29b
hsa-miR-339-3p
hsa-miR-374b
hsa-miR-422a
hsa-miR-454
hsa-miR-484
hsa-miR-590-5p

Figure 1. Differential miRNAs between Elite Controllers (EC) and Viremic Progressors (VP). A) Hierarchical clustering of the differentially expressed miRNAs between EC and VP. Patients are ordered on vertical lines and candidate miRNAs on horizontal lines. For each miRNA, green represents under-expressed and red over-expressed values compared to the average value (median), in dark. Dendrograms (tree graph) between patients and between miRNAs are depicted, where the closest branches of the tree represent patients/miRNAs with the most similar expression pattern. Two blocks of patients (Block 1/Block 2) with an inverse expression profile were segregated. Two groups of miRNAs (Group 1/Group 2) with an inverse expression profile were segregated within each block. B) Fold change (log 2) of the 23 differentially expressed miRNAs in EC. Differential levels are normalized to all assesed miRNAs and relative to VP. Bars represent standard error means (SEM).

Taqman Low-density miRNA arrays reveal differentially expressed miRNAs

All RNAs were suitable (RIN >7) for the miRNA expression profile analysis through the TaqMan Array Human microRNA Cards v3.0. Expression profiles of HIV-, EC, VP, and ART individuals were acquired after adequate normalisation steps for statistical analysis. Finally, 286 (38%) miRNAs were included in the analysis once the exclusion criteria were carried out. Mann-Whitney U test set to a false discovery rate (FDR) of 5% provided a set of miRNAs differentially expressed in each group-pair: 52 miRNAs in HIV- vs ART, 23 miRNAs in EC vs VP, 22 miRNAs in EC vs ART and 25 miRNAs in VP vs HIV-. No differential miRNAs were observed when comparing neither EC vs HIV- nor VP vs ART; EC were statistically similar to HIV- and VP to ART in terms of PHA-activated PBMC miRNA profile (Table S1).

Hierarchical clustering: miRNA profile in Elite Controllers differs from Viremic Progressors

Twenty-three differentially expressed miRNAs resulting from the Mann–Whitney U test (5% FDR) (Table S1) were classified by hierarchical clustering (average linkage clustering constructed on Euclidian distances) (Figure 1A). The analysis segregated the population in two separate blocks (block1/block2). Block 1 included EC and HIV- with no significant differences on miRNA expression. Viremic progressor patient number 3 clustered together within this block, making this block slightly heterogeneous. Block 2 clustered VP and ART patients. A set of 4 miRNAs with an inverse expression profile between the two blocks, subdivided each block of patients into two groups of miRNA (group1/group2). On the one hand, these 4 miRNAs (hsa-miR-221, hsa-miR-27a, hsa-miR-27b and hsa-miR-29b) were down-expressed in VP and ART (block1-group1) and up-expressed in EC and HIV- (block2-group1). On the other hand, these 19 miRNAs (hsa-miR106a, hsa-miR-125a, hsa-miR-140, hsa-miR-146a, hsa-miR-146b, hsa-miR-155, hsa-miR-16, hsa-miR-17, hsa-miR186, hsa-miR-191, hsa-miR-197, hsa-miR-200b, hsa-miR-200c, hsa-miR-339, hsa-miR-374, hsa-miR-422, hsa-miR-422, hsa-miR-454, hsa-miR-484 and hsa-miR-590) were up-expressed in VP and ART (block1-group2) and down-expressed in EC and HIV- (block2-group2). Expression of the differentially expressed miRNAs in EC was measured as fold change (log_2) relative to VP: hsa-miR-221 and hsa-miR-29b were the most highly expressed miRNAs (fold change 1.24 and 1.23, respectively) and hsa-miR-454 showed the lowest expression (fold change -1.95) in EC when compared to VP (Figure 1B).

miRNA profile in Elite Controllers differs from Viremic progressors and treated individuals. Differential miRNA expression between EC and VP was measured as fold change (log_2) relative to ART (Figure 2A). Overall, EC showed a down-expressed miRNA profile compared to the ART group except for hsa-miR-221, -27a, -27b, -29b levels. hsa-miR-29b was the most highly expressed miRNA (fold change 2.1) and hsa-miR-197 the one with the lowest expression level (fold change -2.2) compared to ART. Six miRNAs were statistically similar ($p < 0.05$) between EC and VP when compared to ART: hsa-miR-106a, -140-5p, -17, -27a, -27b and -374b. In summary, VP showed a closer profile (global mean fold change of 0.1) to the ART group than the EC (global mean fold change of -0.69) (Table S2 A).

miRNA profile in Elite Controllers is similar to non-infected individuals. Differential miRNA expression between EC and VP was measured as fold change (log_2) relative to HIV- (Figure 2B). Hsa-miR-221 and hsa-miR-155 were the most highly expressed miRNAs (fold-change 0.9) and hsa-miR-191 and hsa-miR-200c were the ones with the lowest expression levels (fold change -0.3) compared to HIV-. Interestingly, has-miR-155 was the most up-expressed miRNA in both groups compared to HIV- being the expression level significantly higher ($p<0.05$) in VP. Six miRNAs were statistically similar ($p<0.05$) between EC and VP compared to HIV-: hsa-miR-106a, -140-5p, -17, -27a, -27b and -374b. In summary, EC showed a closer profile (global mean fold change of 0.08) to the ART group than the VP (global mean fold change of 0.87) (Table S2 B).

Validation of expression profiles through individual RT-qPCR assays

Differentially expressed miRNAs between EC and VP, with a significance p-value ≤ 0.001 ($n = 5$, 22%), were successfully validated through individual RT-qPCR assays in the same study population (data not shown).

Moreover, in order to strengthen the tendencies observed in the miRNA profiling analysis, four miRNAs of interest were re-assessed in a validation cohort with similar characteristics to the screening cohort (Table 1).

Validation cohort was analysed for the expression levels of hsa-miR-221, -29b, -146a and -155 between EC, VP and ART, relative to HIV- (Figure 3). Although significant differences were only observed for hsa-miR-221 ($p<0.001$) and hsa-miR-29b ($p< 0.05$), the four miRNAs of interest reflected the same expression tendencies observed in the profiling analysis: EC showed up-expressed levels of hsa-miR-221 and hsa-miR-29b and lower levels of hsa-miR146a and hsa-miR-155 compared to VP. However, individual RT-qPCR assay for hsa-miR-146a did not reproduce the expression levels observed in the profiling analysis in any of the three groups of study. Moreover, the ART group from the validation cohort did not imitate the expression levels of hsa-miR-29b and hsa-miR-146a shown in the profiling analysis.

Discussion

The goal of our study was to assess potential miRNAs that are differentially expressed in HIV-1-infected patients who control viremia in the absence of antiretroviral therapy: Elite Controllers. For that purpose, miRNA profile of 29 individuals categorized in EC, VP, ART and HIV-, was obtained from PHA-activated PBMCs. Even though the heterogeneity observed within EC in previous transcriptome studies [17,39], our results show a specific differential miRNA pattern in EC when compared to VP. Our findings revealed 23 differentially expressed miRNAs in EC that are present in similar levels in HIV- but dissimilarly in VP and ART. In order to validate the expression levels observed, those miRNAs with a significance p-value ≤ 0.001 between EC and VP

A)

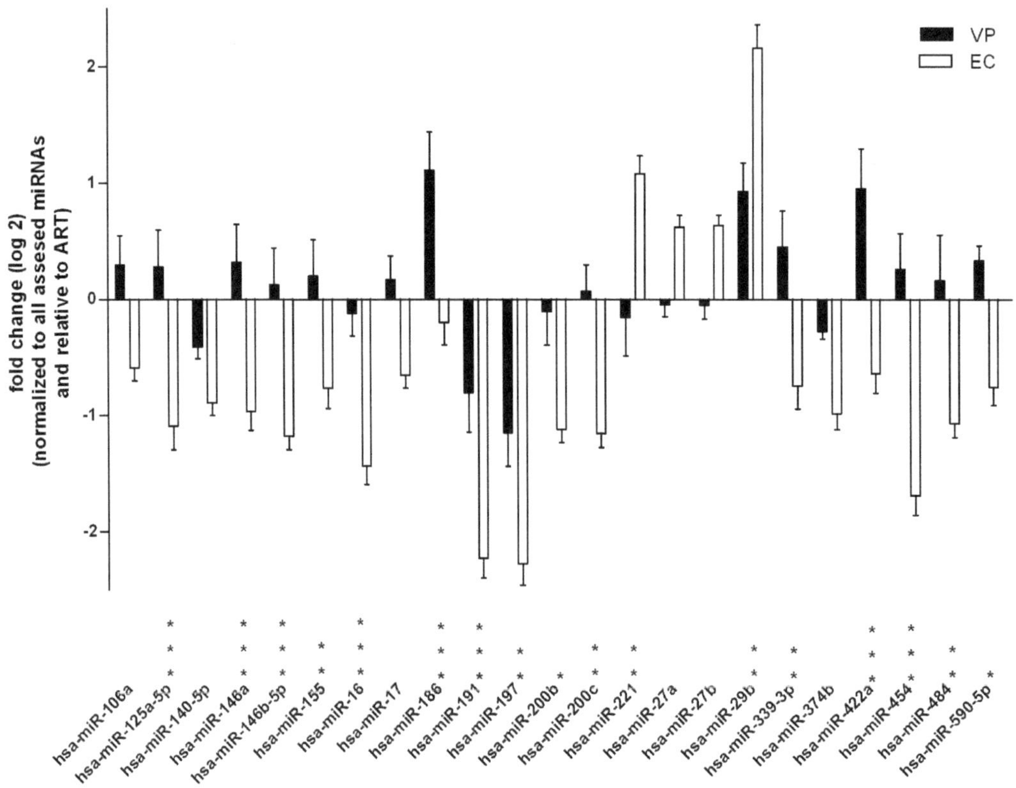
VP
EC
fold change (log 2)
(normalized to all assesed miRNAs
and relative to ART)
2
1
0
-1
-2
hsa-miR-106a
hsa-miR-125a-5p
hsa-miR-140-5p
hsa-miR-146a
hsa-miR-146b-5p
hsa-miR-155
hsa-miR-16
hsa-miR-17
hsa-miR-186
hsa-miR-191
hsa-miR-197
hsa-miR-200b
hsa-miR-200c
hsa-miR-221
hsa-miR-27a
hsa-miR-27b
hsa-miR-29b
hsa-miR-339-3p
hsa-miR-374b
hsa-miR-422a
hsa-miR-454
hsa-miR-484
hsa-miR-590-5p

B)

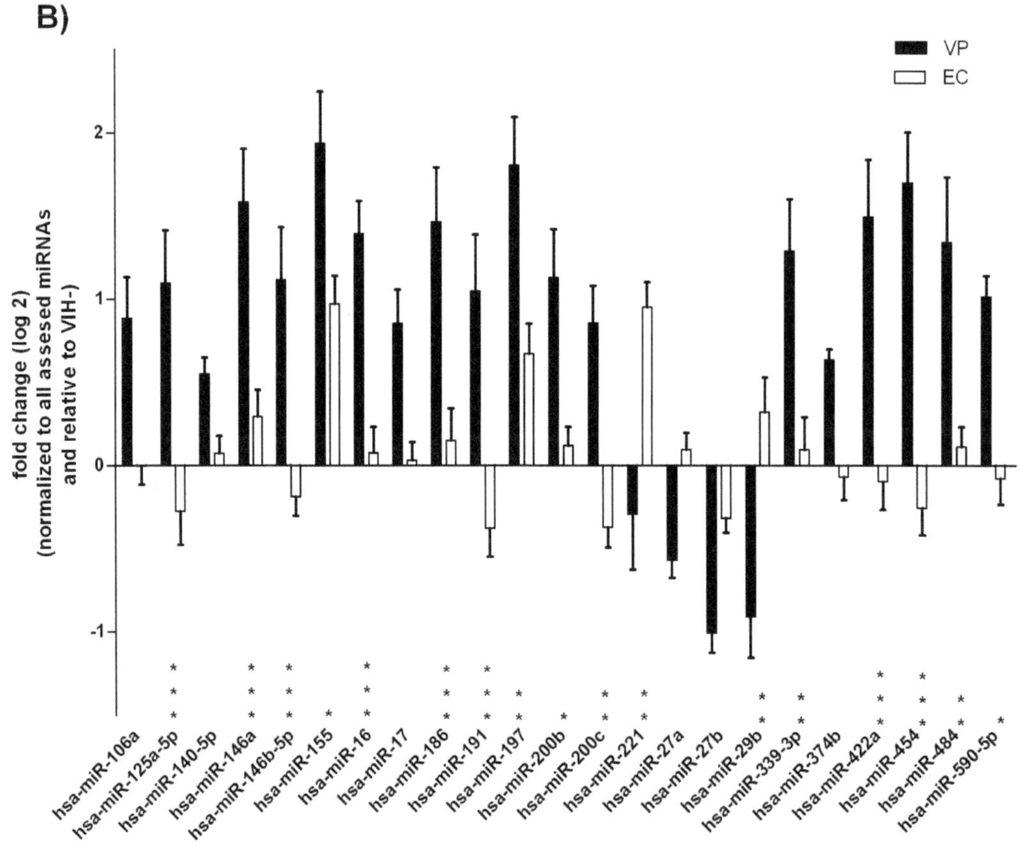
VP
EC
fold change (log 2)
(normalized to all assesed miRNAs
and relative to VIH-)
2
1
0
-1
hsa-miR-106a
hsa-miR-125a-5p
hsa-miR-140-5p
hsa-miR-146a
hsa-miR-146b-5p
hsa-miR-155
hsa-miR-16
hsa-miR-17
hsa-miR-186
hsa-miR-191
hsa-miR-197
hsa-miR-200b
hsa-miR-200c
hsa-miR-221
hsa-miR-27a
hsa-miR-27b
hsa-miR-29b
hsa-miR-339-3p
hsa-miR-374b
hsa-miR-422a
hsa-miR-454
hsa-miR-484
hsa-miR-590-5p

Figure 2. Fold change (log_2) of the 23 differentially expressed miRNAs in EC and VP. A) normalized to all assessed miRNAs and relative to ART, B) normalized to all assessed miRNAs and relative to HIV-. Bars represent standard error means (SEM); *, $p<0.05$; **, $p<0.01$; ***, $p<0.001$; VP, viremic progressors; EC, elite controllers; ART, antiretroviral therapy.

were validated through individual RT-qPCR assays. Our results are consistent with studies reporting that either PBMCs or specific blood cell population miRNA profile of HIV-infected elite controllers, resembles that of HIV- individuals [30,40]. A recent study comparing PBMC miRNA profiles between HIV-infected individuals with low or undetectable viral load and uninfected subjects, conclude that similar patterns are observed across the study groups [32]. However, the suppressed patients used in this last study were all on antiretroviral therapy at the moment of sample collection, a fact that suggest HIV-1 to be able to induce a miRNA dysregulation. Indeed, previously published data showed a major down-regulation of most of the miRNAs in HIV-infected patients [30,31] whereas in the current study, where stimulated PBMCs were used, we observed a trend to a preferential miRNA down-regulation in EC and non-infected subjects as well as a major up-regulation of the differential miRNAs in non-suppressed HIV-positive individuals, probably as a consequence of the effects of the in vitro T-cell stimulation.

On the one hand, EC showed up-expressed levels of hsa-miR-221, hsa-miR-27a, hsa-miR-27b and hsa-miR-29b compared to VP. These miRNAs are highly expressed in PBMCs [41] and are plausible molecular candidates to be involved in HIV replication and infectivity. Human miR-29b has been previously described as one of the profile components of EC [30] and to be related with infected patients with low viral load [31]. Additionally, previous data report the implication of hsa-miR-29b in HIV replication through targeting the virus in the transcribed 3′-LTR region [42] or regulating the viral negative regulatory factor (nef) [43]. Nef highjacks MHC (mayor histocompatibility complex)-class I along with other molecules impeding a correct antigen presentation [44,45]. Moreover, hsa-miR-29b and hsa-miR-27b have been described to repress the translation of cellular cofactor cyclin T1 in resting and activated CD4+ T-cells. Cyclin T1 binds the viral trans-activator of transcription (tat) and activates the transcription of the integrated provirus [46]. Cellular levels of integrated viral DNA have been described to be much lower in elite controllers compared to other patients on and off anti-retroviral drugs [47]. VP and ART patients might express these miRNAs in lower levels in order to avoid cyclin t1 suppression and allow replication of integrated provirus. A second miRNA, newly identified in this work, to be potentially related to the control of viral infectivity is hsa-miR-221. In this case, previous data reports a functionality in the control of Intracellular Adhesion Molecule-1 (ICAM-1) expression levels either through the IFN-alpha pathway or by direct targeting [48,49]. Cellular levels of ICAM-1 influence HIV-1 infectivity and viral dissemination [49-52]. Considering the mentioned functional analyses, up-expression of these two molecules in EC could suggest an improved viral control and antigen presentation through miR-29b and a reduced viral infectivity through miR-221, although this should be more accurately investigated.

On the other hand, 19 miRNAs were significantly down-expressed in EC. Out of these miRNAs, hsa-miR-146a and hsa-miR-155 became of our interest due their important role in a wide spectrum of immune compartments. Both miRNAs were up-expressed in VP and this pattern has already been correlated with high viral load [31,32]. The co-activation of hsa-miR-146 and hsa-miR-155 results in a transcriptional activation of NF-kB target genes that encode various mediators of inflammation, such as cytokines, acute phase proteins and inducible enzymes against a variety of microbial components [53]. Subsequent findings showed that both hsa-miR-146 and -155 targeted mRNAs in the signalling cascade of toll-like receptor 4 (TLR4) and bolstered the link with NFkB-regulated innate immunity, leading to a model in which these two miRNAs facilitate a negative-feedback loop that may protect from an excessive TLR4 response [54]. Other groups have recently found that hsa-miR-155 was strongly expressed in effector/memory Tregs [55]. Levels of effector/memory Tregs are significantly increased in different HIV progression profiles (HIV-infected individuals with progressive infection versus long term non-progressors). Thus, we stress the importance of analysing the expression of these molecules in different T-cell subsets to better understand its role in HIV pathogenesis.

Moreover, hsa-miR-155 has been shown to be involved in the differentiation from naive to effector CD8+ T cells being required for effective CD8+ T cell responses to virus infections through modulation of responsiveness to type I interferon [56-58]. Down-expression of these two molecules in EC would suggest less inflammatory status, a minor activation of the immune system and a better antiviral immune response. In fact, previously data suggested the contribution of miR-155 to the pathogenesis of HIV-1 infection in HIV naïve individuals [29].

In order to give consistency to the tendencies of the miRNA profiles observed, a validation cohort was analysed through individual RT-qPCR assay for four differentially expressed miRNAs of interest: hsa-221, -29b, -146a, -155. Re-assessment of these miRNAs in a new set of patients reflected the same tendencies observed in the profiling analysis between EC and VP, although significant differences were only observed for hsa-miR-221 ($p<0.0001$) and hsa-miR-29b ($p<0.05$). The ART group from the validation cohort did not imitate the expression levels of hsa-miR-29b and hsa-miR-146a shown in the profiling analysis. Intriguingly, ART patients from the two cohorts (screening and validation) differed in the time of exposure to ART [median (IQR)]: 15.1 (1) years in the screening cohort and 6 (10.25) years in the validation cohort and in the time since HIV diagnosis [median (IQR)]: 16 (3) years in the screening cohort and 9 (9.5) years in the validation cohort. This observation leads us to a new hypothesis that questions whether these variables might influence miRNA levels.

The findings described herein should be considered with caution due to the limitations of our study. First of all, although the screening results have been validated by enlarging the number of individuals per group, we are conscious of the degree of variation that could occur by the limited sample size used. Moreover, our experimental design does not allow us to attribute the different pattern of miRNA found to any particular specific cell subset. Lastly, no functional data focused on the differential miRNAs is described in the current manuscript. In order to shed more light to all these questions, new experiments should be performed in the future.

In summary, our study reveals a differentially expressed miRNA profile in Elite Controllers that is similar to non-infected individuals and differs from Viremic Progressors who are closer to treated individuals. Some of these differential miRNAs have been reported to be involved in the control of viral replication, viral infectivity, immune activation, and modulation of both innate and acquired immune responses. Nevertheless, more studies are

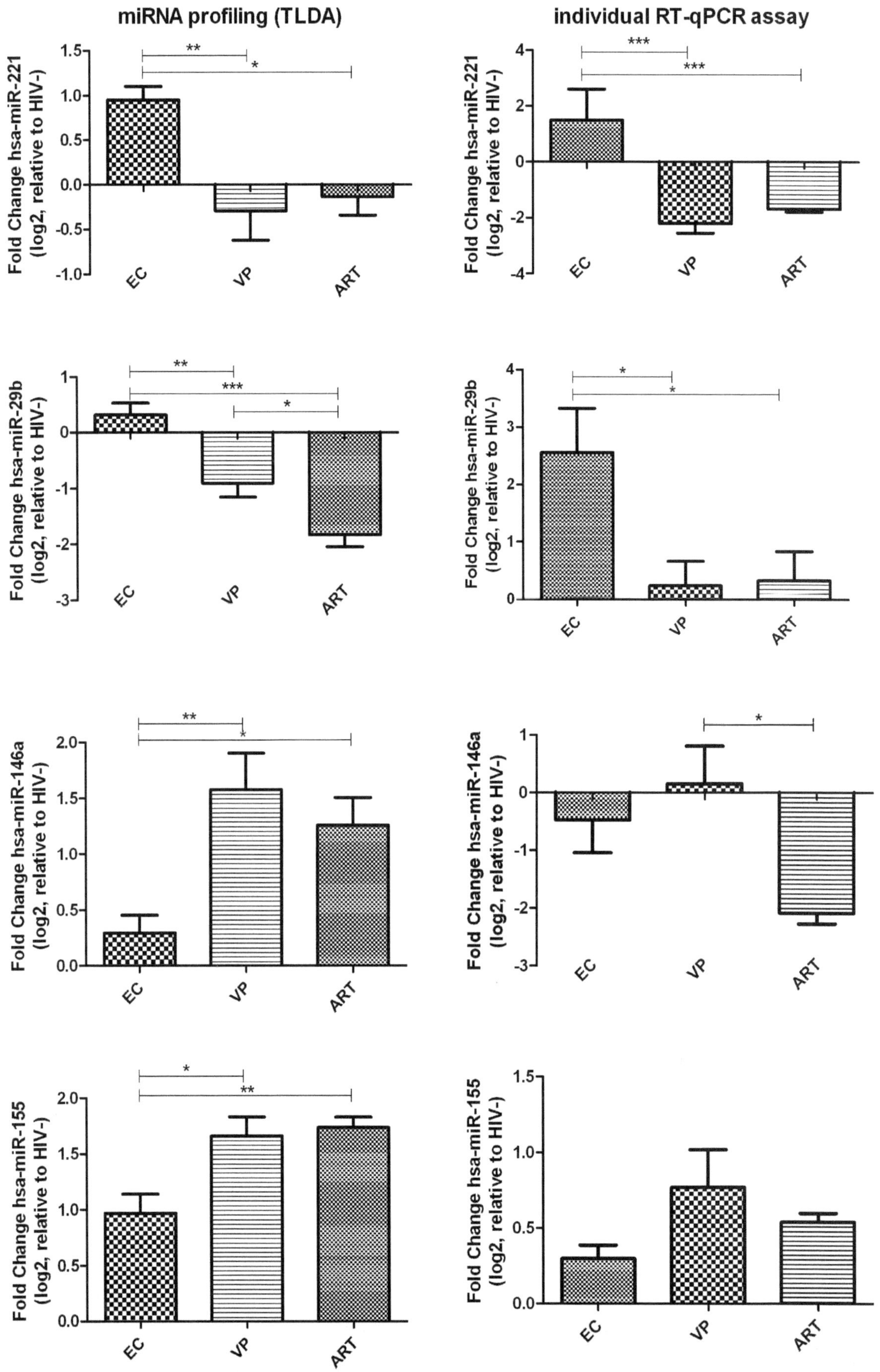

miRNA profiling (TLDA)
individual RT-qPCR assay
Fold Change hsa-miR-221 (log2, relative to HIV-)
Fold Change hsa-miR-29b (log2, relative to HIV-)
Fold Change hsa-miR-146a (log2, relative to HIV-)
Fold Change hsa-miR-155 (log2, relative to HIV-)
EC
VP
ART

Figure 3. Fold change (log_2) of EC, VP and ART, normalized to endogenous control miRNAs and relative to HIV-. One-way analysis of variance (ANOVA) tests were performed for global comparisons and Turkey post-hoc tests for pair comparisons. Bars represent standard error means (SEM); *, $p<0.05$; **, $p<0.01$; ***, $p<0.001$ for Tuckey post-hoc tests; VP, viremic progressors; EC, elite controllers; ART, antiretroviral therapy.

needed in order to dissect the relevant roles of miRNAs in various states of HIV infection and its use as a potential prognostic marker in disease progression or as a future therapeutic approach.

Supporting Information

Table S1 Statistically significant differential miRNAs between analysed group-pairs.

Table S2 Fold change (log2) of differentially expressed miRNAs in Elite Controllers (EC) and Viremic progressors (VP) normalized to all assessed miRNAs and relative to A) VIH- and B) patients under ART.

Acknowledgments

The authors are grateful to all the patients and donors who participated in the study and thank the Retrovirology and Viral Immunopathology Laboratory of the Institut dInvestigacions Biomèdiques August Pi I Sunyer (IDIBAPS). Josep Coromines for his participation in the RT-qPCR assays of the validation cohort. Drs Christian Manzardo, JM Miró and Jose Luis Blanco for helping us complete the different groups of patients.

The members of the HIV Controllers Consortium of the AIDS Spanish Network are: Ruiz-Mateos E[1], Machmach K[1], Ferrando-Martínez S[1], Genebat M[1], Viciana P[1], Leal M[1], Benito JM[2], López M[2], Rallón N[2], Restrepo C[2], López-Galindez C[3], Pernas M[3], Casado C[3], León A[4], Plana M[4], Climent N[4], Arnedo M[4], García F[4], Alcamí P[3]. [1]Laboratory of Immunovirology, Biomedicine Institute of Seville, Clinic Unit of Infectious Diseases, Microbiology and Preventive Medicine, Virgen del Rocío University Hospital, Sevilla, Spain. [2]Infectious Diseases Department, Hospital Carlos III, Madrid, Spain. [3]Centro Nacional de Microbiología, Instituto de Salud Carlos III, Majadahonda, Madrid, Spain. [4]IDIBAPS-Hospital Clínic, AIDS Research Group, Barcelona, Spain.

Author Contributions

Conceived and designed the experiments: MA MP. Performed the experiments: LE TE NB MEB. Analyzed the data: MA LE NB. Wrote the paper: MA LE ACG MP JMG FG. Provided samples and collected data: FG AL. Critically revised and subsequently approved the final version: MA MP LE TE NB MEB ACG JMG FG AL.

References

1. Pantaleo G, Menzo S, Vaccarezza M, Graziosi C, Cohen OJ, et al. (1995) Studies in subjects with long-term nonprogressive human immunodeficiency virus infection. N Engl J Med 332: 209–216.
2. Grabar S, Selinger-Leneman H, Abgrall S, Pialoux G, Weiss L, et al. (2009) Prevalence and comparative characteristics of long-term nonprogressors and HIV controller patients in the French Hospital Database on HIV. AIDS 23: 1163–1169.
3. Okulicz JF, Marconi VC, Landrum ML, Wegner S, Weintrob A, et al. (2009) Clinical outcomes of elite controllers, viremic controllers, and long-term nonprogressors in the US Department of Defense HIV natural history study. J Infect Dis 200: 1714–1723.
4. Deeks SG, Walker BD (2007) Human immunodeficiency virus controllers: mechanisms of durable virus control in the absence of antiretroviral therapy. Immunity 27: 406–416.
5. Saez-Cirion A, Bacchus C, Hocqueloux L, Avettand-Fenoel V, Girault I, et al. (2013) Post-treatment HIV-1 controllers with a long-term virological remission after the interruption of early initiated antiretroviral therapy ANRS VISCONTI Study. PLoS Pathog 9: e1003211.
6. Rodriguez-Garcia M, Climent N, Oliva H, Casanova V, Franco R, et al. (2010) Increased alpha-defensins 1-3 production by dendritic cells in HIV-infected individuals is associated with slower disease progression. PLoS One 5: e9436.
7. Goulder PJ, Watkins DI (2008) Impact of MHC class I diversity on immune control of immunodeficiency virus replication. Nat Rev Immunol 8: 619–630.
8. Lassen KG, Lobritz MA, Bailey JR, Johnston S, Nguyen S, et al. (2009) Elite suppressor-derived HIV-1 envelope glycoproteins exhibit reduced entry efficiency and kinetics. PLoS Pathog 5: e1000377.
9. Pereyra F, Jia X, McLaren PJ, Telenti A, de Bakker PI, et al. (2010) The major genetic determinants of HIV-1 control affect HLA class I peptide presentation. Science 330: 1551–1557.
10. Brennan CA, Ibarrondo FJ, Sugar CA, Hausner MA, Shih R, et al. (2012) Early HLA-B*57-restricted CD8+ T lymphocyte responses predict HIV-1 disease progression. J Virol 86: 10505–10516.
11. Pereyra F, Addo MM, Kaufmann DE, Liu Y, Miura T, et al. (2008) Genetic and immunologic heterogeneity among persons who control HIV infection in the absence of therapy. J Infect Dis 197: 563–571.
12. Dalmasso C, Carpentier W, Meyer L, Rouzioux C, Goujard C, et al. (2008) Distinct genetic loci control plasma HIV-RNA and cellular HIV-DNA levels in HIV-1 infection: the ANRS Genome Wide Association 01 study. PLoS One 3: e3907.
13. Fellay J, Shianna KV, Ge D, Colombo S, Ledergerber B, et al. (2007) A whole-genome association study of major determinants for host control of HIV-1. Science 317: 944–947.
14. Fellay J, Ge D, Shianna KV, Colombo S, Ledergerber B, et al. (2009) Common genetic variation and the control of HIV-1 in humans. PLoS Genet 5: e1000791.
15. Hyrcza MD, Kovacs C, Loutfy M, Halpenny R, Heisler L, et al. (2007) Distinct transcriptional profiles in ex vivo CD4+ and CD8+ T cells are established early in human immunodeficiency virus type 1 infection and are characterized by a chronic interferon response as well as extensive transcriptional changes in CD8+ T cells. J Virol 81: 3477–3486.
16. Chun TW, Justement JS, Lempicki RA, Yang J, Dennis G, Jr., et al. (2003) Gene expression and viral prodution in latently infected, resting CD4+ T cells in viremic versus aviremic HIV-infected individuals. Proc Natl Acad Sci U S A 100: 1908–1913.
17. Rotger M, Dang KK, Fellay J, Heinzen EL, Feng S, et al. (2010) Genome-wide mRNA expression correlates of viral control in CD4+ T-cells from HIV-1-infected individuals. PLoS Pathog 6: e1000781.
18. Bartel DP (2004) MicroRNAs: genomics, biogenesis, mechanism, and function. Cell 116: 281–297.
19. Ambros V (2004) The functions of animal microRNAs. Nature 431: 350–355.
20. Ambros V, Chen X (2007) The regulation of genes and genomes by small RNAs. Development 134: 1635–1641.
21. Petersen CP, Bordeleau ME, Pelletier J, Sharp PA (2006) Short RNAs repress translation after initiation in mammalian cells. Mol Cell 21: 533–542.
22. Yekta S, Shih IH, Bartel DP (2004) MicroRNA-directed cleavage of HOXB8 mRNA. Science 304: 594–596.
23. Pillai RS (2005) MicroRNA function: multiple mechanisms for a tiny RNA? RNA 11: 1753–1761.
24. Griffiths-Jones S, Grocock RJ, van Dongen S, Bateman A, Enright AJ (2006) miRBase: microRNA sequences, targets and gene nomenclature. Nucleic Acids Res 34: D140–144.
25. Bi Y, Liu G, Yang R (2009) MicroRNAs: novel regulators during the immune response. J Cell Physiol 218: 467–472.
26. Lodish HF, Zhou B, Liu G, Chen CZ (2008) Micromanagement of the immune system by microRNAs. Nat Rev Immunol 8: 120–130.
27. Hariharan M, Scaria V, Pillai B, Brahmachari SK (2005) Targets for human encoded microRNAs in HIV genes. Biochem Biophys Res Commun 337: 1214–1218.
28. Triboulet R, Mari B, Lin YL, Chable-Bessia C, Bennasser Y, et al. (2007) Suppression of microRNA-silencing pathway by HIV-1 during virus replication. Science 315: 1579–1582.
29. Bignami F, Pilotti E, Bertoncelli L, Ronzi P, Gulli M, et al. (2012) Stable changes in CD4+ T lymphocyte miRNA expression after exposure to HIV-1. Blood 119: 6259–6267.
30. Witwer KW, Watson AK, Blankson JN, Clements JE (2012) Relationships of PBMC microRNA expression, plasma viral load, and CD4+ T-cell count in HIV-1-infected elite suppressors and viremic patients. Retrovirology 9: 5.
31. Houzet L, Yeung ML, de Lame V, Desai D, Smith SM, et al. (2008) MicroRNA profile changes in human immunodeficiency virus type 1 (HIV-1) seropositive individuals. Retrovirology 5: 118.
32. Duskova K, Nagilla P, Le HS, Iyer P, Thalamuthu A, et al. (2013) MicroRNA regulation and its effects on cellular transcriptome in human immunodeficiency virus-1 (HIV-1) infected individuals with distinct viral load and CD4 cell counts. BMC Infect Dis 13: 250.
33. Swaminathan G, Navas-Martin S, Martin-Garcia J (2014) MicroRNAs and HIV-1 infection: antiviral activities and beyond. J Mol Biol 426: 1178–1197.

34. NCBI Gene Expression Omnibus (GEO). Available: http://www.ncbi.nlm.nih.gov/geo/. Accessed 2014 August 12.
35. D'Haene B, Mestdagh P, Hellemans J, Vandesompele J (2012) miRNA expression profiling: from reference genes to global mean normalization. Methods Mol Biol 822: 261–272.
36. Mestdagh P, Van Vlierberghe P, De Weer A, Muth D, Westermann F, et al. (2009) A novel and universal method for microRNA RT-qPCR data normalization. Genome Biol 10: R64.
37. Saeed AI, Sharov V, White J, Li J, Liang W, et al. (2003) TM4: a free, open-source system for microarray data management and analysis. Biotechniques 34: 374–378.
38. Benjamini Y, Hochberg Y (1995) Controlling the False Discovery Rate: a Practical and Powerful Approach to Multiple Testing. J R Statist 57: 289–300.
39. Vigneault F, Woods M, Buzon MJ, Li C, Pereyra F, et al. (2011) Transcriptional profiling of CD4 T cells identifies distinct subgroups of HIV-1 elite controllers. J Virol 85: 3015–3019.
40. Rossi RL, Rossetti G, Wenandy L, Curti S, Ripamonti A, et al. (2011) Distinct microRNA signatures in human lymphocyte subsets and enforcement of the naive state in CD4+ T cells by the microRNA miR-125b. Nat Immunol 12: 796–803.
41. Hunter MP, Ismail N, Zhang X, Aguda BD, Lee EJ, et al. (2008) Detection of microRNA expression in human peripheral blood microvesicles. PLoS One 3: e3694.
42. Sun G, Li H, Wu X, Covarrubias M, Scherer L, et al. (2012) Interplay between HIV-1 infection and host microRNAs. Nucleic Acids Res 40: 2181–2196.
43. Ahluwalia JK, Khan SZ, Soni K, Rawat P, Gupta A, et al. (2008) Human cellular microRNA hsa-miR-29a interferes with viral nef protein expression and HIV-1 replication. Retrovirology 5: 117.
44. Leonard JA, Filzen T, Carter CC, Schaefer M, Collins KL (2011) HIV-1 Nef disrupts intracellular trafficking of major histocompatibility complex class I, CD4, CD8, and CD28 by distinct pathways that share common elements. J Virol 85: 6867–6881.
45. Schaefer MR, Wonderlich ER, Roeth JF, Leonard JA, Collins KL (2008) HIV-1 Nef targets MHC-I and CD4 for degradation via a final common beta-COP-dependent pathway in T cells. PLoS Pathog 4: e1000131.
46. Chiang K, Sung TL, Rice AP (2012) Regulation of cyclin T1 and HIV-1 Replication by microRNAs in resting CD4+ T lymphocytes. J Virol 86: 3244–3252.
47. Graf EH, Mexas AM, Yu JJ, Shaheen F, Liszewski MK, et al. (2011) Elite suppressors harbor low levels of integrated HIV DNA and high levels of 2-LTR circular HIV DNA compared to HIV+ patients on and off HAART. PLoS Pathog 7: e1001300.
48. Hu G, Gong AY, Liu J, Zhou R, Deng C, et al. (2010) miR-221 suppresses ICAM-1 translation and regulates interferon-gamma-induced ICAM-1 expression in human cholangiocytes. Am J Physiol Gastrointest Liver Physiol 298: G542–550.
49. Zhang C, Han L, Zhang A, Yang W, Zhou X, et al. (2010) Global changes of mRNA expression reveals an increased activity of the interferon-induced signal transducer and activator of transcription (STAT) pathway by repression of miR-221/222 in glioblastoma U251 cells. Int J Oncol 36: 1503–1512.
50. Paquette JS, Fortin JF, Blanchard L, Tremblay MJ (1998) Level of ICAM-1 surface expression on virus producer cells influences both the amount of virion-bound host ICAM-1 and human immunodeficiency virus type 1 infectivity. J Virol 72: 9329–9336.
51. Rizzuto CD, Sodroski JG (1997) Contribution of virion ICAM-1 to human immunodeficiency virus infectivity and sensitivity to neutralization. J Virol 71: 4847–4851.
52. Bounou S, Giguere JF, Cantin R, Gilbert C, Imbeault M, et al. (2004) The importance of virus-associated host ICAM-1 in human immunodeficiency virus type 1 dissemination depends on the cellular context. FASEB J 18: 1294–1296.
53. Schulte LN, Westermann AJ, Vogel J (2013) Differential activation and functional specialization of miR-146 and miR-155 in innate immune sensing. Nucleic Acids Res 41: 542–553.
54. Zhang G, Ghosh S (2001) Toll-like receptor-mediated NF-kappaB activation: a phylogenetically conserved paradigm in innate immunity. J Clin Invest 107: 13–19.
55. Seddiki N, Swaminathan S, Phetsouphanh C, Kelleher AD (2012) miR-155 is differentially expressed in Treg subsets, which may explain expression level differences of miR-155 in HIV-1 infected patients. Blood 119: 6396–6397.
56. Gracias DT, Stelekati E, Hope JL, Boesteanu AC, Doering TA, et al. (2013) The microRNA miR-155 controls CD8(+) T cell responses by regulating interferon signaling. Nat Immunol 14: 593–602.
57. Dudda JC, Salaun B, Ji Y, Palmer DC, Monnot GC, et al. (2013) MicroRNA-155 is required for effector CD8+ T cell responses to virus infection and cancer. Immunity 38: 742–753.
58. Seddiki N, Brezar V, Ruffin N, Levy Y, Swaminathan S (2014) Role of miR-155 in the regulation of lymphocyte immune function and disease. Immunology 142: 32–38.

22

Insignificant Medium-Term Vitamin D Status Change after 25-Hydroxyvitamin D Testing in a Large Managed Care Population

Meng Wei[1], Run Yu[2]*, Stephen C. Deutsch[1]

1 Cedars-Sinai Medical Care Foundation, Beverly Hills, California, United States of America, 2 Division of Endocrinology, Cedars-Sinai Medical Center, Los Angeles, California, United States of America

Abstract

Objectives: To examine the clinical utility of 25-hydroxyvitamin D (25(OH)D) testing in achieving medium-term vitamin D (VD) sufficiency in a managed care population.

Methods: Retrospective study of a continuously-enrolled patient population in a 3-year period between 2011 and 2013. Primary outcome was VD status at ~1 year after 25(OH)D testing. Patient demographics, comorbidities, medications, and 25(OH)D test results were gathered from relevant databases and multivariate logistic regression analysis used to study the risk factors of persistent VD deficiency or insufficiency.

Results: Of 22,784 patients, 7533 (females 69.3%) did 14,563 25(OH)D tests, with an estimated cost of $582,520. Of the 7533 patients, 1126 had another 25(OH)D test at 300–400 days after the first one. Based on the two test results, 234 patients (20.8%) maintained sufficient 25(OH)D levels; 132 (11.7%) turned from VD-sufficient into VD-insufficient or -deficient; 538 (47.8%) remained VD-insufficient or -deficient, and only 222 (19.7%) improved to be VD-sufficient. Overall, only 8.0% more patients were VD-sufficient at ~1 year after 25(OH)D testing. Only younger age and higher BMI were independent risk factors for persistent low 25(OH)D levels and high-dose VD use was not associated with achieving VD sufficiency.

Conclusions: 25(OH)D testing only benefits a small portion of patients thus lacks clinical utility in achieving VD sufficiency in the medium term but incurs a significant cost. A practical strategy to treat VD deficiency or insufficiency is needed; without it, 25(OH)D testing adds little value to most patients' health and should be used with discretion.

Editor: Andrzej T. Slominski, University of Tennessee, United States of America

Funding: The authors have no support or funding to report.

Competing Interests: The authors have declared that no competing interests exist.

* Email: run.yu@cshs.org

Introduction

Extremely low levels of vitamin D (VD), measured by serum 25-hydroxyvitamin D (25(OH)D) levels, are detrimental to bone health and VD supplementation in patients with very low 25(OH)D levels is beneficial in correcting osteomalacia or osteoporosis [1,2]. There have been many studies suggesting that higher 25(OH)D levels are associated with better outcomes of numerous non-skeletal diseases such as cardiovascular diseases and cancers [3,4]. Although there is no consensus on who should undergo 25(OH)D testing and routine screening for VD status is not recommended due to lack of evidence on feasibility, cost-effectiveness, or benefits of such screening [1,2], some physicians may be convinced that it is worthwhile to screen for VD deficiency and to treat patients with VD if they do have it. In developed countries, 25(OH)D testing and the associated cost, mostly for screening purpose, have been dramatically increased over the last decade [5,6]. To justify a screening test, the discovered condition has to be treatable if found earlier in its course. In the case of 25(OH)D testing, the discovered condition, VD deficiency (or insufficiency), is theoretically very treatable by sun exposure and VD supplements. Our clinical experience suggests that treatment of VD deficiency or insufficiency, however, is challenging in current clinical practice, especially if the VD status is followed in longer term [7]. The few prospective randomized clinical trials on VD supplementation, on the other hand, have not demonstrated consistent benefits in fracture risk reduction in community-dwelling individuals [1,2,8–11].

To test our hypothesis that most patients with VD deficiency (or insufficiency) remain VD-deficient (or -insufficient), we did a retrospective review of 25(OH)D testing and its clinical utility in achieving medium-term VD sufficiency in a managed care population in the 3 years between 2011 and 2013. The results of our study demonstrate that 25(OH)D testing lacks clinical utility in achieving VD sufficiency and should not be routinely performed in managed care populations or in other contemporary clinical practice.

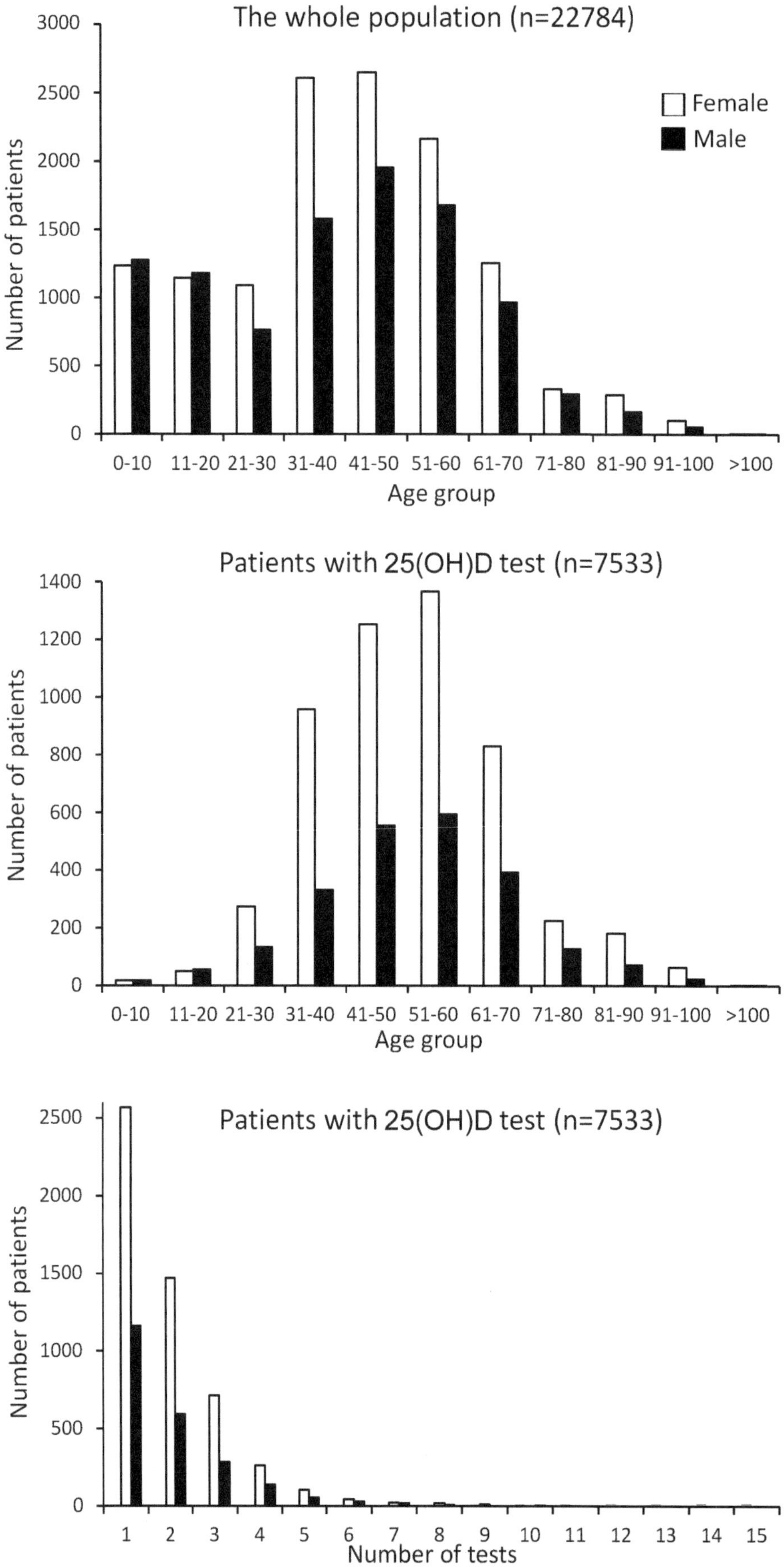
The whole population (n=22784)
Female
Male
Number of patients
3000
2500
2000
1500
1000
500
0
0-10
11-20
21-30
31-40
41-50
51-60
61-70
71-80
81-90
91-100
>100
Age group
Patients with 25(OH)D test (n=7533)
Number of patients
1400
1200
1000
800
600
400
200
0
0-10
11-20
21-30
31-40
41-50
51-60
61-70
71-80
81-90
91-100
>100
Age group
Patients with 25(OH)D test (n=7533)
Number of patients
2500
2000
1500
1000
500
0
1 2 3 4 5 6 7 8 9 10 11 12 13 14 15
Number of tests

Figure 1. Demographics of the managed care population (Top) and the patients who underwent 25(OH)D testing (Middle) over a 3-year period. The numbers of patients who did multiple tests were also shown (Bottom).

Methods

Patients and 25(OH)D tests

This study has been approved by the Cedars-Sinai Institutional Review Board. Requirement of written or verbal consent was waived by the Review Board for this retrospective study. Health records were de-identified prior to use. All managed care patients who were continuously enrolled at a large medical group and an independent physician association from January 1, 2011 to December 31, 2013 were eligible. There were no exclusion criteria for this population-based study. The list of patients was obtained from the managed care enrollment database, race and body mass index (BMI) from the electronic medical records database, and 25(OH)D testing data from the laboratory encounter database. VD status was defined as follows: deficiency (25(OH)D≤20 ng/ml), insufficiency (>20 but <30 ng/ml), and sufficiency (≥30 ng/ml) [2]. The economic burden of 25(OH)D testing was calculated as the total cost of 25(OH)D testing within the study patient population in the 3 years of study period, based on the Medicare rate.

Co-morbidities, procedures, and medications

Data on osteoporosis, pathologic fractures, obesity, fat malabsorption (including Crohn's disease, ulcerative colitis, celiac disease, cystic fibrosis, and history of pancreatectomy, gastrectomy, or small bowel resection), chronic kidney disease, HIV, dual-energy X-ray absorptiometry (DEXA), and bariatric surgery were based on ICD-9 and CPT codes and obtained from encounter database. Medication records and high-dose VD dispensing (50,000 international units or 1.25 mg) data were obtained from pharmacy claim database. To study the risk factors for repeated 25(OH)D testing and failure to improve VD status after testing, the co-morbidities, procedures, and medications for osteoporosis and seizure recorded 6 months before and after the only or the first 25(OH)D test were used as variables. To study the risk factors for failure to improve VD status after testing, high-dose VD dispensed within 350 days after the only or the first 25(OH)D test was used.

Statistics

Student t test was used to compare of the means of continuous data between two groups. Chi square or Fisher's exact test was used to compare the rates of categorical data between groups. Multivariate logistic regression analysis was used to discover independent risk factors associated with a change of VD status [3,12]. All statistical analyses were performed using the JMP Statistical Discovery software (Cary, NC).

Results

Of the 22,784 managed care patients continuously enrolled in the 3-year study period (Fig. 1), 7533 patients did 14,563 25(OH)D tests with valid results, corresponding to an annual test

Table 1. Comparison of patients who did only 1 25(OH)D test and those who did 2 or more 25(OH)D tests in the study period.

	Only 1 25(OH)D test	>=2 25(OH)D tests
n	3,731	3,802
Age (range), yr	48.9 (3–105)***	53.5 (8–100)
Female, %	68.8	69.9
African American, %	22.1	21.5
Results of the only or first test (range), ng/ml	23.8 (0–115)***	26.0 (0–154.9)
Sufficiency/insufficiency/deficiency at the only or first test, %	33.4/29.3/37.3***	31.8/34.3/33.9
Osteoporosis diagnosis, %	5.2***	9.3
Pathologic fractures, %	0.5	0.4
Osteoporosis medications, %	5.2***	8.9
DEXA, %	5.8***	11.1
Obesity diagnosis, %	14.3	15.8
BMI (range)	27.1 (13.4–66.6)***	27.6 (13.4–62.3)
BMI≥30, %	24.8	26.5
History of bariatric surgery, %	1.1**	1.9
Fat malabsorption, %	1.4	1.5
Chronic kidney disease, %	2.0*	2.8
HIV, %	0.9***	2.4
Anti-epileptics, %	0.3	0.2
High-dose VD prescription, %	3.2***	8.2

Statistical analysis was performed to assess the significance of the differences between the two groups.
*$p<0.05$,
**$p<0.01$,
***$p<0.001$.

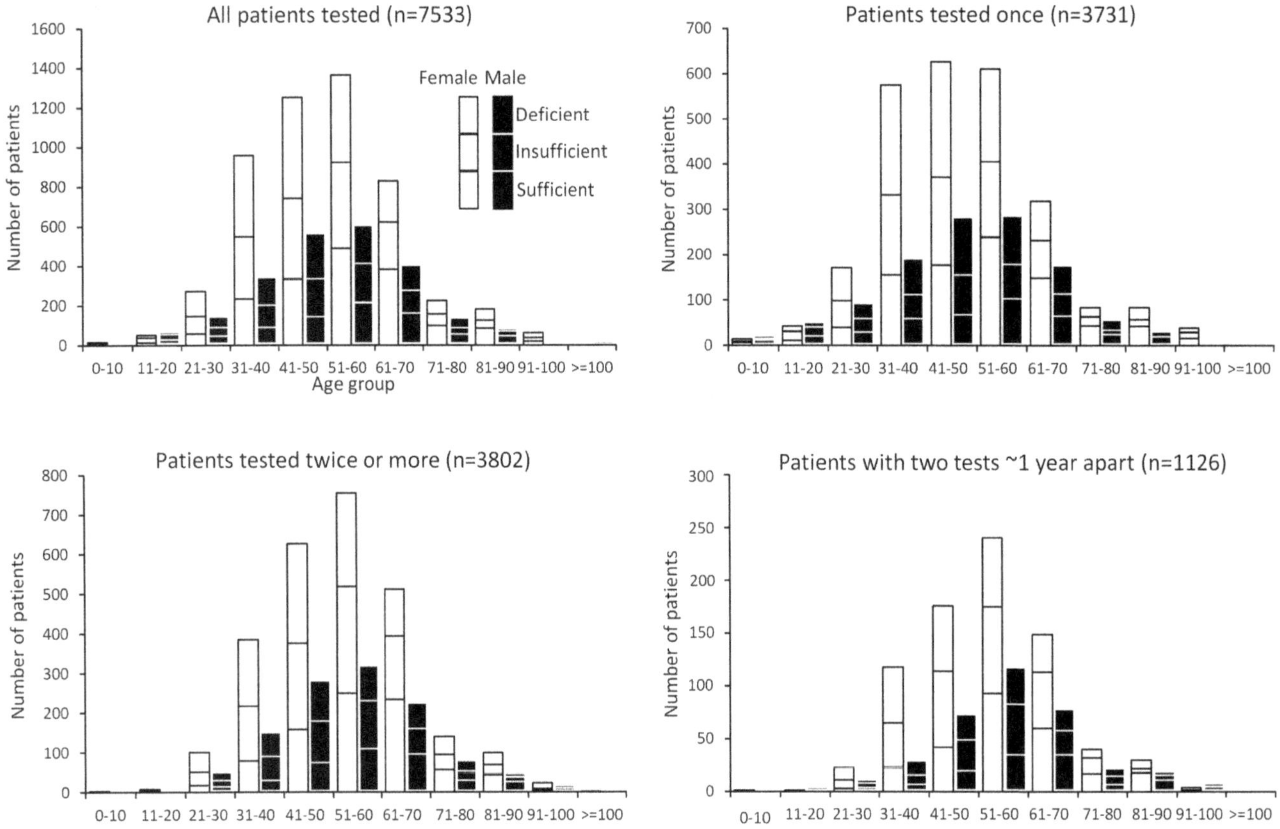

Figure 2. 25(OH)D test results. The results of the only or the first 25(OH)D test were classified into 3 groups: deficiency (≤20 ng/ml), insufficiency (>20 but <30 ng/ml), or sufficiency (≥30 ng/ml). Upper left, results from all patients who underwent 25(OH)D testing. Upper right, results from the patients who had only been tested once. Lower left, results from the patients who had 2 or more 25(OH)D tests. Lower right, results from the patients who had another test at 300–400 days after the first one.

rate of 11.0% of the managed care population and 0.21 25(OH)D test per patient per year. Based on Medicare rates, the total cost of the 25(OH)D tests for the 7533 patients was $582,520. Most tested patients were between 31 and 70 years old (83.4%), and those between 41 and 60 years old made up 50.0%. Females (n = 5224, 69.3%) were tested much more frequently than males (n = 2309, 30.7%) across all age groups. Of the 7533 patients, 3731 (49.5%) had only one 25(OH)D test but 3802 (50.5%) had two or more tests (Fig. 1). Compared with those with only 1 25(OH)D test, patients with more than one 25(OH)D test were 4.6 years older and had slightly higher 25(OH)D levels and BMI; they also had more osteoporosis diagnoses, underwent more DEXA scans, and were more likely on osteoporosis medications (Table 1). Overall, <3% of patients had history of bariatric surgery, fat malabsorption, chronic kidney disease, and HIV, or anti-epileptic use. More patients with more than one 25(OH)D test were dispensed with high-dose VD after the first 25(OH)D test than those with only one test (8.2% V 3.2%, $p<0.001$). Between the two groups, there were no significant differences in patients' sex, race, rates of pathologic fractures, or obesity diagnosis.

Based on the results of the first (or the only) 25(OH)D test, 32.6% of the 7533 patients were VD-sufficient while 31.6% VD-insufficient and 35.7% VD-deficient. Similar results were seen in both sexes across age groups (Fig. 2). Interestingly patients between 21 and 50 years old were less VD-sufficient (25.0% v. 39.2%, $p<0.0001$) but also less frequently tested than people of other ages (45.0% v. 55.2%, $p<0.0001$). There were small seasonal variations in 25(OH)D levels which were highest in July and lowest in December (mean levels 27.7 and 22.7 ng/ml, respectively). In the 21–50-year group, those who were VD-insufficient or -deficient were slightly more likely to be tested again than those who were VD-sufficient (46.3% v. 41.1%, $p = 0.0077$). In other age groups, the repeat test rates were not significantly different between those who were VD-insufficient or -deficient and those who were VD-sufficient (56.2% v. 53.7%, $p = 0.1271$).

To study the impact of 25(OH)D testing on future VD status, we identified 1126 patients who had done another 25(OH)D test at 300–400 days after the first one. The distribution of the results of the first 25(OH)D test of the 1126 patients and that of the 3802 patients were grossly similar to that of the 7533 patients (Fig. 2), suggesting that the 1126 patients were representative of all the patients tested more than once. We also compared the demographics and VD status of the 1126 patients with the rest of the 7533 (6507 patients, the difference of 7533 and 1026) over each decade between 21 and 90 years old. If the 25(OH)D results were divided into the 3 categories of sufficiency, insufficiency, and deficiency, the result distribution was not significantly different in most decades except for in the decades of 41–50 and 71–80 years old ($p = 0.0196$ and 0.0468, respectively). If the 25(OH)D results were divided into 2 groups, sufficiency and abnormally low levels (including insufficiency and deficiency), the 25(OH)D result distribution was not significantly different among any decades ($p = 0.1272$–0.9563).

We compared the second and the first 25(OH)D test results of the 1126 patients and identified 4 patterns of VD status change. As the difference between VD deficiency and insufficiency is

Table 2. Comparison of 4 groups of patients who did another 25(OH)D test at ~1 year after the first one.

Characteristics	Sufficient-to-sufficient	Sufficient-to-low	Low-to-sufficient	Low-to-low	All
n (%)	234 (20.8)	132 (11.7)	222 (19.7)	538 (47.8)	1126 (100)
Age (range), yr	59.2 (30–98)*	55.5 (8–91)	55.4 (21–95)***	51.4 (12–98)	54.3 (8–98)
Female, %	72.6	66.7	70.3	68.4	69.4
African American, %	16.9	18.1	12.6***	26.4	22.1
1st result (range), ng/ml	43.1 (30.0–154.9)***	37.0 (30–87.2)	20.9 (0–29.8)***	19.4 (0–29.9)	26.7 (0–154.9)
Difference between 2nd and 1st results (range), ng/ml	−0.57 (−110.2–38.1)***	−23.4 (−69.8– −0.9)	17.6 (0.5–81)***	−2.7 (−29.7–28.0)	−0.7 (−110.2–81)
Osteoporosis diagnosis, %	17.1*	9.1	5.4	5.8	9.2
Pathologic fractures, %	0.9	0	0	0.2	0.3
Osteoporosis medications, %	17.1	9.8	5.9	6.1	9.5
DEXA, %	20.9*	10.6	6.8	9.3	12.3
Obesity diagnosis, %	10.7	15.9	7.2***	19.1	16.1
BMI (range)	25.1 (14.9–43.5)**	26.8 (14.9–49.0)	26.7 (16.9–47.6)***	28.7 (16.5–62.3)	27.3 (14.9–62.3)
BMI≥30, %	10.2**	21.6	15.2***	32.3	24.6
History of bariatric surgery, %	2.6	3.0	0.9	1.7	2.4
Fat malabsorption, %	3.0	3.0	0.5	1.1	1.6
Chronic kidney disease, %	3.4	3.8	2.3	3.3	3.5
HIV, %	6.4	2.3	2.3	1.1	2.9
Anti-epileptics, %	0	0.8	0	0.2	0.2
High-dose VD prescription, %	1.7*	6.1	5.0**	11.9	8.3

Sufficient-to-sufficient, patients with sufficient VD results from both tests; sufficient-to-low, patients with sufficient results from the first test but abnormally low results (VD-insufficient or deficient) from the second; low-to-sufficient, patients with abnormally low results from the first test but sufficient results from the second one; low-to-low, patients with abnormally low results from both tests. Statistical analysis was performed to assess the significance of the differences between the sufficient-to-sufficient and sufficient-to-low groups, and between the low-to-sufficient and low-to-low groups.
*$p<0.05$,
**$p<0.01$,
***$p<0.001$.

controversial and somewhat arbitrary [13], they were collectively labeled as abnormally low VD levels. Only 234 of the 1126 patients (20.8%) exhibited sufficient VD levels on both tests (sufficient-to-sufficient), indicating maintained VD sufficiency, while 132 (11.7%) who were originally VD-sufficient became VD insufficient or deficient (sufficient-to-low) (Table 2). Interestingly, after the first test, 538 patients (47.8%) remained VD-insufficient or -deficient (low-to-low) and only 222 patients (19.7%) improved to be VD-sufficient (low-to-sufficient). Overall, 67.5% of patients were VD-insufficient or -deficient at the first test and 59.5% were so at the second test. Thus only 8.0% patients benefited from the testing by converting from low to sufficient VD levels at approximately a year after the test. To derive risk factors for inability to maintain VD sufficiency and for persistent low VD levels, we compared the characteristics of the 4 groups of patients (Table 2 and Fig. 3). By univariate analysis, compared with those in the sufficient-to-sufficient group, the patients in the sufficient-to-low group were a few years younger, more obese, and with lower 25(OH)D levels from the first test; they also had fewer osteoporosis diagnoses and underwent fewer DEXA scans. Ironically, a small fraction of both groups of patients were dispensed with high-dose VD but those in the sufficient-to-low group were dispensed with relatively more frequently (6.1% v. 1.7%). Multivariate logistic regression analysis showed that only younger age and lower rate of HIV infection were independent risk factors for inability to maintain VD sufficiency. If only the significant variables identified by univariate analysis ($p<0.05$) were used, younger age remained the sole risk factor for inability to maintain VD sufficiency. Compared with those in the low-to-sufficient group, the patients in the low-to-low group were again a few years younger, more obese, and with lower 25(OH)D levels from the first test; more patients were African Americans. More patients in these two groups were dispensed with high-dose VD than those in the sufficient-to-sufficient and sufficient-to-low groups; however, patients in the low-to-low group were dispensed with relatively more high-dose VD than those in the low-to-sufficient group. Multivariate analysis showed that only younger age, higher BMI, history of bariatric surgery, and lower rate of HIV infection were independent risk factors for persistent low VD levels. If only the significant variables identified by univariate analysis ($p<0.05$) were used, younger age and higher BMI remained risk factors for persistent low VD levels.

Discussion

25(OH)D testing to detect VD deficiency has become a fad in recent years, probably driven by numerous correlational studies connecting low 25(OH)D levels and many human diseases [3–6]. As the literature on benefits of VD sufficiency appears somewhat plausible [1–4], one may presumptively accept that VD sufficiency is beneficial to health in general. The key question then becomes

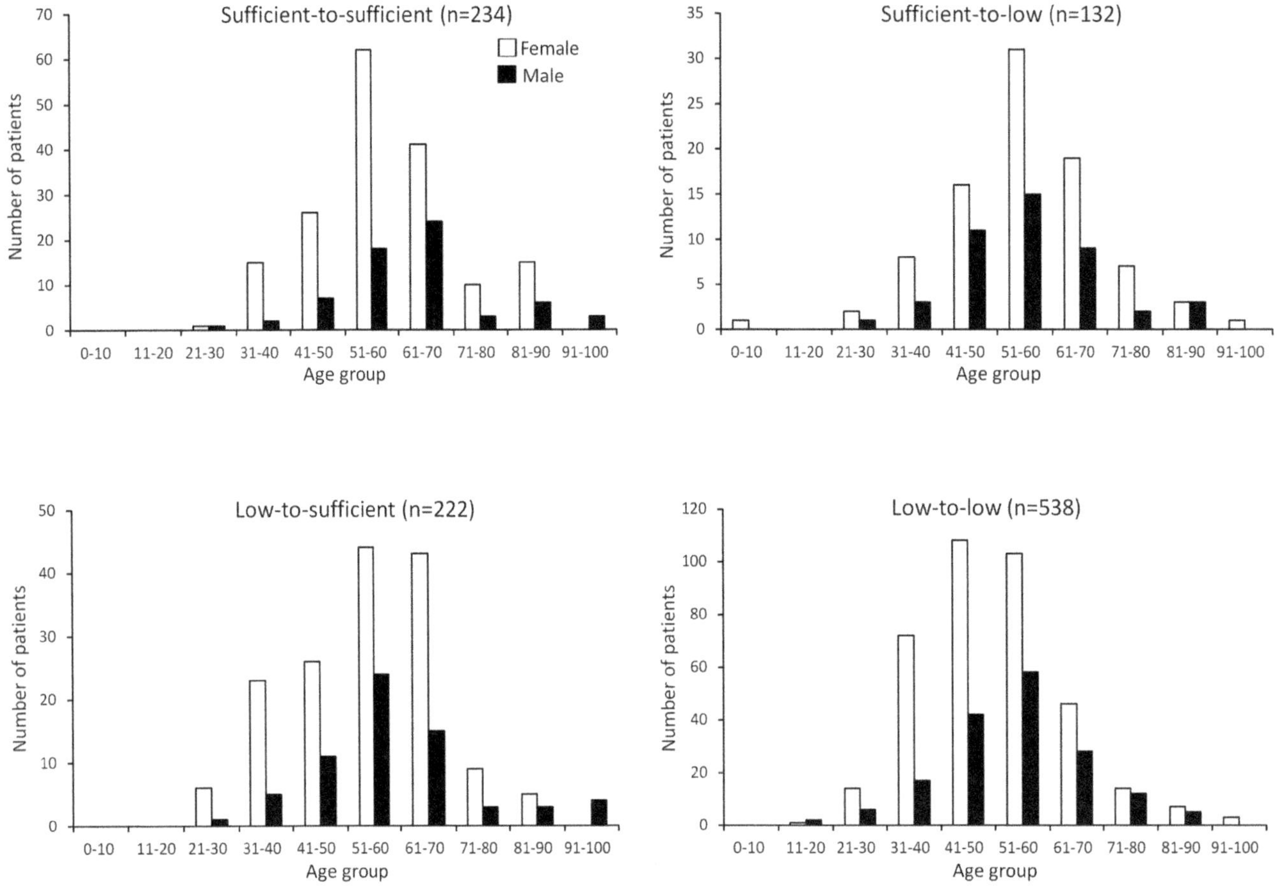

Figure 3. Demographics of the patients who had another 25(OH)D test at about 1 year after the first one. Upper left, the patients with sufficient 25(OH)D results from both tests (sufficient-to-sufficient). Upper right, the patients with sufficient 25(OH)D results from the first test but abnormally low results (VD-insufficient or deficient) from the second (sufficient-to-low). Lower left, the patients with abnormally low results from the first test but sufficient results from the second one (low-to-sufficient). Lower right, the patients with abnormally low results from both tests (low-to-low).

how to effectively help people achieve VD sufficiency. There is no doubt that high-dose VD treatment improves VD status in a few months [2,3,7] (and in years if given every 2 weeks [14]). As VD deficiency or insufficiency is a chronic condition, the key question is whether VD status improves in longer terms after 25(OH)D testing or high-dose VD treatment. Thus in this article, we take a novel approach studying the practical clinical utility of 25(OH)D testing and examine whether 25(OH)D testing helps achieve VD sufficiency in the medium term in a large managed care population.

First of all, the study confirms that VD sufficiency is uncommon (only ~1/3) in the mostly adult managed care population [15]. The most striking finding, however, is that most patients with VD deficiency or insufficiency (~70%) do not achieve VD sufficiency and a portion of patients with VD sufficiency (~40%) lose it at 300–400 days after the first 25(OH)D test. Overall only 8% of the tested patients improve their VD status from deficiency or insufficiency to sufficiency. The true cost of 25(OH)D testing is thus more expensive than the apparent cost because to benefit one patient (to achieve or maintain VD sufficiency after 25(OH)D testing), 12.5 patients (the inverse of 8%) have to be tested. As 1/3 of the entire study population underwent 25(OH)D testing at least once and only <10% of tested patients had osteoporosis diagnosis or history of pathologic fractures, the purpose of the 25(OH)D tests was most likely for screening for VD deficiency. Our results seriously challenge the clinical utility of 25(OH)D testing for screening purpose. First, there does not seem to be a need for screening for VD deficiency or insufficiency if the majority of the population has the condition. Second, the lack of practical and effective treatment of VD deficiency or insufficiency makes VD status screening not worthwhile. Although chronic use of high-dose VD can achieve VD sufficiency for years, this method has not been adopted in clinical practice [14]. Indeed, routine screening for vitamin D status is not recommended by guidelines but the reason for not recommending screening is due to lack of evidence on feasibility, cost-effectiveness, or benefits of such screening [1,2]. Our results provide direct evidence for recommending *against* routine screening for vitamin D status.

Although VD deficiency or insufficiency can be treated in a theoretically straightforward manner by sun exposure and VD supplement, our study clearly shows that it is challenging to be treated in practice. The failure to effectively treat VD deficiency or insufficiency may be either due to lack of counseling on importance and ways to achieve VD sufficiency or due to patients' incompliance. Concern of skin cancer is a known barrier to achieve VD sufficiency [16,17]. Adherence to VD supplementation is an important factor in achieving benefits of VD supplementation on fracture prevention [7,11]. Adherence is satisfactory (60–90%) in elderly populations but unclear in younger populations. If VD sufficiency is indeed critical to health, a practical and effective method is needed to achieve VD sufficiency.

Our study provides novel insights into the potential causes of VD deficiency and failure to improve VD status. In our study, the patients who maintain VD sufficiency are not necessarily healthier than others. They are older and thinner, and tend to have osteoporosis and HIV infection. As most of them do not take high-dose VD supplement, their VD sufficiency is presumably achieved by sun exposure and over-the-counter VD supplement [2,3]. As these measures are dependent on life style, it can be assumed that these patients are highly motivated to achieve VD sufficiency. Although we don't have data on their motivations, their older age and the age-associated osteoporosis in this mostly female population may motivate them to achieve and maintain VD sufficiency. On the other hand, the patients who remain VD-deficient or -insufficient are younger and heavier but fewer of them have osteoporosis or HIV infection. Even though slightly more than 10% of them fill high-dose VD prescriptions, the high-dose VD does not help them achieve VD sufficiency in the medium term. Thus the cause of their persistent VD deficiency or insufficiency is also unconducive life style for VD sufficiency. Their perceived low risk for osteoporosis may give them a disincentive to make life style modifications to achieve VD sufficiency. Compared with other chronic life-style diseases such as obesity, diabetes, and hypertension, VD deficiency can be much more easily treated by simply taking daily 2000–4000 international units of VD without sun exposure [1,2]. The lack of clear evidence that mild VD deficiency or insufficiency indeed causes clear and severe complications is likely the main reason for physicians and patients not to invest in life style modifications to improve VD status. On the other hand, for motivated patients, the physicians should consider the patients' risk factors for persistent low VD levels during counseling; for example, higher doses of VD are likely needed for young and obese patients to achieve VD sufficiency [18–20].

Our study has its strengths and limitations. Because it is based on a population without exclusion criteria, its results more realistically reflect the true characteristics of the population. The defined and stable managed care patient population has several distinct advantages for population studies [21]. As the patients received all their care within the managed care system and their 25(OH)D tests and results, comorbidities, procedures, and medications were all recorded, our study results are accurate and unlikely prone to misinterpretation due to incomplete data. Most importantly, we have followed a cohort of the same patients with 2 25(OH)D tests approximately a year apart so that we can derive specific risk factors for failure to achieve or maintain VD sufficiency. One major limitation is that we do not have data on sun exposure and over-the-counter VD supplement, the main treatments for VD deficiency or insufficiency. Another limitation is that although the cohort of patients we followed appeared to be similar to all patients with 25(OH)D testing, the former has much fewer patients than, and may not represent a random sample of, the latter. The small seasonal variation of 25(OH)D levels should not affect our analysis on medium-term VD status because the second 25(OH)D test was carried out 1 year later, in the same season in which the first test was done.

In summary, this retrospective study of a continuously enrolled managed care population in a 3-year period demonstrates that 25(OH)D testing only benefits a small portion of patients thus lacks clinical utility in achieving VD sufficiency in the medium term but incurs a significant cost. Our data implies that a practical and effective strategy to treat VD deficiency or insufficiency is needed in contemporary managed care practice; without such as strategy, 25(OH)D testing adds little value to most patients' health and should be used with discretion.

Author Contributions

Conceived and designed the experiments: RY SCD. Performed the experiments: MW SCD. Analyzed the data: MW RY. Contributed reagents/materials/analysis tools: MW RY SCD. Contributed to the writing of the manuscript: MW RY SCD.

References

1. IOM (Institute of Medicine) (2011) Dietary reference intakes for calcium and vitamin D. Washington, DC: The National Academies Press; 2011.
2. Holick MF, Binkley NC, Bischoff-Ferrari HA, Gordon CM, Hanley DA, et al. (2011) Evaluation, treatment, and prevention of vitamin D deficiency: an Endocrine Society clinical practice guideline. J Clin Endocrinol Metab 96: 1911–1930.
3. Holick MF (2007) Vitamin D deficiency. N Engl J Med 357: 266–281.
4. Basit S (2013) Vitamin D in health and disease: a literature review. Br J Biomed Sci 70: 161–72.
5. Sattar N1, Welsh P, Panarelli M, Forouhi NG (2012) Increasing requests for vitamin D measurement: costly, confusing, and without credibility. Lancet 379: 95–96.
6. Bilinski KL, Boyages SC (2012) The rising cost of vitamin D testing in Australia: time to establish guidelines for testing. Med J Aust 197: 90.
7. Yu R (2014) Commentary on "Surge in US Outpatient Vitamin D Deficiency Diagnoses: National Ambulatory Medical Care Survey Analysis". South Med J 107: 218–219.
8. Jackson RD1, LaCroix AZ, Gass M, Wallace RB, Robbins J, et al. (2006) Calcium plus vitamin D supplementation and the risk of fractures. N Engl J Med 354: 669–683.
9. Sanders KM1, Stuart AL, Williamson EJ, Simpson JA, Kotowicz MA, et al. (2010) Annual high-dose oral vitamin D and falls and fractures in older women: a randomized controlled trial. JAMA 303: 1815–1822.
10. Bischoff-Ferrari HA1, Willett WC, Orav EJ, Lips P, Meunier PJ, et al. (2012) A pooled analysis of vitamin D dose requirements for fracture prevention. N Engl J Med 367: 40–49.
11. Reid IR, Bolland MJ, Grey A (2014) Effects of vitamin D supplements on bone mineral density: a systematic review and meta-analysis. Lancet 383: 146–155.
12. Looker AC, Pfeiffer CM, Lacher DA, Schleicher RL, Picciano MF, et al. (2008) Serum 25-hydroxyvitamin D status of the US population: 1988–1994 compared with 2000–2004. Am J Clin Nutr 88: 1519–1527.
13. Rosen CJ (2011) Clinical practice. Vitamin D insufficiency. N Engl J Med 364: 248–254.
14. Pietras SM, Obayan BK, Cai MH, Holick MF (2009) Vitamin D2 treatment for vitamin D deficiency and insufficiency for up to 6 years. Arch Intern Med 26: 1806–8.
15. Forrest KY, Stuhldreher WL (2011) Prevalence and correlates of vitamin D deficiency in US adults. Nutr Res 31: 48–54.
16. Reeder AI1, Jopson JA, Gray AR (2012) "Prescribing sunshine": a national, cross-sectional survey of 1,089 New Zealand general practitioners regarding their sun exposure and vitamin D perceptions, and advice provided to patients. BMC Fam Pract 13: 85.
17. Bonevski B, Girgis A, Magin P, Horton G, Brozek I, et al. (2012) Prescribing sunshine: a cross-sectional survey of 500 Australian general practitioners' practices and attitudes about vitamin D. Int J Cancer 130: 2138–2145.
18. Lee P, Greenfield JR, Seibel MJ, Eisman JA, Center JR (2009) Adequacy of vitamin D replacement in severe deficiency is dependent on body mass index. Am J Med 122: 1056–1060.
19. Stratton-Loeffler MJ, Lo JC, Hui RL, Coates A, Minkoff JR, et al. (2012) Treatment of vitamin D deficiency within a large integrated health care delivery system. J Manag Care Pharm 18: 497–505.
20. Drincic A, Fuller E, Heaney RP, Armas LA (2013) 25-hydroxyvitamin D response to graded vitamin D3 supplementation among obese adults. J Clin Endocrinol Metab 98: 4845–4851.
21. Vogt TM1, Elston-Lafata J, Tolsma D, Greene SM (2004) The role of research in integrated healthcare systems: the HMO Research Network. Am J Manag Care 10: 643–648.

23

Retention and Risk Factors for Attrition in a Large Public Health ART Program in Myanmar

Aye Thida[1]*, Sai Thein Than Tun[1], Sai Ko Ko Zaw[1], Andrew A. Lover[2], Philippe Cavailler[3], Jennifer Chunn[4], Mar Mar Aye[5], Par Par[5], Kyaw Win Naing[5], Kaung Nyunt Zan[5], Myint Shwe[6], Thar Tun Kyaw[7], Zaw Htoon Waing[1], Philippe Clevenbergh[1]

1 The Union Office in Myanmar, International Union Against Tuberculosis and Lung Disease, Mandalay, Myanmar, **2** Infectious Diseases Programme, Saw Swee Hock School of Public Health, National University of Singapore, Singapore, **3** Innovation Unit, Médecins Sans Frontières, Geneva, Switzerland, **4** Maths and Statistics Help Centre, James Cook University, Singapore, **5** Medical Care Division, Department of Health, Mandalay, Myanmar, **6** National AIDS Program, Department of Health, Nay Pyi Taw, Myanmar, **7** Disease Control Division, Department of Health, Nay Pyi Taw, Myanmar

Abstract

Background: The outcomes from an antiretroviral treatment (ART) program within the public sector in Myanmar have not been reported. This study documents retention and the risk factors for attrition in a large ART public health program in Myanmar.

Methods: A retrospective analysis of a cohort of adult patients enrolled in the Integrated HIV Care (IHC) Program between June 2005 and October 2011 and followed up until April 2012 is presented. The primary outcome was attrition (death or loss-follow up); a total of 10,223 patients were included in the 5-year cumulative survival analysis. Overall 5,718 patients were analyzed for the risk factors for attrition using both logistic regression and flexible parametric survival models.

Result: The mean age was 36 years, 61% of patients were male, and the median follow up was 13.7 months. Overall 8,564 (84%) patients were retained in ART program: 750 (7%) were lost to follow-up and 909 (9%) died. During the 3 years follow-up, 1,542 attritions occurred over 17,524 person years at risk, giving an incidence density of 8.8% per year. The retention rates of participants at 12, 24, 36, 48 and 60 months were 86, 82, 80, 77 and 74% respectively. In multivariate analysis, being male, having high WHO staging, a low CD4 count, being anaemic or having low BMI at baseline were independent risk factors for attrition; tuberculosis (TB) treatment at ART initiation, a prior ART course before program enrollment and literacy were predictors for retention in the program.

Conclusion: High retention rate of IHC program was documented within the public sector in Myanmar. Early diagnosis of HIV, nutritional support, proper investigation and treatment for patients with low CD4 counts and for those presenting with anaemia are crucial issues towards improvement of HIV program outcomes in resource-limited settings.

Editor: Eduard J. Beck, UNAIDS, Trinidad And Tobago

Funding: Total Yadana, GF round 9 and 3 Diseases Fund have supported the work. The funders had no role in study design, data collection and analysis, decision to publish, or preparation of the manuscript.

Competing Interests: Total Yadana, a commercial source, was among other funders.

* Email: ayethida0612@gmail.com

Introduction

HIV epidemiology and ART coverage in Myanmar

Myanmar has a concentrated HIV epidemic and the global HIV prevalence in adults has been estimated at 0.53% in a recent modelling study [1]. In the same study, the HIV prevalence in high risk groups has been estimated at 9.6, 7.8 and 21.9% in female sex workers (FSW), men who have sex with men (MSM) and injecting drug users (IDU), respectively [1].

There has been a very significant increase in the number of patients receiving ART worldwide, and by the end of 2011, it had reached 20 times the 2003 levels [2]. ART coverage in the Asia-Pacific region increased from 52% in 2009 to 56% in 2011 [3]. By the end of 2011, 40,128 people were receiving ART in Myanmar, which was double the number observed in 2009 [1]. By the end of 2012, 34,733 (65%) patients on ART were followed in the private sector (international NGOs) and 18,976 (35%) patients in the public sector. As per the Asia Epidemic Model (AEM) 2010–2015, the total numbers of people in need of ART in 2013, 2014 and 2015 are estimated at 125,043; 124,286 and 123,915 people respectively. With extended support from the Global Fund against AIDS, Tuberculosis and Malaria for a four-year period, 86% (106,000 patients) of the total affected population is slated to have access to ART by 2016 nationwide [personal communication,

National AIDS Program]. To reach this important goal, the number of patients receiving treatment in the public sector need to be increased to 64,182 people, representing 61% of all patients on ART in Myanmar.

Importance of retention in ART programs

As antiretroviral treatment becomes more readily available [2], the next major challenge for the National HIV Control program and the public sector will be to deliver high quality care [4]. In addition to viral load suppression which remains the key marker of treatment success, several other indicators have been used to measure the quality of HIV programs [5–7]. While retention in care of HIV-infected patients has been shown to reflect individual treatment success [8,9], suboptimal retention is directly associated with negative outcomes including longer time to viral suppression [10], treatment failure and increased mortality [7,8,11,12]. Factors associated with attrition (defined as the occurrence of death or loss to follow up) have been described previously [13–27]; the most common determinants include a late presentation to ART clinics, and a poor nutritional status at baseline.

Previous studies in Myanmar

Determinants of treatment outcomes have been documented within the private sector in an ART cohort administered by Médecins Sans Frontières (MSF)-Holland in Myanmar; in this study the reported retention in care at 60 months reached 72% [95% CI: 70–74] [25]. However, neither the retention rates nor the determinants for attrition have been documented in the public sector. Therefore, the primary objectives in this study are to estimate the retention rates in a large ART program within the public sector in Myanmar, and to determine risk factors for attrition within this setting.

Methods

Ethics statement

Oral inform consent was obtained from all patients enrolled in the cohort; written informed consent was not collected as it was inadvisable to collect written documentation during the time of the military regime in Myanmar. The oral consent was obtained by marking a tick-box on the patient case form at enrollment after full discussion with a trained peer counselor, and kept in the patient's file. The protocol was approved by the Ethical Advisory Group (EAG) committee of the International Union Against Tuberculosis and Lung Disease (hereafter "The Union") (EAG number 4/14). All data were treated confidentially and stored as anonymized data. Biological assays were performed as part of routine follow up and all tests results were anonymized.

Setting

The Union has been implementing an Integrated HIV Care (IHC) program within the public sector in collaboration with the Department of Health, the National TB Program (NTP) and the National AIDS Program (NAP) since 2005. Initially, it was implemented at a single ART clinic in Mandalay. From that starting point, there was a steady expansion of the program so that by mid-2013, more than 15,000 patients were receiving ART in a total of 14 ART centers and 12 ART decentralized sites in 6 regions. The entry points for enrollment in this IHC program include TB clinics, pre-ART clinics run by the NAP, antenatal clinics, and hospitals located in the project area. The IHC program also accepts patients referred from other ART programs. There are no geographical limitations for enrollment in the IHC program (i.e. patients from the entire country have access to the program).

After enrolment, patients went through a standardized process including registration (allocation of a unique IHC code), baseline clinical assessment and laboratory testing, confirmation of eligibility by a selection committee and ART adherence counseling before ART initiation. Once patients are "stabilized", generally 6 to 12 months after ART initiation at district or tertiary hospitals, they are transferred out to the nearest decentralization sites for chronic HIV care. Staff of the Ministry of Health provides clinical care for ART initiation and follow- up. The Union provides support including additional human resources (medical doctors, laboratory technicians ...) comprehensive laboratory investigations (CD4, viral load testing since 2012, and other biochemical tests), drug procurement and supply management, data entry, and program monitoring. Self-management support from the People Living with HIV and AIDS (PLHA) network are deployed in all ART sites and were actively involved in the triage and registration, adherence counseling, and defaulter tracing. They also play an important role in providing financial assistance and social support for patients in distress.

The IHC program follows the national guideline for ART initiation, and uses AZT/3TC or D4T/3TC plus an NNRTI as first-line regimen, and protease inhibitor based regimens for second line treatment. In 2013, the national guidelines were updated to WHO recommendations and adopted TDF/3TC (FTC) as the preferred reverse transcriptase inhibitors. TB/HIV collaborative programs have been well established, and there is a cross-referral system between TB clinics and ART clinics for patients diagnosed at either of these sites. The enrolled patients also get support for necessary drugs for treatment of opportunistic infections (OI) and for required investigations if they are admitted to the hospital.

Study design and population

We retrospectively analyzed a total of 10,413 patients who were enrolled in our program between June 2005 and October 2011 and were followed up until April 2012 when censoring for this analysis occurred. After removing patients with data inconsistencies a total of 10,223 patients were considered for the 5-year cumulative survival analysis. For the logistic regression and survival analyses, patients with missing covariate data (primarily CD4 at initiation) were removed, leaving a final total of 5,718 patients for estimation of risk factors for attrition (Figure 1). The demographics of the full population and those with missing data are compared in table S1 in File S1. The profile of both groups is broadly similar; those with missing information were however less likely to receive a TB treatment at the time of ART initiation, but they were also more frequently reported with a previous ART history. This difference is largely due to the fact that the program absorbed an existing cohort of non-TB HIV-infected patients on ART, and that CD4 testing was only introduced in June 2006, while the program started one year earlier.

Definitions for primary outcomes

The primary outcome of this study was attrition, which included death (all-cause) and loss to follow-up (LTF). Loss to follow-up was defined as patients who did not return to clinic within three months from their last scheduled appointment and who could not be traced by the PLHA network. A system was in place to extract the patient cohort code if they failed to come to the clinic and to allow the PLHA network to trace the patients back within two weeks. A small number of patients have been classified as LTF after referral to non-IHC ART clinics, as we are unable to

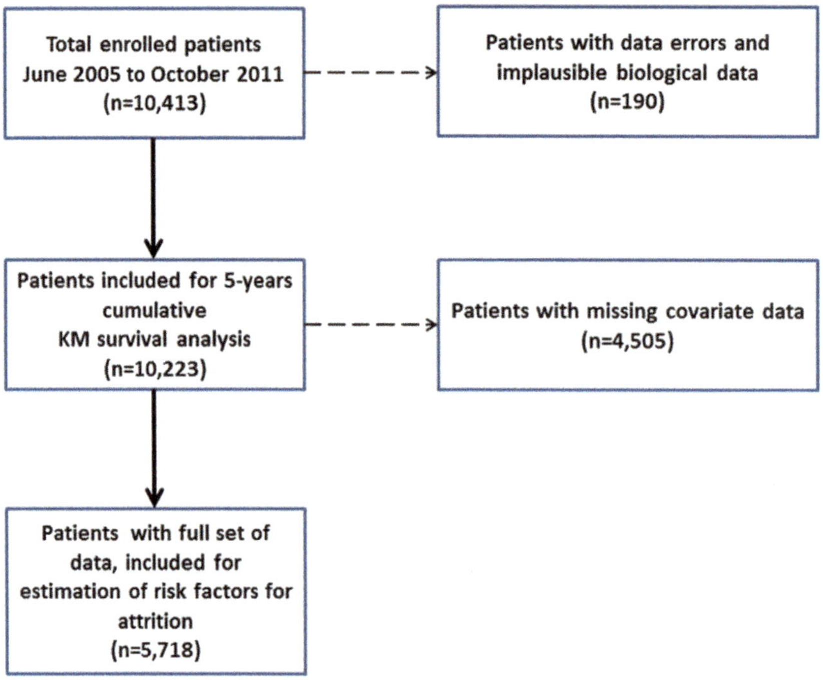

Figure 1. CONSORT diagram for analysis, with a total number of enrolled patients, number of patients for survival analysis and number of patients to estimate risk factors for attrition.

investigate the continuum of care for these patients. The primary survival outcome was defined as those patients who were both alive and still in active follow-up at the end of April 2012. Survival time was measured from date of enrollment to date of death, last recorded clinical visit, or study censoring date.

Data recording and storage

Routine patient medical data are recorded on paper forms by attending clinicians and Union staff. These forms are computerized in a password-protected database. All patient information was entered into the database using a unique coding system and the database is accessible only to data team members. We will make freely available any materials and data described in this publication that may be reasonably requested for the purpose of academic, non-commercial research.

Statistical analysis

In this analysis, the models for attrition utilized recommendations for low-income settings which include CD4 count at baseline, sex, age, ART regimen (NNRTI vs. PI-based) and clinical stage (WHO stage I/II vs. III/IV) as independent predictors [28,29]. Both multivariate logistic regression and survival models were utilized to assess risk factors for attrition.

We included in the multivariate models all variables associated with attrition from the univariate analysis (at $p<0.20$ level). Age was grouped as 18–30, 31–40, 41–50 and 51–60+ years; baseline CD4 cell count was dichotomized using the standard clinical cut-off of 100 cells per mm^3 for HIV to AIDS progression [14,15,18,20,25]. Both the Akaike and Bayesian Information Criteria (AIC/BIC) were used to assess model parsimony. Confounding was also assessed: case-control tabulation and bivariate regression analyses were used to examine potential interactions (defined as 15% change in coefficient of the referent variable), and residual plots were examined for all multivariate models.

For both analyses the predictors examined were: patient characteristics (age, literacy, sex and alcohol consumption), and baseline clinical and laboratory markers (BMI, WHO staging, type of ART regimen, TB diagnosis and Cotrimoxazole prophylactic treatment, CD4 cell count, anaemia, elevated liver transaminase (ALT), prior OIs, and TB, hepatitis B and C serological status).

Proportion surviving was calculated using Kaplan-Meir methods; preliminary survival models used Cox proportional hazard methods. Due to extensive proportional hazard violations in multiple variables (anaemia, low BMI, and CD4<100 at enrollment), Royston-Parmer flexible parametric survival models were used [30]. These alternatives to standard Cox models add in splines to directly model the underlying hazard functions, and allow more comprehensive modeling and predictions.

Data management, exploratory data analyses and logistic regressions models were fit using the software R 2.15; survival analyses were performed using Stata 12.1, (College Station, Texas); all tests were two-tailed with $\alpha = 0.95$.

Management of missing variables

A comprehensive sensitivity analysis of the missing variables was performed and complete case analysis was performed for estimation of risk factors for attrition. The characteristics of the omitted and complete cases were similar with the exception of two variables- those with missing data were more likely to have a history of ART and less likely to have tuberculosis at baseline. As such, we are unable to assume the data are missing completely at random, which may introduce some bias in the estimates.

Our sensitivity analyses had two components. The first used simulated data, whereby data were randomly generated for missing values to assess the potential impact of 'worst-case' scenarios. The simulated data for each missing variable was assigned to one category and then used to compute adjusted odds ratios; this process was then repeated, and re-run with the opposite (for example, if the first set simulated a 'male' for all missing values, then the second set this was reversed, with all missing data coded as a 'female'). The resulting sets of adjusted odds ratios were then compared.

To complement this analysis, the univariate odds ratios for the primary outcome were also compared between full case data and those with missing data (table S2 in File S1).

Results

Baseline Characteristics

The mean (±SD) for age was 36 (±8) years, and 61% of patients were male among a total of 10,413 patients. The demographic characteristics of study population at baseline such as age, sex, literacy, use of alcohol and HIV risk factors are shown in table 1. Clinical baseline characteristics (prior history of ART, WHO clinical Stage at ART initiation, CD4 at baseline, haemoglobin at baseline, HBV and HCV Status at baseline, BMI (baseline), type of ART regimen at baseline, Cotrimoxazole preventive therapy at baseline, tuberculosis treatment at ART initiation) are summarized in tables 2 and 3. Twenty four percent of patients had a prior ART history, 74% were classified as WHO stage III or IV and 46% had CD4 less than 100 cells/µl at ART initiation.

Retention Rate

The cumulative outcomes were death 909 (9%), loss to follow up 750 (7%) and in active follow up 8,564 (84%) for the cohort used for survival analysis (n = 10,223) with the median follow up duration of 13.7 months (interquartile range [IQR] 5.5–28.7). The corresponding retention rates and 95% CI of participants were 12 months (86; 85–87); 24 months (82; 81–83); 36 months (80; 79–81); 48 months (77; 76–78); 60 months (74; 73–76) (figure 2).

Incidence density for attrition

Among 10,223 patients, 1,542 attrition [death or LTF] events occurred over 17,524 person-years at risk, with an annual incidence density of 8.8% (95% CI: 8.4–9.3) in our study. In comparison, 1,061 attrition [death or LTF] events occurred among 5,963 patients over 14,854 person years at risk with an incident density of 7.0% (95% CI: 6.7 to 7.6) per year in the private setting [25] (Table 4). However, we found that the cumulative attrition (death+ default) rate in the very first decentralized sites of IHC program was quite low (3%).

Risk Factors for Attrition

Two complementary analyses were performed to investigate risk factors for attrition. The risk factors identified in logistic regression analysis are shown in Table 5 as odds ratios for primary outcome (death or loss-to-follow-up), and those identified in survival models are shown in Table 6 as hazard ratios from multivariate analysis.

Determinants for Attrition by Logistic Regression

After adjustment in a multivariate model, the significant factors identified were male sex [OR 1.4, 95% CI: 1.21–1.65]; illiteracy [OR 1.47, 95% CI: 1.21–1.79]; prior history of ART [OR 0.73, 95% CI: 0.58–0.90]; WHO stage III or IV at baseline [OR 2.36, 95% CI: 1.90–2.94]; BMI<18.5 kg/m^2 [OR 1.97, 95% CI: 1.71–2.26]; CD4 less than 100 cells/µl at baseline [OR 1.47, 95% CI: 1.29–1.69]; anaemia at baseline [OR 1.67, 95% CI: 1.36–2.05] and protease inhibitor based regimen [OR 4.35, 95% CI: 1.22–15.49].

Determinants for Attrition by Parametric Survival Model

In the adjusted multivariate flexible parametric model, the independent risk factors for attrition were: BMI<18.5 [HR 2.06, 95% CI: 1.76 to 2.40]; WHO stage III or IV at baseline [HR 2.01, 95% CI: 1.58 to 2.57]; anaemia at baseline [HR 1.80, 95% CI: 1.41 to 2.30], and baseline CD4 count <100 cells/µl [HR 1.74, 95% CI: 1.50 to 2.01].

Two factors showed marginally significant increased hazard: Cotrimoxazole treatment at baseline [HR 1.58, 95% CI: 1.10 to 2.25], and male gender [HR 1.37, 95% CI: 1.17 to 1.61].

Several factors showed a protective effect: previous ART at baseline [HR 0.61, 95% CI: 0.42 to 0.86], literacy [HR 0.81, 95% CI: 0.67 to 0.98] and TB treatment at baseline [HR 0.82, 95% CI: 0.71 to 0.94] (figure 3).

Analysis of missing data

The comparison of baseline demographics between full-data cases and those with missing data are presented in table S1 in File S1. All population characteristics are broadly similar with the exceptions of a more frequent ART history and a lower proportion of TB treatment at ART initiation in the group with missing data.

The comparison of the univariate odds ratios between cases with full data and those with missing values (table S2 in File S1), shows small differences in the point estimates between the two groups, but no changes in the substantive conclusions based upon the 95% CIs, with the exception of "PI-based regimen" which becomes not significant in the missing data group (2.39, 95% CI: 0.8 to 7.15) and "not literate" where it becomes not significant in the missing data group (1.15, 95% CI: 0.84 to 1.58).

Finally, the comparison of the multivariate odds ratios with the simulated data found only minor differences in point estimates and confidence intervals of the odds ratios, with the exception of the history of ART, where the odds ratio crosses one in the cases with simulated data (table S3 in File S1).

Discussion

Several studies conducted in low and middle income countries have provided estimates for retention in HIV cohorts; however, most of these studies analyzed a limited number of patients and described only short- to medium-term retention.

Retention in other Asian cohorts

Studies from Cambodia documented the outcomes of ART for short and medium term; the incidence of mortality was 9.1 per 100 person-years which is similar to international standards [31], the two year retention estimate was 85.5% both in a cohort of 416 patients treated in a Médecins Sans Frontières/Ministry of Health program [32], and in a larger cohort of the Sihanouk Hospital Center of HOPE, Phnom Penh [13]. The national program of Vietnam reported retention rates after 6, 12, 24, and 36 months as 88.4% [95% CI: 86.8–89.9], 84.0% [95% CI: 81.8–86.0], 78.8% [95% CI: 75.7–81.6], and 74.6% [95% CI: 69.6–79.0] [27]. In Thailand the survival rates among HIV-TB co-infected patients were 96.1%, 94% and 87.7% at 12, 24 and 36 months, respectively [33]. The retention at 12 month and 24 month of the Chinese National Free Antiretroviral Treatment Program was 92% and 84% [34] and the 12-month retention among eight Asia Pacific countries ranged from 65% to 88% [35].

The National AIDS Program in Myanmar reported a national retention rate of 87% at 12 months after ART initiation for those who received ART in 2010 [1]. The IHC program retention rate at 5 years was 74% [95% CI: 73–76], which is similar to the one reported by MSF Holland in its private sector cohort (72% [95%

Table 1. Demographic baseline characteristics of study population.

		Alive and still in follow-up (N = 8,615)		Negative outcomes: death, lost to follow up (N = 1,798)		Total (N = 10,413)	
		n	**%**	**n**	**%**	**n**	**%**
Age	Mean (SD)	35.95 (7.98)		36.05 (8.52)		35.97 (8.08)	
	Missing					*26*	
Sex	Male	5090	59.1	1243	69.2	6333	60.9
	Missing					*10*	
Alcoholism	Habitual	674	8.7	177	11.0	851	9.1
	Social	1341	17.3	314	19.5	1655	17.7
	Never	5729	74.0	1120	69.5	6849	73.2
	Missing					*1058*	
Literacy	Not literate	798	9.5	210	11.9	1008	9.9
	Literate	7603	90.5	1553	88.1	9156	90.1
	Missing					*249*	
HIV risk factors	Heterosexual	7232	85.8	1510	85.6	8742	85.8
	MSM	141	1.7	32	1.8	173	1.7
	Sex Worker	16	0.2	3	0.2	19	0.2
	IDU	291	3.5	72	4.1	363	3.6
	Blood transfusion	305	3.6	51	2.9	356	3.5
	Mother to child	3	0.0	0	0.0	3	0.0
	Unknown	436	5.2	95	5.4	531	5.2
	Missing					*226*	

SD: Standard deviation; MSM: Men who have sex with men; IDU: Injecting drug user.

Table 2. Clinical baseline characteristics of study population.

		Alive and still in follow-up (N = 8,615)		Negative outcomes: death, lost to follow up (N = 1,798)		Total (N = 10,413)	
		n	**%**	**n**	**%**	**N**	**%**
Prior history of ART	No	6450	74.9	1463	81.4	7913	76.0
	Yes	2165	25.1	335	18.6	2500	24.0
	Missing					*0*	
WHO Clinical Stage at ART Initiation	Stage I/II	2452	28.6	223	12.5	2675	25.8
	Stage III/IV	6127	71.4	1568	87.5	7695	74.2
	Missing					*43*	
CD4 (cells/mm^3) at baseline	Median [IQR]	117 (59–197)		74 (39–132)		109 (55–188)	
	0–100	3426	42.9	1012	62.6	4438	46.3
	>100	4551	57.1	604	37.4	5155	53.7
	Missing					*820*	
Haemoglobin at baseline	Normal	1778	22.8	162	9.9	1940	20.5
	Anaemia	6024	77.2	1477	90.1	7501	79.5
	Mean (SD)	11.0 (2.1)		10.0 (2.2)		10.8 (2.2)	
	Not performed					*972*	
HBV status at baseline	Negative	6552	90.9	1203	89.2	7755	90.7
	Positive	652	9.1	146	10.8	798	9.3
	Not Performed					*1860*	

IQR: Interquartile range.
WHO definition of Anaemia: Haemoglobin concentration <12 g/dL in women and <13 g/dL in men.

Table 3. Clinical baseline characteristics of study population, continued.

		Alive and still in follow-up (N = 8,615)		Negative outcomes: death, lost to follow up (N = 1,798)		Total (N = 10,413)	
		N	**%**	**N**	**%**	**n**	**%**
BMI (baseline)	Underweight (<18.5)	3426	44.7	1029	68.3	4455	48.6
	Normal	4241	55.3	478	31.7	4719	51.4
	Mean (SD)	19.3 (3.5)		17.4 (3.5)		19.0 (3.6)	
	Missing					*1239*	
HCV status at baseline	Negative	6814	94.9	1270	94.6	8084	94.8
	Positive	367	5.1	72	5.4	439	5.2
	Not performed					*1890*	
Type of ART regimen at baseline	NNRTI	8252	99.8	1686	99.4	9938	99.7
	PI	15	0.2	10	0.6	25	0.3
	Missing					*450*	
Cotrimoxazole preventive therapy at baseline	No	749	8.7	117	6.5	866	8.3
	Yes	7866	91.3	1681	93.5	9547	91.7
Tuberculosis treatment at ART initiation	No	5682	66.0	980	54.5	6662	64.0
	Yes	2933	34.0	818	45.5	3751	36.0
	Missing					*0*	

BMI: Body mass index; SD: Standard deviation; NNRTI: Non-nucleoside reverse transcriptase inhibitor; PI: Protease inhibitor.

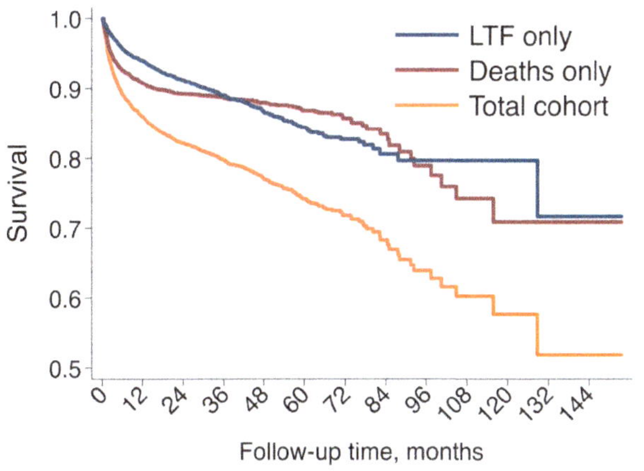

Figure 2. Unadjusted Kaplan-Meier survival curves, full cohort (N = 10,223).

CI: 70–74]) [25]. However, there was a significant difference in the incidence density for attrition between the cohorts: 7.1% [95% CI: 6.7–7.6] per year in MSF versus 8.8% [95% CI: 8.4–9.3] per year in IHC program.

Possible explanations for these differences include the patient to provider ratio, and the corresponding time within the clinic, which can be better in a private setting with greater resources relative to the public sector. While it is extremely challenging to have reliable conclusions on trends in retention rates and to produce consistent nationwide data from many resource-limited countries [2], comparing and combining the results of the two largest cohorts in Myanmar may permit the national AIDS program to track outcomes of ART programs as national figures.

Variations in program definitions

Currently, there is no consensus on how to best assess program retention [9]; although a study that analyzed 111 facilities worldwide suggested defining failure as more than 180 days from the last scheduled appointment [36]. Other methods that have been used include counting missed visits [37], appointment adherence [8] and gaps in care; and the number of gaps within 6, 9, or 12-month periods [9]. Various cohorts have reported various retention rates including 35% in Cameroon [24], 74.6% in Vietnam [27] and 82% in the MSF program in Myanmar [25] at 36 month follow up.

Consideration of missing data

There is considerable debate as to the optimal strategy to handle missing data in cohort studies, and no method is optimal under all circumstances [38].

In this analysis we have focused on cases with full available data (complete case data), to maximize the comparability to studies in similar settings that have appeared in the literature. While this has the potential for introducing biases if the nature of missing data has an influence on the primary outcome, the multiple sets of complementary sensitivity analyses we have performed suggest these effects are likely small. Moreover, the demographics (age, sex, etc.) of the patients with missing data are remarkably similar to the included patients, with two exceptions. A higher proportion of patients with missing data have history of prior ART, while a lower proportion have TB treatment at ART initiation. The broad agreement of our results with prior studies suggests that any biases in our data analysis are likely minor.

Attrition

Many factors have been linked to attrition in various settings, including the type of ART regimen at initiation [39], time to start of ART [16,33], nutritional deficiency and anaemia [13,18,20,22,25], higher education [40] and strategic placing of ART service delivery points [24]. By focusing on modifiable factors in this cohort analysis, we aimed to provide an evidence base to inform policy makers on how to improve outcomes in ART programs implemented in Myanmar and SE Asia.

Comparison with a private sector cohort in Myanmar [25]

Our findings are similar to the results of the MSF cohort analysis. In The MSF cohort, high WHO staging, low BMI, male sex and age were found to be independent risk factors for attrition. Our study did not find a strong impact of age, but also identified that a low CD4 count and anaemia were risk factors for attrition; conversely, TB treatment at ART initiation, ART history and literacy were found to be predictors for the retention in care. The observed differences are likely to be due to differences in program structure, and potentially to some differences between the study populations.

CD4

One of the main risk factors for attrition is low CD4 count at enrollment; this is a common feature which has been found in many other cohort studies [13–23]. Our study found an adjusted hazard ratio for attrition of 1.74 (95% CI: 1.50–2.01), much higher in patients with low CD4 at ART initiation. These finding reinforce the crucial importance of early HIV diagnosis and timely initiation of ART in the broader perspective of increasing survival rates [17,21].

However, pooled data from 13 research cohorts from five sub-Saharan African (Benin, Burkina Faso, Cameroon, Cote d'Ivoire and Senegal) and two Asian (Cambodia and Laos) countries reported a lower survival not only in those patients with low CD4 but also for patients with a high CD4 count [19], which is likely due to the presence of co-morbidities.

Table 4. Attrition Rate at 36-month follow up of the cohort in the public sector comparing with MSF (H) cohort.

Service Delivery Point	Participants (N)	Attrition Cases (N) [death+LTF] during 36 months of follow-up	Person years at risk (to 36 months)	Attrition Rate (%) Per Year	95% Confidence Interval
Private [MSF]	5,963	1,061	14,854	7%	(6.7–7.6) %
Public [The Union +DOH]	10,223	1,542	17,524	8.8%	(8.4–9.3) %

N: Number; LTF: Loss to follow up; MSF (H): Médecins Sans Frontières (Holland); DOH: Department of Health.

Table 5. Prevalence percentages and odds ratios for primary outcome (death or loss-to-follow-up) from the logistic regression analysis.

	Alive and still in follow-up (N = 8615)	Negative outcomes: death, lost to follow up (N = 1798)	Bivariate Analysis	Multivariate Analysis	
			OR (95% C.I.)	OR (95% C.I).	p-value
Age: Mean (SD)	35.9 (8.0)	36.0 (8.5)	-	-	0.980
Sex: male	59.1	69.2	1.55 (1.39–1.73)	1.42 (1.21–1.65)	<0.001
Alcoholism: yes	26.0	30.5	1.25 (1.11–1.40)	0.98 (0.84–1.15)	0.804
Literate	90.5	88.1	0.78 (0.66–0.91)	0.68 (0.56–0.83)	<0.001
Prior history of ART	25.1	18.6	0.68 (0.60–0.78)	0.73 (0.58–0.90)	0.004
WHO Stage III/IV at baseline	71.4	87.5	2.81 (2.43–3.26)	2.36 (1.90–2.94)	<0.001
Underweight (BMI <18.5)	44.7	68.3	2.66 (2.37–3.00)	1.97 (1.71–2.26)	<0.001
CD4 at baseline <100	42.9	62.6	2.23 (1.99–2.48)	1.47 (1.29–1.69)	<0.001
Anaemia at baseline	77.2	90.1	2.69 (2.27–3.19)	1.67 (1.36–2.05)	<0.001
Tuberculosis treatment at baseline	34.0	45.5	1.62 (1.46–1.79)	0.90 (0.78–1.04)	0.140
PI base regimen	0.2	0.6	3.26 (1.46–7.28)	4.35 (1.22–15.49)	0.023
Cotrimoxazole preventive therapy at baseline	91.3	93.5	1.37 (1.12–1.67)	1.12 (0.84–1.50)	0.455

OR: Odds ratio; CI: Confidence interval; BMI: Body mass index; SD: Standard deviation; PI: Protease inhibitor; Anaemia: Haemoglobin concentration <12 g/dL in women and <13 g/dL in men.

BMI, WHO staging and anaemia

Several studies exploring HIV attrition found independent associations between attrition and low BMI [13,18,20,25], WHO staging III/IV [16,18,20,21,25], and anaemia [13,18,20,22]. We found similar associations in our cohort, and these factors are even stronger predictors of attrition than low CD4 count. Our findings support the prioritization of nutritional support and of appropriate management of anaemia as key interventions within the scope of

Table 6. Flexible parametric survival model of potential determinants for attrition among study population (N = 5,718).

		Cox Univariate Analysis	Flexible Parametric Survival Model	
		HR, 95% C.I.	HR, 95% C.I.	p-value
Age	18–30	reference	reference	-
	31–40	0.96 (0.85–1.07)	0.90 (0.77–1.06)	0.201
	41–50	1.03 (0.89–1.20)	0.93 (0.76–1.13	0.466
	51–60 +	1.31 (1.06–1.61)	1.21 (0.90–1.64)	0.194
Enrollment group	Early	reference	reference	-
	Later	1.27 (1.14–1.42)	1.09 (0.94–1.26)	0.250
Sex: male		1.43 (1.29–1.59)	1.37 (1.17–1.61)	<0.001
Alcoholism: yes		1.26 (1.13–1.40)	1.05 (0.90–1.22)	0.542
Literate		0.83 (0.72–0.97)	0.81 (0.67–0.98)	0.031
Prior history of ART		0.52 (0.46–0.58)	0.61 (0.42–0.86)	0.005
Cotrimoxazole at baseline		1.34 (1.07–1.70)	1.58 (1.10–2.25)	0.011
WHO Stage III/IV at baseline		2.35 (2.00–2.76)	2.01 (1.58–2.57)	<0.001
Underweight (BMI<18.5) at baseline		2.55 (2.27–2.85)	2.06 (1.76–2.40)	<0.001
CD4 at baseline <100		2.73 (2.30–3.24)	1.74 (1.50–2.01)	<0.001
Anaemia at baseline		2.27 (1.88–2.75)	1.80 (1.41–2.30)	<0.001
Tuberculosis treatment at baseline		0.65 (0.59–0.72)	0.82 (0.71–0.94)	0.005
PI regimen at baseline		2.03 (1.01–4.07)	(ns #)	0.989

CI: Confidence interval; BMI: Body mass index; PI: Protease inhibitor; WHO definition of Anaemia: Haemoglobin concentration <12 g/dL in women and <13 g/dL in men.
#- not significant in univariate models.
Note: Early enrolment (1 Sep 2005 to 31 Dec 2009), and Late enrolment (1 Jan 2010 to 20 Oct 2011).

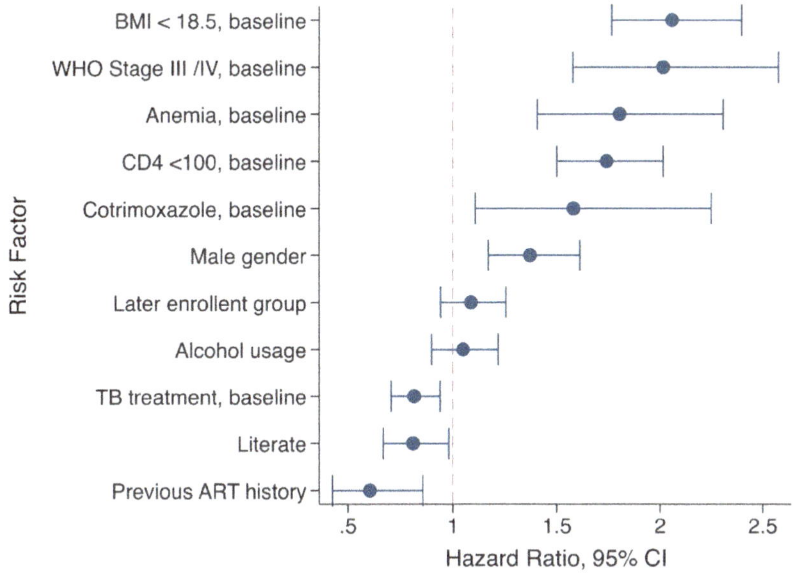

Figure 3. Adjusted hazard ratios from flexible parametric survival analysis (N = 5,718).

the comprehensive care activities proposed in ART clinics in Myanmar. These results also suggest that insufficient nutrition is potentially an important risk factor for attrition in the study population. Further research is needed to more fully explore this association within Myanmar.

Sex and Cotrimoxazole preventive therapy

Although the association is weak, male gender is an independent risk factor for attrition. This is in line with the results from other studies [13,15,23–25].

In contrast to a report from Thailand [26], we have found that cotrimoxazole prophylactic prescription is a risk factor for attrition by parametric survival models. This association is unsurprising as all patients with low CD4 or high WHO staging (both conditions known as strong predictors for attrition), are also treated with cotrimoxazole. This association, however, persisted in the multivariate analysis. This association could be an artifact; the lower range of the confidence interval [HR = 1.58 (95% CI: 1.10 to 2.25)], suggests only a marginal 10% increase in risk of event. This result was not found in logistic regression and may represent a spurious association.

Comparison of first and second line regimens

A review of 18 cohorts in Europe and North America concluded that patients on protease inhibitor had higher probability of treatment interruption or modification; this review also highlighted that those patients receiving tenofovir/emtricitabine based regimens had lower probability of treatment substitutions compared to non-standard regimens [41]. In our cohort, the odds for attrition are higher for those patients receiving protease inhibitor based regimens [OR 4.35, (95% CI: 1.22 to 15.49)] when compared with patients on an NNRTI based regimen. While the number of patients on PI included in the analysis is limited, it is vital to investigate further whether this increased risk is due to delays in referral from non-IHC sites, or instead to the regimen itself in this particular setting.

Like other resource-limited settings, IHC programs in Myanmar used d4T as the main NRTI (67%) followed by AZT (31.2%) and TDF (2.3%) for ART initiation. A recent study from South Africa evaluated the effectiveness of TDF and reported that the adjusted hazard ratio for loss-from-care, when compared to TDF, was 1.5 (95% CI: 1.1–1.9) for d4T and 1.2 (95% CI: 1.1–1.4) for AZT [39]. In our study, only a small number of patients were treated with TDF, and a similar association was not found. However, the retention rate is higher in the unadjusted KM analysis for those on AZT when compared with patient receiving d4T-based regimens ($p<0.0001$), (Figure 4). As the effectiveness of modern cART regimens becomes widely documented it is worthwhile to recommend using those regimens whenever possible in ART programs [34]. In Myanmar, national antiretroviral treatment guidelines have been modified in mid-2013 to take into account the latest WHO recommendations and include the adoption of TDF/3TC as the preferred option for ART initiation.

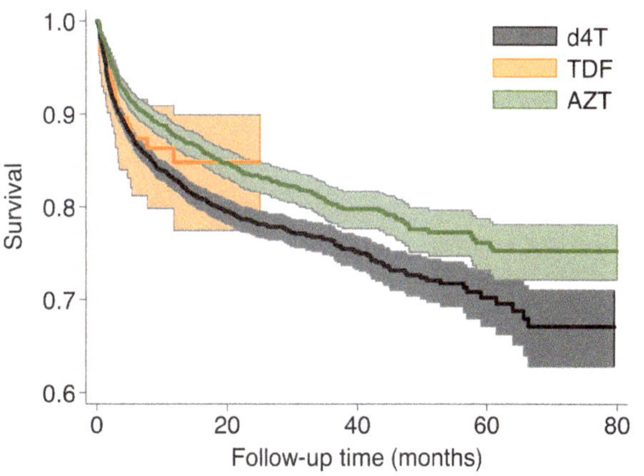

Figure 4. Unadjusted Kaplan-Meier curves, by first-line ART regimen.

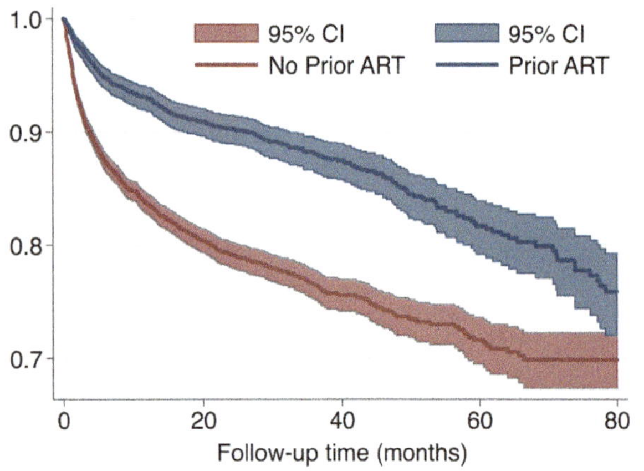

Figure 5. Unadjusted Kaplan-Meier survival curves of non-prior ART group and prior ART group, full cohort (N = 10,223). Log-rank test for equality of survival $\chi 2$ (1 df) = 122.10; p<0.001.

Attrition and TB co-infected patients, previous ART and Literacy

The protective factors for attrition include the administration of a TB treatment at ART initiation and a prior ART history (Figure 5); the better retention in care observed in these two groups can be explained by the more intensive counseling received by these patients in the TB clinics and by earlier ART care providers. In our cohort, 90% of study participants are literate and, not surprisingly, have a higher retention when compared to those with limited literacy. Increased educational attainment has been shown to have a strong positive impact on clinical outcomes [40] and more globally in cohort retention.

Free of charge medical care, adherence support and defaulter tracing

A cluster randomized control trial in Vietnam reported that there was no significant difference in mortality rate between groups who received enhanced adherence versus a control groups without intervention [18]. A study from an ART clinic in Cameroon where patients had to pay for ART, found no difference in retention rates between before and after ART cost reduction [58%, 47% and 35% at 12, 24 and 36 months respectively] [24]. These findings highlight the importance of defaulter tracing in programs apart from the cost of ART. Implementation of support group activities in all project sites, peer involvement in defaulter tracing, and free access to all services are important aspects of the program in Myanmar that may explain these successes.

The modifiable risk factors for attrition we found could motivate attending clinicians to provide more comprehensive care to achieve both increased individual benefit and greater impact at the population level.

ART site and decentralized sites

We found that the attrition remains quite low (3%) in the initial decentralized sites. Patients might have less constraint to come to these sites and better efforts might have been allocated to "stabilize" these patients (including the treatment of co-morbidities) before the transfer.

Strength and limitations

One of the main strengths of this study is the sample size, which allowed us to investigate the retention in care and the risk factors for attrition in a large cohort of patients followed in the public sector in Myanmar. However, there are also some limitations. First, it should be acknowledged that a significant number of patients with missing data were excluded from the analysis, potentially introducing bias. Secondly, the study assessed a limited number of socio-demographic factors; we were not able to include in our analysis other important parameters such as the distance between the patients' residence and the service delivery point [24] and the absorption capacity of the ART clinics [15]. Our study also mainly included patients who had already started ART while it would have also been important to try analyzing attrition before ART initiation [42]. We were also not able to analyze the biological markers after ART initiation [43]. Finally we were not able to capture any secular changes in standards of care and systematic changes within the health sector in Myanmar.

Conclusion

Our study, conducted in a resource-limited setting, provides evidence about the quality and the effectiveness of a large ART program from the public sector in Myanmar. It also advocate for the feasibility of the long-term retention of a large cohort of patients on ART within an Integrated HIV Care program in Myanmar. Our result suggests that key improvements for future programs are early diagnosis of HIV and initiation of ART, comprehensive nutritional support to increase BMI to normal levels, and targeting those patients with low CD4 count and/or haemoglobin for intensive investigation and clinical management. Finally, a comprehensive study of patients in second-line therapy settings would be an important next step in addressing these programs gaps.

Supporting Information

File S1 Contains Tables S1–S3. **Table S1**. Baseline demographics between cases with full data and those with missing predictors (N = 10,413). **Table S2**. Comparison of unadjusted OR for primary outcome between full data and missing case patients. **Table S3**. Comparison of full-case date and data with simulated outcomes to assess the potential impact of missing data.

Acknowledgments

We would like to express our profound gratitude to all physicians from IHC Program who provided medical consultations for the patients and we would like to extend our appreciation to all the patients who agreed to participate in the IHC program.

Author Contributions

Conceived and designed the experiments: AT STTT SKKZ ZHW P. Clevenbergh AAL P. Cavailler JC. Performed the experiments: MMA PP KWN KNZ MS TTK SKKZ P. Clevenbergh. Analyzed the data: AAL P. Cavailler JC STTT AT P. Clevenbergh. Contributed reagents/materials/analysis tools: AT STTT SKKZ AAL P. Cavailler JC ZHW P. Clevenbergh. Wrote the paper: AT AAL P. Cavailler JC P. Clevenbergh.

References

1. National AIDS Program (2012) Global AIDS Response Progress Report Myanmar, 2012. Available: http://www.unaids.org/en/dataanalysis/knowyourresponse/countryprogressreports/2012countries/ce_MM_Narrative_Report.pdf. Accessed 28 April 2013.

2. UNAIDS (2012) UNAIDS report on the global AIDS epidemic: 2012. Geneva: United Nations. Available: http://www.unaids.org/en/media/unaids/contentassets/documents/epidemiology/2012/gr2012/20121120_UNAIDS_Global_Report_2012_with_annexes_en.pdf. Accessed 28 April 2013.
3. United Nations (2013) The Millennium Development Goals Report, 2013. Available at http://mdgs.un.org/unsd/mdg/Resources/Static/Products/Progress2013/English2013.pdf. Accessed 14th August 2013.
4. Fokam J, Billong SC, Bissek AC, Kembou E, Milenge P, et al. (2013) Declining trends in early warning indicators for HIV drug resistance in Cameroon from 2008–2010: lessons and challenges for low-resource settings. BMC Public Health 13: 308. 1471-2458-13-308 [pii];10.1186/1471-2458-13-308
5. Piliero PJ (2003) Early factors in successful anti-HIV treatment. J Int Assoc Physicians AIDS Care (Chic) 2: 10–20.
6. World Health Organization indicators: HIV Drug resistance Early Warning Indicators. World Health Organization indicators to monitor HIV drug resistance prevention at antiretroviral treatment sites. Geneva: World Health Organization indicators; 2010. Available at: http://new.paho.org/hq/dmdocuments/2010/hivdr-early-warning-indicators-updated-april-2010.pdf, accessed on 13 August 2013.
7. Giordano TP, Gifford AL, White AC, Jr., Suarez-Almazor ME, Rabeneck L, et al. (2007) Retention in care: a challenge to survival with HIV infection. Clin Infect Dis 44: 1493–1499. CID41288 [pii];10.1086/516778
8. Mugavero MJ, Lin HY, Willig JH, Westfall AO, Ulett KB, et al. (2009) Missed visits and mortality among patients establishing initial outpatient HIV treatment. Clin Infect Dis 48: 248–256. doi:10.1086/595705
9. Mugavero MJ, Westfall AO, Zinski A, Davila J, Drainoni ML, et al. (2012) Measuring retention in HIV care: the elusive gold standard. J Acquir Immune Defic Syndr 61: 574–580. doi:10.1097/QAI.0b013e318273762f
10. Crawford TN, Sanderson WT, Thornton A (2013) Impact of Poor Retention in HIV Medical Care on Time to Viral Load Suppression. J Int Assoc Provid AIDS Care. 2325957413491431 [pii]; doi:10.1177/2325957413491431
11. Giordano TP (2011) Retention in HIV care: what the clinician needs to know. Top Antivir Med 19: 12–16.
12. Tam LW, Chui CK, Brumme CJ, Bangsberg DR, Montaner JS, et al. (2008) The relationship between resistance and adherence in drug-naive individuals initiating HAART is specific to individual drug classes. J Acquir Immune Defic Syndr 49: 266–271. doi:10.1097/QAI.0b013e318189a753
13. Thai S, Koole O, Un P, Ros S, De MP, et al. (2009) Five-year experience with scaling-up access to antiretroviral treatment in an HIV care programme in Cambodia. Trop Med Int Health 14: 1048–1058. TMI2334 [pii]; doi:10.1111/j.1365-3156.2009.02334.x
14. Castelnuovo B, Manabe YC, Kiragga A, Kamya M, Easterbrook P, et al. (2009) Cause-specific mortality and the contribution of immune reconstitution inflammatory syndrome in the first 3 years after antiretroviral therapy initiation in an urban African cohort. Clin Infect Dis 49: 965–972. doi:10.1086/605500
15. Vella V, Govender T, Dlamini S, Taylor M, Moodley I, et al. (2010) Retrospective study on the critical factors for retaining patients on antiretroviral therapy in KwaZulu-Natal, South Africa. J Acquir Immune Defic Syndr 55: 109–116. 10.1097/QAI.0b013e3181e7744e
16. Fox MP, Sanne IM, Conradie F, Zeinecker J, Orrell C, et al. (2010) Initiating patients on antiretroviral therapy at CD4 cell counts above 200 cells/microl is associated with improved treatment outcomes in South Africa. AIDS 24: 2041–2050. doi:10.1097/QAD.0b013e32833c703e
17. van GJ, Thai S (2011) Predictors of immune recovery and the association with late mortality while on antiretroviral treatment in Cambodia. Trans R Soc Trop Med Hyg 105: 694–703.S0035-9203(11)00168-4 [pii]; doi:10.1016/j.trstmh.2011.08.007
18. Cuong dD, Thorson A, Sonnerborg A, Hoa NP, Chuc NT, et al. (2012) Survival and causes of death among HIV-infected patients starting antiretroviral therapy in north-eastern Vietnam. Scand J Infect Dis 44: 201–208. doi:10.3109/00365548.2011.631937
19. Gabillard D, Lewden C, Ndoye I, Moh R, Segeral O, et al. (2012) Mortality, AIDS-morbidity and loss to follow-up by current CD4 cell count among HIV-1 infected adults receiving antiretroviral therapy in Africa and Asia: data from the ANRS 12222 collaboration. J Acquir Immune Defic Syndr. doi:10.1097/QAI.0b013e3182821821
20. Argemi X, Dara S, You S, Mattei JF, Courpotin C, et al. (2012) Impact of malnutrition and social determinants on survival of HIV-infected adults starting antiretroviral therapy in resource-limited settings. AIDS 26: 1161–1166. doi:10.1097/QAD.0b013e328353f363
21. Biadgilign S, Reda AA, Digaffe T (2012) Predictors of mortality among HIV infected patients taking antiretroviral treatment in Ethiopia: a retrospective cohort study. AIDS Res Ther 9: 15. 1742-6405-9-15 [pii]; doi:10.1186/1742-6405-9-15
22. Duong T, Jourdain G, Ngo-Giang-Huong N, Le CS, Kantipong P, et al. (2012) Laboratory and clinical predictors of disease progression following initiation of combination therapy in HIV-infected adults in Thailand. PLoS One 7: e43375. doi:10.1371/journal.pone.0043375 [doi];PONE-D-12-07448 [pii].
23. Somi G, Keogh SC, Todd J, Kilama B, Wringe A, et al. (2012) Low mortality risk but high loss to follow-up among patients in the Tanzanian national HIV care and treatment programme. Trop Med Int Health. doi:10.1111/j.1365-3156.2011.02952.x
24. Mosoko JJ, Akam W, Weidle PJ, Brooks JT, Aweh AJ, et al. (2011) Retention in an antiretroviral therapy programme during an era of decreasing drug cost in Limbe, Cameroon. J Int AIDS Soc 14: 32. 1758-2652-14-32 [pii]; doi:10.1186/1758-2652-14-32
25. Sabapathy K, Ford N, Chan KN, Kyaw MK, Elema R, et al. (2012) Treatment outcomes from the largest antiretroviral treatment programme in Myanmar (Burma): a cohort analysis of retention after scale-up. J Acquir Immune Defic Syndr. doi:10.1097/QAI.0b013e31824d5689
26. Varma JK, Nateniyom S, Akksilp S, Mankatittham W, Sirinak C, et al. (2009) HIV care and treatment factors associated with improved survival during TB treatment in Thailand: an observational study. BMC Infect Dis 9: 42. 1471-2334-9-42 [pii]; doi:10.1186/1471-2334-9-42
27. Nguyen DB, Do NT, Shiraishi RW, Le YN, Tran QH, et al. (2013) Outcomes of antiretroviral therapy in Vietnam: results from a national evaluation. PLoS One 8: e55750. doi:10.1371/journal.pone.0055750 [doi];PONE-D-12-22705 [pii].
28. Braitstein P, Brinkhof MW, Dabis F, Schechter M, Boulle A, et al. (2006) Mortality of HIV-1-infected patients in the first year of antiretroviral therapy: comparison between low-income and high-income countries. Lancet 367: 817–824. S0140-6736(06)68337-2 [pii]; doi:10.1016/S0140-6736(06)68337-2
29. Keiser O, Anastos K, Schechter M, Balestre E, Myer L, et al. (2008) Antiretroviral therapy in resource-limited settings 1996 to 2006: patient characteristics, treatment regimens and monitoring in sub-Saharan Africa, Asia and Latin America. Trop Med Int Health 13: 870–879. TMI2078 [pii]; doi:10.1111/j.1365-3156.2008.02078.x
30. Royston P, Parmar MK (2002) Flexible parametric proportional-hazards and proportional-odds models for censored survival data, with application to prognostic modelling and estimation of treatment effects. Stat Med 21: 2175–2197. doi:10.1002/sim.1203
31. Morineau G, Vun MC, Barennes H, Wolf RC, Song N, et al. (2009) Survival and quality of life among HIV-positive people on antiretroviral therapy in Cambodia. AIDS Patient Care STDS 23: 669–677. doi:10.1089/apc.2008.0241
32. Ferradini L, Laureillard D, Prak N, Ngeth C, Fernandez M, et al. (2007) Positive outcomes of HAART at 24 months in HIV-infected patients in Cambodia. AIDS 21: 2293–2301. doi:10.1097/QAD.0b013e32828cc8b7 [doi];00002030-200711120-00005 [pii].
33. Manosuthi W, Chottanapand S, Thongyen S, Chaovavanich A, Sungkanuparph S (2006) Survival rate and risk factors of mortality among HIV/tuberculosis-coinfected patients with and without antiretroviral therapy. J Acquir Immune Defic Syndr 43: 42–46. doi:10.1097/01.qai.0000230521.86964.86
34. Zhu H, Napravnik S, Eron J, Cole S, Ma Y, et al. (2012) Attrition among human immunodeficiency virus (HIV)- infected patients initiating antiretroviral therapy in China, 2003–2010. PLoS One 7: e39414. doi:10.1371/journal.pone.0039414 [doi];PONE-D-11-25955 [pii].
35. Srikantiah P, Ghidinelli M, Bachani D, Chasombat S, Daoni E, et al. (2010) Scale-up of national antiretroviral therapy programs: progress and challenges in the Asia Pacific region. AIDS 24 Suppl 3: S62–S71. doi:10.1097/01.aids.0000390091.45435.ea [doi];00002030-201009003-00009 [pii].
36. Chi BH, Yiannoutsos CT, Westfall AO, Newman JE, Zhou J, et al. (2011) Universal definition of loss to follow-up in HIV treatment programs: a statistical analysis of 111 facilities in Africa, Asia, and Latin America. PLoS Med 8: e1001111. doi:10.1371/journal.pmed.1001111 [doi];PMEDICINE-D-11-00857 [pii].
37. Kunutsor S, Walley J, Katabira E, Muchuro S, Balidawa H, et al. (2010) Clinic Attendance for Medication Refills and Medication Adherence amongst an Antiretroviral Treatment Cohort in Uganda: A Prospective Study. AIDS Res Treat 2010: 872396. doi:10.1155/2010/872396
38. Sterne JAC, White IR, Carlin JB, Spratt M, Royston P, et al. (2009) Multiple imputation for missing data in epidemiological and clinical research: potential and pitfalls. BMJ 338: b2393–b2393. doi:10.1136/bmj.b2393.]
39. Velen K, Lewis JJ, Charalambous S, Grant AD, Churchyard GJ, et al. (2013) Comparison of tenofovir, zidovudine, or stavudine as part of first-line antiretroviral therapy in a resource-limited-setting: a cohort study. PLoS One 8: e64459. doi:10.1371/journal.pone.0064459 [doi];PONE-D-12-33991 [pii].
40. Zaragoza-Macias E, Cosco D, Nguyen ML, Del RC, Lennox J (2010) Predictors of success with highly active antiretroviral therapy in an antiretroviral-naive urban population. AIDS Res Hum Retroviruses 26: 133–138. doi:10.1089/aid.2009.0001
41. Antiretroviral Therapy Cohort Collaboration (ART-CC) (2013).Durability of first ART regimen and risk factors for modification, interruption or death in HIV-positive patients starting ART in Europe and North America 2002–2009. AIDS 27: 803–813. doi:10.1097/QAD.0b013e32835cb997 [doi];00002030-201303130-00014 [pii].
42. Clouse K, Pettifor AE, Maskew M, Bassett J, Van RA, et al. (2013) Patient retention from HIV diagnosis through one year on antiretroviral therapy at a primary health care clinic in Johannesburg, South Africa. J Acquir Immune Defic Syndr 62: e39–e46. doi:10.1097/QAI.0b013e318273ac48
43. Neogi U, Heylen E, Shet A, Chandy S, Shamsunder R, et al. (2013) Long-term efficacy of first line antiretroviral therapy in Indian HIV-1 infected patients: a longitudinal cohort study. PLoS One 8: e55421. doi:10.1371/journal.pone.0055421

Permissions

All chapters in this book were first published in PLOS ONE, by The Public Library of Science; hereby published with permission under the Creative Commons Attribution License or equivalent. Every chapter published in this book has been scrutinized by our experts. Their significance has been extensively debated. The topics covered herein carry significant findings which will fuel the growth of the discipline. They may even be implemented as practical applications or may be referred to as a beginning point for another development.

The contributors of this book come from diverse backgrounds, making this book a truly international effort. This book will bring forth new frontiers with its revolutionizing research information and detailed analysis of the nascent developments around the world.

We would like to thank all the contributing authors for lending their expertise to make the book truly unique. They have played a crucial role in the development of this book. Without their invaluable contributions this book wouldn't have been possible. They have made vital efforts to compile up to date information on the varied aspects of this subject to make this book a valuable addition to the collection of many professionals and students.

This book was conceptualized with the vision of imparting up-to-date information and advanced data in this field. To ensure thc same, a matchless editorial board was set up. Every individual on the board went through rigorous rounds of assessment to prove their worth. After which they invested a large part of their time researching and compiling the most relevant data for our readers.

The editorial board has been involved in producing this book since its inception. They have spent rigorous hours researching and exploring the diverse topics which have resulted in the successful publishing of this book. They have passed on their knowledge of decades through this book. To expedite this challenging task, the publisher supported the team at every step. A small team of assistant editors was also appointed to further simplify the editing procedure and attain best results for the readers.

Apart from the editorial board, the designing team has also invested a significant amount of their time in understanding the subject and creating the most relevant covers. They scrutinized every image to scout for the most suitable representation of the subject and create an appropriate cover for the book.

The publishing team has been an ardent support to the editorial, designing and production team. Their endless efforts to recruit the best for this project, has resulted in the accomplishment of this book. They are a veteran in the field of academics and their pool of knowledge is as vast as their experience in printing. Their expertise and guidance has proved useful at every step. Their uncompromising quality standards have made this book an exceptional effort. Their encouragement from time to time has been an inspiration for everyone.

The publisher and the editorial board hope that this book will prove to be a valuable piece of knowledge for researchers, students, practitioners and scholars across the globe.

List of Contributors

Houlin Tang, Yurong Mao, Juan Xu, Jing Han and Zunyou Wu
Division of Integration and Evaluation, National Center for AIDS/STD Control and Prevention, Chinese Center for Disease Control and Prevention, Beijing, China

Cynthia X. Shi
Division of Integration and Evaluation, National Center for AIDS/STD Control and Prevention, Chinese Center for Disease Control and Prevention, Beijing, China
Department of Epidemiology, School of Public Health, Harvard University, Boston, Massachusetts, United States of America

Liyan Wang and Qianqian Qin
Division of Epidemiology, National Center for AIDS/STD Control and Prevention, Chinese Center for Disease Control and Prevention, Beijing, China

Roger Detels
Department of Epidemiology, School of Public Health, University of California at Los Angeles, California, United States of America

Sonia Morales-Miranda, Jerry O. Jacobson, Itzel Loya-Montiel, Ricardo Mendizabal-Burastero and César Galindo-Arandi
Center for Health Studies, Universidad del Valle de Guatemala, Guatemala City, Guatemala

Carlos Flores
National STI/HIV/AIDS Program, Ministry of Public Health, Guatemala City, Guatemala

Sanny Y. Chen
Division of Global HIV/AIDS, Centers for Disease Control and Prevention - Central America Regional Office, Guatemala City, Guatemala

Ujjwal Neogi
Division of Clinical Microbiology, Department of Laboratory Medicine, Karolinska Institutet, Stockholm, Sweden

Amanda Häggblom
Unit of Infectious Diseases, Department of Medicine Huddinge, Karolinska Institutet, Stockholm, Sweden
Department of Infectious Diseases, County Council of Gävleborg, Gävle, Sweden

Michele Santacatterina
Unit of Biostatistics, Institute of Environmental Medicine, Karolinska Institutet, Stockholm, Sweden

Göran Bratt
Department of Clinical Science and Education, Venha¨lsan, Stockholm South General Hospital, Stockholm, Sweden

Magnus Gisslén
Department of Infectious Diseases, University of Gothenburg, Gothenburg, Sweden

Jan Albert
Department of Microbiology, Tumor and Cell Biology, Karolinska Institutet, Stockholm, Sweden

Anders Sonnerborg
Division of Clinical Microbiology, Department of Laboratory Medicine, Karolinska Institutet, Stockholm, Sweden
Unit of Infectious Diseases, Department of Medicine Huddinge, Karolinska Institutet, Stockholm, Sweden

Philippe H. Lagrange
Service de Microbiologie, Hôpital Saint Louis, Paris, France

Satheesh K. Thangaraj and Marc Leportier
BioMérieux, Marcy-l'Etoile, France and New Delhi, India

Rajeshwar Dayal and Amit Singh
SN Medical College, Agra, India

Alaka Deshpande
Sir J.J. Group of Govt Hosp. & Grant Medical College, Mumbai, India

Nirmal K. Ganguly and Deepali Mukerjee
Indian Council of Medical Research, New Delhi, India

Enrico Girardi and Delia Goletti
Department of Epidemiology and Preclinical Research, L. Spallanzani National Institute for Infectious Diseases, Rome, Italy

Beenu Joshi, Kiran Katoch and Vishwa M. Katoch
National JALMA Institute of Leprosy & Other Mycrobacterial Diseases, Agra, India

Manoj Kumar and Sarman Singh
All India Institute of Medical Sciences, New Delhi, India

Vemu Lakshmi and Subbalaxmi V. S. Malladi
Nizam's Institute of Medical Sciences, Hyderabad, India

Christophe Longuet and Guy Vernet
Fondation Mérieux, Lyon, France

Deepthi Nair and Pratibha Sharma
Safdarjung Hospital, New Delhi, India
Alamelu Raja, Balambal Raman and Basirudeen Syed Ahamed Kabeer
National Institute for Research in Tuberculosis (formerly Tuberculosis Research Center), Chetput, Chennai, India

Camilla Rodrigues and Archana Sodha
Microbiology Section, P D Hinduja Hospital & Medical Research Centre, Veer Savarkar Marg Mahim, Mumbai, India

Wenhua Yu, Changping Li, Xiaomeng Fu, Zhuang Cui, Xiaoqian Liu, Linlin Fan, Guan Zhang and Jun Ma
Department of Health Statistics, College of Public Health, Tianjin Medical University, Tianjin, China

Ann Green and Mary-Ann Davies
School of Public Health and Family Medicine, University of Cape Town, Cape Town, South Africa

Virginia de Azevedo
Department of Health, City of Cape Town, Cape Town, South Africa

Gabriela Patten, Mary Ibeto and Vivian Cox
Médecins Sans Frontiéres Khayelitsha, Khayelitsha, South Africa

Laura A. Cooley, Alexandra M. Oster, Charles E. Rose, Cyprian Wejnert and Binh C. Le
Division of HIV/AIDS Prevention, National Center for HIV, Viral Hepatitis, STD and TB Prevention, Centers for Disease Control and Prevention, Atlanta, Georgia, United States of America

Hisashi Eguchi
Department of Public Health, Kitasato University School of Medicine, Sagamihara, Kanagawa, Japan

Koji Wada
National Center for Global Health and Medicine, Tokyo, Japan

Derek R. Smith
School of Health Sciences, Faculty of Health, University of Newcastle, Ourimbah, Australia

Kesetebirhan Delele Yirdaw, Degu Jerene and Zewdu Gashu
Clinical Department, Johns Hopkins University TSEHAI Project, Addis Ababa, Ethiopia

M. E. Edginton
Center for Operational Research, International Union against Tuberculosis and
Lung Disease, Paris, France
Ajay M. V. Kumar
International Union against Tuberculosis and Lung Disease, South-East Asia Regional Office, New Delhi, India

Yohannes Letamo
Health Research and Technology Transfer Support Process, Southern Nations Nationalities and People's Region Health Bureau, Hawassa, Southern Nations Nationalities and People's Region, Ethiopia

Beniam Feleke
Care and treatment branch, TB/HIV unit, Centers for Disease Control and Prevention, Addis Ababa, Ethiopia

Alula M. Teklu
PCM Department, Johns Hopkins University TSEHAI Project, Addis Ababa, Ethiopia

Solomon Zewdu, Bill Weiss and Andrea Ruff
Bloomberg School of Public Health, Johns Hopkins University, Baltimore, Maryland, United States of America

Monde Muyoyeta, Maureen Moyo, Nkatya Kasese, Deborah Milimo, Rosanna Spooner
Department of medicine, School of Medicine, University of Zambia, ZAMBART Project, Lusaka, Zambia

Pragnya Maduskar, Laurens Hogeweg and Bram van Ginneken
Diagnostic Image Analysis Group, Radboud University Medical Center, Nijmegen, The Netherlands

Nathan Kapata
National TB program, Ministry of Health, Lusaka, Zambia

Helen Ayles
Department of medicine, School of Medicine, University of Zambia, ZAMBART Project, Lusaka, Zambia
Clinical research department, Faculty of Infectious and Tropical Diseases, London School of Hygiene and Tropical Medicine, London, United Kingdom

Alison J. Rodger, Andrew Phillips, Andrew Speakman, Richard Gilson, Lorraine Sherr and Fiona C. Lampe
University College London, London, United Kingdom

Martin Fisher
Brighton and Sussex University Hospitals NHS Trust, Brighton, United Kingdom

Ed Wilkins
Pennine Acute Hospitals NHS Trust, Manchester, United Kingdom

Jane Anderson
Homerton University Hospital NHS Foundation Trust, London, United Kingdom

Margaret Johnson
Royal Free NHS London Foundation Trust, London, United Kingdom

Rebecca O'Connell
Newham University NHS Hospital Trust, London, United Kingdom

Simon Collins
HIV i-Base, London, United Kingdom

Jonathan Elford
City University London, London, United Kingdom

Erica H. Layer and Deanna L. Kerrigan
Department of Health, Behavior and Society, Johns Hopkins Bloomberg School of Public Health, Baltimore, Maryland, United States of America

Caitlin E. Kennedy and Sarah W. Beckham
Department of International Health, Johns Hopkins Bloomberg School of Public Health, Baltimore, Maryland, United States of America

Jessie K. Mbwambo and Samuel Likindikoki
Department of Psychiatry, Muhimbili University of Health and Allied Sciences, Dar es Salaam, Tanzania

Wendy W. Davis
Department of Epidemiology, Johns Hopkins Bloomberg School of Public Health, Baltimore, Maryland, United States of America

Heena Brahmbhatt
Department of Population, Family and Reproductive Health, Johns Hopkins Bloomberg School of Public Health, Baltimore, Maryland, United States of America

Ziad Ahmed Memish
Public Health Directorate, Ministry of Health, Riyadh, Kingdom of Saudi Arabia
College of Medicine, Alfaisal University, Riyadh, Kingdom of Saudi Arabia

Elija Afolabi Bamgboye
Public Health Directorate, Ministry of Health, Riyadh, Kingdom of Saudi Arabia
Department of Epidemiology and Medical Statistics, University of Ibadan, Ibadan, Nigeria

Naila Abuljadayel, Hanan Smadi, Mohamed Salamh Abouzeid and Rafat Faisal Al Hakeem
Public Health Directorate, Ministry of Health, Riyadh, Kingdom of Saudi Arabia

Lara Coelho, Sandra Wagner Cardoso, Rodrigo Teixeira Amancio, Ronaldo Ismério Moreira, Dayse Pereira Campos, Valdiléa Gonçalves Veloso, Beatriz Grinsztejn and Paula Mendes Luz
Instituto de Pesquisa Clínica Evandro Chagas, Fundação Oswaldo Cruz, Rio de Janeiro, Brasil

Hongjing Yan and Haitao Yang
Jiangsu Provincial Center for Disease Control and Prevention, Nanjing, China

Min Zhang, Chenchen Wang, Yuanyuan Xu, Li Liu, Susu Wu and Fei Xu
Nanjing Municipal Center for Disease Control and Prevention, Nanjing, China

Jinkou Zhao
Jiangsu Provincial Center for Disease Control and Prevention, Nanjing, China
The Global Fund to fight AIDS, Tuberculosis and Malaria, Geneva, Switzerland

Xiping Huan and Jianping Ding
Jiangsu Provincial Center for Disease Control and Prevention, Nanjing, China
Jiangsu Provincial Preventive Medicine Association, Nanjing, China

Richard Long
Department of Medicine, University of Alberta, Edmonton, Alberta, Canada
Department of Public Health Sciences, University of Alberta, Edmonton, Alberta, Canada

Selvanayagam Niruban
Department of Public Health Sciences, University of Alberta, Edmonton, Alberta, Canada

Courtney Heffernan, Ryan Cooper, Rabia Ahmed and Mary Lou Egedahl
Department of Medicine, University of Alberta, Edmonton, Alberta, Canada

Dina Fisher
Department of Medicine, University of Calgary, Calgary, Alberta, Canada

Rhonda Fur
Alberta Health Services, Alberta, Canada

Annelies Van Rie, Kate Clouse and Colleen Hanrahan
Department of Epidemiology, University of North Carolina at Chapel Hill, Chapel Hill, North Carolina, United States of America

Katerina Selibas and Ian Sanne
Clinical HIV Research Unit, University of the Witwatersrand, Johannesburg, South Africa

Jean Bassett
Witkoppen Health and Welfare Center, Johannesburg, South Africa
Sharon Williams and Peter Kim
National Institute of Allergy and Infectious Diseases, National Institutes of Health, Bethesda, Maryland, United States of America

Thomas A. Odeny
Center for Microbiology Research, Kenya Medical Research Institute, Nairobi, Kenya
Department of Epidemiology, University of Washington, Seattle, Washington, United States of America

Maya Newman
School of Medicine, University of Washington, Seattle, Washington, United States of America

Elizabeth A. Bukusi
Center for Microbiology Research, Kenya Medical Research Institute, Nairobi, Kenya
Department of Global Health, University of Washington, Seattle, Washington, United States of America
Department of Obstetrics and Gynecology, University of Washington, Seattle, Washington, United States of America

R. Scott McClelland
Department of Epidemiology, University of Washington, Seattle, Washington, United States of America
Department of Global Health, University of Washington, Seattle, Washington, United States of America
Department of Medicine, University of Washington, Seattle, Washington, United States of America
Institute of Tropical and Infectious Diseases, University of Nairobi, Nairobi, Kenya

Craig R. Cohen
Department of Obstetrics, Gynecology and Reproductive Sciences, University of California San Francisco, San Francisco, California, United States of America

Carol S. Camlin
Department of Obstetrics, Gynecology and Reproductive Sciences, University of California San Francisco, San Francisco, California, United States of America

Center for AIDS Prevention Studies, University of California San Francisco, San Francisco, California, United States of America

Elisa Mountain, Michael Pickles and Marie-Claude Boily
Department of Infectious Disease Epidemiology, Imperial College London, London, United Kingdom

Peter Vickerman
School of Social and Community Medicine, University of Bristol, Bristol, United Kingdom

Charles Gilks
School of Population Health, University of Queensland, Brisbane, Australia

Sharmistha Mishra
Department of Infectious Disease Epidemiology, Imperial College London, London, United Kingdom
Division of Infectious Diseases, St. Michael's Hospital, University of Toronto, Toronto, Canada
Li Ka Shing Knowledge Institute, University of Toronto, Toronto, Canada

Zhen Li, Lianxian Cui, Yu Hu and Wei He
Department of Immunology, School of Basic Medicine, Peking Union Medical College; National Key Laboratory of Medical Molecular Biology, Institute of Basic Medical Sciences, Chinese Academy of Medical Sciences, Beijing, China

Wei Li, Yanmei Jiao, Dexi Chen and Hao Wu
Center for Infectious Diseases, Beijing You'an Hospital, Capital Medical University, Beijing, China

Ning Li
Beijing You'an Hospital, Capital Medical University, Beijing, China

Lander Egaña-Gorroño, Tuixent Escribà and Mireia Arnedo
Group of Genomics and Pharmacogenomics, AIDS Research Group, Catalan project for the development of an HIV vaccine (HIVACAT), Institut d'Investigacions Biomèdiques August Pi i Sunyer (IDIBAPS), Hospital Clínic de Barcelona, Barcelona, Spain

Nicolas Boulanger
Group of Genomics and Pharmacogenomics, AIDS Research Group, Catalan project for the development of an HIV vaccine (HIVACAT), Institut d'Investigacions Biomèdiques August Pi i Sunyer (IDIBAPS), Hospital Clínic de Barcelona, Barcelona, Spain
Centro Nacional de Análisis Genómico, Scientific Park of Barcelona, Barcelona, Spain

Alberto Crespo Guardo, Manel Enric Bargalló and Montserrat Plana
Immunopathology and Cellular Immunology, AIDS Research Group, Catalan project for the development of an HIV vaccine (HIVACAT), Institut d'Investigacions Biomèdiques August Pi i Sunyer (IDIBAPS), Hospital Clínic de Barcelona, Barcelona, Spain

Agathe León, Felipe Garcia and José María Gatell
Department of Infectious Diseases, Hospital Clínic de Barcelona, University of Barcelona, Barcelona, Spain

Meng Wei and Stephen C. Deutsch
Cedars-Sinai Medical Care Foundation, Beverly Hills, California, United States of America

Run Yu
Division of Endocrinology, Cedars-Sinai Medical Center, Los Angeles, California, United States of America

Aye Thida, Sai Thein Than Tun, Sai Ko Ko Zaw, Zaw Htoon Waing and Philippe Clevenbergh
The Union Office in Myanmar, International Union Against Tuberculosis and Lung Disease, Mandalay, Myanmar

Andrew A. Lover
Infectious Diseases Programme, Saw Swee Hock School of Public Health, National University of Singapore, Singapore

Philippe Cavailler
Innovation Unit, Médecins Sans Frontières, Geneva, Switzerland

Jennifer Chunn
Maths and Statistics Help Centre, James Cook University, Singapore

Mar Mar Aye, Par Par, Kyaw Win Naing and Kaung Nyunt Zan
Medical Care Division, Department of Health, Mandalay, Myanmar

Myint Shwe
National AIDS Program, Department of Health, Nay Pyi Taw, Myanmar

Thar Tun Kyaw
Disease Control Division, Department of Health, Nay Pyi Taw, Myanmar

Index